Arterial Surgery

Arterial Surgery

H H G Eastcott MS (Lond) FRCS (Eng)

*Consultant Surgeon, St Mary's Hospital, Royal Masonic Hospital,
King Edward VII Hospital for Officers, and to the Royal Navy*

Examiner in Surgery, University of Cambridge

Member of the Court of Examiners, Royal College of Surgeons of England

Second Edition

J. B. LIPPINCOTT COMPANY
PHILADELPHIA   TORONTO

*Second edition published in Great Britain by
Sir Isaac Pitman & Sons Ltd in 1973*

*Published and distributed in the United States
and Canada by J. B. Lippincott Company
Philadelphia and Toronto*

ISBN: 0 397 58129 7

Library of Congress No 73-7209

Printed in Great Britain at The Pitman Press, Bath

Preface to the Second Edition

Advances in several areas of interest have been made since the text of the first edition was completed in 1968, and I have tried to choose those that seemed most important for inclusion in this new edition.

In the course of a general follow-up survey of my arterial patients, the work on those with Buerger's disease, carotid stenosis, and abdominal aortic aneurysm was completed, and review of the larger series of notes on those with occlusive disease of the lower limb arteries had begun, when on the night of 5th August 1972 there occurred a major fire in the Records Store at St Mary's Hospital in which many thousands of sets of case notes were lost, including a good proportion of those required for the remainder of the follow-up study. I have decided therefore to leave the figures as they appeared in the first edition. In fact, from the data already in hand there does not seem to have been much change in the methods employed or in the results obtained, except that long endarterectomy in the thigh has been practically given up in favour of reversed femoro-popliteal by-pass, with some improvement in patency rates after the first year.

It is again a pleasure to thank those same friends and colleagues who have helped so much, and to acknowledge the courtesy of fellow authors and their publishers in allowing me to show their work.

4 Upper Harley Street
London NW1
1973

H H G Eastcott

Preface to the First Edition

It was my good fortune to be closely concerned with the surgery of the arteries during those remarkable early years of its transformation from a subject of surgical curiosity to a large, thriving, new addition to the general surgeon's craft. It is for him that this book was written. Nothing here should be outside the range of his needs or skills, nor of the general hospital where most of these patients are first seen. It is hoped, also, that orthopaedic surgeons, general physicians, and cardiologists may find it useful; a fruitful co-operation with other specialists and with general practitioners is one of the continuing pleasures of arterial case-work.

I am grateful to Sir Zachary Cope for suggesting the book in 1963; to my good friends and colleagues Charles Hufnagel and Charles Rob who, long before, gave me the example of their brilliant skill and imaginativeness, and taught me well. Already by then, as registrar to Arthur Dickson Wright, I had seen the results of perfection in surgical technique and was given my big chance to enlarge my own experience by Sir Arthur Porritt whose help and kindness I can never forget. Since those early days two surgical giants, Cid dos Santos and Michael DeBakey, from their opposite poles of excellence and their friendliness to a junior man have provided inspiration which continues undiminished. For his close, strong, and good-humoured support over the past eighteen years I am always grateful to Dr Harry Thornton, whose anaesthetic skill has saved so many of the difficult situations we have had to face together; likewise to the successive residents and members of the nursing team who have given so much to the work. Miss Lindsay Fieldman typed the manuscript from fragments of almost archaeological indecipherability. Miss Gallagher, Head Librarian at St Mary's, has helped me at every stage, and her assistant, Miss Mary Ward, has patiently and accurately checked the hundreds of references.

For many years we have at St Mary's enjoyed the unique advantages of the safe, skilled arteriographic investigations of Dr David Sutton; most of the large selection of X-ray photographs illustrating this book have been his work. I also acknowledge with gratitude the work of Dr Peter Cardew and the members of his Department of Medical Photography at St Mary's whose high standards and swift service have made the illustrations so much less of a task.

It is with much appreciation that I acknowledge the kindness and co-operation of the many authors and publishers who have allowed me to use their material, as cited individually in the figure legends throughout the book.

Lastly, and in so many ways the most important of all, my thanks are due to my own publishers, and especially to Mr S. Whittingham Boothe who has made so rewarding and interesting an arrangement of my efforts. His patience and skill have been my sure guide.

If what we have done should help our colleagues and their patients we shall be well pleased.

March 1969

H H G Eastcott

Contents

For Bobbie and the Girls

1 Causes and Mechanisms of Arterial Disease

Incidence of Degenerative Arterial Disease

Undoubtedly more people each year are developing arterial disease; all the evidence demonstrates a real rise in incidence, greater than can be explained by improved diagnosis or an increased expectation of life. Table 1.1 shows the striking upward trend in mortality from cardiovascular and thromboembolic diseases that took place in England and Wales between 1942 and 1966.

Comparison of the 1961 age-adjusted death rates from arteriosclerotic and degenerative heart disease, also vascular lesions of the central nervous system, shows that England and Wales occupied the middle position between the United States and Sweden, except in cerebrovascular disease in middle-aged and older subjects, for which its figures were the highest of the three (Table 1.2).

It is surprising that differences as striking as these should exist between three developed countries enjoying much the same standards of life and medical care. Even more marked is the difference between most Western countries and Africa and the Far East, where deaths from arteriosclerotic heart disease are rare. We will return to this later when considering the possible effect on dietary habit in causation.

PREVALENCE DURING LIFE
Published reports on silent or subclinical arterial disease are few. In Basle, Switzerland, a survey on 6,400 employees showed that 3 to 7 per cent of men aged forty to sixty-four had occluded limb arteries,

Table 1.1. Rise in Certified Deaths from Cardiovascular Disease, 1942–1966

(Registrar-General's Statistical Reviews)

	1942	1966
Arteriosclerotic and degenerative heart disease	96,953	152,383
Cerebral thrombo embolism	16,143	36,083
Diseases of arteries	11,778	16,679
Aneurysm (non-syphilitic)	586	3,638
Diseases of veins	979	5,319

Table 1.2. Age-adjusted Death Rates per 100,000 Population in 1961 for Both Sexes between 45 and 64 Years of Age

(*From* Burgess, Colton, and Peterson, 1965 [12])

	USA		England and Wales		Sweden	
	M	F	M	F	M	F
Arteriosclerotic and degenerative heart disease	593·2	179·1	339·7	103·7	272·0	83·6
Cerebrovascular disease	94·4	78·4	104·4	87·6	68·3	67·2

two-thirds of whom were unaware of their condition [66, 67]. A survey recently carried out by the London School of Hygiene and Tropical Medicine [60A] on 19,170 civil servants aged 40 or over yielded 0·89 per cent with intermittent claudication and 5 per cent with angina, mostly previously undiagnosed. As to the association of the two conditions: among the men with angina, 3·1 per cent had intermittent claudication, while of the claudicators, 18 per cent had angina.

Comparing the age incidence of peripheral and coronary arterial disease by decades, the Basle and Framingham studies (see p. 3) show a striking parallel (Fig. 1.1), both conditions rising steeply during middle age. Near retiring age, both figures stand at approximately 7 per cent. A fairly high proportion of all these subjects were asymptomatic.

The figures are much higher for peripheral arterial disease in patients with *known symptomatic ischaemic heart disease*. Among 50 British patients with angina pectoris, 12 (24%) showed either intermittent claudication or arterial insufficiency in a limb, as indicated by tonoscillometry [40]. Another series from Oslo [5] had deficient lower limb pulses in 24·3 per cent, although only just over half these patients experienced claudication.

Patients with *known symptomatic peripheral arterial disease* have been examined for evidence of myocardial ischaemia, and similar figures were obtained. Of 79 British patients with intermittent claudication, 23 (29%) showed such evidence [40]. At the Mayo Clinic of 464 patients with aorto-iliac or femoral arterial occlusion, 70 (15%) had either angina or signs of an infarct [32]. In Oslo, 541 such patients, 189 (34·9%) showed signs of ischaemic heart disease [5].

THE EVIDENCE OF THE FOLLOW-UP

At the Manchester Royal Infirmary [6], 1,476 patients who attended with peripheral arterial occlusion were followed up for five years or more, and of these 401 (27%) died from heart disease, accounting for nearly 60 per cent of the deaths. In a more selected group of 520 Mayo Clinic patients with lower limb ischaemia, followed up for 5 years or more, 76 deaths (14·5%) were due to heart disease [32].

EVIDENCE FROM POST-MORTEM STUDIES

Morbid anatomy tells only of the end state, and it may not, except in premature or accidental deaths, allow conclusions about the earlier stages. What it can do, however, is establish the distribution and extent of cardiovascular disease at various sites, and its incidence in patients dying in hospital and in those coming to the coroner's pathologist; all matters of considerable clinical interest.

Among 347 patients dying of non-vascular diseases [59] there was little difference between the sexes in the pattern of arteriosclerosis in patients over forty, and in the elderly members of this 'normal' group there was unexpectedly little cerebral arterial disease. In the same study, 153 patients who had died of some arteriosclerotic catastrophe showed more coronary and aorto-iliac disease, especially the internal iliac in patients over fifty. Obesity was associated with increased severity of arteriosclerosis, though only in the men, in whom hypertension also correlated with increased coronary and cerebral arterial disease and a higher incidence of cardiac infarcts. Patients with nephrosclerosis showed the same pattern.

A post-mortem study of the aorta, and coronary, carotid, and iliac arteries was carried out at Oxford [43] on 293 unselected patients and 116 with large cardiac infarcts. The area of disease and severity of stenosis were measured. The results showed an association in the unselected cases between stenosis of the coronary arteries and in the carotids and iliacs; in the myocardial infarct group there was more aortic disease and, also, more plaque ulceration and stenosis in the carotid and iliac arteries. The length and diameter of the opened aorta in the unselected cases showed a linear relationship with age [44].

Summary
1. The incidence of recognisable coronary and peripheral arterial disease in the middle-aged and elderly section of the general population appears to be in the region of 5 to 7 per cent.
2. The incidence of complications and death from these diseases is rising.
3. There is close association between the severity of the disease in neck, abdomen, and pelvis, and between aortic disease, complicated lesions, and death from myocardial infarctions.

Probable Aetiological Factors

The underlying causes of arterial disease are not yet known, but evidence from social, racial, and epidemiological studies and from the experience of life assurance offices tends to incriminate hypertension, raised serum cholesterol, obesity and the wrong diet, middle age, higher living standards, membership of the male sex, cigarette smoking, lack of exercise, reduced vital capacity, and living in a district with a soft water supply.

Although the composite picture of such a victim which emerges at once suggests the association of his malady with the living conditions of urban life in the Western world, yet, in practice, exceptions to these criteria are frequent, and any conscientious attempt at preventive care is highly frustrating. Because of such doubts, a prospective study, the Framingham Enquiry, was begun in 1950 by the US Public Health Service. The results have been instructive, and though they mainly concern the incidence of ischaemic heart disease, comparison with the Basle study of arterial disease suggests that the two conditions generally go together (*see* Fig. 1.1). Moreover,

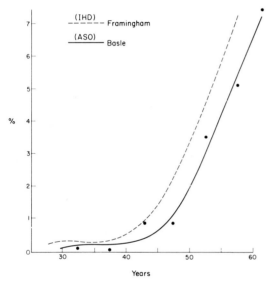

Fig. 1.1. Age incidence of peripheral arterial occlusive disease (ASO), and of ischaemic heart disease (IHD) in two large population surveys. *From Dawber et al.* [16] *and Widmer* [66].

coronary arterial disease, or rather death from it, presents a certain recognisable clinical and pathological end-point with which to test the aetiological factors under suspicion.

Confirmed as significant by the Framingham Study are:

Hypertension. Systolic blood pressures, chosen because they show a wider range and are therefore easier to group, were found to be important. Men aged thirty to fifty-nine with a systolic blood pressure above 160 mm Hg at entry showed a striking increase in coronary morbidity in eight years, and the higher the pressure the greater the risk. The same applied to women aged forty to forty-nine. This agrees with the evidence of post-mortem [59] and of death from strokes (*see* Chapter 8, p. 151), as well as from abdominal aortic aneurysm (*see* Chapter 15, p. 290).

Raised serum cholesterol is important in men under fifty. Those in whom it was over 260 mg per cent showed more than twice the standard risk at eight years. In older men the rise is not so striking, but it is still there.

Cigarette smoking was found by the Survey to carry twice the risk of myocardial infarction and sudden death, comparing all groups of smokers with non-smokers. That there might be little cumulative effect was suggested by the fact that those who had given up cigarettes subsequently had the same lower rate of coronary arterial disease as those who had never smoked.

The case against smoking has been repeatedly made [60B]. In peripheral arterial disease it is now certain that, in men with claudication or other symptoms of arteriosclerosis obliterans, just over 1 per cent are non-smokers compared with 25 to 30 per cent of the normal population [3]. At the Mayo Clinic [32], a follow-up of 520 patients with obliterative arterial disease of the lower limbs for five years or more showed that, of those who gave up smoking when advised, none subsequently required amputation. In the group who continued to smoke, the amputation rate was 11·4 per cent. In the author's experience of over 2,000 patients with lower-limb ischaemia there were less than twenty male non-smokers.

The introduction of machine-made cigarettes in 1880 was followed in Great Britain by a change in smoking habits, away from pipe and cigars towards cigarettes, and also by an increase in the total amount of tobacco consumed. The five-fold increase in mortality from ischaemic heart disease during the years 1930–55 followed the same upward slope (Fig. 1.2), though a fall during the early war years may have been related to dietary restrictions, later reduced by the arrival of lease-lend food from the USA. A fall in tobacco consumption during the post-war decade was not reflected in the mortality figures, again suggesting that dietary freedom was at that time more important, possibly the more so after the period of restriction [9].

Comparison of international mortality figures (Fig. 1.3) shows the same close relationship with cigarette consumption, though complicated here, also, by the effect of diet; those nations who smoked more also ate more [9, 11A, 11B].

Combination of these three factors is shown in Fig. 1.4 for the Framingham men under fifty who had a raised systolic blood pressure, high serum cholesterol, and who smoked: these men had ten times the risk of manifest coronary heart disease as those in which all three were absent.

We will now consider other evidence, outside the scope of the Framingham Survey, but which may

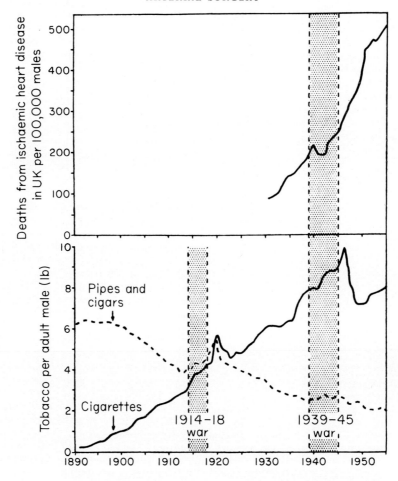

Fig. 1.2. Trends of mortality from ischaemic heart disease and tobacco consumption during the present century. (*From* Bronte-Stewart [9] by courtesy of the author and *British Medical Journal*.)

prove to be of equal preventive significance in the future.

Other Factors

Water Hardness

An inverse relationship between water hardness and the incidence of cardiovascular disease has been shown to exist in Great Britain [4, 15], the USA, and Japan [4]; in other words, using soft water carries a higher mortality. The difference is striking, amounting in England and Wales, for example, to a possible 7,000 deaths yearly among men aged forty-five to sixty-four [20]. Whether hardness in some way protects, or the soft water carries damaging soluble trace constituents is not yet known.

Diet

Though eating too much has been blamed as a likely cause of occlusive vascular disease, it is difficult to prove the relationship. As well as the diet itself there are the associated factors of physical activity, smoking habits, inherited factors and race.

Fat Intake

The case against fats is a very strong one. Though it mainly applies to coronary arterial disease, involvement of the peripheral arteries, though less obvious, is usually there, and any preventive or therapeutic measures based on the fat theory should be used for both because of the high death rate from cardiovascular causes that they share.

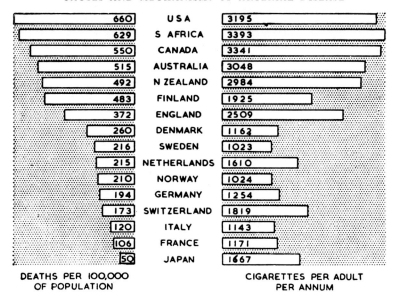

Fig. 1.3. Relationship between cigarette consumption and mortality from ischaemic heart disease in sixteen developed countries. (*From* Bronte-Stewart [9] by courtesy of the author and *British Medical Journal*.)

The Evidence of Animal Experiments

It is over sixty years since atheroma was first produced in rabbits, since when various species have been subjected to a high cholesterol diet and have developed fatty arterial lesions whose severity was directly related to the duration of hypercholesterolaemia, as well as to the level of the blood pressure [10], and to carbon monoxide in the inspired air [2A]. Moreover, rabbits on a high cholesterol regime showed a four-fold prolongation in the time taken to lyse clots in their veins [38].

Study of Plasma Lipid Patterns in Man [11, 26, 53]

Neutral fat from direct intestinal absorption rises soon after a fatty meal to an extent that can easily be seen with the naked eye and under the microscope to be composed of chylomicrons. These can be dispersed by heparin injection. In patients with coronary disease, this lipaemia is prolonged and is less easily cleared by heparin. There is some evidence to suggest that the blood is hypercoagulable in these conditions, at least *in vitro*.

A fat-free plasma loses its power of coagulation with viper venom, and the normal state can be restored by replacing this fat or dairy fat on its own.

The plasma cholesterol level is usually raised in ischaemic heart disease, and can be reduced by a low fat diet, but not if the calories thus lost are replaced by carbohydrate.

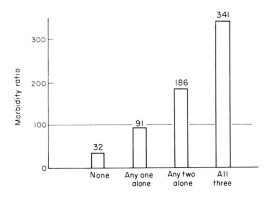

Fig. 1.4. Risk of developing ischaemic heart disease in eight years according to combinations of high serum cholesterol, high blood pressure, and excessive cigarette smoking. Men aged 30–59 at entry. (Framingham Survey—Dawber *et al.* [16])

There is more disturbance of plasma lipid distribution in young than in elderly coronary subjects— as was found with total cholesterol values in the Framingham Survey, suggesting perhaps a premature or heightened change.

Congenital hyperlipidaemia was studied by Fredrickson [24A] who found that plasma lipoproteins varied in their size and concentration in a manner that coincided with the systemic clinical features of the several forms of this disease.

group with a broad beta-band, normal cholesterol and raised triglycerides, showed a higher incidence of lower limb ischaemia which, others have stated, can be improved by low fat diet and clofibrate [70].

Racial and Social Factors [11, 11A, 11B, 33, 44]

By far the most impressive evidence of the importance of fat intake is the close association between national figures for ischaemic heart disease and average fat consumption. The oriental peoples eat less fat and have little arteriosclerotic disease, and when countries are considered in order of progressive Western longitude, generally speaking both these values increase.

Migration studies show that the change can operate during the lifetime of an individual (thus, presumably, excluding genetic factors); for example, the Yemenite Jews, who are little affected by degenerative cardiovascular disease in their traditional home, have a six times greater mortality rate after twenty years in Israel. Differences between male Japanese in Japan, Hawaii, and the USA show the same trend.

Descendants of immigrants from countries with a predisposition to IHD show their national tendency in later generations; thus, Jewish Americans have two to three times the incidence as Italian Americans.

The conditions of war in Europe in 1939–45 brought a fall in the mortality from cardiovascular disease associated almost everywhere with enforced reduction in animal fat intake (though with a restricted use of sucrose as well, *see* below). Among those worst affected, the inmates of concentration camps, the incidence was virtually nil, which suggests that occlusive arterial disease may be reversible where dietary limitation is inescapable [53].

Nutritional factors may be more important before middle age, and may affect the coronary arteries more than the aorta and peripheral arteries [23].

The Seventh Day Adventists, in the USA, take little meat or fat, and are non-smokers. Among their men, the incidence of ischaemic heart disease is 40 per cent below that of the corresponding group of the rest of the population, and the women 15 per cent. Serum cholesterol levels were also lower in both sexes [65].

Calories, Carbohydrate, and Refined Sugar

Much of what has been said about fat would apply equally to total calorie values, and, hence, indirectly to obesity itself, though the connection here is mainly retrospective and is connected with hypertension. Obesity alone is not a significant factor, according to the Framingham study.

The diet of developed countries contains many calories as sucrose, and in close relation to the fat intake [11A]. Even on a low fat diet a high intake of sucrose increases serum cholesterol and glyceride levels [39].

Urine specimens from 25,701 inhabitants of Bedford, England, were tested [34] for sugar, excluding known diabetics, and 1,033 were found to have glycosuria. Of these, 939 attended for glucose tolerance testing and were compared with a control series for evidence of cardiovascular disease, chiefly arterial symptoms and ECG signs. The severity of these was found to bear a direct relationship to the height of the abnormality in the glucose curve. These results suggest a relationship between symptomless impairment of glucose tolerance and arteriosclerotic disease [36]. Carbohydrate intake stimulates insulin release. Recent work on insulin levels in coronary heart disease [62B] suggests that this response raises serum lipids, some of which find their way into the arterial wall. This agrees with the finding of raised insulin and glucose levels in non-diabetic male claudicators [62A].

Physical Activity

An important finding concerned London busmen and the crews of other public transport vehicles; conductors and guards had less ischaemic heart disease than the drivers [45], who were also 'worse' in other ways, e.g. greater body weight, skinfold thickness, systolic blood pressure, and serum cholesterol. A study of 5,000 unselected post-mortems on the general population showed that men in physically active occupations had less disease, and had it less severely and later in life than those in sedentary work [46]. In Finnish men aged thirty to thirty-nine, the capacity to perform measured physical work was inversely related to the serum cholesterol level [27]. In Framingham, a low vital capacity was found to be associated with a higher incidence of heart disease at eight years, and vice versa [16].

Claudication appears to affect most occupations [3], whereas ischaemic heart disease is commoner in the sedentary. In the general population, lesions of both types are about equal. This may mean that some people are protected by their exertions from developing ischaemic heart disease.

Of the several suspected aetiological factors in the development of degenerative cardiovascular disease in its broadest sense, those which at present appear to be significant and potentially controllable include: dietary excess in total calories, fat and refined sugar; cigarette smoking, lack of exercise, hypertension, and, possibly, a high blood cholesterol level.

Genetic predisposition, e.g. when racial factors and a bad family history coincide, may override all other considerations.

Pathology

Traditional Views

The impact of the study of these aetiological factors upon the supposed pathological basis of the disease is now considerable. Until recent years, the 'imbibition theory' of Aschoff [1] was thought to be the one most compatible with observations on fat intake and the widespread distribution of fatty lesions in 'atherosclerosis', it being supposed that lipoid filtrates entering the inner layers of the arterial wall, where they accumulated, degenerated and formed a porridge-like substance which, together with other secondary sclerotic changes in the media, and, later, in the lumen, ending in thrombosis, accounted for the observed morbid anatomical features of the disease.

Duguid in 1946 [18] restated the case for the thrombotic or incrustation theory of Rokitansky [60]. This arose from his observation that serial sections along the length of stenosed coronary arteries showed transition from intralumenal thrombus to lumenal narrowing by organising fibrin and, thence, to arteriosclerotic plaques, some of which showed fatty or atheromatous softening.

Since then, experimental pathologists and others whose interests took them into this field have paid much attention to the possibility that obliterative arterial disease may simply be the result of slow, progressive deposition of thrombus, and that narrowing of the arterial lumen by sheets and plaques of organised deposits of this kind may, in places, go on to actual occlusion, usually the final stoppage being due to a plug of soft thrombus, in most cases quite unlike recent whole clot.

Platelet Adhesiveness

It has been known for many years that the platelet count rises during the first ten days after injury or operation. In 1942, Helen Payling Wright [68] showed that, after operation or childbirth, the platelets are not only increased in number but also in adhesiveness, coinciding with the time at which the tendency to intravascular thrombosis is at its height. The same is true of arterial occlusion, which may then show itself for the first time.

Platelet adhesiveness appears to be increased by collisions between the formed elements of the blood, especially red cells and platelets, due, it is believed to the production of adenosine diphosphate (ADP) from the triphosphate present in large amounts in the cells [7]. This would explain the progressive build-up of thrombus at the site of any irregularity in the vessel, anatomical or from disease. A transferable factor is present in arterial disease [30] which sensitises platelets to ADP.

The following factors are known to affect platelet behaviour:*

Factor	Effects on Platelets
1. Lipaemia	Increased adhesiveness and fall in count [35]
2. High fat diet	Increased deposition in flow chamber [49]
3. Saturated free fatty acids	Increased platelet aggregation *in vitro* [35]
4. Glucose by mouth	Increased adhesiveness [8]
5. Smoking:	
(a) Sustained, with diet controlled	Increased platelet turnover, reduced survival time [50]
(b) Two cigarettes in 20 minutes	Increased platelet adhesiveness [2]

Clot and Thrombus (Fig. 1.5) (thrombus (Gr.)— a plug)

Blood when it clots *in vitro* or in a completely static column, as in an acutely obstructed blood vessel away from collaterals, maintains a recognisable homogeneous microscopic form not very different from fluid blood (Fig. 1.6) but with the cells suspended in fibrin instead of plasma.

When blood is made to clot *in vitro* in a Chandler's tube [13]—a circular loop of plastic tubing kept turning during the experiment—no true clot forms but a solid body with a 'white head' composed of platelets and leucocytes (Fig. 1.7) and a 'red tail' of fibrin and red cells.

A natural thrombus shows much the same structure (Fig. 1.8).

Platelets and Intravascular Thrombosis

Eighty years have passed since it was realised that the blood platelets are primarily concerned with thrombus formation in the living blood vessel, and we must remember that the haemostatic plugs, which seal off the cut ends of the smaller blood vessels or their lumen after injury, in continuity, are mainly made up of platelets; also, that of the many complex changes that go to make up the process of whole blood clotting *in vitro*, platelet aggregation is the first.

Platelets and Factors Responsible for Obliterative Arterial Disease

There is now a very large body of evidence concerning the majority of the suspected aetiological factors

---

* Adhesiveness to a glass surface producing a decrease in the count. Aggregation; a measured change in optical density in platelet-rich plasma. Turnover and survival as estimated using radioactive labelling.

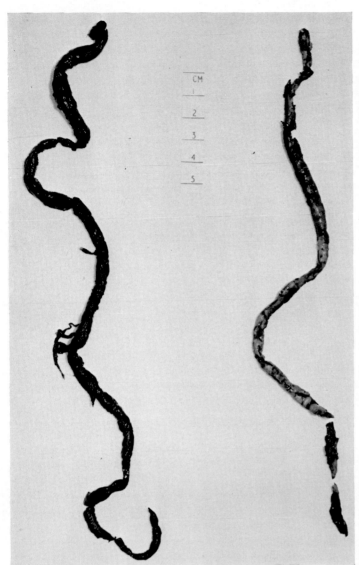

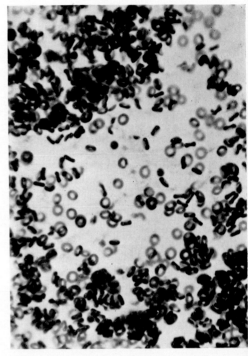

Fig. 1.6. Whole blood clot composed of red blood cells and fibrin (× 640). This and Figs 1.7 and 1.8 are reproduced by courtesy of Dr J. C. F. Poole. *See also* [58].

Fig. 1.5. Occluding material from two patients with obstruction of a femoral artery. The clot lay beyond an embolus and was removed by means of a rubber balloon catheter. The thrombus required dissection with a metal loop stripper.

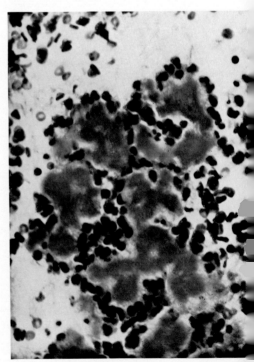

Fig. 1.7. Artificial thrombus from a Chandler's tube. Masses of platelet aggregate surrounded by red and white cells. (× 640)

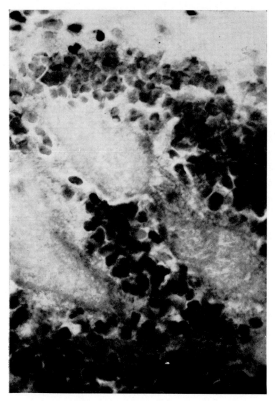

Fig. 1.8. A natural thrombus showing closely similar structure to Fig. 1.7.

already considered, and nearly all of it points to an increase in platelet aggregation as a primary mechanism in the intravascular thrombosis, which is increasingly thought to be responsible for obliterative arterial disease. Thus, most of the aetiological factors considered to play a part in the development of occlusive cardiovascular disease have been shown to exert a stimulating effect upon platelet function (Table 1.3).

Platelet Economy in Cardiovascular Disease [22]

In arteriosclerosis of the occlusive type there is increased platelet turnover and adhesiveness [48]. The latter is also increased in patients with recurring venous thrombosis and pulmonary embolism [29], as well as in cerebrovascular disease and diabetes [42, 8]. Whether these changes are causative or an effect of damage already done is not yet known.

Fibrinolytic Activity [24]

In health, the rates at which fibrin is produced and lysed by the fibrinolytic systems are equal. Heparin favours fibrinolysis, probably by disturbing the formative side of the equilibrium. This effect is not shown after long-term oral phenindione. Fibrinolysis is somewhat reduced after operations, myocardial infarction, in patients with severe angina and or intermittent claudication, also in diabetics, and in heavy smokers [58A]. In obesity [51], a low activity is increased by severe dieting and by exercise, but less than in normal subjects.

Artificial thrombi in a Chandler's tube (*see* p. 7) can be largely dissolved if streptokinase is used as a fibrinolysin activator, though platelet emboli may be released in the process [41].

Table 1.3. Factors Affecting Blood Lipids, Platelet Behaviour and Arterial Occlusive Disease

Genetic predisposition
Hypertension
Excessive calories
Saturated fats
Refined sugars
Reduced glucose tolerance
Lack of exercise
Cigarette smoking
Catecholamines
Adenosine diphosphate
Injury or operation
Androgens and 'the pill'
Increasing age
Menopause
Raised blood viscosity [17]
  (haematocrit)
Raised blood fibrinogen [17]
	PLATELET
	AGGREGATION
	↓
	ARTERIAL
	DEPOSITS
		→ INHIBITION OR
		DISAGGREGATION
			Exercise
			Restricted diet
			Fibrinolysis
			Natural ovarian activity
			Low MW dextrans
			Corticosteroids
			Thyroxine
			Adenosine
			Some vasodilators
			   See Chapter 3, p. 58.

At present the most promising long-term agent for the stimulation of fibrinolysis is to give a sustained dosage of phenformin and a progestogen, ethyl-oestranol [12A], which have also been shown by Fearnley to influence favourably some other factors associated with intravascular thrombosis, i.e. blood cholesterol, fibrinogen and platelet stickiness.

Endocrine Influences

Arterial disease is rare in women before the meno-pause, except for a special form which chiefly affects the central large arteries late in the childbearing period (*see* pp. 141, 234). If her ovaries are removed the premenopausal woman becomes more liable to arterial illness [63]. Normal ovarian function appears therefore to protect, though synthetic oestrogens in high dosage on the other hand are thrombogenic, the best example of this being the greatly increased vascular morbidity in women taking the contraceptive pill [26A, 31, 34A]. Cerebral and coronary thrombosis are serious risks. Fifty per cent of one series of female coronary patients had been on the pill, although almost the whole group showed other predisposing features such as hyper-lipidaemia, hypertension or excessive cigarette smoking [54]. Androgens increase blood lipids, while corticosteroids reduce them. Thyroxine lowers serum cholesterol. Human gonadotrophin administration for ovarian stimulation for infertility has been followed by thrombosis of the femoral vessels and of an internal carotid artery [47], probably from haemoconcentration due to shift of plasma fluid into the peritoneal cavity [64].

Possible Reversibility of Occlusive Arteriosclerosis [21]

The evidence of the war years, and in particular of the concentration camps [53], suggests that this may happen as a result of enforced dietary re-striction. Experimental atheroma in animals can be reversed in this way. Isotope studies in man have confirmed that cholesterol in a diseased artery can exchange with that of the blood; and phospholipid, which can mobilise cholesterol, will also reduce the amount of lipid desposition in rabbit atheroma.

Drug treatments aimed at reducing platelet adhesiveness are under consideration (see above), though no evidence yet exists of any reliable anti-atherogenic agent.

Nomenclature and the Thrombotic Concept of Arterial Disease

It is time to change our usage of the words 'atheroma' and 'atherosclerosis', for though there are lesions in the arterial system that do resemble a lump of por-ridge, or even perhaps a hardened porridge process, which is the literal meaning of these words, this should now be the limit of their use, and the common, diffuse narrowing due to a tubular lining of organ-ised thrombus should be known as arteriosclerosis, adding, as Pickering has suggested, some adjective such as 'nodular' to indicate that change is irregular and that the lumen is concerned more than the arterial wall [57].

Good terms already in common use include:

Arteriosclerosis obliterans (*ASO*): perhaps the best.

Occlusive arterial disease (which would, however, include Buerger's disease and the narrowing dysplasias of young subjects).

Occlusive cardiovascular disease, which is a valu-able descriptive term that takes in the whole range of arteriosclerotic ischaemia, central and peripheral, as well as chronic thrombo-embolic disease, in particular that of the veins.

These names will be used in the sense just des-cribed throughout this text, reserving 'atheroma' for the actual material so often locally encountered between the intimal and medial layers, and 'athero-sclerosis' to the occasional soft, loose, and easy-stripping form, seen particularly at operation in some middle-aged or younger subjects with premature dis-ease, that shows less hardening and more atheroma than the average.

The Natural History of the Lesions in Man [44]

Early Intimal Changes

The first signs appear in youth, even in infancy. The opened aorta shows *fatty streaking* of the intima; histologically the streaks prove to be subendothelial, composed of groups of histiocytes which may have taken up the fat from even earlier, more superficial lesions that are just visible with a hand lens. Fibrin may be associated with the fat, as demonstrated by fluorescein-linked anti-human fibrin [14]. The pos-terior part of the aorta is mainly affected (Fig. 1.9) where the shearing effect of blood flow is greatest; the vicinity of the intercostal branch orifices, a region of blood turbulence, is spared, although, later, *raised arteriosclerotic plaques* nearly always appear here [61]. There seems, therefore, to be a topographic distinction between early streaks and later plaques, though they may have been connected in the actual regions finally affected.

The Arteriosclerotic Plaque, Roll, or Plug

This familiar group of lesions forms the main basis of occlusive arterial disease, and it is found in all parts of the body, causing an eccentric narrowing of the lumen, with a laminar or streamlined leading and

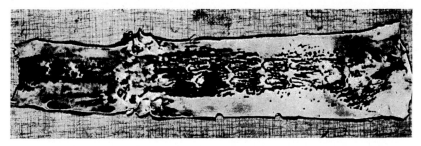

Fig. 1.9. Aorta of a 25-year-old man, stained with Sudan IV, showing fatty streaking posteriorly, except around intercostal orifices. (*From* Mitchell and Schwartz [44] by courtesy of the authors and *Blackwell Scientific Publications.*)

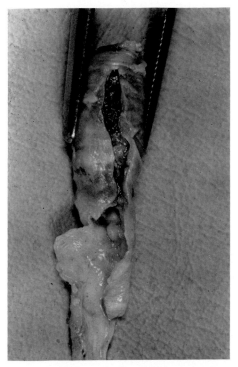

Fig. 1.10. Atheromatous roll with contained plug of more recent thrombus. At the beginning of the patent portion of the lumen beyond the block can be seen two small rounded bodies of the type that may break away producing embolic obstruction of small peripheral branch arteries (Fig. 1.11).

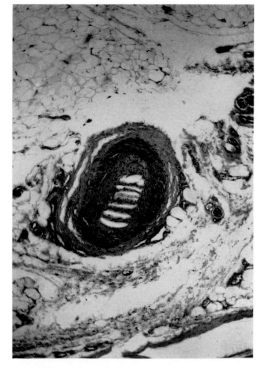

Fig. 1.11. Cholesterol clefts within the obstructed lumen of a small distal artery due to embolisation from a degenerating lesion in a more major proximal artery. (Reproduced by courtesy of Dr Chilton Crane, and the Editor of *AMA Archives of Surgery.*) (*See* Fig. 4.2a, lef.t)

trailing edge which gradually merges into a more normal region where the intima is only slightly thickened. The distal portion of the plaque may, however, rise still more into the lumen, to occlude it either by its own organised substance or by the contained thrombus, the whole lesion when extracted at operation resembling a sausage roll (Fig. 1.10). These were the appearances that led Duguid to revive the thrombotic view of their cause.

Beneath the plaque, a soft atheromatous accumulation is often to be seen, perhaps an end stage of the common 'cholesterol clefts' (Fig. 4.2(a) page 100).

This may separate and migrate to distal branches of the limb or organ, the process being called *athero-embolism* (Fig. 1.11, also Fig. 3.11, p. 38) [13A, 55]; it may be responsible for such varied and serious clinical conditions as blindness, hypertension, pancreatitis, gastrointestinal haemorrhage and cutaneous gangrene away from pressure points or extremities.

Medial and adventitial changes (including calcification) appear, in this form of arteriosclerosis, to increase with age [44], and to coincide with the maximum development of the intimal lesion, probably as a result of mechanical wear and tear over the stiffened segment, and, also perhaps, near a complete occlusion, to the irritative effects of the contained recent thrombus. Cellular infiltration, with cells resembling small lymphocytes, has been found in the aorta and its large branches to be mainly situated over plaques, and particularly over thrombi [62]. In other cases, medial changes are diffuse, and although often very advanced (*see* p. 40) they may bear no relation to occlusion, which may, in fact, be totally lacking.

Complicated Lesions

Ulceration, with fibrin or platelet accumulation, local haemorrhage, or aneurysm formation are seen mainly in older subjects, and are familiar to vascular surgeons in arteries either anatomically or pathologically too wide to have become sealed off earlier by thrombus in the lumen. That the body is able to accommodate for these complications is suggested by their high incidence and extreme severity in both sexes at eighty to ninety years of age, and by the relative ease with which the vascular surgeon may be able to reconstruct such an artery without much risk of postoperative bleeding or thrombosis. Only a minority of such cases with an isolated, locally very advanced lesion and threatening serious clinical complications will reach the surgeon; the rest are seen by the morbid anatomist after death, usually from other cardiovascular causes.

Relationship of the Three Arterial Lesions

Whether there is a relationship between these lesions remains uncertain; it is tempting to conclude that the age-sequence of the three [28] (Fig. 1.12) may mean that they are stages in the same process, although the circumstances of their presentation for study differ so markedly. The stage of inception may be from intra-mural migration of blood lipids, though in fact mainly cholesterol and very little glyceride can be found on electrophoresis of the plaques. Later, raised and complicated lesions are due to thrombosis, probably mediated by hyperlipidaemia [67A].

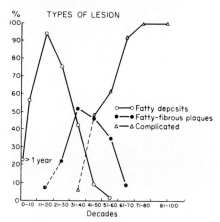

Fig. 1.12. Age incidence of three distinct types of aortic lesion. (*From* Hill *et al.* [28] by courtesy of the authors and *British Medical Journal*.)

THE EFFECTS OF ARTERIAL DISEASE

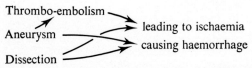

In vascular disease, effects are more readily observed and understood than causes, and their practical importance has concentrated medical attention upon them. The remainder of this chapter is intended as an introduction to the practical themes of the rest of the book.

Thrombo-embolism

We have seen that thrombus forms where there is atheromatous irregularity, ulceration, or marked narrowing or widening of the lumen, conditions

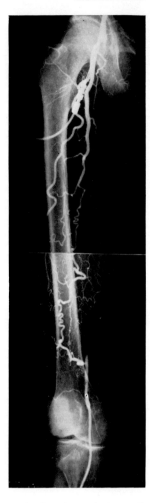

Fig. 1.13. Arteriosclerotic occlusion of the whole length of superficial femoral artery. The profunda femoris artery marks the upper end of the block, and prevents further proximal spread; at the lower end, the occlusion is controlled by a large re-entering collateral trunk from muscular arteries.

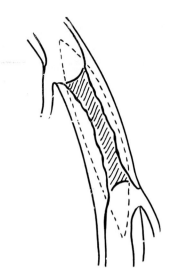

Fig. 1.14. At either end of an arteriosclerotic block, the thrombus is hollowed into a concave shape corresponding with the current of blood across its face to or from the branch opening.

causing turbulence and, locally, favouring thrombus deposition. Eventually, the main artery may become completely occluded over that portion of its length that is marked off at each end by a patent side branch indicating the source and the destination of the collateral circulation (Fig. 1.13). The mouths of these collaterals are often themselves grossly narrowed by atheroma in the main artery and may, in turn, become occluded so that the block in the main artery spreads along until another branch is reached of large enough size to ensure that the rate of flow is sufficient to check the advancing thrombus at this point: here the face of the thrombus is usually concave (Fig. 1.14). A single block may give rise to no symptoms, either because the collateral circulation is sufficient or because the patient's activities are limited. More severe ischaemia will result when additional major arterial occlusion occurs either proximally or beyond the first. This may be caused by local disease or by failure of the heart to maintain perfusion of a previously adequate collateral system. This process is familar when it affects the limbs but it may be overlooked in mesenteric arterial disease.

Sometimes, arterial thrombus becomes detached before it can occlude the lumen, when it becomes an embolus, which will lodge distally at a bifurcation or in a smaller branch. When this process is repeated an extensive and severe ischaemia is caused. Such a sequence of events may, in fact, be a common, important mechanism of the deterioration in chronic, advancing cases, with successive minor emboli which progressively reduce the 'run-off' with their rising resistance, favouring spread of the major proximal thrombotic lesion.

Aneurysm

With age, the arteries lengthen and widen as the elasticity of their medial coat diminishes. A large artery may show gross curving, or even looping,

13

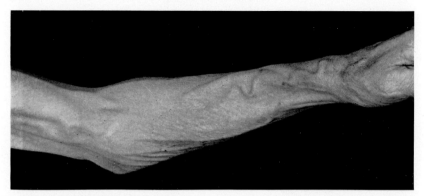

Fig. 1.15. Dilatation, lengthening and tortuosity of the brachial and radial arteries in an elderly man. (Mr Andrew Desmond's patient.)

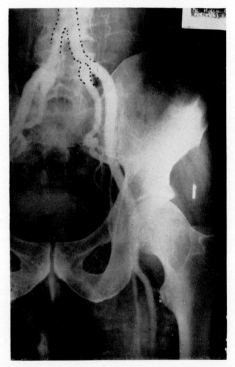

Fig. 1.16. Lengthening and early tortuosity of iliac arteries with early aneurysm formation in both internal iliacs in a man aged fifty-nine.

Dissection

One of the most striking appearances seen in operating for arterial disease is an almost perfect cleavage of the vessel wall into two layers, potentially forming an inner and an outer tube. This plane is sought

AN ILLUSTRATIVE CASE

An aortic bifurcation prosthesis of polyvinyl alcohol sponge removed for late failure due to false aneurysm formation, eight years after implantation. On the posterior surface of the stem of the graft is a 'slick' of occlusive accumulation which just enters the iliac branches. There is a notable symmetry in the shape of this lesion, from its tapering upper limit to the even division of the overhanging lower margins in the iliacs. This formation strongly suggests that in this patient the arteriosclerotic process was independent of factors relevant to any arterial tissues, and that it arose from the deposition of blood elements as a result of flow disturbance at the bifurcation.

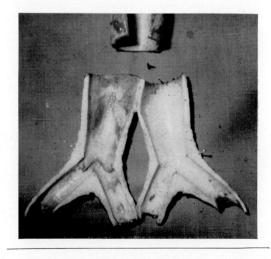

without any functional effect (Fig. 1.15). Sometimes, however, the stretching process becomes more marked in one particular place: this may represent the beginnings of aneurysm formation (Fig. 1.16). Among the known causes of localised arterial dilatation one of the most important is the presence of a proximal stenosis.

during thrombo-endarterectomy, and once found can be followed without much difficulty. It is, in fact, easy to develop it further than intended. There is no regular layer of cleavage in the normal arterial wall.

Even more striking is the dissection that sometimes complicates hypertension with medial degeneration. The inner and outer tubes may appear normal to inspection, with little intimal disease other than the split by which the blood stream enters, and it is difficult to understand why the stripping up of the coats of the artery should be so extensive. Histological examination shows the split to be within a widespread mucoid cystic necrosis partly replacing the middle layers of the media (*see* Chapter 15,

p. 316). Eventually, most cases end with the rupture of the adventitial layer, causing fatal internal haemorrhage.

Conclusions

Degenerative arterial disease in man arises from the lifelong effects of:

1. Occlusive accretion of the arterial lumen by blood elements; in site and extent determined anatomically and haemodynamically.
2. Lengthening of the tissues of the arterial wall with age and continued hypertension.
3. Thrombo-embolic complications of both these.

REFERENCES

1. Aschoff, L. (1924) In *Lectures on Pathology.* New York: Hoeber, p. 131.
2. Ashby, P., Dalby, A. M. and Millar, J. H. D. (1965) Smoking and platelet stickiness. *Lancet*, **ii**, 158.
2A.Astrup, P., Kjeldsen, K. and Wanstrup, J. (1970) Effects of carbon monoxide exposure on the arterial walls. *Ann. N.Y. Acad. Sci.*, **174**, Art. 1, 294.
3. Begg, T. B. (1965) Characteristics of men with intermittent claudication. *The Practitioner*, **194**, 202.
4. Biörck, G., Boström, H. and Widström, A. (1965) On the relationship between water hardness and death rate in cardiovascular diseases. *Acta med. Scand.*, **178**, 239.
5. Bjørnstad, P., Leren, P. and Selvaag, O. (1960) Palpatory examination of arteries in elderly subjects. *J. Oslo City Hospital*, **10**, 249.
6. Bloor, K. (1961) Natural history of arteriosclerosis of the lower extremities. *Ann. Roy. Coll. Surg. Eng.*, **28**, 36.
7. Born, G. V. R. (1965) Platelets in thrombogenesis: mechanism and inhibition of platelet aggregation. *Ann. Roy. Coll. Surg. Eng.*, **36**, 200.
8. Bridges, J. M., Dalby, A. M., Millar, J. H. D. and Weaver, J. A. (1965) An effect of d-glucose on platelet stickiness. *Lancet*, **i**, 75.
9. Bronte-Stewart, B. (1961) Cigarette smoking and ischaemic heart disease. *Brit. med. J.*, **i**, 379.
10. Bronte-Stewart, B. and Heptinstall, R. H. (1954) The relationship between experimental hypertension and cholesterol-induced atheroma in rabbits. *J. Path. Bact.*, **68**, 407.
11. Bronte-Stewart, B. (1965) Epidemiology and dietary factors in occlusive vascular disease. *Ann. Roy. Coll. Surg. Eng.*, **36**, 206.
11A.Brummer, P. (1967) Coronary heart disease and the living standard. *Acta med. Scand.*, **182**, 523.
11B.Brummer, P. (1969) Coronary mortality and living standard. II. Coffee, tea, cocoa, alcohol and tobacco. *Acta med. Scand.*, **185**, 61.
12. Burgess, A. M., Colton, T. and Peterson, O. L. (1965) Categorical programs for heart disease, cancer and stroke. Lessons from international death-rate comparisons. *New Eng. J. med.*, **273**, 533.

12A.Chakrabarti, R., Evans, J. F. and Fearnley, G. R. (1970) Effects on platelet stickiness and fibrinolysis of phenformin combined with ethyloestranol or stanozolol. *Lancet*, **i**, 591.
13. Chandler, A. B. (1958) *In vitro* thrombotic coagulation of the blood: a method for producing a thrombus. *Lab. Invest.*, **7**, 110.
13A.Crane, C. (1967) Atherothrombotic embolism to the lower extremities in arteriosclerosis. *Arch. Surg.*, **94**, 96.
14. Crawford, T. (1960) Some aspects of the pathology of the atherosclerosis. *Proc. Roy. Soc. Med.*, **53**, 9.
15. Crawford, T. and Crawford, M. D. (1967) Prevalence and pathological changes of ischaemic heart-disease in a hard-water and in a soft-water area. *Lancet*, **i**, 229.
16. Dawber, T. R., Kannel, W. B., Revotskie, N. and Kagan, A. (1962) The epidemiology of coronary heart disease—the Framingham Enquiry. *Proc. Roy. Soc. Med.*, **55**, 265.
17. Dormandy, J. A. (1970) Clinical significance of blood viscosity. *Ann. Roy. Coll. Surg. Eng.*, **47**, 211.
18. Duguid, J. B. (1946) Thrombosis as a factor in the pathogenesis of coronary atherosclerosis. *J. Path. Bact.*, **58**, 207.
19. Eastcott, H. H. G. (1962) Rarity of lower-limb ischaemia in non-smokers. *Lancet*, **ii**, 1117.
20. Editorial article: Hardness of water and cardiovascular disease. (1963) *Brit. med. J.*, **i**, 1429.
21. Editorial article: Is atherosclerosis reversible? (1964) *Brit. med. J.*, **ii**, 1477.
22. Entiknap, J. B., Gooding, P. G., Lansley, T. S. and Avis, P. R. D. (1969) Platelet size and function in ischaemic heart disease. *J. Atheroscler. Res.*, **10**, 41.
23. Falconer, G. F. and Adams, C. W. M. (1965) The relationship between nutritional state and severity of atherosclerosis. *Guy's Hosp. Rep.*, **114**, 130.
24. Flute, P. T. (1965) Fibrinolysis in relation to thrombosis. *Ann. Roy. Coll. Surg. Eng.*, **36**, 225.
24A.Fredrickson, D. S. (1971) Mutants, hyperlipoproteinaemia, and coronary artery disease. *Brit. med. J.*, **2**, 187.

25. French, J. E. (1965) The structure of natural and experimental thrombi. *Ann. Roy. Coll. Surg. Eng.*, **36**, 191.

26. Greenhalgh, R. M., Lewis, B., Rosengarten, D. S., Calnan, J. S., Mervart, I. and Martin, P. (1971) Serum lipids in peripheral vascular disease. *Lancet*, **ii**, 947.

26A. Hall, R. and Bunch, G. A. (1971) Aorto-iliac occlusion in women using oral contraceptives. A report of 2 cases. *Brit. J. Surg.*, **58**, 508.

27. Hernberg, S. (1964) Serum-cholesterol and capacity for physical work. *Lancet*, **ii**, 441.

28. Hill, K. R., Camps, F. E., Rigg, K. and McKinney, B. E. G. (1961) Atherosclerosis: results of a pilot survey in a North London area. *Brit. med. J.*, **i**, 1190.

29. Hirsh, J. and McBride, J. A. (1965) Increased platelet adhesiveness in recurrent venous thrombosis and pulmonary embolism. *Brit. med. J.*, **ii**, 797.

30. Hampton, J. R. and Mitchell, J. R. A. (1966) A transferable factor causing abnormal platelet behaviour in vascular disease. *Lancet*, **ii**, 764.

31. Inman, W. H. W., Vessey, M. P., Westerholm, B. and Engelund, A. (1970) Thromboembolic disease and the steroidal content of oral contraceptives. A report to the Committee on Safety of Drugs. *Brit. med. J.*, **2**, 203.

32. Juergens, J. L., Barker, N. W. and Hines, E. A. (1960) Arteriosclerosis obliterans: review of 520 cases with special reference to pathogenic and prognostic factors. *Circulation*, **21**, 188.

33. Kagan, A. (1960) Atherosclerosis of the coronary arteries—epidemiological considerations. *Proc. Roy. Soc. Med.*, **53**, 18.

34. Keen, H., Rose, G., Pyke, D. A., Boyns, D., Chlouverakis, C. and Mistry, S. (1965) Blood-sugar and arterial disease. *Lancet*, **ii**, 505.

34A. Keown, D. (1969) Review of arterial thrombosis in association with oral contraceptives. *Brit. J. Surg.*, **56**, 486.

35. Kerr, J. W., Pirrie, R., MacAulay, I. and Bronte-Stewart, B. (1965) Platelet-aggregation by phospholipids and free fatty acids. *Lancet*, **i**, 1296.

36. Kingsbury, K. J. (1966) The relation between glucose tolerance and atherosclerotic vascular disease. *Lancet*, **ii**, 1374.

37. Kinmonth, J. B., Rob, C. G. and Simeone, F. A. (1962) In *Vascular Surgery*. London: Arnold, p. 30.

38. Kwaan, H. C. and McFadzean, A. J. C. (1957) Inhibition of fibrinolysis *in vivo* by feeding cholesterol. *Nature*, **179**, 260.

39. Macdonald, I. and Braithwaite, D. M. (1964) The influence of dietary carbohydrates on the lipid pattern in serum and in adipose tissue. *Clin. Sci.*, **27**, 23.

40. McDonald, L. (1953) Ischaemic heart disease and peripheral occlusive arterial disease. *Brit. Heart J.*, **15**, 101.

41. McNicol, G. P., Bain, W. H., Walker, F., Rifkind, B. M. and Douglas, A. S. (1965) Thrombolysis studied in an artificial circulation. *Lancet*, **i**, 838.

42. Millar, J. H. D. and Dalby, A. M. (1965) Platelet stickiness in cerebrovascular disease. *Proc. 8th Internat. Cong. Neurology, Vienna, 5th–10th September, 1965*, Vol. 4, p. 483.

43. Mitchell, J. R. A. and Schwartz, C. J. (1962) Relationship between arterial disease in different sites. A study of the aorta and coronary, carotid and iliac arteries. *Brit. med. J.*, **i**, 1293.

44. Mitchell, J. R. A. and Schwartz, C. J. (1965) *Arterial Disease*. Oxford: Blackwell Scientific Publications.

45. Morris, J. N., Heady, J. A., Raffle, P. A. B., Roberts, C. G. and Parks, J. W. (1953) Coronary heart-disease and physical activity of work. *Lancet*, **ii**, 1053.

46. Morris, J. N. and Crawford, M. D. (1958) Coronary heart disease and physical activity of work. *Brit. med. J.*, **ii**, 1485.

47. Mozes, N., Bogokowski, H., Antebi, E., Lunenfeld, B., Rabau, E., Serr, D. M., David, A. and Salomy, M. (1965) Thromboembolic phenomena after ovarian stimulation with human gonadotrophins. *Lancet*, **ii**, 1213.

48. Murphy, E. A. and Mustard, J. F. (1962) Coagulation tests and platelet economy in atherosclerotic and control subjects. *Circulation*, **25**, 114.

49. Mustard, J. F., Rowsell, H. C., Murphy, E. A. and Downie, H. G. (1963) Diet and thrombus formation: quantitative studies using an extracorporeal circulation in pigs. *J. Clin. Invest.*, **42**, 1783.

50. Mustard, J. F. and Murphy, E. A. (1963) Effect of smoking on blood coagulation and platelet survival in man. *Brit. med. J.*, **i**, 846.

51. Ogston, D. and McAndrew, G. M. (1964) Fibrinolysis in obesity. *Lancet*, **ii**, 1205.

52. Oldham, J. B. (1964) Claudication: the case for conservatism. *J. Roy. Coll. Surg. Edin.*, **9**, 179.

53. Oliver, M. F. (1960) Plasma lipids and atherosclerosis. *Proc. Roy. Soc. Med.*, **53**, 15.

54. Oliver, M. F. (1970) Oral contraceptives and myocardial infarction. *Brit. med. J.*, **2**, 210.

55. Perdue, G. D. and Smith R. B. (1969) Atheromatous microemboli. *Ann. Surg.*, **169**, 954.

56. Philp, R. B. and Wright, H. P. (1965) Effect of adenosine on platelet adhesiveness in fasting and lipaemic bloods. *Lancet*, **ii**, 208.

57. Pickering, G. W. (1964) Pathogenesis of myocardial and cerebral infarction: nodular arteriosclerosis. *Brit. med. J.*, **i**, 517.

58. Poole, J. C. F. (1960) Methods of observing thrombosis *in vitro*. *Proc. Roy. Soc. Med.*, **53**, 22.

58A. Pozner, H. and Billimoria, J. D. (1970) Effect of smoking on blood-clotting and lipid and lipoprotein levels. *Lancet*, **i**, 1318.

59. Roberts, J. C., Moses, C. and Wilkins, R. H. (1959) Autopsy studies in atherosclerosis. *Circulation*, **20**, 511, 520, 527.

60. Rokitansky, C. (1852) *A Manual of Pathological Anatomy*, Vol. 4. London: Sydenham Society.

60A. Reid, D. D. and Rose, G. (1971) Incidence of intermittent claudication and angina. Personal communication.

60B. Royal College of Physicians (1971) *Smoking and Health Now*. London: Pitman Medical and Scientific.

61. Schwartz, C. J. and Mitchell, J. R. A. (1962) Observations on localisation of arterial plaques. *Circulation Res.*, **11,** 63.
62. Schwartz, C. J. and Mitchell, J. R. A. (1962) Cellular infiltration of the human arterial adventitia associated with atheromatous plaques. *Circulation,* **26,** 73.
62A.Sloan, J. M., Mackay, J. S. and Sheridan, B. (1970) Glucose tolerance and insulin response in atherosclerosis. *Brit. med. J.,* **4,** 586.
62B.Stout, R. W. and Vallance-Owen, J. (1969) Insulin and atheroma. *Lancet,* **i,** 1078.
63. Sznajderman, M. and Oliver, M. F. (1963) Spontaneous premature menopause, ischaemic heart-disease and serum-lipids. *Lancet,* **i,** 962.
64. Tysak, A. J. and Ellis, J. D. (1971) Management of severe ovarian hyperstimulation. *Brit. med. J.,* **2,** 263.
65. Walden, R. T., Schaefer, L. E. and Lemon, F. R. (1964) Effect of environment on the serum cholesterol-triglyceride distribution among Seventh-Day Adventists. *Amer. J. Med.,* **36,** 269.
66. Widmer, L. K. (1963) Periphere Atherosklerose. Ihre frühzeitige Erfassung und Bedeutung in der Praxis. *Schw. med. Woch.,* **93,** 1583.
67. Widmer, L. K., Greensher, A. and Kannel, W. B. (1964) Occlusion of peripheral arteries: a study of 6,400 working subjects. *Circulation,* **30,** 836.
67A.Woolf, N. (1970) Aspects of the pathogenesis of atherosclerosis. In *Modern Trends in Vascular Surgery,* **1** (Ed. Gillespie, J. A.) London: Butterworth, p. 1.
68. Wright, H. P. (1942) Changes in the adhesiveness of blood platelets following parturition and surgical operations. *J. Path. Bact.,* **54,** 461.
69. Wuest, J. H., Dry, T. J. and Edwards, J. E. (1953) The degree of coronary atherosclerosis in bilaterally oophorectomised women. *Circulation,* **7,** 801.
70. Zelis, R., Mason, D. T., Braunwald, E. and Levy, R. I. (1970) Effects of hyperlipoproteinemias and their treatment on the peripheral circulation. *J. clin. Invest.,* **49,** 1007.

2 Acute Ischaemia

The Early Picture

The effects of sudden loss of blood supply are shown in their simplest form when an arterial tourniquet is tightened. The first obvious change is the total disappearance of all peripheral pulses beyond the obstruction. Skin colour and warmth are not much affected during these early moments, and there is no pain or discomfort except from the constriction of the cuff. The first visible effects are pallor at the periphery, with collapse of the superficial veins; these occur within a few moments of the obstruction, and are more marked if the limb has just been exercised. Venous emptying is due to draining of blood from the superficial vessels into those of the deep tissues whose blood requirement, even at rest, is greater than that of the skin, and much more so after exercise. Wide, static vasodilatation soon develops in muscle vessels, and pallor therefore becomes progressively more marked, with a 'waxen' appearance of the skin when its vessels are almost completely empty.

Release of the tourniquet after a few minutes of total ischaemia is followed by a conspicuous reactive hyperaemia, proving that vasodilatation develops early during ischaemia. Plethysmograph tracings show that the first in-rush of blood after release takes a few moments to reach the measuring chamber; it must first 'take up slack' in the dilated vascular bed between it and the tourniquet cuff. Then, almost at once, the tracing shows a flow rate of up to ten times the resting level. At the same time the skin becomes brightly flushed. In the normal lower limb this flush should reach the toes within 5 to 10 seconds. If any arterial obstruction remains, it takes much longer (Table 2.1) and the plethysmograph shows that the returning pulse waves are damped [6].

It is clear, therefore, that the effects of acute ischaemia, though extensive and almost immediate, are at first clinically somewhat inconspicuous, which accounts for difficulties often experienced in recognising this serious condition and in assessing its probable duration.

EARLY SIGNS OF STRUCTURAL DAMAGE
Within fifteen minutes of the onset of total ischaemia of a limb, numbness develops in the tips of the digits, and Lewis found that it spreads proximally at the rate of 3 to 4 cm a minute [18]. It is probably due to

Table 2.1. Reactive Hyperaemia Skin Test [21]
Time taken for skin flushing to reach a stated point after removal of an arterial tourniquet from the warm limb.

	Patellar tubercle	Ankle malleoli	Toes
A normal limb	immediate	immediate	2–5 sec
Limb with an occluded popliteal artery	8 sec	28 sec	47 sec
Same limb after reconstruction of arterial block	2 sec	6 sec	8 sec

N.B. Exercise of a limb without a tourniquet but with an existing occlusion of its main artery frequently reproduces this cycle of transient acute ischaemia and delayed skin flushing (see Chapter 3, p. 48). The diagnosis of acute limb ischaemia should take this phenomenon into account.

18

a direct effect on sensory nerve endings in the skin. About the same time, weakness begins in the short intrinsic muscles of the extremity and soon spreads upwards to involve the long muscles. That this is an effect upon their nerve supply, and not upon the muscles themselves, is shown by the fact that the muscle bellies will respond to an electrical stimulus long after all voluntary movement and reflex activity have disappeared. Damage to the muscles comes later, taking several hours to become complete.

ISCHAEMIC MUSCLE CONTRACTURE

This is a selective muscle infarction affecting the forearm and hand, or the calf and foot, due to ischaemia, often combined with compression, not at first sufficient to kill the other tissues of the limb.

The typical deformity produced in the hand is shown in Fig. 2.1.

The skin and supporting tissues remain viable, being better adapted to withstand damaging conditions, and having a lower resting blood requirement. Within this living envelope, irreversible changes, which will, in these first few hours, decide the fate of the limb as a useful appendage, soon establish themselves. Seddon [27] has defined ischaemic contracture as a circumscribed, deep-seated affection of voluntary muscle encased in normal tissue. The lesions may be localised within one or more muscles, and are ellipsoidal in shape, being composed, at first, of more or less infarcted tissue, partly or completely necrosed, and, later, by fibrous tissues mixed with unharmed muscle fibres in the marginal zones, but merging with amorphous material in the depths of the lesion, which may later liquefy or even become calcified. This explains why milder cases may show full recovery over weeks or months as the surviving

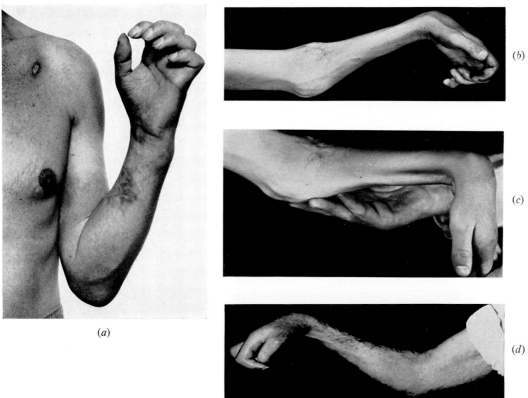

Fig. 2.1.

(a) Early ischaemic contracture of the forearm muscles in a man aged thirty-two following compression under the body for 36 hours after a drug overdose. (Mr A. J. Harrold's case.)

(b) and (c) Late forearm contracture in a boy aged twelve who, two years previously, sustained the condition within 48 hours of a fracture dislocation of the elbow. Note that wrist flexion enables the fingers to be straightened. (Sir Herbert Seddon's case.)

(d) Late contracture complicating wrist fracture in a haemophilic. (Mr H. R. I. Wolfe's case.)

19

muscle fibres recover and overcome the limitation of fibrous lesions running through them, and also why, in the more severe cases, excision of these strips from the centre of otherwise healthy muscle may be rewarded by the return of much useful movement. When nerves are affected, it is not by fibrous compression but much earlier, during the ischaemic phase. The median is more affected than the ulnar, for it lies deeply in the most ischaemic region of the forearm, though if, on exploration, it shows clear signs of returning circulation, recovery of function is likely. In the worst cases, tendon, cartilage, bone, and even subcutaneous fat may be affected.

The early recognition of the start of ischaemic contracture is, therefore, a matter of the utmost urgency and importance, for reversibility of the damage depends wholly upon the duration of the ischaemia. The earliest signs of certain muscle involvement are weakness of the digits, and above all, pain on passive extension. To these must be added the visible effects of mild to moderate skin ischaemia, namely pallor and cyanosis with diminished sensation; also, almost always, loss of the distal pulses. We consider the operative measures necessary to correct this terrible condition in the chapter on arterial injuries, but it must be said at once that the least suspicion of these appearances in a vulnerable case, such as a child with a supracondylar fracture of the humerus, should warn the surgeon that he must remove the plaster, or

any other obvious cause of compression, and be prepared to explore the artery without delay if there is not an immediate improvement. Indirect methods such as stellate block and body heating have no place, for they only delay the essential step, which is operative decompression of the obstructed circulation, with wide fasciotomy, which releases the constriction of the swollen muscle bellies within their compartments [1]. Ischaemic muscle contracture may be caused by conditions other than limb fractures, for example: penetrating arterial wounds, peripheral arterial embolism, compression of the limb by the body weight in coma from head injury, diabetes or barbiturates; or from coal-gas poisoning, in which tissue hypoxia from lack of oxy-haemoglobin aggravates the ischaemic effect of the body pressure upon the limb [14]; also, from acute arterial thrombosis following an accidental injection; and quite often from sudden arterial occlusion in injury or disease, part or the whole of the calf being most commonly affected (Fig. 2.2). Fractures about the knee region, like those of the elbow, are specially

Fig. 2.2.
(a) Typical flexion and inversion ankle deformity due to ischaemic contracture of the calf, in a woman aged 68, following a femoral embolism and its removal. Note oedema of revascularisation (Chapter 3, p. 68).
(b) Massive segmental infarction, necrosis, and gas formation in the calf. One month previously, the popliteal artery had been divided by a pane of glass.

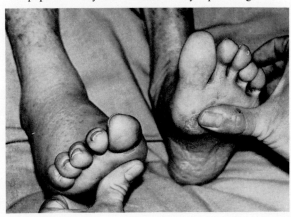

(a)

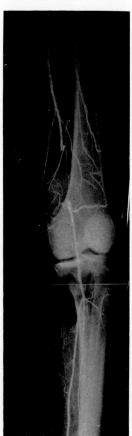

(b)

likely to damage the popliteal artery (*see* Chapter 12, p. 250) in young adults, the flexor longus hallucis being the most frequently affected muscle, then the anterior tibial group [28].

A special form is seen in the anterior tibial compartment in young people following over-exercise, and in older patients as a result of thrombosis or embolism of the anterior tibial artery, either on its own or as a secondary complication of an earlier occlusion of the main artery proximally.

SIGNS OF RECOVERY

1. *In the Skin*

These are well shown towards the end of an operation for resection of an abdominal aortic aneurysm, during which the aorta and common iliac arteries have been clamped for one to two hours, or more. While the clamps are in place, the patient's feet show the typical waxy pallor of acute ischaemia, being far beyond the range of the small collateral from the lumbar region. After removal of the clamps, the pallor, which at first extends over most of the limb, will be replaced by an even *cyanosis which gradually spreads down the limb*, to reach the heel, then the forefoot, and finally the toes, in much the same way as the flush of reactive hyperaemia though much more slowly, perhaps because of aggregation or sedimentation of red cells in small vessels. This cyanosis bears no resemblance to the static form seen in early irreversible ischaemia, from which it can readily be distinguished by its slow downward spread, whereas *the cyanosis of early gangrene extends upwards*. The blueness of recovery is an active process in moving blood whose oxygen is quickly removed by the anoxic tissues. The stationary, mottled cyanosis of severe, unrelieved ischaemia in a dying limb is due to local pooling of blood with reduced haemoglobin in paralytic, anoxic vessels, with pallor in the still-constricted areas between. In the recovering limb, as the blue tinge passes into the pale peripheral skin, behind it the skin becomes pinkish in colour, and perceptibly warmer as its circulation returns*. Finally, as further confirmation, the *superficial veins begin to refill*, and the stroking test shows that blood is entering them from their distal end.

A sure sign of recovery in a conscious patient is the return of sensation progressively down the limb, tending, in fact, to precede the visible skin changes. When both these evidences are present the limb prognosis is good.

2. *The Pulses*

Return of the peripheral pulses is an obvious sign of recovery, though, at first, they will be small in volume and tend to vary with the general condition, particularly in cardiac or postoperative patients. The skin signs may precede the reappearance of pulses, no doubt because the widely dilated peripheral bed offers so little resistance to the pulse wave that it will remain small or impalpable for many hours.

It cannot be overemphasised that the strength of a peripheral arterial pulse is no certain index of the flow through the artery at that point; the most bounding pulse may be present immediately above a recent complete block such as an embolus or a distally occluded graft.

During an operation, this failure of pulse volume on release of the arterial clamps can be investigated by the simple expedient of restoring peripheral resistance by occluding either the main artery, or one of its large branches, e.g. the profunda femoris, when at once the pulse volume rises sharply. Partial release may allow the appreciation of a high-flow state by generating a thrill between the fingers on either side of the artery.

Severe, Irreversible Acute Ischaemia

The Imminent Condition

Danger signs $\begin{cases} \text{Waxy pallor} \\ \text{Sensory loss} \\ \text{Hand or foot much colder than} \\ \quad \text{other extremities} \\ \text{Muscle weakness, tenderness or} \\ \quad \text{rigidity} \end{cases}$

To be able to recognise with certainty the irreversibility of this serious condition in time to institute effective treatment is one of the heaviest responsibilities any clinician can be called upon to bear, yet there is often confusion, unjustified optimism, and delay, or, what may be as bad, an ill-timed operative intervention upon a limb that has begun to recover.

Quite simply, the diagnosis of irreversible acute ischaemia depends upon the lack of signs of early improvement, which have been stated at length for this reason. *Unless within two hours of the recognition of acute ischaemia there is a return of some skin circulation and sensation, centrifugally and beyond all doubt progressive, there is little chance of limb survival* [16].

This does not mean that there is a two-hour limit within which active treatment must be undertaken,

---

* The cycle of skin changes: waxy pallor—cyanosis—pink warmth is precisely that of the Raynaud phenomenon of the digits (*see* Chapter 11, p. 202) on a larger and somewhat slower scale.

but rather that unless spontaneous improvement is unmistakably taking place by that time, it probably never will, and in these circumstances there can be no hope of avoiding loss of some part of the limb unless something effective can be done to the circulation before irreversible damage occurs. This period of grace may vary a great deal and can be extended by medical treatment, but with massive ischaemia it will not often be longer than eight hours.

Established Gangrene

Cases such as the one shown in Fig. 2.3 are familiar to all who treat elderly hospital patients with cardiovascular disease, in whom neither the cardiac nor the peripheral condition responds to treatment. Collateral supply to such limbs depends to a large extent on cardiac function, as does the outcome of surgical attempts to improve the blood supply locally. Figure 2.4 shows the lower limbs of a second patient who was in hospital at the same time, and whose first presentation was practically identical, but who rallied in his general condition and responded well to unorthodox arterial surgery (*see* Chapter 3, p. 83) to by-pass his occluded left iliac arteries. These two cases are good examples of 'moist' and 'dry' gangrene, respectively.

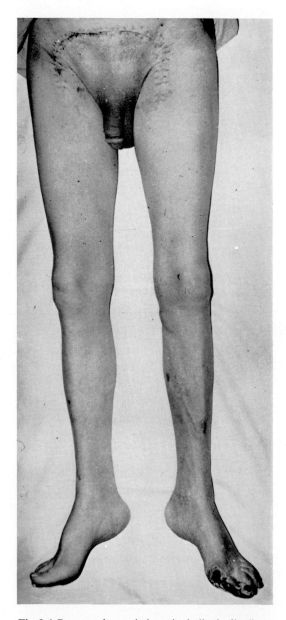

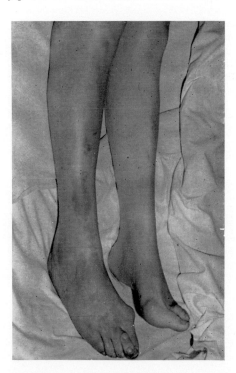

Fig. 2.3. Cold, mottled and flexed right ankle and foot during irreversible acute ischaemia. (An elderly woman with acute femoro-popliteal arterial thrombosis.)

Fig. 2.4. Recovered acute ischaemia similar in distribution to that of Fig. 2.3, but here due principally to occlusion of the left iliac artery. Reconstruction by dacron femoro-femoral cross-over graft, combined with repair of two large inguinal herniae becoming incarcerated. Note also thrombosed varicose vein below left medial tibial condyle, another sign of recent acute ischaemia.

(a) *Moist gangrene* is a massive necrosis of a limb, purplish-white, with rigidity giving place to softening of the muscles, blistering, and peeling of the skin and, proximally, a region of dying tissue, patchily ischaemic, and often extending upwards as the patient's conditions further deteriorates. Death soon brings an end to the story, an all too-common one, regrettably still to be seen after unsuccessful elective arterial surgery, constituting a major arterial injury without effective repair.

(b) *Dry gangrene* as an end result of acute ischae-mia indicates that slow mortification, confined as a rule to the foot or hand, though sometimes extending higher up the limb, has taken place during the time required for the collateral circulation, or restored flow after arterial surgery such as embolectomy, with the paradox that just above this the skin may be hot, yet beyond it, black and mummified. Spontaneous, painless separation of the tissues will follow, in the absence of spreading infection, until only the bones remain to hold the extremity (Fig. 2.5).

Causes of Acute Limb Ischaemia and Their Diagnosis

Local and systemic factors must both be considered in a seriously ill patient if it is difficult to decide which may be the more important.

Any of the following causes, separately or together, can account for the appearance of acute ischaemia in an extremity. Likely associations between the two groups will suggest themselves.

1. Thrombosis in obliterative arterial disease: (arteriosclerosis, thrombo-angiitis obliterans, and the collagen diseases)

2. Arterial embolism

3. Damage to artery: (injury, injection or operation)

4. Pathological dissection of the arterial wall

5. Raynaud's disease and phenomenon

6. Frostbite

7. Ergot poisoning

1. Reduced peripheral blood flow due to:
   (a) Shock from injury or operation
   (b) Heart failure or myocardial infarction
   (c) Senility, recumbency

2. Blood conditions:
   (a) anaemia (reduced O_2 capacity)
   (b) haemoconcentration (dehydration, diuresis polycythaemia)
   (c) thrombophilic and hyperco-agulable states
   (d) leukaemia, sickle-celled haemoglobin-C disease

3. Advanced carcinoma

Most cases of acute ischaemia are due to occlusion of the arterial lumen from local physical damage or disease, in many instances aggravated by one or more of the general factors listed above, which on occasion are sufficient to cause ischaemic occlusion of a normal artery, e.g. in early childhood [24] (Fig. 2.6) though in normal health this probably never occurs.

Diagnosis

The local appearances of acute ischaemia are quite non-specific with little to distinguish between cases due to such widely differing causes as frostbite and emboli from an artery damaged by a cervical rib, or ergotism and Buerger's disease, and much less again when arteriosclerotic thrombosis and major embolism are both considered possible in elderly subjects who develop serious ischaemia.

Most guidance can be provided by the patient's general condition, with the previous history and the systematic examination almost certain to provide the information upon which the diagnosis can be based.

Conditions often leading to acute ischaemia are considered in detail in other chapters; here only a brief summary need be given.

1. *Thrombosis* most commonly affects an artery already sclerotic and narrowed or aneurysmal, as evident on local palpation. More often, the signs of arterial disease in other limbs suggest this, the most usual cause of acute ischaemia (*see* Chapter 3, p. 43 and Chapter 4, p. 102).

2. *Embolism* is suggested by the finding of signs of serious heart disease, most of all when there is atrial fibrillation (*see* Chapter 14, p. 259).

3. *Recent acute injury, injection or arterial operation* are obviously to blame when the affected limb shows acute ischaemia shortly afterwards (*see* Chapter 13, p. 238).

4. *Pathological dissection* occurs mainly with severe hypertension and in cases of congenital connective tissue defect (*see* Chapter 15, p. 319).

5. *Raynaud's disease and phenomenon*, themselves difficult to distinguish between, nevertheless present a somewhat different picture from other types of ischaemia in their repeated and cyclical features (*see* Chapter 11, p. 202).

6. *Frostbite*, like injury or operation, should be clearly due to the physical conditions recently endured. It is less obvious when it occurs in lonely old people sitting still, indoors, or after

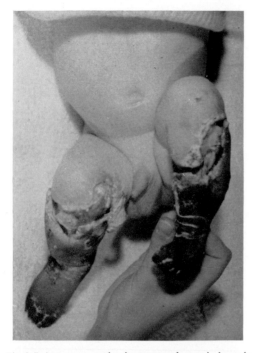

Fig. 2.5. Auto-amputation in recovered acute ischaemia due to neo-natal aorto-iliac thrombosis. (Professor Charles Rob and Dr Langridge's case.)

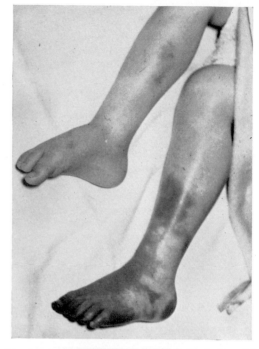

Fig. 2.6. Acute ischaemia of both lower limbs in a girl of 2½ years developing during extreme dehydration from gastro-enteritis. (Mr David Bolt's case.)

unexpected cold exposure as in youth mountain-training exercises, or sail-plane flying (*see* Chapter 11, p. 206).
7. *Ergot poisoning* in migraine sufferers, or women attempting to procure abortion is usually preceded by a phase of sensory impairment longer in duration than with most other causes of acute ischaemia, and venous spasm precedes arterial (*see* Chapter 11, p. 207).

SYSTEMIC FACTORS IN ACUTE ISCHAEMIA
These are important in diagnosis and, also, have a profound bearing upon treatment. A reduction in limb blood flow due to some general cause can, in itself, be sufficient to cause acute ischaemia. Two main groups of conditions may do this:
1. *Cardiovascular insufficiency*, either peripherally as in shock of all kinds (traumatic, metabolic, or toxic), or from cardiac causes (heart failure, or myocardial infarction) or where both factors occur together, e.g. after major heart or arterial surgery. Acute mesenteric ischaemia is particularly likely to occur in these circumstances in elderly subjects (*see* Chapter 17, p. 370), and by the same type of mechanism the extremities may show symmetrical acute ischaemia as a complication of acute myocardial failure without actual peripheral occlusions [7,20,31].
2. *Blood conditions* readily aggravate structural and haemodynamic causes of the above kinds:

(*a*) Anaemia, from a further reduction in the effectiveness of the remaining circulation;
(*b*) Dehydration, with increased blood viscosity such as may occur in cholera, or in severe gastro-enteritis of children (Fig. 2.6) or after operation; or from the effects of diuretic treatment of heart failure, in which blood viscosity tends to rise with the haematocrit, and also the fibrinogen content, as the body weight falls [10], so that the critical period may occur during the restoration of cardiac compensation, a time incidentally, when emboli are specially common (*see* Chapter 14, p. 259).
(*c*) Blood diseases, which also increase blood viscosity and thereby reduce blood flow through smaller vessels, particularly if there is also a structural cause for stagnation; polycythaemia, sickle-cell haemoglobin-C disease, and leukaemia are haematological causes regularly met with in limb ischaemia patients in a large hospital population.

Malignant disease of various kinds is frequently complicated by the development of spontaneous intravascular thrombosis, chiefly of the veins, but also sometimes of large arteries, e.g. the popliteal (Fig. 2.7) while smaller ones, such as the digitals, not infrequently thrombose, causing a severe form of secondary Raynaud phenomenon with gangrene (*see* Chapter 11, p. 208).

Treatment: General and Medical Measures

Each case should pose the question: can this obstruction be removed? It is an emergency situation that calls for immediate action. The penalties of delay and indecision are known to every doctor. The following active measures to conserve and promote the circulation should be considered whether or not surgery is in prospect.

1. Rest and the relief of pain
2. Exposure of the limb
3. Correct positioning of the patient
4. Warmth to the rest of the body
5. Correction of general circulatory impairment, (e.g. shock, heart failure)
6. Anticoagulants, fibrinolysins
7. Low molecular weight dextrans
8. Hyperbaric oxygen.

Important though these medical measures are, they must never be allowed to hold up the arrangements for surgical restoration of the blood supply; when operation is possible it must have first priority; these supporting forms of treatment are then accorded their useful place in postoperative care.

REST
Unless kept at rest, the patient will waste his strength in unnecessary movements; potential blood flow will be diverted from the ischaemic region to other parts of the body. Relief of pain is essential, and effective analgesics must be freely given. The affected limb must also be kept at complete rest, for in most cases some muscle activity is still possible and will be detrimental, for it creates further metabolic demands. Alcohol is a most useful sedative and analgesic, which also prevents vasoconstriction.

EXPOSURE OF THE LIMB
The object is to maintain an equable air temperature around the limb, avoiding thermal injury, which will result either from heating or cooling the affected skin. A low level of circulation renders a limb incapable of conducting calories to or from itself. Even mild local heat can cause severe damage (Fig. 2.8). Electric fans or other vigorous means of cooling should be avoided, for the cold may cause further physical injury to the already devitalised tissues. A normal extremity cooled continuously in such a way would soon register discomfort or pain.

Only in massive or irreversible necrosis may there be a case for deliberate refrigeration or freezing, with ice or solid CO_2 respectively. Time may be gained in this way, during which the patient's general condition may be improved, and the spread of a collateral circulation down towards the dead zone may ensure better conditions for the healing of amputation flaps.

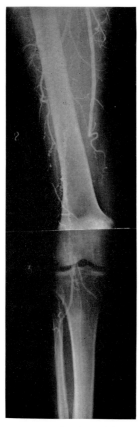

Fig. 2.7. Acute thrombosis of the right popliteal artery occurring in a man aged thirty-six with Hodgkin's disease, successfully removed using arterial balloon catheter.

CORRECT POSITIONING OF THE PATIENT
The aim should be to utilise gravity to improve the in-flow of blood to the affected limb, by keeping it a little below the rest of the body, e.g. in the lower

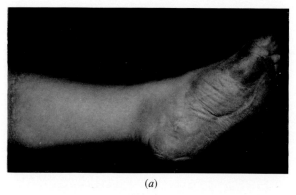 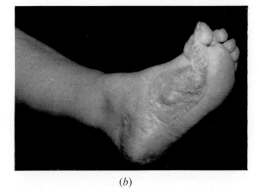

(a)   (b)

Fig. 2.8. (*a*) Full thickness burn of left sole produced by a 'comfortably warm' hot-water bottle during acute ischaemia with anaesthesia of foot following popliteal embolism.

(*b*) Final extent of damage after excision and skin graft replacement also shows resolving flexion contracture of calf.

limb by slightly raising the head of the bed. Patients with acute-on-chronic ischaemia will usually have learnt to hang their leg out of bed or to sleep in an armchair. Often the limb is oedematous as a result.

If the occlusion is located in one of the iliac or common femoral arteries it may be useful to turn the patient partly on to his sound side, to prevent compression of important collaterals in the gluteal region. In upper limb ischaemia, elevation of the legs may improve blood flow to the arms [29].

WARMTH TO THE BODY
Reflex heating is a physiological term meaning the release of vasoconstrictor tone to an extremity by the application of heat elsewhere [13] (Fig. 2.9).

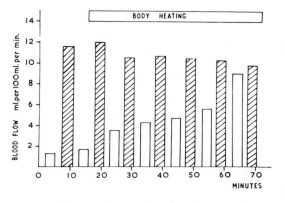

Fig. 2.9. Increase of foot blood flow (open columns) during body warming. Within one hour, blood flow almost equals that of the sympathectomised opposite limb.

When a single, normal limb is the subject of study, this proves to be a most effective mechanism, but its clinical use in the case of an ischaemic limb presupposes that the affected vessels are capable of such a response. Excessive room heat, bedding, gloves, and socks are sometimes prescribed with the object of opening up the circulation in the obstructed limb. Apart from the manifest discomforts of this regime, it may possibly do harm by tending to draw blood away from the affected region, as pharmacological vasodilatation is known to do (*see* Chapter 3, p. 31) because of the relatively higher resistance there compared with the rest of the body.

Body warming should be limited to that sufficient for comfort and to prevent vasoconstriction in cool weather or draughty surroundings, which may be difficult in an open ward at certain times.

CARE OF THE GENERAL CIRCULATION
After major injury or operation, with uncorrected hypovolaemia, peripheral vasoconstriction attempts to compensate for loss of circulating blood volume. At such a time a diseased, traumatised or recently operated artery may thrombose. A good clinical guide to the general level of the circulation is the skin temperature of the extremities, e.g. the tip of the nose. More precisely, blood volume measurement with simple isotope techniques is becoming routine, and central venous pressure is easily monitored in the theatre and recovery room. Vasopressors, it is becoming increasingly realised, should not be used for falling blood pressure due to low blood volume, for they merely elevate the pressure at the expense of the periphery, and in an ischaemic zone this may be decisive against tissue survival. Adequate blood replacement is the correct way in which to maintain

both pressure and flow. Gentle, expeditious surgery, with careful control of blood loss is even better.

Cardiac failure can produce ischaemia of the limbs [7, 20, 31]. Recognition of this factor may save a limb, even though it may not have been possible to remove the arterial occlusion. Supportive treatment to the heart, like replacement of blood volume in shock, assumes a critical importance in the postoperative period in arterial surgery where there is ischaemia or the risk of its occurrence.

ANTICOAGULANTS

Heparin is invaluable in acute limb ischaemia and should be given as soon as the diagnosis has been made. It in no way affects the surgical management, for the action can be quickly reversed at any time. It prolongs the period of grace by its certain prevention of the spread of occluding thrombus across the mouths of patent collateral branches, particularly in the stagnant column of blood beyond the block. Heparin is contra-indicated:

(a) in the very aged in whom there is the risk of cerebral haemorrhage;
(b) where ischaemia is due to structural failure of the arterial wall, as in dissecting aneurysm, or leakage from or compression by a peripheral aneurysm.
(c) after arterial reconstructive operation whether undertaken for acute ischaemia or itself the cause of it: bleeding is almost certain after the first few hours, and hypotension may actually encourage platelet thrombus accumulation, upon which heparin has very little effect (see Chapter 3 [113]).

With these exceptions most cases are likely to be helped by heparin.

Details of dosage are given in Chapter 14, p. 265, and, also, of the use of phenindione, mainly in reducing secondary deep venous thrombosis, which often complicates limb ischaemia.

LOW MOLECULAR WEIGHT DEXTRAN (LMDX) [8, 11, 12, 23]

Reservations have been expressed as to the rationale and mode of action of this type of treatment [5, 26], and suggestions have been made that plasma volume expansion is their main effect. Nevertheless, vascular surgeons are in general agreement as to their useful-

ness in limb ischaemia, for the clinical response is, in most cases, very favourable. Early claims for LMDX to have reduced viscosity (other than by haemodilution), and platelet and red cell aggregation in stasis zones have some support [2]. It now seems more likely that viscosity-lowering effects of dextran are due to plasma volume expansion alone, this haemodilution lasting longer than that which follows the infusion of considerably greater amounts of electrolyte solutions [11, 26].

The normal dosage of LMDX is 500 ml each twelve hours by intravenous infusion at a steady rate. Excretion is fairly rapid, and very high urine specific gravities are recorded.

Special care must be taken when administering dextran to patients with cardiac failure, as in peripheral arterial embolism (see Chapter 14, p. 266). It is even more dangerous in patients with incipient or established renal failure, or other serious antecedent general illness, or if given for longer than three days in elderly or arteriosclerotic subjects. In any of these conditions the highly viscous urine in the renal tubules may damage them severely from a type of 'osmotic nephrosis' [19].

HYPERBARIC OXYGEN [3, 15]

If oxygen is breathed at an ambient pressure of two atmospheres, the proportion in simple solution in the plasm increases from 0·25 vol % to 4·2 vol %. The combined oxygen with haemoglobin remains the same at 19·5 vol %. Thus, an increase in the oxygen-carrying capacity of the blood in these conditions of about 25 per cent is provided, which might prove decisive to tissues in marginal ischaemia. Certain provisions must be made, however: there must be an effective remaining circulation for any of this increase to reach the ischaemia area, and there should be no reduction in total blood flow as a result of the increased oxygen tension. This however, has been shown to happen in the cerebral [17], retinal [9] and limb [22] circulations. The place of hyperbaric oxygen treatment in limb ischaemia is not yet established, though it may tide the recovering extremity over, pending a return of better circulatory conditions [3, 15].

Frost bite responds well to hyperbaric oxygen at two atmospheres pressure. Rapid 'pinking', relief of pain and resolution of blistering have been reported after two hours daily for up to nineteen days [32].

SURGICAL TREATMENT

Of the important common causes of acute ischaemia, most are concerned with the main artery of the limb, and most are potentially curable by arterial surgery, the limiting factors being:

1. Established, irreversible damage to the limb tissues.
2. When the artery containing the occluding thrombus or the branches (the 'run-off') is extensively

and irregularly narrowed by previous arteriosclerotic disease.

3. When the cardiac and general condition cannot support the patient through surgery, or maintain the restored peripheral circulation afterwards.

Sympathetic block or denervation are virtually useless in the treatment of acute ischaemia, for there is no lack of local vasodilatation, which metabolism has already provided. What is missing is the force and flow of the arterial supply to perfuse this open distal vascular bed. Operative sympathectomy or any other fruitless surgical intervention can do positive harm, by placing further strain on the patient's reserves. It may also damage useful collaterals. The benefits of heparin are practically precluded by operations upon the body cavity.

Late surgical intervention in protracted acute ischaemia is sometimes worth while, so long as the limb remains viable, when there is a barely sufficient collateral supply, but enough to keep the distal arteries from becoming blocked by consecutive thrombus. Otherwise, late reconstruction, although technically possible, may perfuse blood through a large section of dying muscle, with fatal consequences (*see* Chapter 14, p. 268).

Once it is clear that the time for arterial restoration is past, it is better to postpone amputation for a while, to allow the improvement in proximal soft tissue blood supply, which can be expected to take place and which may mean that it will shortly be possible to conserve more of the limb, or at least with better prospects for the skin flaps decided upon. Infection will overrule any such plan; an early amputation then becomes mandatory. A patient who is too ill for surgery may be helped by refrigeration or freezing of the dead portion (*see* p. 126) until sufficiently recovered for the ordeal.

Technical Details of Arterial Operations for Acute Ischaemia

These and any special indications and contra-indications are discussed under their respective causes:

1. Arterial injury—Chapter 13, p. 239.
2. Peripheral embolism—Chapter 14, p. 266.
3. Dissecting aneurysm—Chapter 15, p. 325.
4. Leaking peripheral aneurysm—Chapter 15, p. 314.

REFERENCES

1. Benjamin, A. (1957) The relief of traumatic arterial spasm in threatened Volkmann's ischaemic contracture. *J. Bone and Jt. Surg.*, **39B**, 711.
2. Bennett, P. N., Dhall, D. P., McKenzie, F. N. and Matheson, N. A. (1966) Effects of dextran infusion on the adhesiveness of human blood-platelets. *Lancet*, **ii**, 1001.
3. Boerema, I. (1964) Hyperbaric oxygen. *Proc. Roy. Soc. Med.*, **57**, 817.
4. Breckenridge, I. M. and Walker, W. F. (1963) Blood-loss in open heart surgery with low-molecular-weight dextran. *Lancet*, **i**, 1190.
5. Collins, G. M. and Ludbrook, J. (1966) The rheologic properties of low molecular weight dextrans: fact or fancy? *Amer. Heart J.*, **72**, 741.
6. Cooper, D., Hill, L. T. and Edwards, E. A. (1967) Detection of early arteriosclerosis by external pulse recording. *J. Amer. med. Assn.*, **199**, 499.
7. Cotton, R. T. and Bedford, D. R. (1956) Symmetric peripheral gangrene complicating acute myocardial infarction. *Amer. J. Med.*, **20**, 301.
8. Couch, N. P. (1965) The clinical status of low molecular weight dextran: a critical review. *Clin. Pharmacol. Ther.*, **6**, 656.
9. Dollery, C. T., Hill, D. W., Mailer, C. M. and Ramalho, P. S. (1964) High oxygen pressure and retinal blood-vessels. *Lancet*, **ii**, 291.
10. Eisenberg, S. (1964) Changes in blood viscosity, hematocrit value, and fibrinogen concentration in subjects with congestive heart failure. *Circulation*, **30**, 686.
11. Folse, R. and Cope, J. G. (1965) A comparison of the peripheral and central hemodynamic effects of regular and low molecular weight dextran in patients with ischemic limbs. *Surgery*, **58**, 779.
12. Gelin, L-E. and Ingelman, B. (1961) Rheomacrodex, a new dextran solution for rheological treatment of impaired capillary flow. *Acta Chir. Scand.*, **122**, 294.
13. Gibbon, J. H. and Landis, E. M. (1932) Vasodilatation in the lower extremities in response to immersing the forearms in warm water. *J. Clin. Invest.*, **11**, 1019.
14. Howse, A. J. G. and Seddon, H. (1966) Ischaemic contracture of muscle associated with carbon monoxide and barbiturate poisoning. *Brit. med. J.*, **i**, 192.
15. Illingworth, C. (1962) Treatment of arterial occlusion under oxygen at two-atmospheres pressure. *Brit. med. J.*, **ii**, 1271.
16. Jacobs, A. L. (1959) In *Arterial Embolism in the Limbs*. Edinburgh & London: E. & S. Livingstone, p. 94.
17. Jacobson, I., Harper, A. M. and McDowall, D. G. (1963) The effects of oxygen under pressure on cerebral blood flow and cerebral venous oxygen tension. *Lancet*, **ii**, 549.
18. Lewis, T. (1946) In *Vascular Disorders of the Limbs*. London: Macmillan, 2nd edition, p. 17.
19. Matheson, N. A. (1970) Renal failure after the administration of dextran-40. *Surg. Gynec. Obstet.*, **131**, 661.
20. Perry, C. B. and Davie, T. B. (1939) Symmetrical peripheral gangrene in cardiac failure. *Brit. med. J.*, **i**, 15.

21. Pickering, G. W. (1933) On the clinical recognition of structural disease of the peripheral vessels. *Brit. med. J.*, **ii**, 1106.
22. Pollock, J. G. and Ledingham, I. McA. (1967) The relationship between arterial oxygen tension, peripheral blood-flow and tissue oxygenation. *Brit. J. Surg.*, **54**, 236.
23. Powley, P. H. (1963) Rheomacrodex in peripheral ischaemia. *Lancet*, **i**, 1189.
24. Raffensperger, J. G., D'Cruz, I. A. and Hastreiter, A. R. (1964) Thrombotic occlusion of the bifurcation of the aorta in infancy: a case with successful surgical therapy. *Paediatrics*, **34**, 550.
25. Ratcliff, A. H. C. (1963) Low-molecular-weight dextran (Rheomacrodex) in the treatment of severe vascular insufficiency after trauma. *Lancet*, **i**, 1188.
26. Replogle, R. L., Kundler, H. and Gross, R. E. (1965) Studies on the hemodynamic importance of blood viscosity. *J. Thor. Cardiovasc. Surg.*, **50**, 658.
27. Seddon, H. (1964) Volkmann's ischaemia. *Brit. med. J.*, **i**, 1587.
28. Seddon, H. J. (1966) Volkmann's ischaemia in the lower limb. *J. Bone and Jt. Surg.*, **48B**, 627.
29. Shepherd, J. T. (1963) In *Physiology of the Circulation in Human Limbs in Health and Disease*. Philadelphia and London: W. B. Saunders Company, p. 45.
30. Tsapogas, M. J. (1964) The role of fibrinolysis in the treatment of arterial thrombosis: experimental and clinical aspects. *Ann. Roy. Coll. Surg. Eng.*, **34**, 293.
31. Wade, O. L. and Bishop, J. M. (1962) In *Cardiac Output and Regional Blood Flow*. Oxford: Blackwell.
32. Ward, M. P., Garnham, J. R., Simpson, B. R. J., Morley, G. H. and Winter, J. S. (1968) Frostbite: general observations and a report of cases treated by hyperbaric oxygen. *Proc. Roy. Soc. Med.*, **61**, 787.

3 Chronic Ischaemia

A part of the body is in a state of chronic ischaemia when its arterial inflow is reduced to a level at which normal function is impaired. If further reduction takes place the vitality of the tissues is threatened. Chronic ischaemia is, thus, a relative term, with several possible degrees of severity. Deterioration is by additional arterial occlusions, each of which tends to induce a further temporary episode of acute ischaemia, and during one of these some of the tissues may die.

This chapter will be mostly concerned with arteriosclerosis obliterans. Other important causes such as embolism, Buerger's disease and arteritis are the subject of separate chapters; also fibromuscular hypertrophy (*see* pp. 153 and 358) and malignant disease (Fig. 2.7, p. 25) or its treatment by radiation (Fig. 3.78.)

Effects on Tissue Function and Viability: the Anatomy of Deterioration

The disturbance produced by chronic ischaemia is proportional to the extent and number of arterial occlusions and to the rate at which they form. Many patients never notice much loss of exercise capacity; in some active people the limitation becomes troublesome, while in about 10 per cent peripheral blood flow continues to fall with each fresh spread of their occlusion, eventually reaching a low level at which pain is present at rest. In these, there is considerable risk of gangrene, which can follow quite minor local damage or some sudden general illness, though the ischaemia is still chronic. At any stage in the history a large added occlusion may precipitate severe acute-on-chronic ischaemia with imminent massive gangrene and the need for urgent surgical treatment.

CLAUDICATION (Claudicare = Gr. to limp)
Bouley, in Paris in 1831 [10], reported his findings in the case of a six-year-old bay mare, who, after a fall, went lame in the right hind leg, and later in the left; she appeared normal, however, when at rest.

Finally, both limbs became cold and devoid of sensibility. At post-mortem both femoral arteries were found to be occluded by a long thrombus, adherent at its upper end. In 1846, Sir Benjamin Brodie [13] showed that the same lesion in man could cause pain on walking. We now regard claudication

early childhood [41]. Sometimes the symptom dates back to a previous 'silent' or 'quiet' embolus to the affected limb in a relatively fit patient with mitral disease (*see* Chapter 14, p. 258). The aortic bifurcation may obstruct in this way without the acute features usually associated with this diagnosis

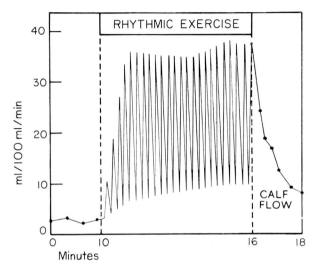

Fig. 3.1. Calf blood flow during rhythmic exercise. Hyperaemia is generated, but it can only perfuse the muscle during relaxation. When inflow is restricted there may be too little time for the muscle vessels to refill during these intervals; claudication pain is then experienced. (*From* Barcraft and Swan's *Sympathetic Control of Human Blood Vessels* by kind permission of the authors and publishers, Edward Arnold.)

as a muscular pain or discomfort within the distribution of an obstructed artery, regularly occurring after a certain constant amount of exertion of the affected muscles, relieved by rest, but recurring with further activity, usually of the same extent though sometimes more, and often less. In man, the calf of the leg is most affected because the commonest site for an arterial occlusion is at the femoro-popliteal junction, and the calf muscles take their blood supply below this point. Foot claudication occurs in patients with Buerger's disease (*see* Chapter 4) when the lower tibial or plantar arteries are blocked.

Less commonly the upper limb claudicates. Arteriosclerosis is seldom responsible: most often it is due to thrombosis from compression damage to the artery at the limb root, typically a cervical rib (*see* Chapter 12), or follows long-continued crutch pressure in cripples or amputees [111].

Not all occlusions responsible for claudication are from thrombosis and local disease. The main artery may be absent, congenitally, or from thrombosis in

[126]. Claudication may be aggravated by anaemia (Fig. 3.16), which may even be the only evident cause; also by polycythaemia, which increases the resistance effect of any vascular occlusion.

Haemodynamic Aspects. It used to be thought that vascular spasm played a leading part in the production of claudication because the main arterial occlusion was constant, whereas the pain was only intermittent. Blanching of the toes of the affected limb often accompanies the pain of claudication (*see* Fig. 3.27), which led to the concept of 'angiospastic claudication'. Such reasoning may explain the tendency, even today, to prescribe vasodilators for claudication. Yet, in all probability, there is no shortage of metabolic vasodilators within ischaemic muscle, and the administration of generally acting vasodilator drugs may 'steal' some of the limited inflow away from the zone of increased resistance to other parts of the body [62, 64].

By 1931, Lewis *et al.* [93] had already shown that pain identical to intermittent claudication is produced

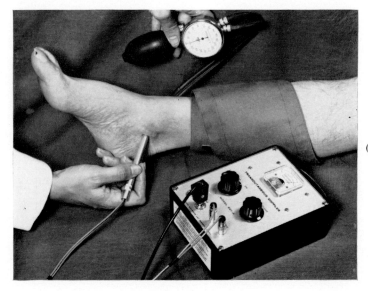

(a) Apparatus

(b) Results in 326 patients (Pressure index = Ankle pressure ÷ Brachial pressure)

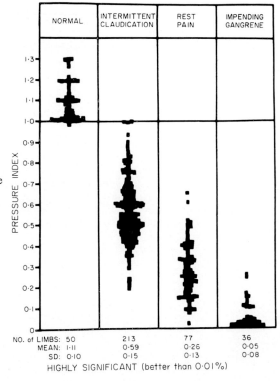

Fig. 3.2. Measurement of ankle systolic pressure by Doppler ultrasound [151]. (By courtesy of Dr S. T. Yao and the *British Journal of Surgery*.)

by exercise during arterial arrest with a tourniquet. There could be no question of vasoconstriction, because wide dilatation of the vessels in the ischaemic limb must have been present to have allowed an immediate development of reactive hyperaemia on release of the arterial obstruction. Neither could oxygen lack on its own be the cause of the pain, for if both limbs were exercised during ischaemia, one having already been subjected to tourniquet ischaemia for ten minutes, the onset of claudication was simultaneous on the two sides. From this it was deduced that the pain was due to a product of the

at 32°C an equally sustained rise was recorded. With the limb circulation arrested, these changes were abolished, proving that the tendency to 'normalise' the muscle temperature in a relatively short time, provided the circulation was open, was a result of a hyperaemia accompanying the muscular work.

When the same observations were made *during sustained strong contraction, the picture changed to one of ischaemia*: both the 'hot' and the 'cold' muscle heated up slightly. This was due most probably to the metabolic effect of the contraction. The probable reason for the ischaemia in this type of contraction is that the muscular vessels were themselves compressed by the forces of the surrounding contracting muscle. A similar state occurs intermittently in strong rhythmic exercise (Fig. 3.1) [2].

Measurement of the post-exercise calf blood flow (Fig. 3.3*a*) [122] shows a pattern of immediate

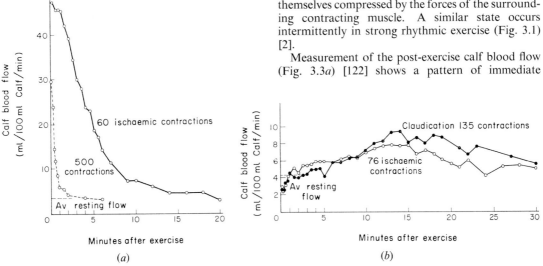

Fig. 3.3. Shepherd's experiments on post-exercise calf-blood flow measurement. (From Shepherd's *Physiology of the Circulation in Human Limbs in Health and Disease* by permission of the author and publishers, W. B. Saunders Company.)

(*a*) In normal subjects, the hyperaemia is immediate and unless conducted under ischaemic conditions, the debt is low and quickly paid off. With coincident ischaemia, however, there is a greater deficit, which requires a more prolonged and conspicuous hyperaemia to satisfy it. This may have some bearing on the severity of arterial injury after exercise, *see* pp. 242, 250.

(*b*) The same experiment in a patient with intermittent claudication shows only a poor and delayed hyperaemia with little difference between the ischaemic and free contractions.

exercise and not to anoxia. Relief of the pain occurred at once when the circulation was restored.

Direct evidence of vasodilatation in human muscle during sustained weak contraction was obtained by Barcroft and Millen [1A] with heat measurements, using a thermocouple inserted into the muscle. When the muscle had been previously warmed in a bath at 42°C it showed a steady cooling during contraction; however, with the bath temperature

hyperaemia, and early return to normal resting level which closely corresponds to that following a temporary arterial arrest (Fig. 3.4*a*, *b*). Thus, quick filling of the wide open arterial bed of the exercising muscle is essential if ischaemic pain is to be avoided. Normally, the pressure reaching the muscle arteries is sufficient to achieve this during the pauses between rhythmic contraction, as in walking or running. But an occlusion in the main artery supplying these

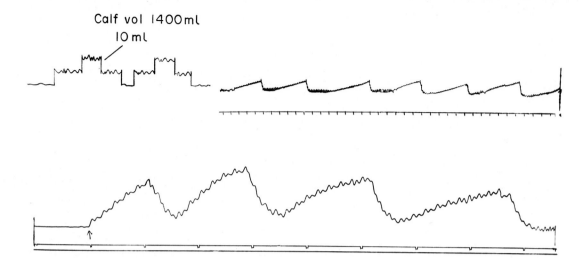

Calf vol 1400ml

10 ml

(*a*) A typical plethysmographic tracing showing striking and immediate increase in calf flow at the point of release of five minutes arterial arrest at the thigh. Within a few seconds, the slopes begin to flatten. This is a normal response. (Dr P. H. Fentem's case.)

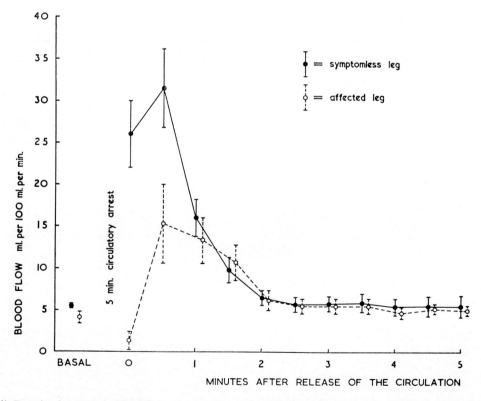

(*b*) Reactive hyperaemia blood-flow measurements comparing symptomless and claudicating legs. Delay is present on both sides, but much more severe on the occluded side.

Fig. 3.4. Reactive hyperaemia calf flow. (Reproduced by courtesy of the Editor of *Lancet* [125].)

muscular branches may mean that the pressure in them (Fig. 3.2) will have fallen below the minimum level required to perfuse the muscle against the contractions quickly enough to satisfy its needs.

This is what appears to happen in claudication. Both the reactive hyperaemia and the post-exercise inflow to muscle are slower and smaller than in normal subjects (Figs. 3.4*b*, 3.3*b*). A minute or more may elapse before the flow rate builds up to a higher level than at rest [122]. Maximum flow rates are not reached until five minutes in a severe case. Generally speaking, the higher the initial inflow rate the sooner is the maximum level reached. This would seem to be the purpose of the rest period in intermittent claudication. It also agrees with the finding that cardiac output is a significant factor in determining exercise flow in arteriosclerotic subjects [56].

Further evidence of the haemodynamic disturbance in the claudicating limb can be obtained by observing the *changes produced by operation* to restore the main arterial channel [125]. Using reactive hyperaemia calf-blood flow as the parameter, it was shown that in twelve cases a nearly normal pattern of post-ischaemic flows had returned (Fig. 3.5). When other patients, treated by lumbar sympathectomy, were studied by ergo-plethysmography [122], none showed any increase in calf-blood flow after exercise, and none appeared to have gained any increase in performance. This is in keeping with the clinical fact that the only consistently effective treatment for intermittent claudication is a successful arterial reconstruction.

Oxygen utilisation and lactate formation in claudicating lower limbs have been studied [5] by means of arterial and venous samples before and after exercise. Higher than normal values for both items were found, indicating a greater extraction of oxygen from the slowed blood flow and that the

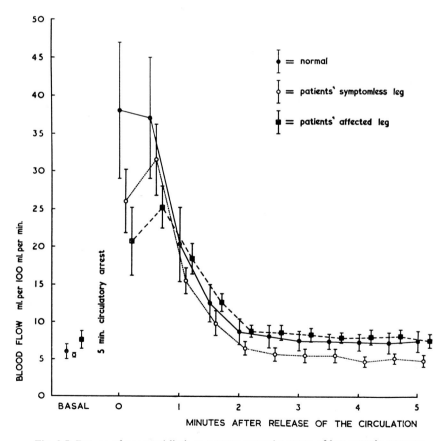

Fig. 3.5. Return of operated limb to a more normal pattern of hyperaemia response.

It will be noted that the symptomless leg in patients with arteriosclerosis occupies an intermediate position between this and the normal upper curve. (Reproduced by courtesy of the Editor of the *Lancet* [125].)

lactate produced by muscle work was likewise being added to a smaller volume of blood per unit time. Three patients whose tests were repeated after femoro-popliteal by-pass grafting showed a rise in the venous oxygen saturation, both at rest and after exercise, and a reduced venous-arterial lactate difference, both findings suggesting that the former restriction in blood flow had been abolished by the operation, and that the oxygen extraction and lactate addition were now being spread over a larger circulating volume of blood in the muscle bed.

PAIN AT REST

When the resting blood flow falls below a level at which it can provide for the whole needs of the resting limb, pain develops. In the foot, this means a circulation of well under 1 ml/100 ml/minute. Such low flow rates are difficult to measure plethysmographically; and readings for the whole foot do not necessarily apply to the toes, where really severe ischaemia is first shown. Digital artery pressures, measured with toe cuffs and strain gauges [18A, 66A] are found to fall to 20 mmHg or less in patients with severe ischaemia. Skin can tolerate extremes of environment, and will survive a very low flow rate, but nerve requires an assured blood supply, which explains why the first effects of severe ischaemia, acute or chronic, are upon the peripheral nerves. Biopsy of sural nerves from patients with rest pain showed degeneration and repair [41B].

The clinical picture is all too well known (Fig. 3.6). Pain in the toes and across the metatarsal heads at first troublesome only at night. During sound sleep, with wide generalised vasodilatation over the rest of the body, and the affected leg horizontal there may (as with drug-vasodilatation) be gradual shunting of blood away from the obstructed limb, which then 'drains away' until the pain threshold is reached. The patient awakes and, to refill the blood vessels and relieve his pain, hangs the affected leg over the side of the bed. Walking about the room also gives comfort, no doubt also because of the vertical position; and the process of waking, rising, and cooling the body reduces general vasodilatation; locally the act of walking on the cool floor removes excessive warmth from the tissues of the ischaemic foot. (This is the most likely explanation of the ischaemic form of erythromelalgia.)

Later, rest pain becomes practically continuous. Drugs are required and cigarette smoking often becomes excessive. The appearance of the forefoot deteriorates, the toes tapering and shiny with thin skin and rubor at the pressure points; the nails become thick and dry and cease their growth (*see* Fig. 3.28).

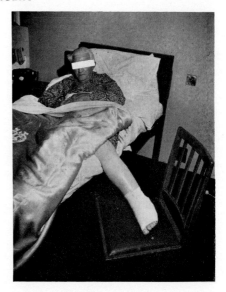

Fig. 3.6. Rest pain with dependent oedema.

Relief often follows *operative sympathectomy* (*see* Chapter 10). Though immediate, its mechanism is probably not neurological but haemodynamic. By permitting the maximum available flow into the obstructed zone at all times, irrespective of any periods of vasoconstriction which might affect the remainder of the body, the balance of the blood flow mechanism is persistently tipped in favour of the ischaemic tissues whose marginal supply is thus augmented, not by any spectacular increase such as that which follows arterial reconstruction, but steady maintenance and conservation, which can at rest amount to an increase in the total twenty-four hour flow.

Rest pain is nearly always immediately and completely relieved by *reconstruction of the main artery*. Discomfort and minor pain sometimes persist for a while during gradual recovery from ischaemic neuropathy. The outlook depends upon the extent of the nerve damage; if pain is still transmitted, function is still present and recovery is usual, though it may take several weeks.

Muscle wasting and weakness, as well as that which is due to direct ischaemic damage, may also be neuropathic, the pain causing disuse atrophy. The ankle jerks may be prolonged and slowed in calf ischaemia [59].

Flexion contracture of the knee (Fig. 3.7) is a common and troublesome feature in patients with rest pain, and may persist after amputation, though pain is no longer present. This late type is due to fibrous

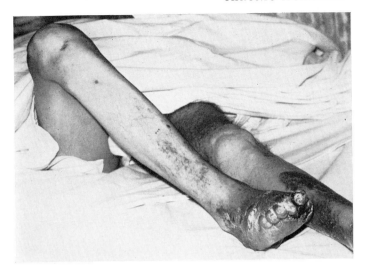

Fig. 3.7. Flexion contracture of the knee due to rest pain.

This patient's subsequent response to arterial grafting and conservative foot amputation is shown in Fig. 6.7, p. 128 (Mr J. R. Kenyon's case.)

contraction of the muscles and joint capsule, and may require open operation, dividing the contracted posterior structures in order to straighten the knee.

GANGRENE

Gangrene in chronic ischaemia is at first usually *confined to a small area* at a pressure point (Fig. 3.8) over a prominent toe joint, or on the heel. Some minor additional damage, chiropody or infection entering a crack in the interdigital web, cannot now be repaired by the defective local circulation. A necrotic patch forms and slowly spreads until it reaches a region where the blood supply is better; thus, if the ischaemia is chiefly due to a local arterial block, gangrene tends to limit itself to this area (Fig. 3.9).

Spreading gangrene is caused by anything that upsets this stability:

(a) Additional proximal arterial occlusion; or loss of nearby branches.
(b) Local infection spreading proximally.
(c) Venous thrombosis.
(d) Cardiac failure or other causes of general circulatory depression such as hypovolaemia, or serious intercurrent illness such as pneumonia.
(e) Worsening of diabetes, collagen disease or other condition underlying the arterial disease.

Double Blocks, Multiple and Venous Occlusions

In severe or massive gangrene, the process may be locally more advanced in certain areas as when, for

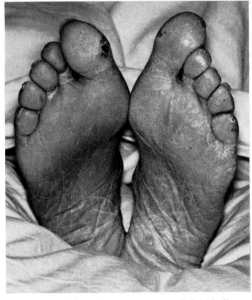

Fig. 3.8. Ischaemic pressure sore of right hallux.

example, the anterior tibial region is worse affected than the back of the calf, which may appear intact as far as the heel or sole. A strip of necrotic skin surrounded by rubor lies over the front of the damaged muscle compartment. This is a common presentation in elderly subjects (Fig. 3.10) and is a combined effect of anterior tibial occlusion, in its tight compartment with few collateral connections, and a major proximal block. Either may come first, and either or both may be thrombotic or embolic.

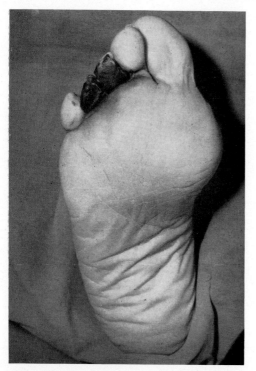

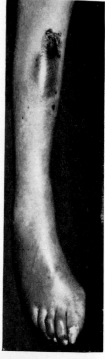

Fig. 3.10. Early massive gangrene of foot, ischaemic calf contracture, and necrotic anterior tibial syndrome in an elderly man who sustained an unrecognised right common femoral embolus during a left lumbar sympathectomy (*see* Fig. 10.7, p. 197).

Fig. 3.9. The third and fourth toes have a poorer collateral supply than the marginal toes, which are closer to the major skin supply of the distal foot.

Embolic secondary blocks have been established as a common cause of severe local ischaemia in the upper limb (*see* Chapter 12). It now seems probable that the same is true for the lower limb, and the multiple small vessel involvement so often seen in amputation specimens [35, 36, 47] may also be the result of small emboli [22, 110B]. The fact that the source of these is less obvious than the conspicuous lesions due to subclavian compression at the thoracic outlet has no doubt led to the possibility being overlooked that, in the lower limb also, embolic detachment of portions of the softer inner layers of the occluding material in the narrowed but still patent main artery may gradually scatter a series of small blocks throughout the terminal distribution. These areas of the toes and the heel, like the anterior tibial compartment, are structurally in some isolation [47] and here selective, premature necrosis may occur long before the main artery has closed off (Fig. 3.11). This can easily be recognised, when it happens, as a fairly major event in some patients with popliteal aneurysm (Fig. 3.12), and there seems every reason to believe that smaller platelet or cholesterol emboli can originate in, and repeatedly migrate down the

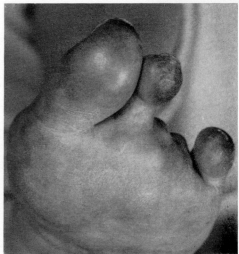

Fig. 3.11. Ischaemic toes with strong ankle pulses—almost certainly due to atherothrombotic embolism from diseased proximal main artery. (*See* Figs 1.10 and 1.11, p. 11.)

lower limb artery, as they are known, retinoscopically, to do from the stenosed internal carotid.

This rising peripheral resistance may determine the final closure of the main artery, as it is known to

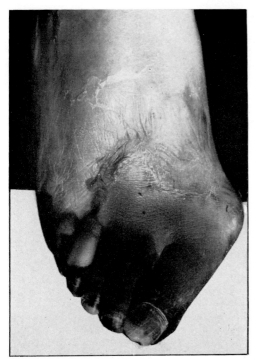

do after some grafting operations. Stasis, sludging in capillaries, and the additional embarrassment of venous thrombosis most likely complete the picture, regional gangrene then becoming massive and, usually, moist.

Venous occlusion on its own can, though usually only in patients with carcinoma or other serious underlying disease, cause gangrene [55] by obstructing the capillary circulation. The rising tension and swelling in such a limb produce a dusky, hot, blistered extremity (Fig. 3.13) quite unlike gangrene from arterial obstruction, though a few small arteries do undergo secondary closure, a fact that can be confirmed later when a distal type of amputation is performed. Major arterial occlusion may also complicate circulatory stasis from the venous side. The aorto-iliac segment may thrombose after vena caval ligation, or, if an aneurysm is present, the rising pressure may cause it to rupture [15].

Infection

Bacteria may gain entry to the deeper tissues through some local skin deficiency such as a crack or small ulcer, or under the margin of a small gangrenous patch. With an insufficient blood supply to overcome this added damaging factor, the infection tends eventually to spread and, when once pus reaches the fascial planes of the sole of the foot and the tendon sheaths leading to the calf, a calamitous spread of

Fig. 3.12. Dry gangrene of distal half of foot from a larger embolus originating in a right popliteal aneurysm. Good response to transmetatarsal amputation after sympathectomy and grafting of the aneurysm.

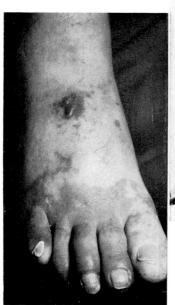
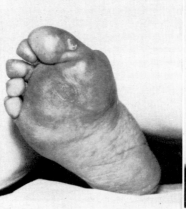
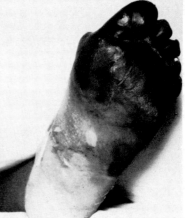

Fig. 3.13. Venous gangrene.

ABOVE. A more advanced case with early involvement on the opposite side.

LEFT. An early case. The foot is hot, suffused with patchy cyanosis and blistering. Pulses may be obscured by oedema. Heparin and elevation at this stage may save the limb.

gangrene is almost certain, particularly in diabetic subjects whose low resistance to infection, multiple, small arterial and arteriolar occlusions and tendency to sensory neuropathy (*see* Chapter 5) aid the hidden spread until infection is sufficiently massive on its own to threaten the patient's life.

Even at this late stage the skin over the gangrenous part of the limb may be warm and pink, for most of the remaining life and circulation is contained in this layer. Thus, the line of demarcation produced by infective skin necrosis is sharply defined, the surviving areas deceptively healthy in appearance.

Anatomy of Arterial Occlusions causing Chronic Ischaemia

LOCAL FACTORS

The topography of occlusive disease is remarkably constant. Local factors of probable importance include:

1. *Extrinsic pressure*, e.g. at the adductor opening and beneath the inguinal ligament.
2. *Change of direction of the blood flow*, as in the aortic arch and round the mouths of its large branches, and at the bifurcations of the abdominal aorta and common iliac.*
3. *Sites of repeated bending*, e.g. the common femoral at the groin, and the popliteal a little above the knee-joint line.

It is usual to classify patients with lower limb disease as aorto-iliac or femoro-popliteal. In practice, after lumbar aortography, about a quarter of each group show obstruction in the other territory [68].

Aorto-iliac Occlusive Disease [146]

Approximately one in four patients with claudication or more severe lower limb ischaemia show narrowing or occlusion of one or both iliac arteries, the lower aorta particularly at its bifurcation and sometimes extending upwards to the level of the inferior mesenteric origin, or higher still in some late cases. Most of these are men in their early fifties, with femoral arteries which, at aortography, appear to be relatively free from the disease, though whether from a protective effect [124] or because the femoral arteries are usually not affected until later in life is not yet clear. Both possibilities are compatible with the thrombo-embolic hypothesis of occlusive arterial disease (*see* Chapter 1). In older people with aorto-iliac disease the irregularity is more diffuse and often shows heavy calcification (Fig. 3.14). Aneurysmal

changes may also be present (Fig. 3.15). They may be accelerated by distal iliac obstruction (*see* p. 292).

Women before the menopause sometimes develop a localised narrowing of the abdominal aorta between its bifurcation and the level of the inferior mesenteric origin (Fig. 3.16). A cause other than occlusive arteriosclerosis should be suspected (as in any other patient who is young, female, or a non-smoker). The author has seen this lesion in premenopausal women with subclavian and renal arterial obstruction, some of whom later developed features of systemic lupus erythematosus.

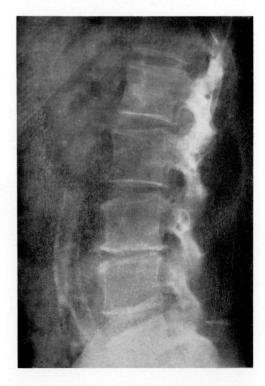

Fig. 3.14. Calcified aorta and iliac arteries in a patient with occlusive disease. Such calcification may, however, be present in a fully patent artery.

---

* The area ratio of the aortic bifurcation (stem/branches), normally 1·1, becomes less with age; with this comes an increase in pulse wave reflection that may be responsible for localised disease in the lower aorta [65A, 86A].

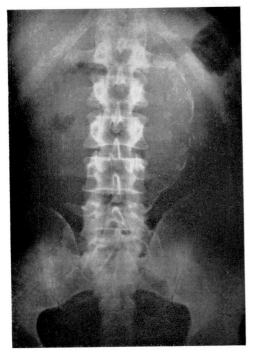

Fig. 3.15. Calcification of aorta and iliac arteries with aneurysm formation. A symptomless patient of sixty-eight who died three years later from coronary thrombosis.

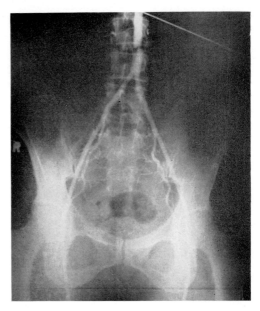

Fig. 3.16. Localised stenosis of the abdominal aorta in a woman of forty whose claudication responded well to treatment of anaemia due to menorrhagia from fibroids. Well and fully active ten years following thrombo-endarterectomy.

Clinical Features

Symptoms. In the early stages these may be confined to the calf, for example in a patient with unilateral common iliac stenosis. Later, the discomfort becomes more extensive and severe, the 'whole-leg' type of claudication which is the usual accompaniment of bilateral iliac or aortic occlusion (*see* Fig. 3.21). For a long while the patient manages to carry on his activities, but within a few months to a year the disability is reported. Spontaneous improvement is less common than with femoro-popliteal type claudication. On the other hand, severe ischaemia is slow to develop [135], perhaps because in these early years there is little disease in the more peripheral branches.

When the muscles of the buttock, hip, and lumbar region are affected the patient experiences a greater disability. Pain may now be quite severe, though it is still fully relieved by rest. Sometimes, however, a patient with iliac occlusion has an ache in the thigh at rest.

In men, the loss of flow in both internal iliac arteries, as in aortic bifurcation occlusion, causes failure of erection. Not all patients have this symptom, perhaps because a low aortic obstruction may permit wide lumbar collateral supply to the pelvic arteries. The combination of bilateral high-type claudication and impotence constitutes the 'Leriche syndrome' [90]. Others complain of abdominal pain, or the desire to defaecate, after walking.

Physical Signs. Most patients with aorto-iliac occlusion show wasting of the muscles in the area of distribution of the arterial branches below the block. Thin legs, thighs, and buttocks are usual in the fully developed case (Fig. 3.17). The male genitals may be smaller than normal.

The skin colour and warmth of the feet and toes are often normal at rest in the younger patients. Later, there is atrophy of the whole extremity with cool bluish discoloration, the toes becoming thin, tapered, hard and sometimes clawed; eventually ulceration develops, though not always at the tips.

Gangrene of the foot is uncommon with chronic iliac occlusion alone, but it soon develops when the femoro-popliteal becomes occluded as well (Fig. 3.18) and a major amputation will be required (*see* Fig. 6.1, p. 124) unless some effective flow can be restored.

Absence of the pulses at the groin confirms what the history may have already suggested, that the

Fig. 3.17. Wasting of the buttocks and lower limbs in a patient with Leriche syndrome. More general wasting is common with juxta-renal occlusion and may signify mesenteric involvement.

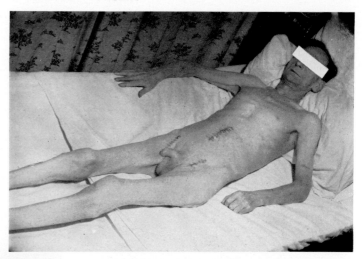

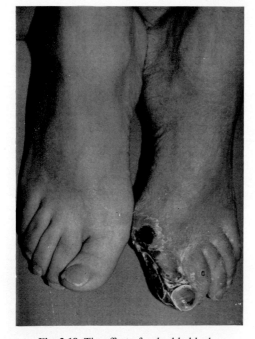

Fig. 3.18. The effect of a double block.

Both femoral arteries were occluded, and on the left side, the iliac also. Relief of pain and healing of great-toe amputation following crossover femoro-femoral graft. (*See also* p. 21.)

occlusion is higher than usual. The external (Fig. 3.19) and common iliac pulses should then be examined; in a patient of average build these should be readily palpable if the arteries are normally patent, while aortic pulsation should be even in an obese subject. If it is absent, the lower abdominal aorta is probably occluded.

Reduced or unequal common femoral pulses are also good evidence of aortic or iliac disease, even though the distal limb pulses may still be palpable at rest. A bruit is usually present, higher in pitch on the worse-affected side. *Auscultation of the common femorals* is therefore important. If no bruit is heard there is less likelihood of narrowing or irregularity in the iliacs, exceptions to this general rule being:

(*a*) in some cases with severe or complete obstruction in which the pulse wave is coming via collaterals instead of the main channel;

(*b*) in the presence of a major femoral occlusion, preventing iliac flow from reaching the velocity needed to generate the murmur while building up the femoral pulse pressure to a falsely high level against the distal obstruction [136].

Femoro-popliteal Occlusion

Commonest in patients over sixty, this lesion accounts for over two-thirds of all cases of claudication, and is the major factor also in most problems of severe ischaemia. It is recognisably bilateral in about a quarter of those affected [145] though with claudication only on the worse affected side. Likewise severe ischaemia due to femoro-popliteal occlusion is seldom bilateral at any one time, though the second limb often goes the way of the first.

The focal point in 60 to 75 per cent of these lesions [11, 145] is the opening in the adductor magnus, where the tendon is closely applied to the artery at the femoro-popliteal junction (Fig. 3.20) and where the local mural and haemodynamic

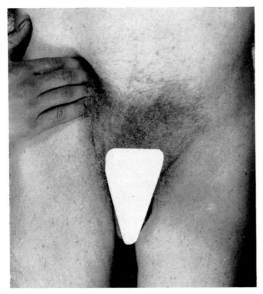

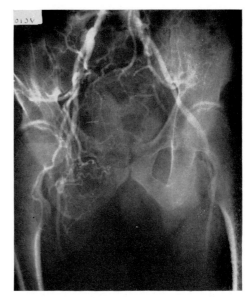

Fig. 3.19. Palpation of the external iliac pulse.

(*a*) Gentle deep pressure above the groin shows the external iliac to be patent in this patient whose common femoral was palpably occluded and thickened and tender.

(*b*) The arteriogram confirms the diagnosis. Note rich collateral network around the groin and hip compared with the left side. This may confirm the suspected diagnosis in arteriograms of poorer quality, where the common femoral itself cannot be clearly seen.

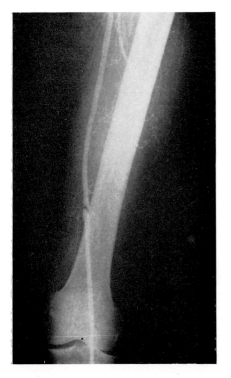

stresses caused by several large branch orifices may tend to concentrate the occlusive disease. Here, also, the straight, fixed femoral becomes the bending, mobile popliteal, whose curve may cause the deposition of obstructive material [137].

From this starting point the occlusive process tends to spread proximally [118] up the superficial femoral where branches are few and small; the main stagnant channel may soon thrombose, lengthening the occlusion until it reaches the wide and fast-flowing stream at the profunda origin. This branch is almost never seriously affected and usually remains patent even when the whole artery from which it arises has occluded.

Extension downwards from the adductor opening is slower, and seldom completely occludes the popliteal, except in its upper part. Large re-entering collaterals from the geniculate anastomosis pour their blood into the patent popliteal under considerable pressure, they can often be seen to be pulsating

Fig. 3.20. The usual starting point for arteriosclerotic occlusion in the thigh. The tendon of the adductor magnus is closely applied to the artery at this point.

A good result was obtained following local thrombo-endarterectomy.

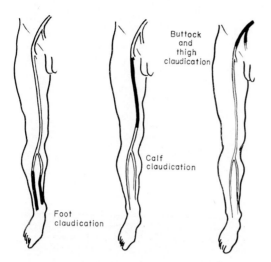

Fig. 3.21. Common sites for intermittent claudication and the arterial occlusions which cause them.

Buttock and thigh claudication

Calf claudication

Foot claudication

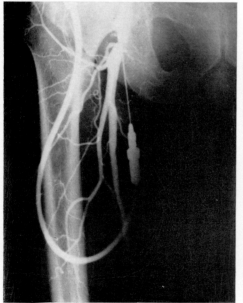

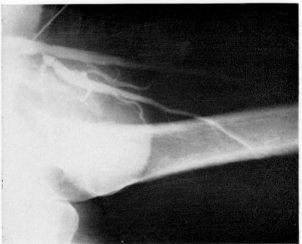

Fig. 3.22. Stenosis of the profunda femoris artery, visible only in the lateral view.

at operation, and the lumen of the main artery receiving them may become a post-stenotic expansion chamber.

Claudication is typically felt in the middle of the back of the calf (Fig. 3.21) though the level of the pain depends upon which of the muscular arteries may still be receiving a sufficient blood supply. Thus, a purely popliteal occlusion may not involve the upper gastrocnemius arteries; claudication then affects the lower soleus fibres, or the peronei.

The popliteal bifurcation is another common site for plaques and narrowing, and when this occludes, the femoral already having done so, severe ischaemia is certain to occur, and if secondary tibial blocks are also present gangrene is highly probable [36].

Occlusion of the Common Femoral Artery (Fig. 3.19)

Though fewer than 10 per cent of cases of lower limb ischaemia are due to this lesion, it is important because symptoms are severe (thigh as well as calf claudication, with a high incidence later of pain at rest, then minor gangrene) and, also, because in this accessible position reconstruction is simple and highly effective.

Moreover, the block is easily localised clinically, sometimes without the need for an arteriogram, for the short occlusion can be palpated clearly as a hard and, if recent, tender segment just beyond the inguinal ligament, above which the external iliac pulse can be distinctly felt (*see* Fig. 3.19).

Not infrequently, on exploration, the artery is found to be aneurysmal as well as occluded. Strip resection is then indicated, as in the post-stenotic subclavian at the thoracic outlet (*see* Chapter 12).

The Obstructed Profunda Femoris

In the past this artery was thought to be immune from the encroachments of occlusive disease; perhaps because its origin, the site of greatest risk, is obscured in routine femoral arteriograms. Lateral films are needed to show it clearly (Fig. 3.22). However these add to the duration and discomfort of the examination and also to the stray radiation, so there should be definite clinical suspicion for the extra examination to be requested. Points of importance include:

(a) Severe ischaemia with a strong pulse at the groin.
(b) Induration of the common femoral artery.
(c) Strong pulsation just above the inguinal ligament, with a localised bruit at the groin, not heard above, and not conducted distally.

If on routine arteriography poor profunda filling is noted a lateral view should be taken [4].

The importance of the profunda femoris flow into the lower limb has long been appreciated [88, 107], particularly for its provision of a good 'run-off' for an ilio-femoral reconstruction in cases of severe ischaemia in the elderly. Recently Martin has stressed the value of investigating and treating this type of patient (*see* profundaplasty, p. 68).

Popliteal Thrombosis [11]

The term 'primary popliteal thrombosis' was originally applied to any localised, unexplained occlusion of the popliteal artery, of probably mechanical or traumatic origin, due to the vulnerable position of the vessel. It is now believed that most cases are secondary to some recognisable lesion, including localised arteriosclerotic plaque or stenosis, Buerger's disease, thrombosis of a popliteal aneurysm, cystic adventitial disease, and anatomical anomaly of the relation of the artery to the gastrocnemius muscle.

CYSTIC ADVENTITIAL DISEASE
8, 45, 45A, 66B, 92, 106] (Fig. 3.23)

This uncommon cause of popliteal arterial narrowing occurs mostly in active young men, nearly all of whom show a marked, localised constriction at or ust above the upper level of the femoral condyles.

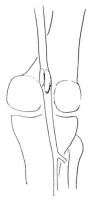

Fig. 3.23. Cystic adventitial disease of the popliteal artery at the intercondylar level.

Rarely is the obstruction complete, though flexion of the knee may produce a temporary acute ischaemia with pallor, pulselessness, and cooling of the feet. Arteriography will be required to distinguish this condition from Buerger's disease, though it may be suspected if the man is a non-smoker, as in the case shown in Fig. 3.24. Surgical treatment is by incision and evacuation of the jelly-like content of the cyst or cysts, or may have to include endarterectomy if the lumen is much narrowed. In the

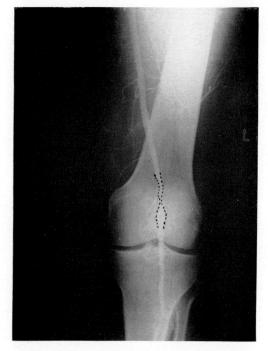

Fig. 3.24. Narrowing of left popliteal artery due to cystic adventitial disease showing post-stenotic dilatation. Patient was a master builder aged forty-seven, of strong muscular development, who had played much rugby football earlier in life. Clinically diagnosed from the murmur of the stenosis in a life-long non-smoker [45].

Fully relieved following endarterectomy ten years ago.

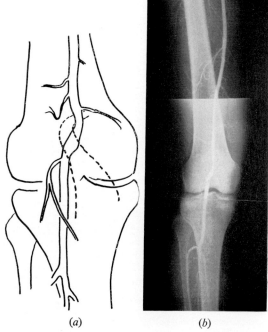

(a)   *(b)*

Fig. 3.25. Popliteal entrapment syndrome.

(*a*) The tendinous origin of the medial head of the gastrocnemius passes lateral to the artery, and compresses it against the outer side of the medial femoral condyle.

(*b*) The effect of this is well seen in this arteriogram upon which a diagnosis of the condition was confidently made. Relief of symptoms following correction of the deformity.

occluded case, an arterial replacement is necessary, preferably with a length of saphenous vein.

Bilateral cases are rare, for the cause is probably traumatic, resembling a common ganglion.

POPLITEAL ENTRAPMENT SYNDROME
(anomalous position of artery and of gastrocnemius muscle) [18, 72, 96, 120]

Clinically similar, though quite different in its cause, is the obstruction resulting from an abnormality that has been known to anatomists for many years; in fact, the first description was in 1879 on a specimen of a leg amputated for popliteal aneurysm. The usual fault is for the artery to run first over, and then beneath, the medial head of the gastrocnemius (Fig. 3.25*a*), and sometimes also the popliteus. Clinically, it presents with claudication on severe exercise in a youth or young man. Dorsiflexion of

the ankle produces paraesthesia of the foot, and arteriograms show the medial displacement of the artery (Fig. 3.25*b*) with perhaps a localised occlusion also (Fig. 3.26). Exploration is essential and, if not unduly delayed by diagnostic uncertainty, nothing more is required than division of the abnormal origin of the compressing muscle and its reattachment to a correct position on the capsule over the medial femoral condyle. In the late case, grafting may be necessary for occlusion or post-stenotic aneurysm. The condition, being congenital, is often bilateral.

Clinical Assessment of a Patient with Chronic Lower-limb Ischaemia

GENREAL CONDITION
Twenty-five per cent or more of patients with intermittent claudication have angina pectoris or other evidence of ischaemic heart disease (*see* Chapter 1,

p. 2), and about the same number die in five years, almost all from cardiovascular disease. These facts should be given fair consideration in the patient's general assessment before planning his treatment.

The exercise potential assumes meaning only when related to the individual patient, considering age, general condition, and social status. An elderly retired professional man may have extensive

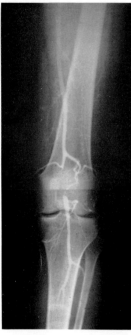

Fig. 3.26. The left knee of the same patient as Fig. 3.25, with a complete occlusion at the point of compression, previously diagnosed as Buerger's disease.

The left popliteal block was restored with a saphenous vein by-pass graft.

bilateral superficial femoral arterial occlusions without leg symptoms other than cold feet 'for years', whereas a young, active working man will experience serious limitation of his activities with a short block or stenosis.

The physiological age, an impression soon gained during the history taking from the patient's powers of memory and expression, his general state of preservation, liveliness of movement, the time taken to undress, and his co-operation during the examination: all these are more important than the date of birth. In general, these arteriosclerotic subjects may be reckoned 'to be ten years older than they should be' [9].

Obesity, cyanosis, easy dyspnoea, arcus senilis, nicotine staining of the fingers, lips or hair, are unfavourable features.

The blood pressure should be taken in both arms at the beginning of the examination, and at the end, if the level is raised.

An ECG is routine, and should be available because hidden ischaemic heart disease is common, and it will also elucidate any chest pain or arrhythmia of uncertain origin. Likewise, no final decision on treatment can be made until a normal chest X-ray film has been seen.

In a case of doubtful fitness or suspected ischaemic heart disease a cardiological opinion is essential.

The Peripheral Arterial Examination

The room should be warm and well lighted. Daylight is preferable. With the patient completely undressed and covered with a small blanket the following observations are noted:

1. *The Appearance of the Limbs*
Pallor of the affected extremities usually means that the patient has recently exercised (Fig. 3.27a). Later in the examination a more normal colour should be regained, though, with a recent occlusion in an ambulant patient, slight pallor may persist at rest with the limb horizontal even though the ischaemia is evidently neither acute nor severe.

Dependent congestion, rubor, or cyanosis of the affected limb (Figs. 3.27b and 3.43) mean that ischaemia is fairly severe. It quickly changes to pallor on elevation or exercise, and a useful test is to ask the patient either to walk about, or to exercise both limbs in elevation. When they are lowered and rested the ischaemic one will appear much paler. If all four extremities appear congested in a man of middle age or older, polycythaemia should be suspected; sometimes primary, though more often secondary to cardio-pulmonary disease, both types being haemodynamically important (*see* p. 57).

The limb may be held in flexion in a patient with rest pain, or be swollen at the foot and ankle from prolonged dependency.

Wasting and fasciculation are common in ischaemic muscle groups and may show the extent of the occlusion. The toes and foot may be shrunken. The skin may be thin and dry, with many fine superficial cracks and wrinkles in the epidermis. Bruising in the web or beneath the nail may indicate recent severe ischaemia with partial recovery. The nails are often thick and narrowed (Fig. 3.28).

Hair may be missing from the dorsum of affected toes, and indolent, infected cracks be present in the webs when the toes are parted. Pressure points such as the 'bunion' region and the heel are examined for rubor or necrosis.

Persistent scabbing sores, scattered over the

extensor area of the calf and ankle represent athero-matous microemboli in the skin arteries (Fig. 3.29) [110B].

Visible pulsation along the course of the main artery often means there is well-established medial disease causing lengthening of the artery, which when the limb is slightly flexed shows marked tortuosity. There may also be obvious aneurysmal dilatation, often at the groin and sometimes be-hind the lower thigh and knee, but unless large, aneurysms here are less often seen than palpated.

2. Palpation of the Limb

(a) *The Temperature of the Skin.* The feet are warm in a young subject with occlusive disease even though there may be complete occlusion as high as the aorta. In most elderly patients the affected extremity is cool, though it is essential to compare the temperature of the other limbs, for such coolness may be due to generalised vasoconstriction following recent exposure to cold, or to nervousness at the interview. It follows that the unaffected limbs must be perceived to be warm or, if any useful purpose is served by observing the temperature of the affected one, the examination must wait until they have become so.

In a patient with a previous history of hospital treatment for ischaemia, a warm, dry foot on the affected side usually signifies that a lumbar sym-pathectomy was performed on the earlier occasion. The same sign is sometimes shown in the left foot after resection of an abdominal aortic aneurysm.

The skin temperature over the patella is a useful sign of the course of the blood flow at knee level:

paradoxically, in femoro-popliteal occlusion it is almost invariably *warmer on the affected side*, whereas the foot on this side is cooler. This is because the collateral arteries run nearer the surface than the main artery; medial to the patella, or over

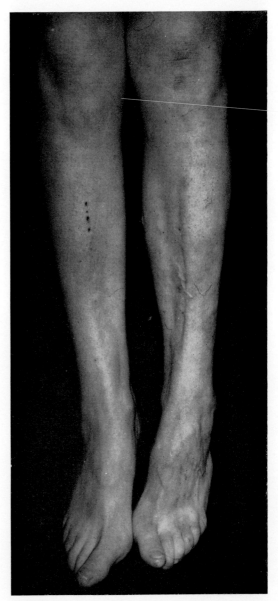

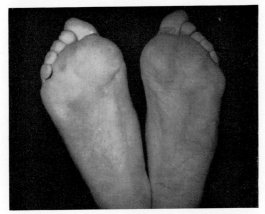

Fig. 3.27. Skin colour at rest in the ischaemic lower limb.

LEFT. Pallor of the right foot on recumbency after mild exercise; a 'steal' effect (*see* pp. 31 and 171).

RIGHT. Congestion of the right foot a few minutes later with the patient hanging her legs over the side of the couch.

A case of right femoro-popliteal occlusion in a woman aged sixty. (A further example of dependent rubor is shown in Fig. 3.43.)

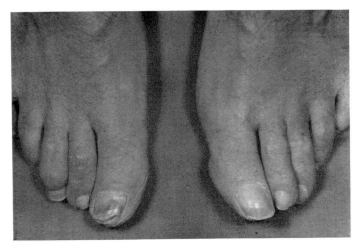

Fig. 3.28. Ischaemic changes of skin and nail of right great toe in an elderly patient with a short popliteal occlusion on the right side.

either femoral condyle, a large pulsating branch may often be felt.

(*b*) *The Pulses.* A systematic examination of all the accessible pulses is the most important part of the physical examination. Some typical findings have already been described (p. 42). Figure 3.30 shows those that should always be palpated, and a simple and convenient system of notation.

False findings may be due to the following circumstances:

(i) *Observer error* is the most important [97]; if the examiner's hands are warm, he may feel his own pulses. If this is suspected he could count his own and the patient's radial pulse and compare the timing, or obliterate his own pulse during palpation of the patient's.

(ii) *The patient may be cold* or tired and vasoconstricted, with all his pulses diminished, including those in question. Anatomical variations are common. The dorsalis pedis may be absent, and the radial arteries may cross the back of the wrist. Obesity or oedema from venous insufficiency may obscure both ankle pulses. Ankle tendons may be contracting involuntarily from nervousness, cold, or fasciculation, and may resemble a fibrillating pulse.

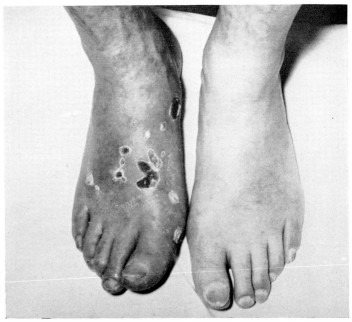

Fig. 3.29. 'Cholesterol scabs,' another feature of athero-embolism and, like the commoner digital lesions, painful and slow to heal.

49

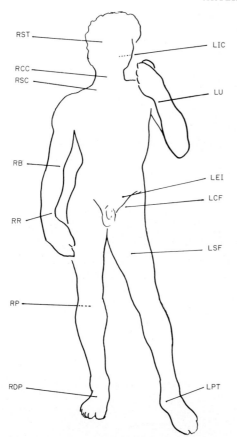

Fig. 3.30. All these accessible pulses should be palpated and recorded in the routine peripheral arterial examination. A system of notation is suggested.

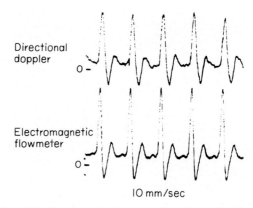

Fig. 3.31. Tracing of pulse wave taken from directional Doppler apparatus. It has an identical form with the actual flow curve made with the quantitative electromagnetic flowmeter. (*From* Yao, S. T. [151] by courtesy of the author and the *British Journal of Surgery*.)

(iii) *Shortly after exercise the ankle pulses may disappear*, returning later at rest. This valuable evidence of proximal arterial obstruction may be missed unless the examiner is on the look out for it. If the skin colour improves during the examination the pulses should be palpated again before the patient is allowed to dress.

Auscultation along the artery may locate a stenosis at a point of maximum systolic bruit, which will increase after exercise.

(*c*) *Oscillometry.* Where conditions such as these lead to uncertainty over the strength of the pulses, or where a measure of comparison is required between the two sides or serial readings on several occasions, oscillometry provides visual evidence with a numerical value for the case records. The instrument should be checked against a normal limb if the readings are in doubt. No absolute value can be attached to them and no comparison made between different instruments.

(*d*) *Determination of Blood Velocity by Ultrasonic Doppler Effect.* Frequency shift of a reflected ultrasonic wave by the blood stream in a limb artery can be detected and amplified on an audio-frequency circuit. This simple apparatus (Fig. 3.2(*a*)) is now used in all cases for arterial assessment, not only to measure systolic pressure at the ankle or wrist (*see* p. 36), but for the clear information it gives on the wave form. Unobstructed arterial pulses have a small flow reversal after the systolic thrust, followed by a third, still smaller onward wave (Fig. 3.31); these signals are identical in the Doppler output to that of the electromagnetic flowmeter. The three phases can be clearly heard in the headphones or speaker. Obstructed pulses have a damped, monophasic signal. The frequency of the sound is proportional to the velocity of blood flow [129A].

Other Information from Palpation
(*a*) *The width of the artery* can be compared with what the normal should be, or with other arteries in

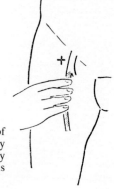

Fig. 3.32. Palpable thrombosis of the right superficial femoral artery below the profunda. The artery may be tender if the thrombus is recent.

the same patient. The common femoral arteries should not be larger than a finger's breadth. They may be two or three times this diameter in a patient with abdominal aneurysm. Wide arteries mean degenerative disease and support the suspicion of peripheral occlusive lesion elsewhere.

(b) *The artery may be hard and cordlike,* a most useful finding in the groin and thigh, where the extent of a superficial or common femoral, or even a low popliteal thrombosis can be made out with an accuracy almost equal to that of an arteriogram (Fig. 3.32).

(c) *Tenderness, hardness, or swelling* together suggest either a recent arteriosclerotic thrombosis, a recent embolism, spontaneous thrombosis of a small aneurysm, or perhaps the early stages of a mycotic aneurysm (*see* Chapter 7, p. 136).

(d) The whole course of a patent main artery may be traced by palpation along it; this is a simple and useful test that can readily be applied in most thin or hypertensive subjects.

Exclusion of Other Painful Conditions of the Lower Limb

In the middle-aged and elderly, causes of pain in the lower limb, sometimes mistaken for arterial insufficiency, include:

Lumbosacral root irritation
Osteoarthritis of hip or knee   } 'pseudo-claudication'
Venous insufficiency
Myxoedema claudication

Peripheral neuritis   } rest pain
Glomus tumour of the foot

The diagnostic problem is made particularly difficult if there is doubt about the state of the lower limb pulses.

Low lumbar and sacral root irritation [6] (Fig. 3.33), often due to disc protrusion or a narrow lumbar canal [80A], may cause pain in the buttocks, thighs and calves on exertion, as well as tingling of the toes at rest. The full cauda equina syndrome, with saddle anaesthesia and sphincter involvement, is less common than the unilateral and more peripheral type, though the latter is more difficult to distinguish from true intermittent claudication of arterial origin. Anoxia of the compressed nerve roots with exercise may explain the consistent relationship of pain to a regular amount of exercise; relief may be effected by breathing oxygen [54]. Unlike true arterial claudication, which passes fairly quickly with standing at rest, the pain of root compression requires stooping, sitting or lying for its relief, and takes longer to go [81D].

Spondylosis, and secondary carcinoma, most often from the prostate, are common causes of this

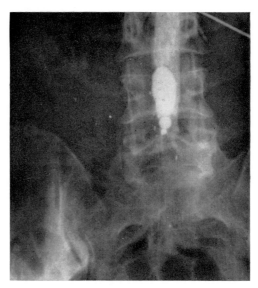

Fig. 3.33. Aortic bifurcation occlusion in a patient with severe bilateral whole-limb claudication. Note myodil from previous examination for suspected prolapsed lumbar intervertebral disc.

type of 'pseudo-claudication'. As in simple lateral disc protrusion, the relationship to exercise is not so clear cut as in the cauda equina type, for though there often seems to be a 'claudication distance', on further questioning the patient usually admits to having had the same pain at rest or standing. His movements on the examination couch are sometimes typically stiff. If, however, these features are present in a patient of middle age or over, who also happens to have coincidental lack of some lower limb pulses, or in whom they are obscured by soft tissue swelling, there may be real difficulty over the diagnosis. Root pain affects the peroneal region more than the calf, and is often more severe than in true claudication. Closer consideration shows that the symptoms and signs are incompatible: for example, in a patient with whole-leg claudication whose common femoral pulses are strong and without bruit, a root pain is much more likely to be the cause. The condition of gluteal claudication from isolated internal iliac occlusion must be very rare; the writer has not yet seen a case. Most patients with significant ischaemia will, on exercising to the point of pain, show either blanching of the foot on the affected side, or distal pulses, which previously were easily palpable at rest, will disappear. It is essential to make a rectal examination and to elicit the full mobility of the spine. The reactive hyperaemia skin test may be useful to avoid arteriography. Sensory disturbance due to root lesion conforms to a segmental neurological pattern. For example, the outer toes, or the first interdigital cleft may be numb to pin prick. In claudication, sensory loss is rare except perhaps immediately after the exercise. With ischaemia at rest there is some sensory blunting over most of the

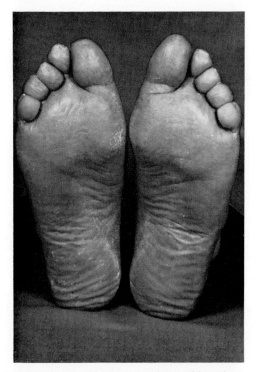

Fig. 3.34. Dry cool feet in myxoedema. This patient, a senior naval officer, had slow speech, a slow pulse, slow ankle jerks, and typical bilateral intermittent claudication. All his peripheral pulses were normally present, and he quickly improved on thyroid treatment, losing all his symptoms within six weeks.

toes, which by then are obviously ischaemic in appearance.

In osteoarthritis of the hip and knee, both common causes of painful limitation of lower limb activity, claudication may be suspected because the pain on walking may be nowhere near the affected joint, with 'muscular pain' as the chief complaint. Pain and spasm on *passive movement* should suggest that osteoarthritis is the cause, especially if the same pain occurs on exertion, or on arising from rest. When both conditions are present, good judgement is needed to determine which is the cause of pain. In case of doubt, pallor developing on exercise is the decisive factor in ischaemia.

Venous insufficiency, superficial or deep, may cause pain in the calf and ankle after 'a long day on the feet', though, typically, the pain is worse when standing than it is after walking, which tends to relieve it. Absent pulses at the ankle are of uncertain significance in venous occlusive disease because of swelling and thickening of the soft tissues, by which normal pulses may be obscured. Oscillometry finds one of its best uses in correcting this common error. In acute venous insufficiency, oscillations are often greater than on the normal side.

Myxoedema claudication in no way differs from ischaemic claudication. Typical calf symptoms, tending to be severe and progressive, occur in the familiar pattern, no doubt due to interferences with muscular energy exchanges. Peripheral pulses are likely to be normal but slow, and the skin of the feet is dry (Fig. 3.34). Diagnostic is the marked slowing of the ankle jerks. Early and complete relief follow thyroxine treatment.

Peripheral Neuritis (Fig. 3.35). Severe night pain of lancinating type in the elderly subject, with incidental absence of the tibial pulses, may suggest arterial disease when, in fact, diabetes, bronchial

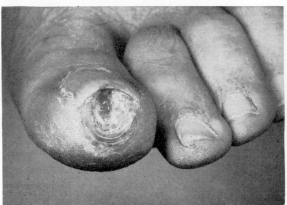
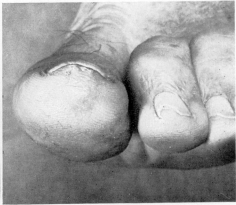

Fig. 3.35. Neuropathic pressure sore of left great toe in a middle-aged man with alcoholic neuritis. Healing complete within six weeks with abstinence and vitamin B treatment.

neoplasm, alcohol, megalocytic anaemia or other common cause for neuritis is responsible. The complaint of 'walking on gravel', or 'upon cotton wool' is usual, and absence of vibration sense and deep reflexes almost the rule. A blood count should include examinations of the red cell picture.

Glomus Tumour of the Toe. Severe pain, at rest, worse at night and at other times when the foot is warm, may suggest ischaemia, especially when the lesion is sub-ungual and shows an area of discoloration. Pulses should be present. Pain is abolished by the inflation of a proximal sphygomanometer cuff above systolic arterial pressure, and not worsened, as would be expected. The diagnosis in any of these conditions may remain in doubt, and if no firm conclusion can be reached on the clinical evidence arteriography will be required.

Arteriography in Peripheral Occlusive Disease

The importance of arteriography in the management of peripheral arterial disease of every kind will be evident from the large number of arteriograms illustrating this book. This examination is now integral in our practice at St Mary's, and study of the findings in several thousand cases has provided a clearer concept of the natural progress of these diseases, as well as valuable guidance in diagnosis and case management. Complications are so rare with the contrast dilutions recommended* that the investigation has become routine in any case likely to require active treatment or continued observation.

Precautions to be Observed before Arteriography
(*a*) Enquiry as to any allergic or sensitive conditions, particularly asthma or iodinism.
(*b*) Renal insufficiency must be excluded.
(*c*) If anticoagulants have been given, these should be discontinued from the day before the examination.
(*d*) A test dose will exclude sensitivity, also extrathecal or intramural injection.

1. *Indications*
(*a*) Arteriography helps to distinguish between arterial insufficiency and other causes of painful limb.
(*b*) In a patient with chronic ischaemia of uncertain origin, the cause can usually be established, e.g. arteriosclerosis obliterans, Buerger's disease, aortic arch syndrome, the arterial basis of secondary Raynaud's disease, thrombosed aneurysm, or the relation of an arterial occlusion to a recent or an old

---

* The following strengths and average dosage were employed by Dr David Sutton [130] in the majority of the arteriograms illustrating this book:
(*a*) Femoral arteriography: Urografin 60 or Hypaque 45. 20 ml (maximum 60).
(*b*) Lumbar aortography: Urografin 60 or Hypaque 45. 15–20 ml (maximum 40).
(*c*) Brachial arteriography: Urografin 60 or Hypaque 45. 15 ml (maximum 45).
(*d*) Arch aortography: Urografin 60 or Hypaque 45. 20–30 ml (maximum 60).

bony injury or gunshot wound. Findings in typical cases of each of these kinds are described in the appropriate chapters.
(*c*) In the assessment of a patient with cerebrovascular insufficiency.
(*d*) In suspected visceral ischaemia, particularly of the kidney or mid gut loop.

2. *Choice of Method*
Aortography is generally the most suitable [68, 136]. Experience of over 5,000 cases at St Mary's Hospital has given us confidence in the safety of the *translumbar injection* for routine use. Provided the test dose is tolerated, and can be seen not to have entered an important branch (visceral, or lumbar to the spinal cord), there is no danger of complications of any significance. *Trans-femoral catheter* aortography is less safe in patients with occlusive disease (*see* Chapter 13, p. 247). For selective studies it is preferable. With both methods it is advisable to stop any anticoagulant treatment at least a day before the examination.

Percutaneous femoral arteriography is less used now that it is better known that aorto-iliac involvement occurs in about 25 per cent of femoro-popliteal cases [68], and that the proximal bruit that would be expected may be checked by the obstructed distal outflow [136]; also the need in every case to examine both lower limbs. Yet the femoral arteriogram is preferable for any detailed examination of a lower limb, e.g. for Buerger's disease or arteriovenous fistula. Warm conditions or a general anaesthetic will help to obtain good small vessel pictures. Otherwise local analgesia is routine for all angiography. Lateral views are required if profunda obstruction is suspected (*see* p. 44).

3. *Interpretation of the Findings
in Lower-limb Ischaemia*

(*a*) *The main artery only is filled*, and its major branches (Fig. 3.36*a*, *b*). This is a normal examination, with exposures taken at an early stage, or with the patient vasoconstricted.

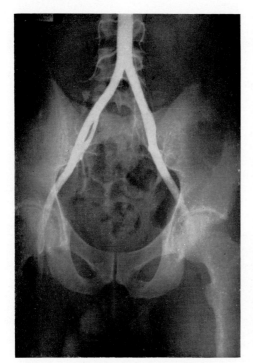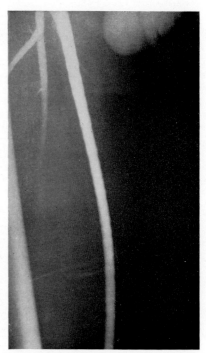

Fig. 3.36. Normal arteriograms with fast flow in the main arteries.

The regular, beaded appearance in the femoral is transient and is determined by a flow artefact, probably a standing wave, which might be generated either by vibrations within the injecting syringe, by shear between contrast medium and blood, or by intrinsic wave forms due to arterial resonance (*see* Chapter 15, p. 281). It is rather common in Buerger's disease (*see* p. 103).

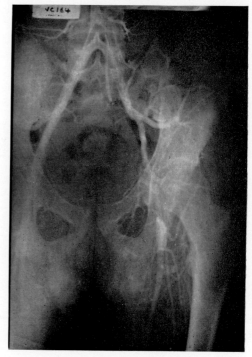

Fig. 3.37. Traumatic left external iliac block in a young subject, whose right iliac filling is mostly confined to the main channel. On the obstructed left side, though there is not much delay and the block itself is hidden by the overfilled internal iliac, an obstruction must be present because of the striking development of collaterals over the whole hindquarter area. (*See also* Fig. 13.9, p. 246.)

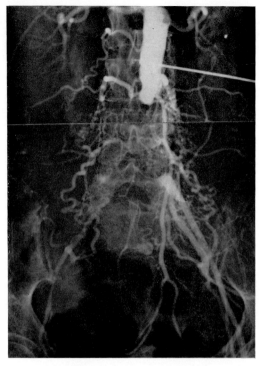

Fig. 3.38. Intense, rich screen of fine collaterals indicates that the aorto-iliac obstruction in this elderly woman is causing severe lower-limb ischaemia.

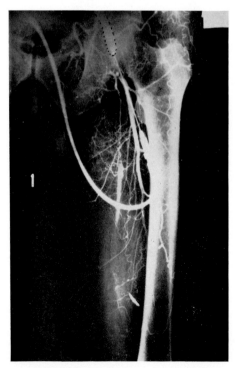

Fig. 3.39. Multiple femoral arterial occlusions in severe lower-limb ischaemia. Note the dense mesh of fine collaterals around the principal blocks and relatively unaffected profunda femoris artery.

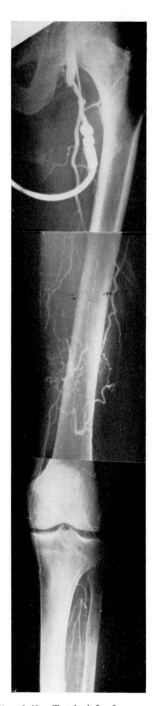

Fig. 3.40. Total left femoro-poplitcal occlusion with collaterals extending as far as the tibial arteries, in a patient with severe ischaemia. The profunda origin is stenosed.

(*b*) *A block is present in the main artery with a few large collaterals* and little delay in the onward passage of medium, as for example when compared with the opposite lower limb in a lumbar aortogram (Fig. 3.37). This is a well-compensated occlusion either in a young patient or of longstanding in an older subject.

(*c*) *A block is present, but with a richly filled screen of fine branched and convoluted collaterals* throughout the soft tissues of the part (Fig. 3.38). The distal main artery may be filled, but it often shows considerable irregularity or further blocks (Fig. 3.39). These are the findings in severe chronic ischaemia, usually in an older patient.

(*d*) *The lower end of the main artery occlusion is not seen*, while the collaterals extend well beyond the point at which the lower end of the block would be expected to lie (Fig. 3.40). This nearly always means that the lesion is inoperable to any direct arterial operation, though, on occasion, a delayed film may show a slow retrograde filling of the segment in question [84, 98] (Fig. 3.41).

(*e*) *Early venous filling* is sometimes noticed [67, 82], as with an arteriovenous fistula. The explanation for this phenomenon is not yet known (*see also* Chapter 4, p. 107).

4. *Use as a Progress Checking Examination*

This application is of occasional use as a guide to conservative treatment, or in the evaluation of persistent symptoms after an operation which appears to have restored arterial patency to a patient who previously has had claudication or painful aneurysm.

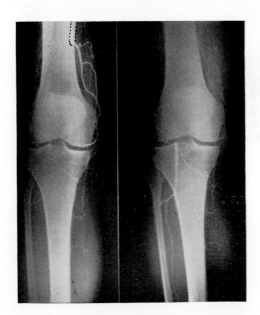 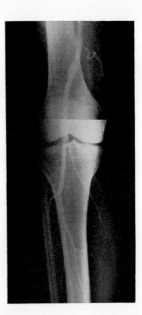

Fig. 3.41. The value of a delayed film in recent ischaemia.

Late distal filling; with a good result of thrombo-endarterectomy.

Prognosis in Untreated Chronic Ischaemia

Many patients are untreated because they are never diagnosed. These are elderly people who live quietly and do not claudicate, though they later die from cardiovascular causes at approximately the same age as others die from other diseases.

In patients who are still active, claudication remains static or may often improve with the passage of time. It is common to obtain a history of previous mild claudication of the opposite limb which passed off without treatment. Nearly 60 per cent of the 1,476 patients studied at the Manchester Royal Infirmary improved considerably, even up to three years from the onset of claudication [9].

Severe ischaemia develops only in quite a small

minority. In a series of 3,735 patients with occlusive disease of the lower limb arteries from five large hospitals [9, 81, 89, 116, 118, 135] in Europe and the United States, the amputation rate was 10 per cent in five years. Factors tending to worsen the limb prognosis include:

(a) diabetes (25 per cent amputations) [89, 118].
(b) failure to stop smoking (11·4 per cent amputations, compared with 0 per cent in those who stopped) [81].

The life prognosis was worse: approximately 20 per cent of the whole group had died within five years of diagnosis.

The presence of ischaemic heart disease does not influence the amputation rate but it does increase the mortality [139]. This is higher in patients with aorto-iliac than in those with femoro-popliteal disease [46, 81].

In severe chronic ischaemia, it is an axiom that old or diabetic patients do less well than the young and non-diabetic, and that the outlook is below average in those whose hygiene and home conditions are poor.

Patients who have already had a lower limb amputation seldom do well if the opposite side becomes affected; history tends to repeat itself (Fig. 3.42).

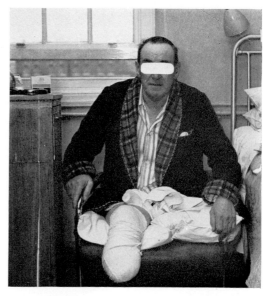

Fig. 3.42. This man could not give up cigarettes after undergoing a left mid-thigh amputation following a failed arterial graft for severe ischaemia. When a similar ischaemia developed on the right, a below-knee amputation failed to heal, and he subsequently required a further amputation on this side also. Good rehabilitation by the Roehampton Limb Fitting Unit with satisfactory bilateral prostheses.

Treatment: General Measures

There is, at this time, no effective medical treatment for intermittent claudication, the commonest feature of chronic ischaemia. None of the standard 'remedies' has been shown to have any measurable effect either upon exercise tolerance or measured blood flow in the affected limb. Vasodilator drugs may simply shunt the blood away from where it is needed [62]. Induced hypertension has been shown to reverse this 'steal' into a 'donation', by means of angiotensin infusion which supposedly constricts the vessels of the normal peripheral vascular bed more than those of the atonic ischaemic area [24A, 81C].

(a) Exercise and physical training are better than rest for these patients. Controlled studies with blood flow estimations in treated and untreated groups have established this fact [52, 87]. Over a shorter period bed rest may be followed by an improvement, which may gain credit for an operation such as lumbar sympathectomy, or even an arteriogram, though such benefit seldom lasts.

(b) Anaemia may contribute to muscle anoxia in occlusive arterial disease, and its correction may improve exercise capacity in a striking way (see Fig. 3.16, p. 41).

(c) Polycythaemia (Fig. 3.43), a common accompaniment of occlusive vascular disease, also aggravates its effects by increasing the haemodynamic resistance of peripheral obstructive lesions. True polycythaemia with haemoglobin levels of 120 to 140 per cent will require full medical treatment, including antihaemopoietic drugs. Lesser degrees will not be acceptable to most physicians for active treatment unless the full significance of their effect upon blood flow is agreed. Blood viscosity rises rather steeply at haematocrit values above 50 per cent. Venesection to reduce these to below 43 per cent was effective in patients with lower limb ischaemia [23] on three criteria: (i) improvement in symptoms and signs; (ii) increased digital pulsations and skin temperature; and (iii) improvement in cardiac function as suggested by ballistocardiography. Untreated, such patients have in the author's experience later developed coronary thrombosis, stroke and graft occlusion.

now so strong that it can be accepted without question (*see* Chapter 1, p. 3). Dietary restrictions are discussed on p. 6. Their value remains unproven. Weight reduction should be encouraged, however. Blood cholesterol levels (Fig. 3.44), and cholesterol absorption can be reduced by ileo-colic bowel shunting [14]. Treatment of the Type III lipoprotein disorder of Fredrickson (*see* Chapter 1, p. 6) by diet and clofibrate increased the reactive hyperaemia calf blood flow [152].

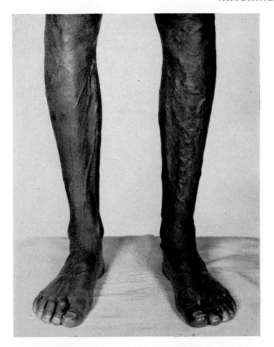

Fig. 3.43. Dependent rubor and rest pain in a patient with polycythaemia vera and a left femoro-popliteal occlusion. Good response to left lumbar sympathectomy and treatment of the blood condition.

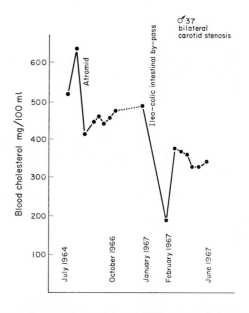

Fig. 3.44. Lowering of blood cholesterol level reduced by partial ileo-colic intestinal by-pass.

(*d*) Long-term anticoagulants, while they may possibly protect the claudicator from some other thrombo-embolic complications, do not appear to benefit the limb condition, though repeated arteriography over a mean period of three years in another group of patients receiving this treatment suggested that fewer occlusions developed in stenosed femoral arteries in the treated group, compared with controls [119].

Anticoagulants in use today exert little or no effect on platelet function. Active investigation of other therapeutic methods of preventing the formation of intravascular platelet aggregates suggests that several popular vasoactive drugs may have this effect [73].

Trials of oestrogen administration have not yet established their place in preventive treatment (Chapter 1, p. 10).

Probably the most important preventive measure in chronic ischaemia, particularly in younger patients, is *total cessation of cigarette smoking*. Unless the patient accepts this there is no firm basis for hopes of future improvement. The evidence is

Palliative Measures. Complete freedom from the discomforts of claudication of the milder kind can be achieved by modifying the patient's mode of life: he should avoid walking farther or faster than his limit, particularly on stairs and inclines; he should ride rather than walk; cycling is often well tolerated; raising the shoe heels may help by reducing the work of the calf muscles. If the patient accepts the need for limitations, understanding that no simple means exist for relief of his difficulties, the surgeon will less often be pressed to take an active line. *Hyperbaric oxygen* gives temporary relief from rest pain but in the long term no significant benefit has been shown from its use [65].

SURGICAL TREATMENT

Lumbar Sympathectomy and Other Indirect Operations

Lumbar sympathectomy is still the most valuable of the standard methods of treatment because it is simple and can be safely applied to most patients; benefit is nearly always experienced, though much less often for claudication [108] than for rest pain. It improves the general hygiene and well-being of the limb, and is definitely a favourable factor in prognosis [135]. The subject will be considered in detail in Chapter 10.

Indirect measures such as achilles tenotomy [12, 111B] and section of the motor nerves of the calf [101, 111A] have been tried with no convincing benefit to most patients. They act by an enforced limitation of walking, nerve section being more effective in this respect.

Arterial Reconstruction

Direct arterial surgery stands alone as the only potentially certain and wholly effective form of curative treatment in ischaemia due to major arterial obstruction. It should be accepted that the good prognosis of 75 per cent of patients with early chronic ischaemia excludes them from this type of operation. Nevertheless, there are many who qualify for its positive benefits. Firm indications for operation arise from long experience of its end results, and we will now examine the factors that make for success and failure, realising, nevertheless, that sometimes operation may be needed even though unfavourable factors exist. In these the risks are higher and the outcome less certain.

Success or Failure in Arterial Surgery for Occlusion

Favourable Factors (indications)	*Unfavourable Factors* (contra-indications)
Large artery	Small artery
Localised disease	Diffuse disease
Free from calcification	Heavily calcified
Good general condition	Poor general condition
Compelling disability	Tolerable disability
Young patient	Elderly patient
Bad prognosis untreated	Good prognosis untreated
Clean field	Infected field
Non diabetic	Diabetic
Experienced operator	Limited experience
Autogenous reconstruction	Foreign material

Factors For and Against Reconstruction

1. *Disability*

Reconstruction should not be undertaken if the ischaemic disability is slight. Failure of the operation, either early or late, may well leave the patient worse off than before (Fig. 3.45). In other patients, although the main object of the surgery may have been achieved, complications such as nerve damage or venous thrombosis may dominate the postoperative picture, and any improvement in the original symptoms may be quite overshadowed.

Where symptoms are the cause of serious physical or economic distress, the surgeon is free to do all he can to improve matters; even a small improvement will be gratifying.

Acute deterioration in chronic ischaemia usually demands urgent surgery, though the results are uncertain.

2. *The Local Lesion*

Paradoxically, the natural prognosis is inversely related to the therapeutic value of direct arterial surgery. This simply means that a patient whom we

Table 3.1. Case Selection for Reconstructive Operation for Occlusion of the Lower Limb Arteries: 1964–68

	Patients investigated	Patients operated
Aorto-iliac	144	126
Femoro-popliteal	350	
unilateral	225*	42
bilateral	125**	8

*27 had severe ischaemia (12·2%).
**17 had one side with severe ischaemia (13·4%).

know to be likely to do well without operation, has less to gain and much more to lose from an arterial reconstruction which, in these circumstances, would clearly be ill advised. Most patients with superficial femoral occlusion fall into this group. Some with aorto-iliac obstruction can also be regarded in this way (Fig. 3.46).

Fig. 3.45. A man of fifty, referred after popliteal reconstruction with a teflon prosthesis for moderate claudication. Primary failure of the reconstruction produced the severe condition shown in the left-hand picture. Good result with regrafting using a stored homograft. (By permission of the Hon. Editor, *Proc. Roy. Soc. Med.* [44].)

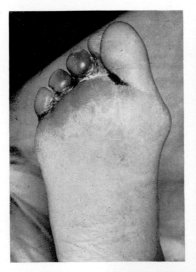
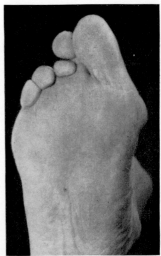

Double blocks. A patient who already has a deficient arterial supply to a limb, with the prospect of losing what remains because of imminent further occlusion, should always be advised to undergo operation. For example:

(*a*) Bilateral superficial femoral occlusions, with an iliac stenosis on one side. The iliac lesion must be dealt with, for completion of the double occlusion may lead to gangrene (*see* Fig. 3.18).

(*b*) Subclavian stenosis due to compression at the thoracic outlet tends to give rise to repeated embolisation of the upper limb, and with each episode the ischaemia becomes more severe (*see* Fig. 12.4, p. 221).

(*c*) Arteriosclerotic popliteal aneurysm also does this in the later stages (*see* Fig. 3.12), an important prognostic feature because the condition is so often bilateral, and the earlier, smaller member of the pair may be treated expectantly while the other must be corrected at the earliest opportunity.

3. *The Patient's General Condition*

This mainly affects the decision to operate for extensive aorto-iliac occlusion. Multiple exposures, wide retraction, the risk of severe blood loss, with the upper limit of the lesion close to the renal origins, all weigh against operation in patients of uncertain fitness, particularly in those with reduced cardio-respiratory reserve. A history of ischaemic heart disease or chronic bronchitis should restrict the scope of the procedure to something simpler. This is one of the indications for aorto-femoral by-passing which, though open to greater reservations

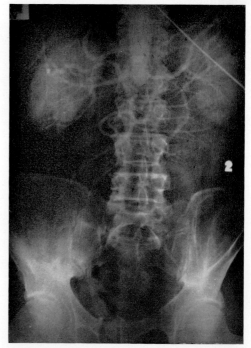

Fig. 3.46. Complete aorto-iliac occlusion in a man of sixty whose mode of life was hardly affected by his disability. Operation not advised for this patient, whose lesion closely approached the renal arterial origins. He remains well seven years after retirement.

over late results, then an endarterectomy, does offer a limited operation well suited to the poor-risk patient. The same applies even more to the femoro-femoral cross-over procedure (*see* p. 82).

4. *Infection*

This is the most serious single risk factor in arterial surgery, particularly if a cloth prosthesis is to be used (*see* p. 86). In combination with the extensive haematoma formation that commonly follows the use of post-operative anticoagulants, it goes on to cause repeated and, often, disastrous secondary haemorrhages [44], frequently requiring proximal ligation and, later, amputation.

5. *Diabetes*

In diabetes, the course of occlusive arterial disease tends to be unusually severe. Small vessel lesions are multiple and the 'run-off' may be poor. Extensive and multiple lesions, frequently with heavy calcification, are difficult to repair. Obesity and the risk of infection are other factors weighing against success in arterial surgery, as well as the general hazards of any operation in a diabetic patient.

Diabetic gangrene (*see* Chapter 5) is a special problem in which chronic ischaemia is often complicated by neuropathy and infection. Both these are helped by medical treatment. Thus, the presence of severe neuropathy often means that an arterial operation will not be needed, and severe infection that it is contra-indicated until local drainage and antibiotic treatment has brought the infection under control.

It is not surprising that the proportion of good results after arterial restoration has been found to be lower (54 per cent) in diabetics than in non-diabetics (77 per cent), and that their operative mortality rate is much higher (6·2 per cent and 1·6 per cent) [61].

The Artery

The critical diameter is 5 to 6 mm. Arteries smaller than this are often reconstructed but with uncertain results. The reasons are not all technical: suturing is not unduly difficult if the vessel wall is in fair condition. Probably more important is the volume of flow which, in the abdominal aorta below the renals, is three times greater than in the superficial femoral.

Some patients, particularly women and small slender men have a generalised arterial narrowing (Fig. 3.47). They do less well after arterial reconstruction: early and late failures are common. Patients with wide arteries are good subjects for arterial restoration, unless, as is sometimes shown at arteriography, the flow rate is much reduced as a

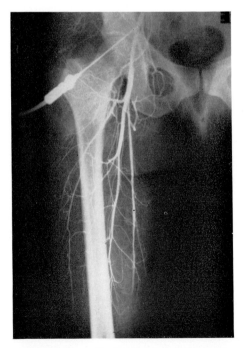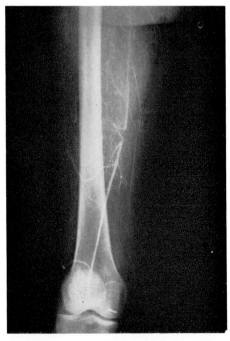

Fig. 3.47. Generalised arterial narrowing of anatomical or constitutional origin in a middle-aged woman who also has localised arteriosclerosis with a femoro-popliteal block. Such cases seldom do well with arterial reconstruction.

result of the dilatation. This mainly applies to the lower-limb arteries and is another potent cause of failure after arterial reconstruction [50].

Well-localised atheromatous narrowing is a common and favourable lesion in the large arteries of the trunk, the limb roots, and the neck, where operation provides the maximum improvement in blood flow over large and important areas of distribution for the least extensive type of procedure.

Diffuse narrowing is commonest in the lower-limb arteries, where the adverse factor of a low regional flow rate also prejudices the results of the necessarily incomplete and imperfect clearance, which is often the best the surgeon can obtain. Extensive endarterectomy of the femoro-popliteal artery has been advised because of this [20].

Much calcification is usually a sign of advanced disease (see Fig. 3.14). It is common in elderly and diabetic subjects, and in chronic renal failure. Endarterectomy is difficult, for the artery is adherent to important neighbouring structures—in particular the main vein—and the atheromatous plug may, in places, be inseparable from the inner surface of the thin medio-adventitial remnant. Closed loop-stripping may easily perforate the wall. The aortic bifurcation may be so brittle that no clamp can be applied or, if this difficulty can be overcome, there may not be sufficient good material for suturing.

Revision-endarterectomy is a dangerous operation for most of these reasons, and by-pass grafting should always be preferred.

THE IMPORTANCE OF TECHNIQUE
Given good case selection, the determining factors for success in this type of surgery are mainly technical [24]. For the less-experienced operator the work bristles with difficulties and pitfalls. A wide general surgical capability is essential; access and exposure must be easy. Patience and a special inclination towards fine work, and a readiness to re-operate at inconvenient times, often soon after the main procedure; these attributes are essential in operating for occlusive arterial disease. Judgement in the timing and dosage of heparin and protamine is crucial in the difficult case. The type of reconstruction chosen is often decisive. There is now very general agreement that, as in most other forms of reconstructive surgery, autogenous tissues are a better and more durable basis for repair than any foreign material. Whenever possible, endarterectomy and autogenous vein grafting are preferable to plastic cloth prostheses.

Finally, anaesthesia must be perfect, with full relaxation and blood pressure and flow maintained at normal level by synchronous replacement of the blood loss as estimated by swab weighing.

Methods of Reconstruction in Occlusive Arterial Disease

Thrombo-endarterectomy (disobliteration)
This operation was introduced by Cid dos Santos in 1946 [37]. It has since become the most important and widely used procedure in reconstructive arterial surgery, and shares with lumbar sympathectomy the merits of a well-tried and long-proved method with clear limitations and high factor of safety. There are several variations in technique, but common to all is the basic step of finding the correct plane of cleavage.

1. THE BASIC OPERATION
(a) The mobilised artery is incised longitudinally over a completely blocked portion.

(b) Clamps need not yet be applied, nor heparin be given.

(c) A Watson Cheyne probe-pointed dissector (Fig. 3.48) is a good instrument with which to define the plane of dissection between the arteriosclerotic plug and the cleanly separating remnant of the arterial wall. This plane is always outside the internal elastic lamina, so that the specimen will include some of the media (Fig. 3.49). Once entered, the layer is easily and quickly opened up. It is

important to keep to the same plane all round the plug. This can be ensured by passing the end of the probe across the front of the specimen at either end of the arteriotomy (Fig. 3.50). Then the dissection can be developed to meet from both sides on the deep surface of the plug.

(d) It is now time to enter the patent part of the artery, where the lesion tends to thin itself out into a tongue or sleeve (Fig. 3.51) which will be divided with scissors, taking care not to lift the remnant from the media more than can be helped.

(e) Clamps are first applied, and heparin is given into the distal artery (25 to 50 mg according to the probable duration of the occlusion phase).

2. TECHNICAL ADAPTATION TO BLOCKS OF VARIOUS LENGTHS AND DIFFERENT POSITIONS
The following are in general use:

(a) Open thrombo-endarterectomy (for short blocks, e.g. carotid, common iliac, common femoral, and those limited to the femoro-popliteal junction). The whole of the obstructed segment is fully exposed and opened up through a single arteriotomy (Fig. 3.52).

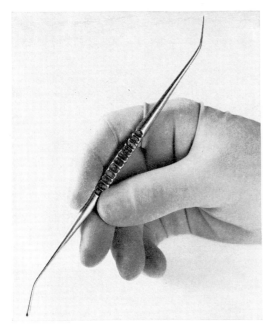

Fig. 3.48. The Watson Cheyne probe pointed dissector, an indispensable instrument in thromboendarterectomy.

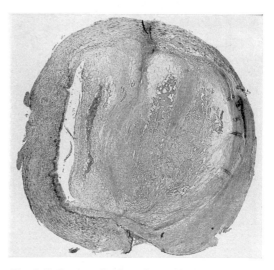

Fig. 3.49. Section of a thrombo-endarterectomy plug, showing a considerable portion of the media wrapped around the laminated, almost occluding, thrombus containing cholesterol clefts in its deeper layers (Photomicrograph by Dr. A. Knudsen).

Fig. 3.50. Method of keeping to the same endarterectomy plane at the limits of the arteriotomy.

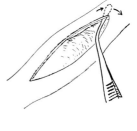

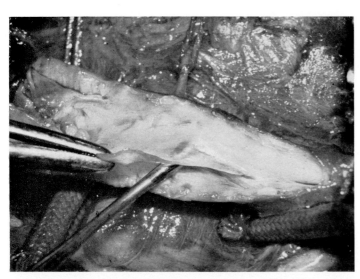

Fig. 3.51. Delicate tapering lamination at distal end of occluding plug. (The same lesion is shown in Fig. 1.10, p. 11.)

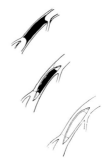

Fig. 3.52. Open endarterectomy exposing the whole extent of the occluding plug with control of the two limiting collaterals.

(*b*) *Semi-closed* (Fig. 3.53) (for aorto-iliac obstruction which is not too extensive). The whole length of the blocked artery is exposed through one operative wound. The upper and lower ends of the

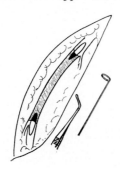

Fig. 3.53. Semi-closed endarterectomy by means of dissector and loop stripper between two arteriotomies, but with whole obstructed segment exposed. A good method for moderately limited occlusions at the femoro-popliteal junction.

occlusion must be freely visualised, so that an arteriotomy can be safely made at each end, between which the endarterectomy can be developed instrumentally (*see* below). Sometimes digital squeezing from the proximal end clears the upper limit of the block, and the upper clamp can be reapplied to this now pulsating segment.

(*c*) *Closed* (for a long femoro-popliteal occlusion in which the plane of cleavage is found to be very free). This simple technique, almost as small an operation as the pull-through by-pass shunt and, like it, requiring only a limited exposure of the upper and lower limits of the block, was made possible by the introduction by Cannon in 1955 [16] of the loop stripper (Fig. 3.54). As a rule, two

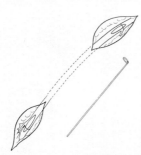

Fig. 3.54. Closed femoro-popliteal endarterectomy, by means of the loop stripper. A minor operation compared with saphenous vein by-passing, though the late results are less good.

arteriotomies are required, though sometimes it is sufficient to break the tube of occluding material at the upper end, just beyond a large branch such as the profunda femoris, after which it may be possible to withdraw the whole plug from the lower end arteriotomy. CO_2 injection may be used for stripping [115].

Endarterectomy is less satisfactory for patients in whom the occlusion extends into the popliteal segment. For these, a vein by-pass is preferable (*see* p. 65).

3. COMPLETION AND CLOSURE

Common to all methods is the need for thoroughly flushing both ends (by momentary unclamping) and of the intervening segment, open or closed, by a vigorous irrigating stream of isotonic saline.

The loose flap or tube of intimal material can be trimmed and left unsutured at the proximal arteriotomy, for the arterial stream will keep it against the wall, but at the lower end the greatest care must be taken to ensure that either the line of division is at a point where the plug has thinned out completely (Fig. 3.51), as often happens in the carotid and profunda femoris, or that the remaining diseased material is closely adherent, or can be safely secured with sutures of the type shown in Fig. 3.55.

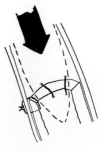

Fig. 3.55. Distal securing sutures placed axially to secure the cut end of the intima after thrombo-endarterectomy. The patch graft should 'over-pass' this point, as dos Santos has recommended.

PATCH GRAFTING

Patch Graft Closure (Figs 3.56 and 3.57)

For any artery less than 6 mm diameter, a simple linear repair tends to narrow the lumen excessively, and thrombosis is common. An exception is the internal carotid which, perhaps because of its local widening at its origin in the carotid sinus, or the high flow rate through it, can usually be closed with a simple suture. All other narrow arteries, and many that are wide but diseased, and which become narrowed at their bifurcation, e.g. the common iliac, require a patch graft to prevent narrowing, particularly at the distal end where the 'step' of the cut intimal layer (Fig. 3.55) may create further obstruction and turbulence.

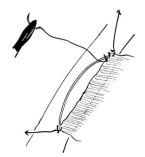

Fig. 3.56. Securing the patch graft.

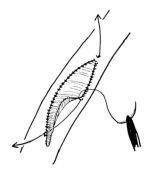

Fig. 3.57. Completing the patch graft.

Autogenous Vein Patch Grafts
Small arteries with low flow in relatively superficial sites are ideally closed with this material; 5/0 or 6/0 suture material should be used. Sometimes a large tributary in the operative field is sufficient, when opened out, to make good a normal arterial diameter or slightly greater. Too wide a channel is a disadvantage, especially in the longer patches, as Edwards, the originator of this type of repair, later showed [50]. A convenient donor site is the main internal saphenous in the lower calf or ankle region, but not when there is severe ischaemia or when there is infection in the foot.

Dacron Patches
Larger arteries, with higher stretching forces along their wall, will require a stronger material. Flat, uncrimped knitted dacron material is suitable for these. Being deeply placed, there is less objection to the use of foreign material here.

Comment: Open endarterectomy, though tedious, has considerable advantages. Closed endarterectomy, though attractive, is less often completely satisfactory.

BY-PASS GRAFTING
Advantages of this widely used technique, in comparison with thrombo-endarterectomy are: its relative simplicity, and the fact that a less extensive exposure of the diseased artery is usually sufficient; often, only the two segments containing the limits of the block need be inspected, incompletely mobilised, laterally clamped (Fig. 3.58), and the graft inserted. For these reasons its value as a

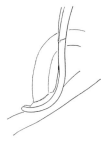

Fig. 3.58. Lateral clamping during end-to-side anastomosis.

'rescue operation' in a poor risk case (*see* Fig. 5.10 p. 120) should be remembered, when thrombo-endarterectomy might be too much for the patient.

The method is highly adaptable to various unusual and opportune circuit arrangements, for example the femoro-femoral cross-over graft (*see* p. 82) and for the addition of side arms which permit secondary revascularisation of other parts, including abdominal viscera or the branches of the arch of the aorta (*see* Chapters 8 and 17).

Plastic Cloth Tube Prostheses
The late results of dacron and other plastic tube grafts are not yet known, although they appear to be entirely satisfactory in situations with high flow, and where the receiving artery is reasonably wide and healthy. In smaller arteries, and particularly in the lower limb, there have been very general reports of late closure [48, 80, 128, 131, 149]. Cloth grafts function by conducting blood through a tube of fibrous tissue reinforced against scar tissue stretching by the inert mesh of the polymer. False aneurysms are proving to be rather common, particularly at femoral anastomoses at the groin (*see* Fig. 3.71). True graft failure has also been described [83] but seems to be rare. Dissatisfaction with cloth grafts in the limbs is witnessed by the growing number of papers on veins as arterial substitutes.

Autogenous Vein Grafts

These grafts were first used in obliterative arterio-sclerosis by Kunlin, of Paris [86]. Grafts from the saphenous, cephalic or external jugular give satisfactory results in small limb arteries [27, 70]. Early failure is common, no doubt because of the technical difficulty sometimes experienced in suturing a small thin-walled vein to a thickened, friable, and deeply placed artery. A few more failures occur during the first six months, but the late failure rate is low [29].

These grafts do not arterialise. Those recovered from patients have shown fibrous thickening of their wall [34], and experimentally this and some muscle hypertrophy are the only changes of note.

Recanalisation of vein grafts is known to occur [26], perhaps because veins contain large amounts of fibrinolysin activator [140]. The same reason may apply to their good record in positions with slow blood flow, or with temporary stasis, as must often happen to the normal veins in life.

Arterial Homografts

Although these homografts have fallen from favour in recent years, the story of their introduction into clinical use by Gross [66] and Hufnagel [77] represents the crowning achievement of the pioneer work of Carrel and Guthrie, fifty years before; it ensured the growth and development of the new specialty of vascular surgery, and led directly on to the larger field of organ transplantation.

Although of the many hundreds of homografted peripheral arteries of the 1950s few still function, in the thoracic aorta late results remain excellent [30B, 57], while in the abdominal aorta and iliacs late complications are commoner [105, 132A].

The failure of the arterial homograft came not with this first, important though only occasional application, but in the common problem of femoro-popliteal grafting for lower limb ischaemia. As many as 50 per cent thrombosed within the first year, and of those that remained patent three years, approximately half of them became aneurysmal along their course [3, 80]. The reasons for this are still not clear, but they may relate to the more exacting and controlled conditions, in the early days, of banking of the shorter aortic segments in their smaller numbers; in contrast, the later indictments of limb homograft performance seldom give details of banking technique [31]. Other possibilities include the larger proportion of cellular tissue, especially muscle, in limb arteries, in comparison with the almost wholly elastic structure of the aorta, a difference that could explain the greater durability of thoracic aortic homografts—at least equal to that of synthetic prostheses [57, 105]; and, finally, the mechanical and haemodynamic conditions of the peripheral site which may predispose to failure of both kinds.

BANKING TECHNIQUE [43]

It is of fundamental importance to ensure freedom from protein denaturation, as always applies to the storage of biological materials. The early aortic grafts, which gave such good results, were in fact stored alive, and thus their freshness was ensured. Later, homostatic grafts deep frozen or freeze-dried could, if conditions were imperfectly controlled, deteriorate seriously without visible sign. Optimum standards for accepted methods of artery banking are given in Table 3.2.

The importance of these standards cannot be over-stressed. Now that aortic valve homografts are proving satisfactory in clinical use, the techniques of the artery bank may find new application. All material must be taken as soon as possible after death, nevertheless, in practice, the next morning has been found satisfactory. Sterile precautions are desirable, but disinfection with ethylene oxide or beta-propiolactone is a good alternative.

Table 3.2. Methods of Artery Banking

Fresh-refrigerated	*Deep-frozen*	*Freeze-dried*
0–4°C in separate refrigerator	−79°C in solid CO_2	Room temperature, in sealed evacuated tube, regularly tested for fluorescence.
Discard after 4–6 weeks	Indefinite storage	Indefinite storage.
Preparation: Placed in Hanks' solution [74] with added 10 per cent homologous serum and antibiotics	Rapid initial freezing to −79°C or −195°C (liquid nitrogen)	Rapid initial freezing in same way. Drying in high vacuum system, one or two stage, to final moisture content of not more than 1 per cent of dry weight.
Use: Direct, with bacteriological culture as safeguard	Rapid thaw in isotonic saline at 40°C	Reconstitution by adding cool saline *in vacuo*.

The Hyperaemia of Successful Reconstruction

Pulses may not return immediately following removal of the clamps. We have seen (Chapter 2) that wide dilatation of the distal vessels occurs in acute ischaemia, for example, during clamping for resection of a previously patent (aneurysmal) aorta. Until these vessels take up slack, no pulse pressure can be held by them. Pulses later return, and an obvious reactive hyperaemia may establish itself, though the process is usually more gradual and less conspicuous, perhaps because of stasis and sludging in the large peripheral vascular bed. In clamping and reconstructing an artery that is already occluded there is no such effect, for no extra ischaemia has been imposed. Yet there is often a delay in the return of peripheral pulses. The reason is probably that the vessels beyond the block have previously undergone a general dilatation [35, 36, 79A, 123] with atrophy of their muscle from intraluminal pressure. Restoration of the blocked main artery will allow a high rate of flow into these dilated and perhaps atonic channels and, as after acute clamping ischaemia, the pulse pressure is temporarily lost, in this case to be regained only after some hours or even a day or more, at the receiving vessels regain their tone and their diameter returns towards normal. During the operation, on removing the clamps this sudden loss of pulse pressure beyond the graft can be disconcerting. Lacking a practical method of measuring blood flow in the main artery through and beyond the reconstructed segment there will be uncertainty as to the success of the operation and the possible need to re-explore the artery. A useful simple test is to occlude the artery gradually between the finger and thumb, at first against only soft resistance with the pulse pressure so low, then, as occlusion is nearly complete, a thrill of high blood flow may be palpable, and as occlusion is completed the proximal pulse against the fingers will become strong and comparable with that in other parts of the body. This is a sure sign that the reconstruction has succeeded, and such a patient will be almost certain to regain strong peripheral pulsations after operation.

At the conclusion of the operation, when the skin towels are removed, though the ankle pulses may still be absent, the foot itself is bright pink or red, with a better 'capillary return' than the unoperated side.

The *hot foot syndrome* (Fig. 3.59) is shown most typically in just this type of patient. The more severe the preceding chronic ischaemia the more conspicuous is the hyperaemia after reconstruction [42, 60, 123, 125, 148]. It may be so intense as to resist the effect of reflex sympathetic vasoconstriction

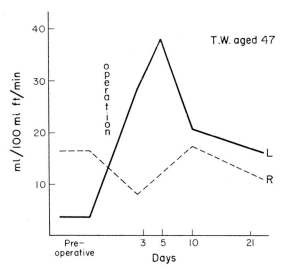

Fig. 3.59. An early example of the postoperative hyperaemia phenomenon after reconstruction of the left popliteal artery in one of the author's first cases in 1952 [42]. Note the coincident fall in blood flow on the symptomless side. A good example of the phenomenon of haemometakinesia or the 'borrowing-lending syndrome'. (*See* Chapter 10, [6].)

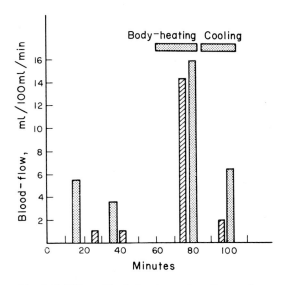

Fig. 3.60. Effect of body heating and cooling on foot blood flow during postoperative hyperaemia. On the operated side (dotted columns) there is still the capacity for further release of sympathetic tone. Vasoconstriction by body cooling, however, does not equalise the flow on the two sides. At all stages, the flow on the operated side is greater.

[125] (Fig. 3.60). The phenomenon lasts from one [42] to four [60] weeks, and may cause oedema [79].

We shall consider a closely similar problem in Chapter 7, p. 134, in the patient who, after repair of an aortic coarctation, develops an acute hyper-aemia of the lower aortic distribution, leading to a necrotising arteritis.

Aorto-iliac Reconstruction for Occlusive Disease

Between a quarter and a third of all claudicating patients can be considered for operations of this type. Operability is higher and contra-indications far fewer than in the larger, femoro-popliteal group. The chief concern is the patient's fitness for major surgery, perhaps because of a history of coronary disease or from the evidence of the ECG. Local factors such as the state of the adjoining arteries are less important than in operations for distal occlusion. Of the patients seen with aorto-iliac obstruction during the years 1960–68, 224 received surgical treatment aimed at restoring the blood flow past the lesion, of whom 132 were found to be suitable for thrombo-endarterectomy. This is the experience of others early in the field [132]. Aorto-femoral by-pass grafting is preferable for the extensive occlusion involving the aorta above the inferior mesenteric and the iliacs beyond their bifurcation, also those with heavy calcification of the aortic bifurcation and adjoining arteries. Mostly, these are old or pre-maturely aged, poor-risk patients in whom the surgical exposure and operating time must be limited. Reconstruction in these is justifiable only when symptoms are severe, for in patients with high aorto-iliac occlusion, rest pain and early gangrene are seldom relieved by lumbar sympathectomy. If the disability is only moderate and there is no deterioration, surgery of any kind is better avoided if the investigation shows extensive disease, but in a similar condition in middle age the operation may be safely advised for its preventive value.

The Problem of External Iliac Arterial Occlusion. Although in theory this simple, mainly unbranched, artery should be suitable for closed endarterectomy, its deep position beneath the lower end of the abdominal wound and the inguinal ligament, where three important collaterals hinder the dissection and haemostasis, its tendency to become grossly nar-rowed, thickened, tortuous and calcified in places, all make for undue difficulty when attempting to reconstruct it in this way. Primary failures are common, which may be evident on removing the clamps. Immediate recourse should then be had to common iliac-to-common femoral by-passing.

The Importance of the Profunda Femoris Artery. In severe ischaemia due to iliac and femoral occlu-sion, though the common femoral may be hard and pulseless, and fail to fill on the arteriogram, there is still a chance for success if the profunda femoris is used. It is usually patent; occlusive disease often seems to overlook it. In a series of 910 femoral arteriograms, non-filling of the profunda was seen in only 3 patients [88]. In these elderly patients with severe chronic ischaemia it may hardly show any contrast at aortography, and then only on delayed films; yet in most cases this good potential 'run-off' can be used. It is safe to assume, without radiological confirmation, that only the mouth of the artery is occluded by the material in the common femoral. This, often only recently deposited, can be removed without difficulty; good back-bleeding then shows itself from the profunda, and some form of re-construction can be brought down to this level, usually an ilio-femoral by-pass graft, or sometimes one from the opposite femoral. Occasionally, the procedure can be limited to the occluded common femoral (*see* Fig. 3.19) if the external iliac is still patent.

Profunda revascularisation has a high success rate [107]. Severe ischaemia with the imminent prospect of major amputation is at once reduced to a moderate or mild degree of claudication, or in the elderly, no disability at all.

A Note on Profundaplasty (Fig. 3.61)

This invaluable addition to arterial surgery is required in two main circumstances: (*a*) to provide adequate run-off for an ilio-femoral or common femoral reconstruction (and exceptionally for an aortic bifurcation graft); and (*b*) as an individual procedure confined to the course of the profunda itself. Exposure is the same for both. A free longi-tudinal incision across the groin finds the common femoral and the profunda origin. The inguinal ligament is divided if necessary [112A]. The pro-funda can be traced downwards behind and lateral to the superficial femoral, first by exposing its upper surface, taking care to identify large venous tribu-taries that often cross it, and dividing these after ligation in continuity. Larger arterial branches of the profunda mostly run laterally and deeply. If the main trunk divides soon after its origin the operation is more difficult.

The widening stage of the profundaplasty is made either with the long tongue of the tubular or patch graft that comes down from above, or—for a pure profundaplasty—with the superficial femoral throm-bosed; this artery is transected at the lower limit of the profunda arteriotomy; the plug of atheroma is removed; and the artery is slit up posteriorly to make a pedicled patch graft.

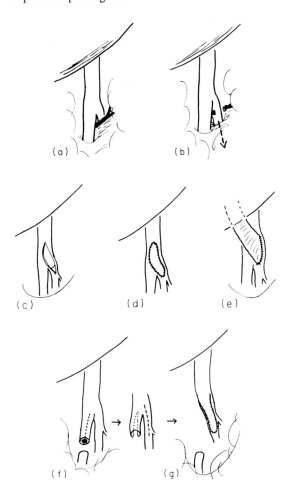

Fig. 3.61. Profundaplasty. (a and b, exposure; c–e, widening the profunda. f and g, arterial flap graft from occluded superficial femoral.)

TECHNIQUE

Thrombo-endarterectomy

Exposure must be adequate (Fig. 3.62). Most cases are well suited to a left paramedian laparotomy with evisceration occasionally needed if the upper limit of the block is juxtarenal (*see* Chapter 15, p. 295). Recovery, however, is smoother and quicker if the procedure can be made extraperitoneal, the method of choice in a significant minority.

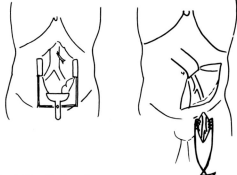

Fig. 3.62. Choice of exposure for aorto-iliac operations.

Paramedian transperitoneal	Lateral oblique extraperitoneal
Bilateral disease of uncertain extent	Unilateral aorto-iliac lesion preferably limited
High upper limit easily reached	Not above inferior mesenteric
Poor exposure of external iliac	Good view of external iliac
Right sympathectomy difficult	Sympathectomy easy on either side
Laparotomy acceptable	Laparotomy inadvisable
Ileus common	Little ileus
Tension sutures for 14 days	Early removal of sutures

In either case the incision is centred over the lowest palpable pulse or the upper arteriographic limit of the block. The bowels or the mobilised peritoneal sac are packed away medially, and the exposure is completed and maintained by the insertion of the three-bladed Goligher self-retaining retractor, with extra packs laterally, above, and below.

Lumbar sympathectomy should be considered [85] at this stage, before heparin has been given. It is advisable in most cases with severe ischaemia or concomitant distal occlusions. With well-localised central lesions and good patency of the lower limb arteries (i.e. most claudicators) it can be dispensed with, for the reconstruction alone will be sufficient.

The arterial assessment is mainly by palpation, with aortograms in sight, feeling for the hard, adherent zone of the block, the strong pulsation above it, and the soft patent main artery below. Calcification, already noted on the arteriograms, may now be found to be so extensive as to rule out the safe completion of endarterectomy. The plan should then be changed to by-passing between healthy segments, or in the worst cases instrumental dilatation from below (*see* p. 85).

The dissection may be easy or very difficult. In the average patient it is soon possible to free the blocked segment and to pass a tape around it, using a cholecystectomy forceps, taking care not to injure any lumbar vessels that cross the dissection space; these can usually be gently felt with the instrument or the index finger before completing the mobilisation and taping. Lifting up on the tape, the artery is now freed, using gentle stroking with a mounted dental cotton roll or Lahey swab. The vena cava or common iliac veins usually separate without much difficulty. The lumbar vessels may now be secured with bulldog clips or thick thread loops. Any serious difficulty or setback at this stage, or continued uncontrollable oozing with general adherence of the artery to its bed, should lead to a consideration of the abandonment of the procedure before heparin has been given. It will usually be possible to change the plan and to insert an aorto-iliac or aorto-femoral by-pass graft.

Endarterectomy

This should normally be immediately preceded by the intra-arterial administration of heparin distal to the occlusion, 25 to 50 mg being given according to the severity of the disease, the amount of oozing already encountered, and the speed with which clots have been forming in blood already shed. In simple, localised procedures on one iliac artery, in young patients with ample back-flow, it is now the writer's practice sometimes to omit heparin. However, any tendency to lose the back flow will change this plan.

A short longitudinal incision is made in the completely occluded part of the artery, before applying the clamps. The free plane of the endarterectomy is sought and entered with a Watson Cheyne dissector and, generally, this is easily developed so that it encircles the atheromatous plug and its contained thrombus (*see* p. 62). Often, it is now possible, using the finger and thumb, to squeeze out the proximal portion of the obstruction, and when at this point the full gush of arterial blood enters the wound, swiftly to place the proximal (aortic or common iliac) clamp on the segment of artery already prepared for it. The distal end of the block may be exposed separately or through the same arteriotomy, according to the length of the block (*see* p. 63), and a place is then chosen for the division, with fine curved scissors, of the lower end of the sclerotic sleeve of material where it is thinnest and most adherent to the arterial wall. Axially-placed mattress stitches (Fig. 3.55) are often needed to secure the end of the divided layer if it is at all thick or loose, in order to hold it out to the arterial

wall. This is a most important step towards preventing early postoperative re-occlusion from dissection of the blood into the distal endarterectomy plane.

Repair of the Artery. Unless the lumen is wide and smooth, a patch graft should be inserted. Part of a knitted dacron arterial graft or, better, an uncrimped piece of the same material, is cut to size and sutured into place with arterial silk or dacron, 4 or 5/0, according to the thickness of the remaining arterial wall.

The heparin is reversed with intravenous protamine (in 2:1 dosage) during the conclusion of this stage.

Removal of the Clamps. There should be little bleeding if the repair has been satisfactory, provided sufficient time has been allowed for the protamine to take effect (5 to 15 minutes). Extra sutures are required only for vigorous spurting leaks. Swab pressure or the application of a piece of crushed muscle or haemostatic gauze will quickly check most bleeding. Clamps should be reapplied only if loss is excessive or if the patient's general condition gives cause for concern. The anaesthetist should by now have replaced the measured blood loss. Mannitol may be infused if the operation has been unusually long or difficult, or if a clamp has been placed near the renal arteries.

Closure of the posterior peritoneum, using a 2/0 atraumatic catgut suture, after removal of all tapes, clips, etc. covers the reconstructed artery. The anterior peritoneum is then closed, using a stronger catgut, after a final review of the abdomen for packs, and for intestinal ischaemia, and the rectus sheath is repaired with continuous 34 gauge stainless steel wire, having previously placed stout nylon tension sutures at one inch intervals beneath the sheath but not including muscle. When the skin has been closed, these should be tied over a sterile sanitary towel. Wound complications are unusual if this compressing support is left in place for the full fourteen days after operation.

BY-PASS GRAFTING (Figs. 3.63, 3.64)
Special indications include:

(*a*) extensive, advanced and calcified disease;

(*b*) some acute cases (the 'rescue operation', *see* p. 119);

(*c*) involvement of the external iliac artery (*see* p. 68); and

(*d*) any question of renal or mesenteric arterial insufficiency to which extended endarterectomy is likewise ill adapted, though it has been successfully undertaken [127]; ordinarily, the branching by-pass method of DeBakey and his colleagues [30] offers a more practical solution.

Steps in the procedure are essentially the same as in aorto-iliac thrombo-endarterectomy which, in fact, may serve as a preliminary stage in the construction of the proximal anastomosis (as in by-passing the external iliac, described above).

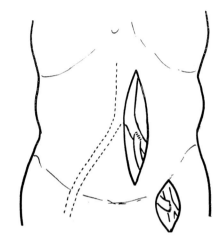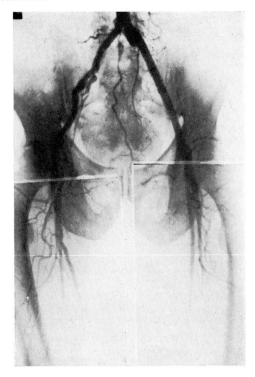

Fig. 3.63. Ilio-femoral by-pass.

LEFT. The abdominal exposure is shown larger than would normally be used, for purposes of clarity. It may be extra-peritoneal if desired. The graft is always brought extra-peritoneally, through the femoral canal to the common femoral anastomosis. Thrombo-endarterectomy may be a necessary preliminary to either anastomosis, though more often, the iliac.

RIGHT. Lumbar aortogram five years after such an operation showing knitted dacron graft free from kinking and with a smooth, regular lumen.

Practical differences from thrombo-endarterectomy include:

(a) *Limited exposure* of the aorta and common femoral arteries (Fig. 3.17) may suffice if an elective by-pass operation has been decided on. Only a sufficient length for the two or three anastomoses need be dissected. The retroperitoneal course of the graft can easily be tunnelled using gentle dissection with the two index fingers between the abdominal and inguinal wounds.

(b) *Lateral clamping* of the three arteries may permit the construction of end-to-side anastomoses without interruption of the blood flow, further limiting the amount of dissection necessary before applying the clamps. Because of this and the shorter clamping and operating time, heparin may sometimes be avoided, or used in low dosage, e.g. 25 mg.

(c) *Transection of the aorta* with an end-to-end anastomosis to the stem of the bifurcation graft is preferable when the aorta is thrombosed, or the inferior mesenteric origin is occluded. It is also valuable in the event of difficulty with bleeding from lumbar vessels, or a split occurring in the posterior surface of the aorta during its preparation for an anterior anastomosis.

A note on the operative management of juxtarenal aortic occlusion by temporary renal artery clamping (Fig. 3.65).

There is grave danger of renal embolisation during manipulations of the thrombosed, atheromatous aorta close to the renal orifices [138]. Fatal renal ischaemia may follow. To avoid this disaster use a long upper extension of the normal paramedian laparotomy incision, mobilise the left renal vein and

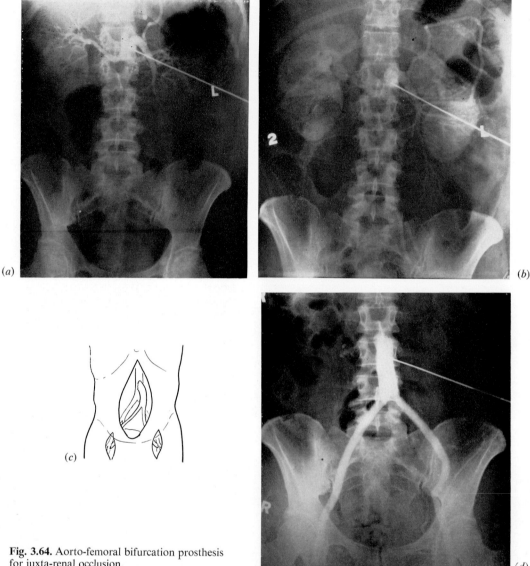

Fig. 3.64. Aorto-femoral bifurcation prosthesis for juxta-renal occlusion.

(*a*) First phase of high lumbar aortogram showing upper limit of thrombus level with the lower margin of the renal orifice; superior mesenteric filling well with early passage of medium into middle-colic artery.

(*b*) Later film showing conspicuous dilatation of the marginal artery of the left colon, and good collateral filling of the left iliac arteries.

(*c*) Trans-peritoneal operation with all three anastomoses made end-to-side. The limbs of the bifurcation are brought retroperitoneally through the femoral canals. A much smaller abdominal incision is normally used (*see* Fig. 3.17). It is often necessary, as in the case shown, to perform a cautious thrombo-endarterectomy of the juxta-renal stump of the aorta; using heparin and taking great care not to displace loose material into the renal arteries. If necessary, these may be temporarily clamped during the clearance of this vital segment.

(*d*) Postoperative low aortogram into endarterectomised segment showing good filling of both femorals. In this case, the external iliac artery was used for the left anastomosis. It is more difficult to apply the necessary tension when this is done, and the left branch of the graft is a little longer than it should be.

(This woman, aged forty-four, was grafted ten years ago for claudication at a few yards accompanied by a febrile illness subsequently recognised as disseminated lupus. She remains well and active on low dosage steroids.)

body of pancreas from the aorta at renal level, then free and tape the two renal arteries. Now the gently mobilised infra-renal aorta is divided across *without any clamps being applied*. There will be no bleeding from this pulseless occluded lumen except perhaps a small amount if there is a channel through the thrombus leading to the inferior mesenteric. The plug of obstructing material is now gently freed, using a Watson Cheyne dissector. The two

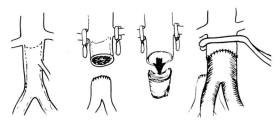

Fig. 3.65. Grafting for juxta-renal aortic occlusion.

renals are now clipped and the plug is eased out by fingers of the right hand, pressing firmly from in front of the stump. After two or three short, wide-open flushings the aorta is formally clamped just below the renals and the two renal clips are removed. The whole process takes 2 to 3 minutes. End to end anastomosis of the stump to the graft is then completed.

POSTOPERATIVE CARE

Serious early complications are few. Operative blood loss should seldom exceed 500 ml and must have been replaced before the patient leaves the operating theatre.

In a few patients the distal pulses do not immediately reappear. As a rule they soon do, and show a rapid improvement during the early hours of recovery. Rarely there may be severe acute ischaemia which tends to affect the limb that was the better of the two. In such a patient the foot circulation will

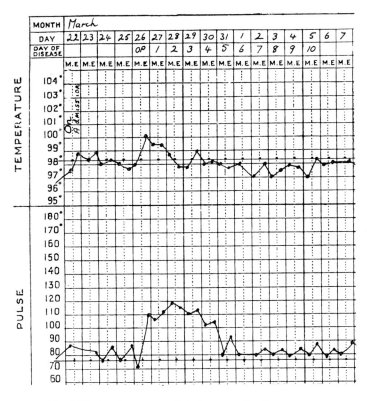

Fig. 3.66. Another aspect of the hyperaemia phenomenon.

From the chart of a man aged 46 undergoing aortic bifurcation reconstruction who developed tachycardia in the region of 120 beats/min on the second postoperative day, probably as a result of the low resistance in the distal-vascular bed now being perfused by the graft. Gradual fall in pulse rate as tone returns.

have been obviously impaired from the clamping period onwards. In operations for chronic occlusive disease, clamping of the blocked segment should make little difference to the resting foot circulation. Unless the aorta has been clamped above its bifurcation, one limb of which was previously patent and with a normal flow; or there has been dislodgement of aortic thrombus into the patent branch; or stasis thrombus has formed, due to insufficient heparin dosage: then there should be no pallor or venous collapse in the lower limbs beyond the aortic clamp. This is in absolute contrast to the effect of aortic clamping for abdominal aneurysm, in which acute ischaemia always develops.

Gastric intubation, hourly suction, and controlled intravenous fluid replacement are as essential as in other major abdominal operations. Ileus is common, but not usually severe or prolonged. Tension sutures prevent early strain on the healing wound.

Any prolonged or serious gastro-intestinal difficulties should raise the suspicion of mesenteric arterial occlusion, whose mechanism may partly be that of aorto-iliac 'steal' [140A]. Here the hyperaemia into the lower half of the body may divert blood from the splanchnic sector, with fatal results if there is already any significant disease there.

Hourly pulse and blood pressure readings are kept up for the first twenty-four hours, and four-hourly for the next two to three days, according to the state of the patient.

Urine output must be carefully watched. Manipulation of the upper abdominal aorta may have displaced thrombus or atheromatous material into the renal arteries [138]. Neurogenic interference with renal blood supply has been postulated but never proved. Anuria from these causes or from blood loss or transfusion complications must be vigorously treated (see Chapter 15, p. 303) for the mortality is high.

Tachycardia without fever or shock is fairly common (Fig. 3.66). It may be a response to the hyperaemic phase of revascularisation, as is commonly noticed after restoration of the obstructed circulation in one lower limb (see p. 67).

Chest complications are common in heavy smokers.

Burst abdomen was common in the experience of the early years of this work. Shorter operating time, better technique, and meticulous wound closure with stainless steel wire, using tension sutures, have almost eliminated this setback.

Femoro-popliteal Reconstruction for Occlusive Disease

We have already seen that the indications for this type of arterial surgery should be strictly limited by the uncertain late results, with present-day methods.

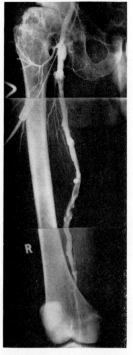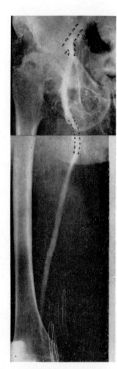

Fig. 3.67. Late patency in a femoro-popliteal homograft, inserted in September 1956, after storage at −79°C. In 1964, his claudication returned, bruits were heard along the graft, which this arteriogram shows to be grossly arteriosclerotic. Successfully regrafted with knitted dacron and condition maintained.

In recent years, many limbs have been lost after attempts to reconstruct the femoral artery for claudication mostly using imperfect technique and unsuitable grafts. In the writer's own experience there were 3 such cases in a total of 238 femoro-popliteal reconstructions, since 1951.

Axial replacement homografts (1951–55) [43] nearly all failed within a year; the early by-pass homografts (1955–59) first used in Britain by Cockett [20] proved much better (Fig. 3.67) but were hopelessly unpractical as routine treatment for such a common condition, and late complications, principally occlusion and aneurysm formation, have been common [3, 80]. Cloth prostheses (1959–63) although easy to obtain, sterilise, and insert have been disappointing in most experience (see p. 88). This was soon found to be true of the woven teflon cloth tube, which as its originator, Sterling Edwards, showed in 1960 [48], is not only impervious to blood but also to cellular incorporation by the body, as a result of which loose amorphous and partly cellular debris accumulated within its lumen, became detached, and formed an embolus that obstructed the lower anastomosis or its 'run-off'. Late patency rates of 10 to 20 per cent after three years are obviously unsatisfactory.

In the uncommon event of a cloth prosthesis remaining patent for five years or more it, too, appears to become affected by the complications of arterial disease. The patient shown in Fig. 3.68 had a teflon femoro-popliteal graft, still patent in 1968 after nine years, that showed marked lengthening and convolution, though under full tension when originally inserted. Arteriosclerotic narrowing is a common feature in late cases [133], and aneurysmal dilatation of a dacron graft has been reported at six years [84]; much more often the sac forms at the groin anastomosis (Fig. 3.69).

In 1960, the writer abandoned the cloth prostheses for the reconstruction of the femoro-popliteal artery, except for an occasional 'rescue operation', and began to use endarterectomy in selected cases, as described by Cockett [20] some years earlier. The results have proved more satisfactory than those achieved by any method previously used (*see* Table 3.6), and this technique is now standard practice for limited femoro-popliteal occlusions. Nevertheless, for more extensive distal or irregular disease it is now believed that saphenous vein by-pass grafting is more satisfactory [1, 27, 34A]. The two operations can often be combined, using the wide upper part of the saphenous vein for the distal part of the reconstruction [94A] (*see* p. 82).

TECHNIQUE

Operating Position

(*a*) *Sims' position* (Fig. 3.70*a*). Lying on the affected side with the sound leg flexed forward gives the best exposure of the femoro-popliteal junction where most limited blocks are situated. Extension distally is simple, but there is no view of the upper femoral, and lumbar sympathectomy is not possible.

(*b*) *Cockett's position* (Fig. 3.70*b*). Similar to (*a*) but with the sound limb towelled and suspended out of the way, so as to expose the whole femoral artery if necessary. This is effective, though somewhat cumbersome, and if there should be ischaemia of the opposite limb, any prolonged elevation might be harmful.

(*c*) *Rob and Owen's position* [110] (Fig. 3.70*c*). In this the patient is lying on his 'good' side. A combined synchronous exposure of the femoral origin and the back of the popliteal gives excellent conditions for a pull-through graft between these

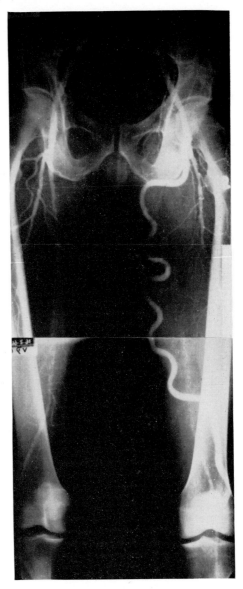

Fig. 3.68. Marked lengthening and tortuosity of a left teflon femoro-popliteal graft inserted in November 1959, and still patent. This behaviour is characteristic of teflon grafts, and is usually considered to be an important reason for their common early failure. In this case, however, most of the tortuosity is away from the limb flexures. Several other teflon grafts inserted at about the same time are still patent, although shortly after this the material was abandoned for this purpose.

This fifty-three-year-old diabetic patient recently received a right femoro-popliteal saphenous vein graft by Mr R. C. Shepherd, with satisfactory results.

Fig. 3.69. False aneurysm at the common femoral anastomosis of a plastic femoro-popliteal prosthesis, itself inserted in replacement of an aneurysmal deep-freeze homograft. Both aneurysmal conditions were symptomless. This patient had been free from claudication since his first operation. Subsequently died of coronary thrombosis.

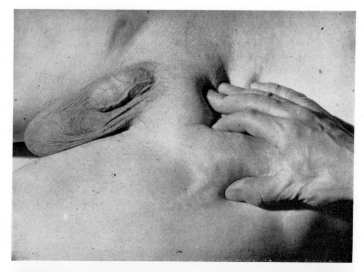

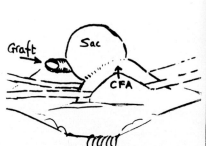

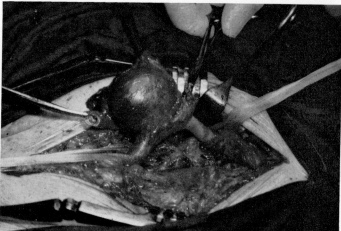

two arteries, as when inserting a homograft or cloth prosthesis, but it is totally unsuitable for the autogenous vein graft or long endarterectomy operations since the middle and lower part of the thigh is obscured.

(*d*) *The dorsal position* (Fig. 3.70*d*). Described by Henry [72] and widely used in the United States, this is probably the best position for general use. The medial approach to the popliteal artery is not as easy as from behind, but with it there is less risk of damage to the medial popliteal nerve, and there is no need to divide the large arterial branch to the medial head of the gastrocnemius. The whole of the femoro-popliteal artery and saphenous vein can be exposed, and lumbar sympathectomy carried out without moving the patient.

The Operation

In some operations, planned limited exposure of part of the femoro-popliteal can be based on recent arteriograms, with the object of mobilising and reconstructing a short segment of the stenosed or obstructed artery locally in one of three sites:

(*a*) The common femoral and profunda origin.
(*b*) The superficial femoral in Hunter's canal.
(*c*) The femoro-popliteal junction beneath the adductor magnus tendon, and the proximal popliteal.

More often, two or all three regions will require direct inspection. This is possible with the patient in the dorsal position. The upper and lower limits of the obstructing lesion are inspected and assessed,

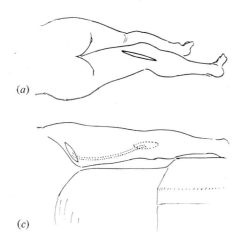
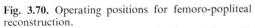
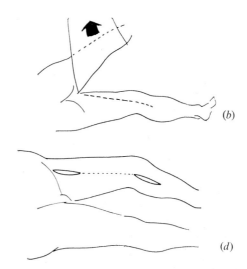

Fig. 3.70. Operating positions for femoro-popliteal reconstruction.

(*a*) Sims' position: (*b*) Cockett's position: (*c*) Rob and Owen's position: (*d*) Henry's or the dorsal position, probably the most generally useful.

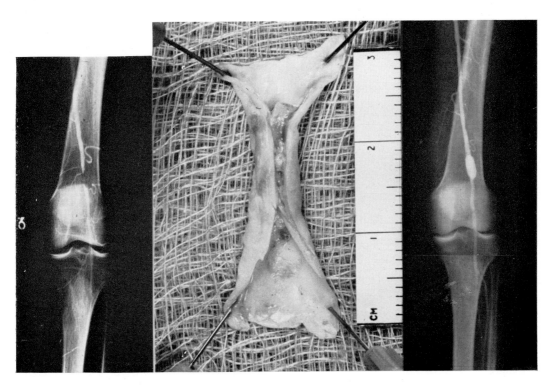

Fig. 3.71. A good case for a short, open endarterectomy. Note the thin limits of the plaque, and the short, dense nature of the occluding material.

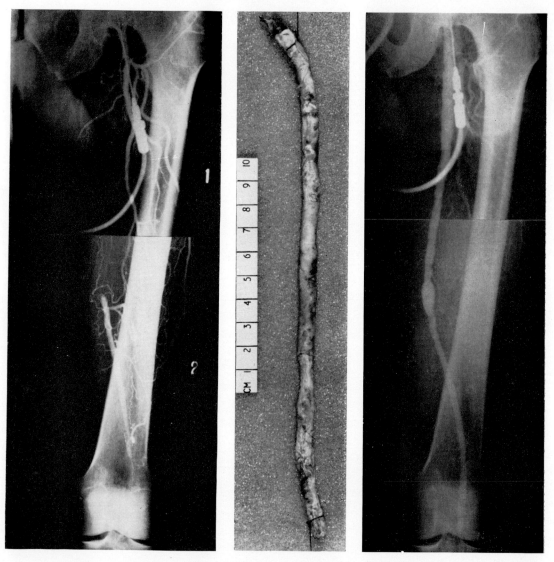

Fig. 3.72. Full-length superficial femoral thrombo-endarterectomy by closed method.

with any necessary extension or joining up of the initial incisions along the line of the artery. The type of reconstruction best suited can then be decided.

Exposure. (*a*) *The common femoral* is easily reached through a longitudinal incision across the groin, the line being chosen after palpation of the artery at this point. With the pulsation or the thickened thrombosed vessel as a ready guide, the superficial tissues are divided freely, there being no

important structure over the artery in this dissection. A self-retaining retractor is used early, and the artery is soon seen. At its upper and lower limits, and deeply in its middle portion, there are small to medium-sized branches, which should be preserved if possible.

(*b*) *The superficial femoral* lies beneath the sartorius, which is dissected free and displaced posteriorly, and the aponeurotic fascia beneath the muscle. The only structure of importance in the superficial

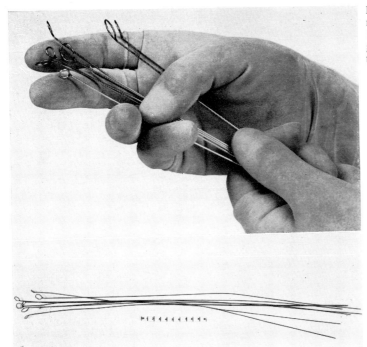

Fig. 3.73. Vollmar's ring strippers with non-cutting, obliquely inclined head [144A]. This simple instrument has greatly simplified closed endarterectomy, in the author's experience.

dissection is the saphenous vein. It is helpful to mark this on the skin before operation, and to plan the incision so as to avoid crossing the vein, if possible keeping the vein in the posterior flap, otherwise it will have to cross the upper end of the wound to gain the medial side of the artery. When the artery is being mobilised, care should be taken not to injure the deep vein.

(c) *The adductor opening and upper popliteal region.* Again, avoiding the saphenous vein, the sartorius is displaced backwards. A sheet of tendinous fibres beneath includes the adductor tendon, and through it passes the saphenous nerve, which is the guide to the artery that lies close beneath. Often, it is hard and pulseless at this point, and so may be difficult to distinguish from the tendon so closely applied to it. Beneath is the deep vein, which, like the nerve that runs over the artery, can easily be damaged unless special care is taken over the tendon division and artery mobilisation.

Procedure. The block can readily be felt as a hard, cord-like adherent segment with a normal pulse pressure at its proximal end (though this may be reduced by anaesthesia or blood loss). Distally, the artery becomes softer, compressible, and may have a weakened pulse. The limits of the block are also marked off by the leaving and re-entering collateral branches. Both may be pulsating strongly. Being dilated and thin walled, they are easily damaged, particularly where they join the main artery.

ENDARTERECTOMY

Trial endarterectomy. The artery is mobilised, and whichever type of endarterectomy appropriate to the site and length of the lesion is attempted. *Open endarterectomy* is preferable for a short lesion with good patency above and below (Fig. 3.71). The method has been extended to clear out the whole superficial femoral [48], using a long opened-out strip of saphenous vein as a closing gusset graft, but the long suture line is a serious objection, though good results have been obtained, no doubt because of the thoroughness of the endarterectomy under direct vision.

Closed femoro-popliteal endarterectomy offers a much simpler means of dealing with the common, full-length block in the thigh, via two small exposing incisions. Provided there is little calcification in the hidden part of the artery, and the best plane of stripping is carefully sought, the whole length of the occluding plug can usually be removed in one piece (Fig. 3.72). Vollmar's oblique non-cutting strippers (Fig. 3.73) have proved easy and safe to use.

A third arteriotomy may occasionally be required, through a separate skin incision over the middle region of the artery.

Loose atheromatous material is cleared out by passing a smaller non-cutting stripper several times, and the operation is completed with distal intimal securing stitches and patch grafts, as required.

Wound closure in the thigh is with fine catgut to

the fascial layers, and interrupted 36-gauge stainless steel wire to the skin. A vacuum drain is normally used.

By-pass Grafting

In the event of difficulty during any stage of an attempt at a long, closed endarterectomy, the correct course is to convert the operation to a vein by-pass procedure. Experience is proving that this is the best method for any extensive femoro-popliteal obliteration in which the lower limit involves the popliteal segment [20].

Endarterectomy often fails in such a case because the lower end is so small and inaccessible. A good many successful operations are now on record in which the lower anastomosis has been made to the posterior tibial artery well beyond the popliteal bifurcation [25, 70].

Two methods are now in use:

1. The free, reversed saphenous vein graft [29] (Fig. 3.74(b), (e)).
2. The *in situ* saphenous vein graft with destruction of its valves [21, 41A, 69] (Fig. 3.74(c)).

The point at issue mainly concerns the diameter of the graft. Experience has shown that one of the several technical difficulties [94A] of the standard reversal operation is the tendency of the vein to contract, making it difficult to construct a wide sound anastomosis at the upper end.

Figure 3.74(c) suggests a point in haemodynamics that may be important. With the narrow end of the graft at the distal anastomosis, the velocity of flow (though not, of course, its volume) is considerably greater than in its wider proximal portion. This may protect the continued patency of the graft, from the smaller tendency to platelet accumulation from the fast stream over the lower suture line.

For really long grafts, especially those ending beyond the knee joint, the *in situ* technique is preferred by some surgeons [21, 41A, 69, 70], because the vasa vasorum of the middle segment of the graft are intact. For severe ischaemia, where secondary blocks in the distal vessels will reduce 'run-off', the vein graft has shown its superiority in saving limbs [99], and flow studies in some of these patients revealed that patency was maintained with blood flow as low as 15 ml/minute through the graft [100], a finding that agrees with the known facts of venous blood flow, as well as with the capacity of veins and vein grafts to recanalise thrombus [26]. Hall [17] recommends an injection into the graft of tolazine (Priscol) 5 mg, or papaverine 40 mg, and has shown a striking increase in graft-flow, especially in cases in which the lower anastomosis was not excessively far down the limb. Lumbar sympathectomy to the grafted limb may do the same [100]. The form of the pulse wave tracing by an electromagnetic flow meter has been shown to be important for graft prognosis. In actual measurement this method indicates that graft-flow greater than 100 ml per minute is highly favourable; less than this carried a 50 per cent risk of occlusion [17A, 136A].

With the patient in the dorsal position, the whole femoro-popliteal obstruction and the proximal superficial femoral, whether or not it is patent, and the corresponding extent of the internal saphenous vein, are exposed. Only the two ends are fully mobilised.

If a reversal graft is planned, the entire vein is dissected free, ligating the tributaries with silk on the graft side, and catgut on the wound side. The graft is then distended with cool isotonic saline solution which detects leaks and helps to enlarge its contracted lumen. The lower opening can be further enlarged by gentle bouginage, using the moistened end of the Watson Cheyne dissector. Vein grafts should not be left to soak in saline, it is better to wrap them in a saline swab.

For an *in situ* graft, a close search is made for tributaries without freeing the vein, and as each one is found it is tied as above. Should a tributary be left intact, its valve may become incompetent and a small arterio-venous fistula will be established, which can cause delay in wound healing in this region [104]. The upper and lower two or three inches of the vein are fully mobilised, and the sapheno-femoral junction is transected over a lateral clamp; the femoral vein is then repaired by a longitudinal vascular suture. Care must be taken to avoid tension when dividing the vein to size at the two ends, for the *in situ* graft has less freedom to stretch than a free graft, particularly proximally.

The anastomoses are fine and exacting, especially at the lower end which, because the knee is flexed during the operation, should not be cut too short. 6/0 suture is preferable here. It is useful to leave a short segment of the lower anastomosis open, for subsequent patency testing by saline irrigation from above, when the upper anastomosis is nearly complete. The upper anastomosis is simpler, and 5/0 material is suitable. Before it is completed a small Cannon stripper, or bullet-headed vein stripper [21] is passed down the vein several times: the valves are felt to break as they catch the stripper. Hall [69], the originator of the method, has preferred to excise each valve through a venotomy. After a final test irrigation the anastomoses are closed, protamine is given and the clamps are removed. If there is doubt over patency an operative arteriogram is done [112]. Closure is as described in the section on femoral endarterectomy.

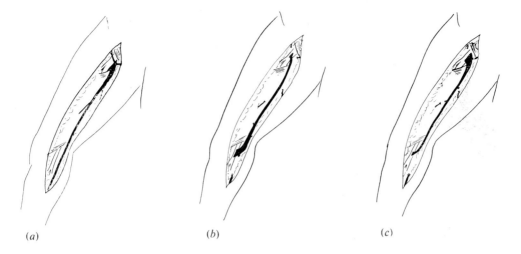

(a)   (b)   (c)

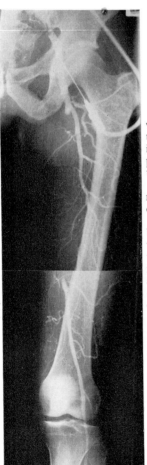

(*a*) The long exposure necessary to visualise all tributaries, and to extract the vein without damage. It is better to interrupt the skin incision in several places. Skin edge necrosis in the mid-thigh can be minimised in this way.

(*b*) Graft inserted by the reversed technique with a narrow proximal and wide distal anastomosis.

(*c*) Grafting by the *in situ* method with branches ligated and valves destroyed with a sharp Cannon loop stripper. This technique ensures that the lower anastomosis should not be too wide, thus avoiding slowing of the velocity of flow over the vulnerable segment of the reconstruction.

(*d*) Superficial femoral occlusion resulting from the late thrombosis of a long thrombo-endarterectomy, in a fisherman aged fifty-six.

(*e*) Reversed saphenous vein graft restores patency. Late mortality from coronary occlusion.

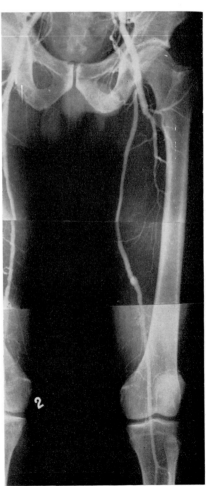

(*d*)   (*e*)

Fig. 3.74. Femoro-popliteal saphenous vein by-pass graft.

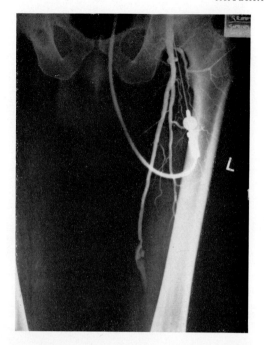

Fig. 3.75. Atheromatous obstruction in a short endarterectomy segment at the femoro-popliteal junction. The medium can be seen cascading over the obstruction and into the dilated chamber covered by the vein graft, in which there are two further filling defects—probably thrombi.

Re-operation will usually correct such a situation.

Combined proximal femoral endarterectomy and distal femoro-popliteal vein by-pass grafting is useful when the popliteal, though patent, is too badly diseased for safe reconstruction by endarterectomy, or when only the upper half of the saphenous vein is sufficiently wide to use as a graft [28, 50, 94A]. The cephalic vein has also proved useful in patients whose saphenous vein has already been stripped out [81A].

POSTOPERATIVE CARE

It is unnecessary and inadvisable to allow the action of heparin to continue after the release of the arterial clamps. If more heparin is given, considerable oozing may occur during the first night after the operation. Delayed primary closure [20, 42] answers this difficulty, though a second operation is unwelcome to the patient. A more important consideration, however, is the finding that anticoagulants (even heparin) do little to prevent thrombosis in a moving arterial blood stream, however effective they may be *in vitro* and in static blood *in vivo*

(during clamping or other acute ischaemia). The lowered peripheral blood flow caused by heparin-induced hypovolaemia precipitate arterial occlusion from platelet aggregation, which heparin does nothing to prevent [113].

Low molecular weight dextran is beneficial, promoting the blood flow in a severely ischaemic limb, and is also valuable after reconstruction. It can be stopped as soon as the ankle pulses on the operated side become strongly palpable, which may not be until late on the first postoperative day.

Failure of distal pulses to reappear at this time means there has probably been a primary failure of the reconstruction (Fig. 3.75), and, the patient's condition permitting, a re-exploration should be undertaken without delay. The Fogarty catheter is most useful. The thrombus is removed and its cause is sought and corrected. Loose atheroma material, or a kink or twist, or an intact valve cusp are the usual reasons, though a poor 'run-off' is often responsible, and cannot be remedied though it can usually be recognised at arteriography during operation.

Oedema of the operated limb is common: 12 per cent in one series [34], and may be due to hyperaemia (*see* p. 67), to extravasation, or to phlebothrombosis (Fig. 3.76*a*); the latter may require anticoagulant treatment, or operative thrombectomy with repair of the venotomy (Fig. 3.76*b*). Swelling also occurred in 12 per cent of a similar series of femoro-popliteal cloth grafts [80]. Lymphangiography after such operations indicated that the degree of swelling was related to the extent of damage to the lymph channels [141]. The apparently low incidence of deep venous thrombosis may be due to the use of heparin during operation, which is when most thrombi begin to form [81B].

Weight-bearing can be started quite soon after a limited endarterectomy (on the third day for the common femoral, the fifth for the adductor opening operation) and at one week the patient with a full femoro-popliteal reconstruction may resume restricted hospital activities.

Before and after re-ambulation the physiotherapist should treat as though for meniscectomy.

The Cross-over Graft [103, 110A, 143, 144] (Fig. 3.77)

This useful expedient is freely indicated for unilateral iliac obstruction in elderly, poor-risk patients, often with heavy aorto-iliac calcification, further precluding abdominal arterial surgery. Provided there remains a patent ilio-femoral on the sound side, the two common femorals are connected by using a dacron or saphenous vein graft drawn through a low supapubic subcutaneous tunnel. An endarterectomy may be required on the ischaemic side in order to open up the profunda femoris, for this may be occluded at its origin by the obstruction in the common femoral (*see* p. 78).

Close attention should be paid to the bladder function after this operation: with any history of delay or nocturia it is wise to insert a fine Gibbon catheter at the end of the operation, for the graft may interfere with subsequent retropubic prostatic surgery. In one case of the writer's, however, this was possible less than two weeks after the graft operation, using a transverse incision 2 cm above the pulsating shunt, transurethral resection having previously failed.

Other Unorthodox and 'Unanatomical' Shunts
These include:

1. *Splenic-femoral*, said to be 'fraught with difficulties' [58] and probably never indicated for occlusive disease.
2. *Subclavian-bilateral femoral* [91] has been used for extensive aneurysm with dissection.

3. *Axillo-femoral*, for bilateral iliac occlusion, in which only one side requires reconstruction [7, 95]. Saphenous vein is the material of choice.
4. *Axillary-bilateral femoral* [114] which may provide the only safe solution to the serious and not uncommon problem of the failed, high aortic bifurcation reconstruction. Patency with cloth prostheses of over eighteen months has been reported, but there is a risk of a 'steal' effect from the upper limb while exercising the legs.

The construction of these unorthodox, superficial shunts requires minimal anaesthesia and is well adapted to a synchronous technique with two surgeons. The proximal take-off point is from the axillary, splitting the pectoralis major just below the middle of the clavicle [7].

This technique has yet to establish its value. Most surgeons with early experience of the method have been disappointed by the high failure rate [106A, 110A], though up to twelve months the results are often good [100A].

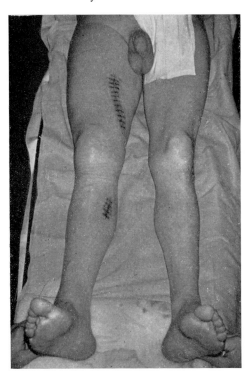 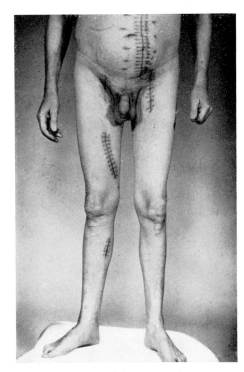

Fig. 3.76. Ilio-femoral phlebo-thrombosis complicating bilateral arterial reconstruction.

LEFT. Femoral thrombo-endarterectomy two weeks before, and a recent ilio-femoral by-pass, since which the previously operated right thigh has swelled greatly with an effusion in the knee joint, and a palpable tender thrombus in the common femoral vein at the groin.

RIGHT. Early complete resolution of swelling and pain following ilio-femoral thrombectomy through the short, right inguinal incision, using Fogarty balloon catheters.

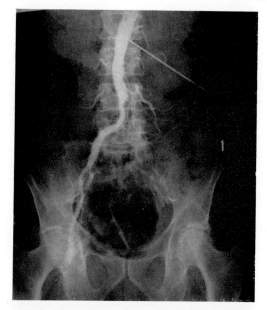

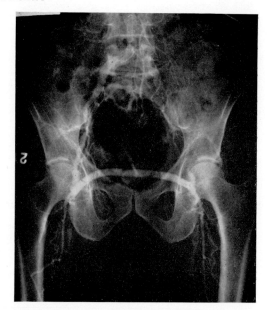

(a)

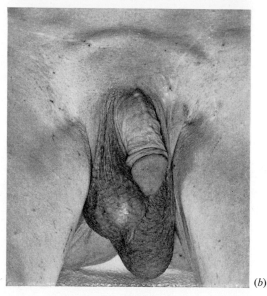

(b)

Fig. 3.77. Femoro-femoral cross-over graft.

(a) Calcified, occluded left iliac arteries in a severely bronchitic patient of sixty-three, with severe left lower limb ischaemia. Dacron shunt between the femorals has made patency for the past two years. There is the risk that, as in this case, the grafted limb may 'steal' blood from the donor side. On the whole, however, the results of this operation are better than would be expected with a low primary failure rate, and well maintained patency, though the period of trial is still under three years for the earliest of cases. (Courtesy the Editor, *Scand. J. Clin. Lab. Invest.* [46].)

(b) Supra-pubic course of the graft in another patient, also still patent, after two years.

Summary of Operative Methods for Chronic Lower-limb Ischaemia

1. Lumbar sympathectomy should be used for early, slow gangrene of the toes, in support of an arterial reconstruction involving an abdominal exposure, and in distal operations in the limb if the ischaemia is severe.

2. Thrombo-endarterectomy is ideal for short occlusions at any point along the main artery. It is good in many cases of extensive femoral obliteration. Patch widening should be freely used.

3. For extensive occlusion or in an artery with much diffuse patchy disease or calcification (or inaccessible, such as the external iliac), the by-pass principle gives better results.
(a) Saphenous vein is preferable for long lower limb by-pass.
(b) Vein or flat dacron knit appear to be equally suitable for arterial patching, with preference for the vein in small or thin-walled arteries.

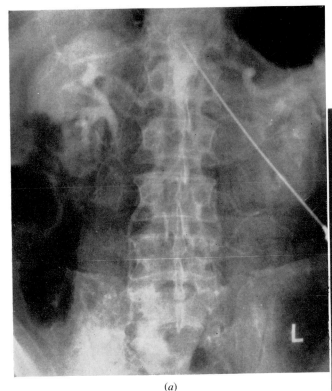

(a)

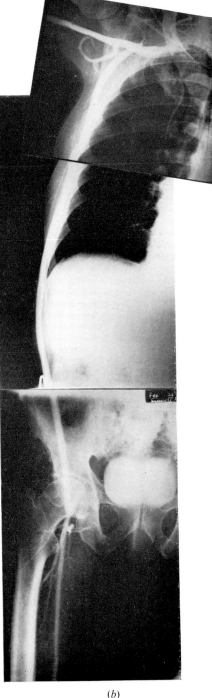

(b)

Fig. 3.78. Subclavian common femoral shunt for inoperable abdominal aortic occlusion.

(a) Complete aortic and juxta-renal thrombosis following radiotherapy for seminoma of the testis. Multiple interventions for radionecrosis and faecal fistula preclude any direct aortic surgery.

(b) An 8 mm knitted dacron prosthesis was placed between the third part of the right subclavian and the right common femoral artery, and functioned well for a while with relief of pain from a severely ischaemic right foot. With occlusion of the graft a few weeks later, a major amputation became necessary.

(c) The knitted dacron tube remains ideal for the more proximal by-pass operations, e.g. aorto-iliac, ilio-femoral, aorto-femoral, as well as for some of the unorthodox shunts.

Unorthodox routes should be considered when simpler than accepted anatomical restoration through the depth of the body cavities.

Instrumental and Other Non-operative Methods
Percutaneous Dilatation with Graded Catheters over a Seldinger Guide. This technique was developed by Dotter and Judkins [38, 39] who, during the course of arteriography for severe ischaemia, noticed

85

that there was, sometimes, considerable improvement in the peripheral circulation after examination, and they were able to confirm clinically and radiologically that patency had been restored to a segment previously blocked. They followed this discovery by a deliberate instrumentation of the same kind, using progressively larger arterial catheters, and at

the time of a further report had treated 155 patients in this simple way with improvement in 80 per cent of those with stenosis, but they had less good results with complete obstruction. Others have reported similar results [40]. The author has had a limited but favourable experience, mostly with the artery exposed at operation.

The Problem of the Failed Arterial Reconstruction

1. EARLY FAILURE (Table 3.3)

An early relapse in the distal circulation after initial improvement is shown by the extremity cooling, and disappearance of the peripheral pulses.

Thrombosis of the reconstructed segment is generally due to some technical difficulty at operation, with the displacement of loose obstructing material (Fig. 3.75), or obstruction by external pressure from other structures, twisting or kinking, or from the

Table 3.3. Early Failures in 475 Cases

A/I claudication	F/P claudication
4/190	16/151
A/I severe ischaemia	F/P severe ischaemia
3/47	17/87

accumulation of a large wound haematoma and clot, particularly in patients who are being maintained on anticoagulant treatment. In most of these instances an immediate re-exploration, on the same day, will correct the complication and late patency can be achieved [32]. Vein grafts are particularly liable to early thrombosis, figures as high as 25 per cent being reported [34A].

A poor 'run-off' will have been appreciated before and during the operation and little can be done to improve this, but re-exploration may show some other reason for the failure and should never be omitted, except when the patient's condition precludes further surgery.

Infection is the most serious of all causes. Apart from fever and local pain there may be little sign that anything is wrong until the patient has a secondary haemorrhage. Patency is maintained with distal pulses still palpable, even while a false aneurysm may be forming at the site of the infected suture line. Local repair should not be attempted. The safest course is to perform proximal ligation, though where there has been previous chronic ischaemia, a massive gangrene may follow.

Revision of the reconstruction, using a fresh, uninfected bed for the graft [30A, 121], may sometimes succeed, for example an infected femoropopliteal graft can be by-passed, using the obturator foramen as a clean route from the iliac to the lower popliteal. Another example, an abdominal aortic graft lying in an abscess, was by-passed between the supra-coeliac aorta and common femoral [142]. Though some cases have responded to massive disinfection and antibiotic treatment [19], nowadays this situation would constitute the strongest of indications for an axillo-femoral by-pass graft.

2. LATE FAILURE

Much the most important factor is the condition for which the reconstruction was originally performed. Reasons for success or failure have already been discussed (p. 58). Imponderables such as the body tolerance to foreign materials [149], or the activity or status of the occlusive disease [53], and cigarette smoking [64A, 149A] are difficult to assess, and more so to control.

Many failures are the result of technical faults or difficulties at the time of operation [24]. Their elimination should certainly improve late patency. Late revision operations using better prostheses and with close attention to every detail of operative technique often succeed [28].

Revision of endarterectomy operations is difficult to the point of impossibility, for the thin fraction of remaining arterial wall is densely adherent to its surroundings, which are often highly vascular from collaterals and easily damaged. By-passing is always preferable, though it is often better to do nothing.

Failure of the graft structure, or of suture material is uncommon but when it does occur, it mostly affects situations of high mechanical stress such as the upper aortic suture line or the groin anastomosis [129]. Ivalon and woven teflon grafts, impervious to fibrous invasion tend eventually to separate and a false aneurysm forms (Fig. 3.69). Late infection is always possible with an implanted foreign body

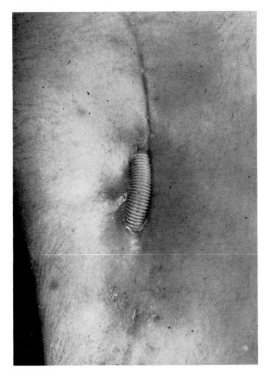

Sepsis not involving an anastomosis does not readily travel along a graft, hence the same anastomosis sites may be used when re-grafting along a fresh course when only the middle portion of the graft lies in the infected zone.

A note on sexual function in men following aorto-iliac surgery. (Fig. 3.80)

Part of the disability in high aorto-iliac occlusion is impotence from failure of erection. Hopes may be raised of a return to normal after operation and indeed it often is so. Yet defects are still likely [104A]; either from stagnant thrombosis of the by-passed, diseased internal iliacs, with continued failure of blood supply to the corpora cavernosum; or, with endarterectomy in particular, a loss of ejaculation due to division of the presacral sympathetic nerves as they cross the aortic bifurcation. Otherwise the sexual act is normal. Impairment is common after any major operation in older men, but these may recover. The aorto-iliac difficulties described tend, however, to persist.

Fig. 3.79. Extrusion of an infected teflon graft through the scar on the patient's thigh. This graft had thrombosed, but cases are described in which it presented still pulsating [117].

(Fig. 3.79) but the problem posed is less acute than with early infection, and there have even been instances [117] in which the exposed, pulsating fabric graft, was obviously lying in chronically infected granulation tissues, yet these eventually closed over the graft, either spontaneously or, more often, with the help of surgically mobilised soft tissue cover, and antibiotics.

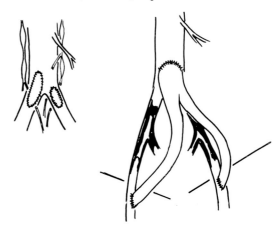

Fig. 3.80. Mechanisms of sexual impairment after aorto iliac reconstruction.

Results of Reconstruction for Chronic Ischaemia

Hospital Mortality. This is now between 0 and 1 per cent according to the operative site (Table 3.4).

Late Mortality. Nothing in the operative procedure could be expected to improve the outlook for life, except perhaps the capacity for a more active existence, and willingness, after major surgery, to accept the need to give up smoking and to follow advice on dietary restriction. Operative mortality over all types of cases now stands at 4 per cent [46]. Survivors might have a shorter time to live if the operative ordeal were severe, though there is no evidence to suggest this. Table 3.5 shows the late mortality in 440 of the author's series of surgically treated cases of chronic ischaemia, all of whom received a reconstructive operation. The cardiovascular mortality of the aorto-iliac group was slightly higher than the femoro-popliteal, though the latter were on the average five years older, which agrees with the Mayo Clinic findings in 520 patients not treated by reconstruction [81].

Table 3.4. Mortality of Reconstruction of Occluded Lower Limb Arteries

	(1951–68) Whole series		Last 100 cases
F/P	2·1%	(5/240)	0%
	*1° haemorrhage	1	
	*2° haemorrhage	1	
	Anuria	1	
	Staph. enteritis	1	
	Amputation	1	
A/I	4·0%	(10/250)	1%
	Anuria	3	
	Coronary infarction	2	
	Haemorrhage {(1°)	1	
	{(2°)	2	
	Colon necrosis	1	
	Senility	1	

* 1° hge from heparin or other primary clotting defect.
2° hge from oral anti-coagulant and staph. infection.

Table 3.5. Late Mortality in 440 Patients 1–16 years following Arterial Reconstruction for Lower Limb Ischaemia

Aorto-iliac 22/212 (average age at operation: 57)		Femoro-popliteal 20/228 (average age at operation: 62)	
Cardiac causes	18	Cardiac causes	15
Stroke	3	Malignant disease	4
Malignant disease	3	By violence	2
Chronic bronchitis	1	Stroke	1
Opposite side sympathectomy	1	Old age	1

Annual cardiovascular mortality 4·3 per cent; comparable with most untreated series.

RECURRENT OCCLUSION (Tables 3.6 and 3.7)

With no means yet of controlling occlusive disease, it is not surprising that reconstructed segments, after prolonged patency and normal function, eventually show recurring obliterative changes, though not necessarily any sooner than other arteries in the same patient. Figure 3.67 shows a femoro-popliteal (frozen stored) homograft, eight years after implantation, severely affected by occlusive

Table 3.6. Results of 212 Initially Successful Operations for Aorto-iliac Occlusive Disease (1–16 Years)

Late deaths (several patent)	22
Late patency	138/190

i.e. an overall patency rate of 72 per cent for an average of 4·1 years (including 10 over 10 years)

Table 3.7. Late Results of 173 Initially Successful Operations for Femoro-popliteal Occlusion

Operated for claudication: 52/116 patent for an average of 3 years.
Operated for severe ischaemia: 24/57 patent for an average of 3 years.
i.e. an overall patency rate of 44 per cent at an average period of three years.

arteriosclerosis. Vein grafts also show these later changes [4, 51].

Occlusion six months to two years after operation is common, particularly with cloth prostheses, and more so when part or the whole of the graft lies distal to the groin. All case series agree upon this. Closure at this stage may be due to a thrombotic tendency of the patient [53] plus factors relating to the suitability of the graft [149], and other technical aspects such as suture material and tension.

Conclusions

Though figures from the published series do not lend themselves to statistical comparison, trends have emerged that should guide future work.

1. *Aorto-iliac reconstruction* for occlusive disease gives good results over the first seven years, equally so for prosthetic by-pass or thrombo-endarterectomy [131, 132]; 80 per cent would be a representative figure. Fifteen- to twenty-year patencies are confirmed (Figs. 3.81 and 3.82).

2. *Femoro-popliteal reconstruction* gives generally poorer results (Table 3.7). First-year failures are so common with all types of plastic cloth prostheses that most surgeons have given them up. However, the late results of methods employing autogenous tissue, i.e. thrombo-endarterectomy and also autogenous vein by-pass grafting, are much better, even after allowing for a generally somewhat high initial failure rate, especially with the latter method.

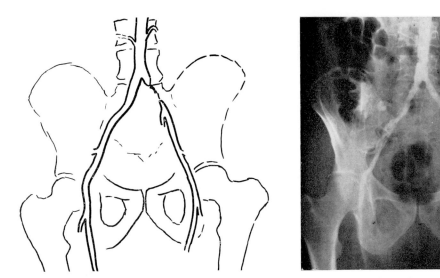

Fig. 3.81. A twenty-year patency following common iliac thrombo-endarterectomy.

Left. The patient whose aortogram this drawing represents was a retired naval commander aged forty-seven at the time of his operation in 1952.

Right. Lumbar aortogram eight years later for a recurrence of pain, subsequently diagnosed as sciatica. All pulses have remained palpable since.

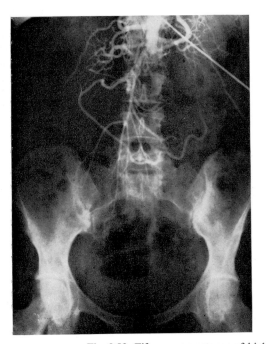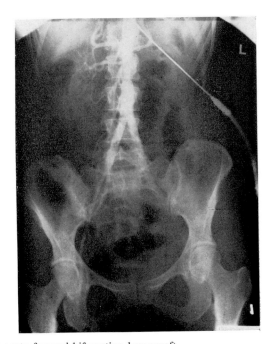

Fig. 3.82. Fifteen-year patency of high aorto-femoral bifurcation homograft.

(*a*) Juxta-renal occlusion in a woman of 40 requiring mobilisation and clamping of superior mesenteric and both renal arteries under hypothermia, in January 1954.

(*b*) Early postoperative patency of frozen aortic homograft.

This patient was seen in 1968. All her lower limb pulses were fully patent and free from murmurs or sign of aneurysm formation.

The Contribution of Arterial Reconstruction to Limb Salvage

Really worthwhile results can be obtained in patients with advanced ischaemia in whom the only alternative is amputation. Of 304 severely ischaemic limbs seen at St Bartholomew's Hospital in 10 years, only 74 had amputation as their first treatment; 230 were grafted. At the end of the first year three-quarters of all patients, whether aorto-iliac or femoro-popliteal, had kept their affected limb, though actual patency in the latter group was only 59 per cent. Even at 5 years a half of all patients still enjoyed a useful limb [5A]. The same approximate figures apply to other series, both of femoro-popliteal

vein grafts in Britain and the U.S.A. [1, 34A], and of aorto-iliac restorations of several types at the Mayo Clinic [64A]. Late deaths, almost all from cardiovascular disease, ended the follow-up in 13 per cent and 21 per cent respectively.

Even in the aged there is much to be said for an attempt at a femoro-popliteal graft. Of 54 such patients whose average age was 74·5 years, mostly with end-stage ischaemia and an early prospect of amputation, operative mortality was 9 per cent compared with 25 per cent of the amputed group, and limb salvage at two years was 22 per cent. By that time 25 per cent of the operative survivors had died, many with the limb intact [125A].

REFERENCES

1. Baddeley, R. M., Ashton, F., Slaney, G. and Barnes, A. D. (1970) Late results of autogenous vein by-pass grafts in femoro-popliteal arterial occlusion. *Brit. med. J.*, **1**, 653.

1A. Barcroft, H. and Millen, J. L. E. (1939) The blood flow through muscle during sustained contraction. *J. Physiol.*, **97**, 17.

2. Barcroft, H. and Dornhorst, A. C. (1949) The blood flow through the human calf during rhythmic exercise. *J. Physiol.*, **109**, 402.

3. Barner, H. B., DeWeese, J. A., Dale, W. A. and Mahoney, E. B. (1966) Aneurysmal degeneration of femoropopliteal arterial homografts. *J. Amer. Med. Assoc.*, **196**, 631.

4. Beales, J. S. M., Adcock, F. M., Frawley, J. S., McLachlan, M. S. F., Martin, P. and Steiner, R. E. (1971) The radiological assessment of disease of the profunda femoris artery. *Brit. J. Radiol.*, **44**, 854.

5. Bellman, S. Pernow, B. and Zetterquist, S. (1962) Effects of arterial reconstruction in arteriosclerosis obliterans evaluated on a metabolic basis. *Acta. chir. Scand.*, **124**, 54.

5A. Birnstingl, M. and Taylor, G. W. (1970) Results of reconstructive surgery in severe ischaemia. *J. Cardiovasc. Surg.*, **11**, 447.

6. Blau, J. N. and Logue, V. (1961) Intermittent claudication of the cauda equina. *Lancet*, **i**, 1081.

7. Blaisdell, F. W. and Hall, A. D. (1963) Axillary-femoral artery bypass for lower extremity ischemia. *Surgery*, **54**, 563.

8. Bliss, B. P., Rhodes, J. and Rains, A. J. H. (1963) Cystic myxomatous degeneration of the popliteal artery. *Brit. med. J.*, **ii**, 847.

9. Bloor, K. (1961) Natural history of arteriosclerosis of the lower extremities. *Ann. Roy. Coll. Surg.*, **28**, 36.

10. Bouley, (1831) Claudication intermittente des membres postérieurs, déterminée par l'oblitération des artères fémorales. *Recueil de méd. vétér.*, **8**, 517.

11. Boyd, A. M., Ratcliffe, A. H., Jepson, R. P. and James, G. W. H. (1949) Intermittent claudication: clinical study. *J. Bone Jt. Surg.*, **31B**, 325.

12. Boyd, A. M. and Bloor, K. (1960) Results of tenotomy of the tendo achillis in intermittent claudication. *Brit. med. J.*, **i**, 548.

13. Brodie, B. C. (1846) *Lectures Illustrative of Various Subjects in Pathology and Surgery*. London: Longman, p. 360.

14. Buchwald, H. and Varco, R. L. (1967) Partial ileal by-pass for hypercholesterolemia and atherosclerosis. *Surg. Gynec. Obstet.*, **124**, 1231.

15. Calem, W. S. and LeVeen, H. H. (1962) Arterial thrombosis complicating inferior vena cava ligation. *Surgery*, **52**, 613.

16. Cannon, J. A. and Barker, W. F. (1955) Successful management of obstructive femoral arteriosclerosis by endarterectomy. *Surgery*, **38**, 48.

17. Cappelen, C. and Hall, K. V. (1964) The great saphenous vein used *in situ* as an arterial shunt after vein valve extirpation. An evaluation of its properties of conducting blood by the use of an electromagnetic square wave flowmeter. *Acta chir. Scand.*, **128**, 517.

17A. Cappelen, C. and Hall, K. V. (1967) Electromagnetic flowmetry in clinical surgery. *Acta chir. Scand. Suppl.*, **368**, 3.

18. Carter, A. E. and Eban, R. (1964) A case of bilateral developmental abnormality of the popliteal arteries and gastrocnemius muscles. *Brit. J. Surg.*, **51**, 518.

18A. Carter, S. A. and Lezack, J. D. (1971) Digital systolic pressures in the lower limb in arterial disease. *Circulation*, **43**, 905.

19. Carter, S. C., Cohen, A. and Whelan, T. J. (1963) Clinical experience with management of the infected dacron graft. *Ann. Surg.*, **158**, 249.

20. Cockett, F. B. and Maurice, B. A. (1963) Evolution of direct arterial surgery for claudication and ischaemia of legs. *Brit. med. J.*, **i**, 353.

21. Connolly, J. E. and Stemmer, E. A. (1970) The non-reversed saphenous vein by-pass for femoro-popliteal occlusive disease. *Surgery*, **68**, 602.

22. Crane, C. (1967) Atherothrombotic embolism to lower extremities in arteriosclerosis, *Arch. Surg.*, **94**, 96.

23. Cranley, J. J., Fogarty, T. J., Krause, R. J., Strasser, E. S. and Hafner, C. D. (1963) Phlebotomy for moderate erythrocythemia. Improvement in peripheral circulation and myocardial function in patients with obliterative arterial disease of the lower extremities. *J. Amer. Med. Assoc.*, **186**, 206.

24. Crawford, E. S., DeBakey, M. E., Morris, G. C. and Garrett, E. (1960) Evaluation of late failures after reconstructive operations for occlusive lesions of the aorta and iliac, femoral, and popliteal arteries. *Surgery*, **47**, 79.

24A. Dahn, I., Hallböök, T., Larsen, O. A., Nilsen, R. and Westling, H. (1969) Treatment of acute ischaemic pain in the leg by induced hypertension. *Acta chir. Scand.*, **135**, 391.

25. Dale, W. A. (1963) Grafting small arteries: experience with nineteen shunts below the knee. *Arch. Surg.*, **86**, 22.

26. Dale, W. A. (1966) Chronic ilio-femoral venous occlusion including seven cases of cross-over vein grafting. *Surgery*, **59**, 117.

27. Dale, W. A. (1966) Autogenous vein grafts for femoropopliteal arterial repair. *Surg. Gynec. Obstet.*, **123**, 1282.

28. Darling, R. C. and Linton, R. R. (1964) Management of the late failure of arterial reconstruction of the lower extremities. *New Eng. J. Med.*, **270**, 609.

29. Darling, R. C., Linton, R. R. and Razzuk, M. A. (1967) Saphenous vein bypass grafts in femoro-popliteal occlusive disease: a reappraisal. *Surgery*, **61**, 31.

30. DeBakey, M. E. (1963) Basic concepts of therapy in arterial disease. *J. Amer. Med. Assoc.*, **186**, 484.

30A. Deithrich, E. B., Noon, G. P., Liddicoat, J. E. and DeBakey, M. E. (1970) Treatment of the infected aorto-femoral arterial prosthesis. *Surgery*, **68**, 1044.

30B. Deterling, R. A. and Clauss, R. H. (1970) Long term fate of aortic and arterial homografts. *J. Cardiovasc. Surg.*, **11**, 35.

31. DeWeese, J. A., Woods, W. D. and Dale, W. A. (1959) Failures of homografts as arterial replacements. *Surgery*, **46**, 565.

32. DeWeese, J. A. (1962) Early failures in arterial reconstruction. *Arch. Surg.*, **85**, 901.

33. DeWeese, J. A., Dale, W. A., Mahoney, E. B. and Rob, C. G. (1963) Thromboendarterectomies and autogenous venous by-pass grafts distal to the inguinal ligament. *Circulation*, **34**, Supp. 171.

34. DeWeese, J. A., Terry, R., Barner, H. B. and Rob, C. G. (1966) Autogenous venous femoropopliteal bypass grafts. *Surgery*, **59**, 28.

34A. DeWeese, J. A. and Rob, C. G. (1971) Autogenous venous by-pass grafts five years later. *Ann. Surg.*, **174**, 346.

35. Dible, J. H. (1964) The ageing and collateral peripheral artery. *Lancet*, **i**, 520.

36. Dible, J. H. (1966) *The Pathology of Limb Ischaemia*. Edinburgh and London: Oliver and Boyd.

37. dos Santos, J. C. (1947) Sur la désobstruction des thromboses artérielles anciennes. *Mém. Acad. Chir.*, **73**, 409.

38. Dotter, C. T. and Judkins, M. P. (1965) Percutaneous transluminal treatment of arteriosclerotic obstruction. *Radiol.*, **84**, 631.

39. Dotter, C. T., Rösch, J. and Judkins, M. P. (1968) Transluminal dilatation of atherosclerotic stenosis. *Surg. Gynec. Obstet.*, **127**, 794.

40. Dow, J. and Hardwick, C. (1966) Transluminal arterial recanalisation. *Lancet*, **i**, 73.

41. Dumanian, A. V., Frahm, C. J., Benchik, F. A. and Wooden, T. F. (1965) Intermittent claudication secondary to congenital absence of iliac arteries. *Arch. Surg.*, **91**, 604.

41A. Dundas, P. (1970) The 'in-situ' vein by-pass. *J. Cardiovasc. Surg.*, **11**, 450.

41B. Eames, R. and Lange, L. (1967) Ischaemic neuropathy. *J. Neurol. Neurosurg. Psychiat.*, **30**, 215.

42. Eastcott, H. H. G. (1953) Arterial grafting for the ischaemic lower limb. *Ann. Roy. Coll. Surg. Eng.*, **13**, 177.

43. Eastcott, H. H. G. (1961) 'The storage of tissues for grafting'. *Surgical Progress*. London: Butterworth's, p. 332.

44. Eastcott, H. H. G. (1962) Obstruction of the lower limb arteries: chronic ischaemia. *Proc. Roy. Soc. Med.*, **55**, 596.

45. Eastcott, H. H. G. (1962) Rarity of lower-limb ischaemia in non-smokers. *Lancet*, **ii**, 1117.

45A. Eastcott, H. H. G. (1963) Cystic myxomatous degeneration of the popliteal artery. *Brit. med. J.*, **2**, 1270.

46. Eastcott, H. H. G. (1967) Experience of vascular surgery with special regard to late results. *Scand. J. Clin. Lab. Invest. Suppl.*, **99**, 172.

47. Edwards, E. A. (1959) Postamputation radiographic evidence for small artery obstruction in arteriosclerosis. *Ann. Surg.*, **150**, 177.

48. Edwards, W. S. (1960) Late occlusion of femoral and popliteal fabric arterial grafts. *Surg. Gynec. Obstet.*, **110**, 714.

49. Edwards, W. S. (1960) Composite reconstruction of the femoral artery with saphenous venous after endarterectomy. *Surg. Gynec. Obstet.*, **111**, 651.

50. Edwards, W. S., Holdefer, W. F. and Mohtashemi, M. (1966) The importance of proper calibre of lumen in femoro-popliteal artery reconstruction. *Surg. Gynec. Obstet.*, **122**, 37.

51. Ejrup, B., Hiertonn, T. and Moberg, A. (1961) Atheromatous changes in autogenous vein grafts. Functional and anatomical aspects. Case report. *Acta. chir. Scand.*, **121**, 211.

52. Ericsson, B., Haeger, K. and Lindell, S. E. (1970) Effect of physical training on intermittent claudication. *Angiology*, **21**, 188.

53. Evans, G. and Irvine, W. T. (1966) Long-term arterial-graft patency in relation to platelet adhesiveness, biochemical factors, and anticoagulant therapy. *Lancet*, **ii**, 353.

54. Evans, J. G. (1964) Neurogenic intermittent claudication. *Brit. med. J.*, **ii**, 985.

55. Fogarty, T. J., Cranley, J. J., Krause, R. J., Strasser, E. S. and Hafner, C. D. (1963) Surgical management of phlegmasia cerulea dolens. *Arch. Surg.*, **86**, 256.

56. Folse, R. (1965) Alterations in femoral blood flow and resistance during rhythmic exercise and sustained muscular contractions in patients with arteriosclerosis. *Surg. Gynec. Obstet.*, **121**, 767.

57. Foster, J. H., Collins, H. A., Jacobs, J. K. and Scott, H. W. (1965) Long term follow-up of homografts used in the treatment of coarctation of the aorta. *J. Cardiovasc. Surg.*, **6**, 111.

58. Freeman, N. E. and Leeds, F. H. (1953) Resection of aneurysms of the abdominal aorta with anastomosis of the splenic to the left iliac artery. *Surgery*, **34**, 1021.

59. Galpin, O. P. and O'Brien, P. K. (1964) Prolongation of tendon reflexes in ischaemia. *Lancet*, **i**, 209.

60. Gaskell, P. (1956) The rate of blood flow in the foot and the calf before and after reconstruction by arterial grafting of an occluded main artery to the lower limb. *Clin. Sci.*, **15**, 259.

61. Gensler, S. W., Haimovici, H., Hoffert, P., Steinman, C. and Beneventano, T. C. (1965) Study of vascular lesions in diabetic, nondiabetic patients. *Arch. Surg.*, **91**, 617.

62. Gillespie, J. A. (1959) The case against vasodilator drugs in occlusive vascular disease of the legs. *Lancet*, **ii**, 995.

63. Gillespie, J. A. and Douglas, D. M. (1961) *Some Aspects of Obliterative Vascular Disease of the Lower Limb*. Edinburgh and London: E. & S. Livingstone.

64. Gillespie, J. A. (1967) Vasodilator properties of alcohol. *Brit. med. J.*, **ii**, 274.

64A. Gomes, M. R., Bernatz, P. E. and Juergens, J. L. (1967) Aorto-iliac surgery. *Arch. Surg.*, **95**, 387.

65. Gorman, J. F., Stansell, G. B. and Douglass, F. M. (1965) Limitations of hyperbaric oxygenation in occlusive arterial disease. *Circulation*, **32**, 936.

65A. Gosling, R. G., Newman, D. L., Bowden, N. L. R. and Twinn, K. W. (1971) The area ratio of normal aortic junctions. Aortic configuration and pulse-wave reflections. *Brit. J. Radiol.*, **44**, 850.

66. Gross, R. E., Bill, A. H. and Peirce, E. C. (1949) Methods for preservation and transplantation of arterial grafts. *Surg. Gynec. Obstet.*, **88**, 689.

66A. Gundersen, J. (1971) Diagnosis of arterial insufficiency with measurement of blood pressures in fingers and toes. *Angiology*, **22**, 191.

66B. Haid, S. P., Conn, J. and Bergan, J. J. (1971) Cystic adventitial disease of the popliteal artery. *Arch. Surg.*, **101**, 765.

67. Haimovici, H., Steinman, C. and Caplan, L. H. (1966) Role of arteriovenous anastomoses in vascular diseases of the lower extremity. *Ann. Surg.*, **164**, 990.

68. Haimovici, H. and Steinman, C. (1969) Aorto-iliac angiographic patterns associated with femoro-popliteal occlusive disease: significance in reconstructive arterial surgery. *Surgery*, **65**, 232.

69. Hall, K. V. (1964) The great saphenous vein used *in situ* as an arterial shunt after vein valve extirpation. The method and the immediate results. *Acta chir. Scand.*, **128**, 365.

70. Hall, K. V. (1965) The great saphenous vein used *in situ* as an arterial shunt after vein valve extirpation. A follow-up study. *Acta chir. Scand.*, **129**, 33.

71. Hamilton, M. and Wilson, G. M. (1952) The treatment of intermittent claudication. *Quart. J. Med.*, **21**, 169.

72. Hamming, J. J. and Vink, M. (1965) Obstruction of the popliteal artery at an early age. *J. Cardiovasc. Surg.*, **6**, 516.

73. Hampton, J. R., Harrison, M. J. G. Honour, A. J. and Mitchell, J. R. A. (1967) Platelet behaviour and drugs used in cardiovascular disease. *Cardiovasc. Res.*, **1**, 101.

74. Hanks, J. H. and Wallace, R. E. (1949) Relation of oxygen and temperature in the preservation of tissues by refrigeration. *Proc. Soc. Exp. Biol. Med.*, **71**, 196.

75. Henry, A. K. (1957) *Extensile exposure*. Edinburgh and London: E. & S. Livingstone (2nd ed.), p. 214.

76. Hiertonn, T. (1960) Reconstruction surgery in peripheral arterial occlusion. *Acta chir. Scand.*, **119**, 129.

77. Hufnagel, C. A. (1954) Experimental and clinical observations on the transplantation of blood vessels. In: *Preservation and Transplantation of Normal Tissues*. A Ciba Foundation Symposium. (Ed. Wolstenholme, G. E. W. and Cameron, M. P.) London: J. & A. Churchill, p. 196.

78. Humphries, A. W., Young, J. R., deWolfe, V. G., LeFevre, F. A. and Beven, E. G. (1963) Severe ischemia of lower extremity due to arteriosclerosis obliterans. *Arch. Surg.*, **87**, 175.

79. Husni, E. A. (1967) The Edema of arterial reconstruction. *Circulation*, **35**, Supp. I–169.

79A. Husni, E. A. and Manion, W. C. (1967) Atrophy of the arterial wall incident to localised chronic hypotension. *Surgery*, **61**, 611.

80. Irvine, W. T., Kenyon, J. R. and Stiles, P. J. (1963) Early results in ninety-five patients undergoing femoro-popliteal by-pass graft. *Brit. med. J.*, **i**, 360.

80A. Jones, R. A. C. and Thomson, J. L. G. (1968) The narrow lumbar canal. *J. Bone Jt. Surg.*, **50B**, 595.

81. Juergens, J. L., Barker, N. W. and Hines, E. A. (1960) Arteriosclerosis obliterans; review of 520 cases with special reference to pathogenic and prognostic factors. *Circulation*, **21**, 188.

81A. Kakkar, V. V. (1969) The cephalic vein as a peripheral vascular graft. *Surg. Gynec. Obstet.*, **128**, 551.

81B. Kakkar, V. V., Field, E. S., Nicolaides, A. N., Flute, P. T., Wessler, S. and Yin, E. T. (1971) Low doses of heparin in prevention of deep vein thrombosis. *Lancet*, **ii**, 669.

81C. Kane, S. P. and Gillespie, J. A. (1970) Induced hypertension in the treatment of the ischaemic foot. *Ann. Roy. Coll. Surg. Eng.*, **47**, 287.

81D. Kavanaugh, G. J., Svien, H. J., Holman, C. B. and Johnson, R. M. (1968) 'Pseudoclaudication' syndrome produced by compression of the cauda equina. *J. Amer. med. Ass.*, **206**, 2477.

82. Köhler, R. and Viljanen, V. (1964) Angiographically demonstrated arteriovenous shunting in circulatory obstructions in the lower extremities. *Acta Radiologica Diagnosis*, **2**, 473.

83. Knox, W. G. (1962) Aneurysm occurring in a femoral artery dacron prosthesis five and one half years after insertion. *Ann. Surg.*, **156**, 827.

84. Knox, W. G., Finby, N. and Moscarella, A. A. (1965) Limitations of arteriography in determining operability for femoropopliteal occlusive disease. *Ann. Surg.*, **161**, 509.

85. Kountz, S. L. and Cohn, R. (1963) Aortic blood flow following lower aortic resection and sympathectomy. *Surgery*, **53**, 173.

86. Kunlin, J. (1951) Le traitement de l'ischaemia artéritique par la graffe veineuse longue. *Rev. Chir. Orthop.*, **70**, 206.

86A. Lallemand, R. C., Brown, K. G. E. and Boulter, P. S. (1972) Vessel dimensions in premature atheromatous disease of aortic bifurcation. *Brit. med. J.*, **2**, 255.

87. Larsen, O. A. and Lassen, N. A. (1966) Effect of daily muscular exercise in patients with intermittent claudication. *Lancet*, **ii**, 1093.

88. Leeds, F. H. and Gilfillan, R. S. (1961) Importance of profunda femoris artery in the revascularization of the ischemic limb. *Arch. Surg.*, **82**, 25.

89. LeFevre, F. A., Corbacioglu, C., Humphries, A. W. and DeWolfe, V. G. (1959) Management of arteriosclerosis obliterans of the extremities. *J. Amer. Med. Assoc.*, **170**, 656.

90. Leriche, R. and Morel, A. (1948) The syndrome of thrombotic obliteration of the aortic bifurcation. *Ann. Surg.*, **127**, 193.

91. Lewis, C. D. (1961) A subclavian artery as the means of blood-supply to the lower half of the body. *Brit. J. Surg.*, **48**, 574.

92. Lewis, G. J. T., Douglas, D. M., Reid, W. and Watt, J. K. (1967) Cystic adventitial disease of the popliteal artery. *Brit. med. J.*, **iii**, 411.

93. Lewis, T., Pickering, G. W. and Rothschild, P. (1931) Observations upon muscular pain in intermittent claudication. *Heart*, **15**, 359.

94. Linton, R. R. and Darling, R. C. (1962) Autogenous saphenous vein bypass grafts in femoropopliteal obliterative arterial disease. *Surgery*, **51**, 62.

94A. Linton, R. R. and Wilde, W. L. (1970) Modifications in the technique for femoro-popliteal saphenous by-pass autografts. *Surgery*, **67**, 234.

95. Louw, J. H. (1963) Splenic-to-femoral and axillary-to-femoral bypass grafts in diffuse atherosclerotic occlusive disease. *Lancet*, **i**, 1401.

96. Love, J. W. and Whelan, T. J. (1965) Popliteal artery entrapment syndrome. *Amer. J. Surg.*, **109**, 620.

97. Ludbrook, J., Clarke, A. M. and McKenzie, J. K. (1962) Significance of absent ankle pulse. *Brit. med. J.*, **i**, 1724.

98. Madejski, T. and Tobik, S. (1964) Arteriographic errors in occlusive diseases of lower limbs. *Surgery*, **55**, 210.

99. Mannick, J. A. and Hume, D. M. (1964) Salvage of extremities by vein grafts in far-advanced peripheral vascular disease. *Surgery*, **55**, 154.

100. Mannick, J. A. and Jackson, B. T. (1966) Hemodynamics of arterial surgery in atherosclerotic limbs. I. Direct measurement of blood flow before and after vein grafts. *Surgery*, **59**, 713.

100A. Mannick, J. A. (1971) Are there practical alternatives to aorto-iliac reconstruction? *Amer. J. Surg.*, **122**, 344.

101. Marston, A. and Cockett, F. B. (1962) Total gastrocnemius and soleus denervation in the treatment of intermittent claudication. *Lancet*, **i**, 238.

102. McCabe, M., Cunningham, G. J., Wyatt, A. P. and Taylor, G. W. (1965) Vein grafts. Changes in phospholipid structure due to storage in saline solution. *Lancet*, **ii**, 109.

103. McCaughan, J. J. and Kahn, S. F. (1960) Crossover graft for unilateral occlusive disease of the iliofemoral arteries. *Ann. Surg.*, **151**, 26.

104. May, A. G., DeWeese, J. A. and Rob, C. G. (1965) Arterialized *in situ* saphenous vein. *Arch. Surg.*, **91**, 743.

104A. May, A. G., DeWeese, J. A. and Rob, C. G. (1969) Changes in sexual function following operation on the abdominal aorta. *Surgery*, **65**, 41.

105. Meade, J. W., Linton, R. R., Darling, R. C. and Menendez, C. V. (1966) Arterial homografts. A long-term clinical follow-up. *Arch. Surg.*, **93**, 392.

106. Mentha, C. (1965) Dégénérescence kystique adventitielle ou bursite de l'artère poplitée. *J. Chir. (Paris)*, **89**, 173.

106A. Moore, W. S., Hall, A. D. and Blaisdell, F. W. (1971) Late results of axillo-femoral by-pass grafting. *Amer. J. Surg.*, **122**, 148.

107. Morris, G. C., Edwards, W., Cooley, D. A., Crawford, E. S. and DeBakey, M. E. (1961) Surgical importance of profunda femoris artery: analysis of 102 cases with combined aortoiliac and femoropopliteal occlusive disease treated by revascularization of deep femoral artery. *Arch. Surg.*, **82**, 32.

108. Myers, K. A. and Irvine, W. T. (1966) An objective study of lumbar sympathectomy. 1. Intermittent claudication. *Brit. med. J.*, **i**, 879.

109. Nunn, D. B., Chun, B., Whelan, T. J. and Martins, A. N. (1964) Autogenous veins as arterial substitutes. A study of their histologic fate with special attention to endothelium. *Ann. Surg.*, **160**, 14.

110. Owen, K. and Rob, C. G. (1956) Technique for by-pass operations in femoral arterial disease. *Brit. med. J.*, **ii**, 273.

110A. Parsonnet, V., Alpert, J. and Brief, D. K. (1970) Femoro-femoral and axillo-femoral grafts—compromise or preference. *Surgery*, **67**, 26.

110B. Perdue, G. D. and Smith, R. B. (1969) Atheromatous microemboli. *Ann. Surg.*, **169**, 594.

111. Platt, H. (1930) Occlusion of the axillary artery due to pressure by a crutch. *Arch. Surg.*, **20**, 314.

111A. Pollock, A. V. and Jackson, D. W. (1970) Calf

denervation in the treatment of intermittent claudication. *Brit. J. Surg.*, **57**, 344.

111B. Powis, S. J. A., Skilton, J. S., Ashton, F. and Slaney, G. (1971) Place of Achilles tenotomy in the treatment of severe intermittent claudication. *Brit. med. J.*, **3**, 522.

112. Renwick, S., Royle, J. P. and Martin, P. (1968) Operative angiography after femoro-popliteal arterial reconstruction—its influence on early failure rate. *Brit. J. Surg.*, **55**, 134.

112A. Rosengarten, D. S., Knight, B. and Martin, P. (1971) An approach for operations upon the iliac arteries. *Brit. J. Surg.*, **58**, 365.

113. Salzman, E. W. (1965) The limitations of heparin therapy after arterial reconstruction. *Surgery*, **57**, 131.

114. Sauvage, L. R. and Wood, S. J. (1966) Unilateral axillary bilateral femoral bifurcation graft. A procedure for the poor risk patient with aorto-iliac disease. *Surgery*, **60**, 573.

115. Sawyer, P. N., Kaplitt, M. J., Sobel, S. and DiMaio, D. (1967) Application of gas endarterectomy to atherosclerotic peripheral vessels and coronary arteries: clinical and experimental results. *Circulation*, **35**, Supp. I., 163.

116. Schadt, D. C., Hines, E. A., Juergens, J. L. and Barker, N. W. (1961) Chronic atherosclerotic occlusion of the femoral artery. *J. Amer. Med. Assoc.*, **175**, 937.

117. Schramel, R. J. and Creech, O. (1959) Effects of infection and exposure on synthetic arterial prostheses. *Arch. Surg.*, **78**, 271.

118. Selvaag, O., Myren, J., Thorsen, R. K. and Bjørnstad, P. (1960) Progressive tendency of arteriosclerosis obliterans of the lower extremities. *Acta chir. Scand. Supp.*, **253**, 187.

119. Selvaag, O. (1962) Long-term anticoagulant treatment in atherosclerosis obliterans of the lower extremities. *J. Oslo City Hosp.*, **12**, 89.

120. Servello, M. (1962) Clinical syndrome of anomalous position of the popliteal artery. *Circulation*, **26**, 885.

121. Shaw, R. S. and Baue, A. E. (1963) Management of sepsis complicating arterial reconstructive surgery. *Surgery*, **53**, 75.

122. Shepherd, J. T. (1950) The blood flow through the calf after exercise in subjects with arteriosclerosis and claudication. *Clin. Sci.*, **9**, 49.

123. Simeone, F. A. and Husni, E. A. (1959) The Hyperemia of reconstructive arterial surgery. *Ann. Surg.*, **150**, 575.

124. Singer, A. (1963) Segmental distribution of peripheral atherosclerosis. *Arch. Surg.*, **87**, 384.

125. Snell, E. S., Eastcott, H. H. G. and Hamilton, M. (1960) Circulation in lower limb before and after reconstruction of obstructed main artery. *Lancet*, **i**, 242.

125A. Sogocio, R. M. and Gorman, J. F. (1971) Femoro-popliteal reconstruction in the aging. *Arch. Surg.*, **103**, 345.

126. Starer, F. and Sutton, D. (1960) Aortic occlusion (Leriche's Syndrome) in mitral stenosis. Report of six cases. *Brit. med. J.*, **ii**, 644.

127. Starzl, T. E. and Trippel, O. H. (1959) Reno-mesentero-aorto-iliac thromboendarterectomy in patient with malignant hypertension. *Surgery*, **46**, 556.

128. Stokes, J. M., Sugg, W. L. and Butcher, H. R. (1963) Standard method of assessing relative effectiveness of therapies for arterial occlusive diseases. *Ann. Surg.*, **157**, 343.

129. Stoney, R. J., Albo, R. J. and Wylie, E. J. (1965) False aneurysms occurring after arterial grafting operations. *Amer. J. Surg.*, **110**, 153.

129A. Strandness, J. R., Schultz, R. D., Sumner, D. S. and Rushmer, R. F. (1967) Ultrasonic flow detection. *Amer. J. Surg.*, **113**, 311.

130. Sutton, D. (1962) *Arteriography*. Edinburgh and London: E. & S. Livingstone.

131. Szilagyi, D. E., Smith, R. F., Elliott, J. P. and Allen, H. M. (1965) Long-term behavior of a dacron arterial substitute. Clinical, roentgenologic, and histologic correlations. *Ann. Surg.*, **162**, 453.

132. Szilagyi, D. E., Smith, R. F. and Whitney, D. G. (1964) The durability of aorto-iliac endarterectomy; a roentgenologic and pathologic study of late recurrence. *Arch. Surg.*, **89**, 827.

132A. Szilagyi, D. E., Rodriguez, F. J., Smith, R. F. and Elliot, J. P. (1970) Late failure of arterial allografts. Observations 6 to 15 years after implantation. *Arch. Surg.*, **101**, 721.

133. Tarizzo, R. A., Alexander, R. W., Beattie, E. J. and Economou, S. G. (1961) Atherosclerosis in synthetic vascular grafts. *Arch. Surg.*, **82**, 826.

134. Taylor, G. W. (1962) Arterial grafting for gangrene. *Ann. Roy. Coll. Surg.*, **31**, 168.

135. Taylor, G. W. and Calo, A. R. (1962) Atherosclerosis of arteries of the lower limbs. *Brit. med. J.*, **i**, 507.

136. Taylor, G. W. (1966) Personal communication.

136A. Terry, H. J., Allan, J. S. and Taylor, G. W. (1972) The relationship between blood-flow and failure of femoro-popliteal reconstructive arterial surgery. *Brit. J. Surg.*, **59**, 549.

137. Texon, M., Imparato, A. M. and Lord, J. W. (1960) The hemodynamic concept of atherosclerosis. *Arch. Surg.*, **80**, 47.

138. Thurlbeck, W. M. and Castleman, B. (1957) Atheromatous emboli to the kidneys after aortic surgery. *New Eng. J. Med.*, **257**, 442.

139. Tillgren, C. (1965) Obliterative arterial disease of the lower limbs iii: Prognostic influence of concomitant coronary heart disease. *Acta. Med. Scand.*, **178**, 121.

140. Todd, A. S. (1959) The histological localisation of fibrinolysin activator. *J. Path. Bact.*, **78**, 281.

140A. Trippel, O. H., Jurayj, M. N. and Midell, A. I. (1972) The aorto-iliac steal: a review of this syndrome and a report of one additional case. *Ann. Surg.*, **175**, 454.

141. Vaughan, B. F., Slavotinek, A. H. and Jepson, R. P. (1970) Edema of the lower limb after vascular operations. *Surg. Gynec. Obstet.*, **131**, 282.

142. Veith, F. J., Hartuck, J. M. and Crane, C. (1964)

Management of aortoiliac reconstruction complicated by sepsis and hemorrhage. *New Eng. J. Med.*, **270**, 1389.

143. Vetto, R. M. (1962) The treatment of unilateral iliacartery obstruction with a transabdominal, subcutaneous, femorofemoral graft. *Surgery*, **52**, 342.

144. Vetto, R. M. (1966) The femorofemoral shunt. An appraisal. *Amer. J. Surg.*, **112**, 162.

144A.Vollmar, J., Trede, M., Laubach, K. and Forrest, H. (1968) Principles of reconstructive procedures for chronic femoro-popliteal occlusions. Report on 546 operations. *Ann. Surg.*, **168**, 215.

145. Watt, J. K. (1965) Origin of femoro-popliteal occlusions. *Brit. med. J.*, **ii**, 1455.

146. Watt, J. K. (1966) Pattern of aorto-iliac occlusion. *Brit. med. J.*, **ii**, 979.

147. Weale, F. E. (1966) *An Introduction to Surgical Haemodynamics*. London: Lloyd-Luke (Medical Books) Ltd.

148. Wellington, J. L., Olszewski, V., and Martin, P. (1966) Hyperaemia of the calf after arterial reconstruction for atherosclerotic occlusion. *Brit. J. Surg.*, **53**, 180.

149. Wesolowski, S. A. (1962) *Evaluation of Tissue and Prosthetic Vascular Grafts*. Springfield, Illinois: Charles C. Thomas.

149A.Wray, E., DePalma, R. G. and Hubay, C. H. (1971) Late occlusion of aorto-femoral by-pass grafts: influence of cigarette smoking. *Surgery*, **70**, 969.

150. Wylie, E. J. (1952) Thromboendarterectomy for arteriosclerotic thrombosis of major arteries. *Surgery*, **32**, 275.

151. Yao, S. T. (1970) Haemodynamic studies in peripheral arterial disease. *Brit. J. Surg.*, **57**, 761.

152. Zelis, R., Mason, D. T., Braunwald, E. and Levy, R. I. (1970) Effects of hyperlipoproteinemias and their treatment on the peripheral circulation. *J. clin. Invest.*, **49**, 1007.

4 Buerger's Disease

This is a disease of misconceptions. For years it was a popular diagnosis for any problem of gangrenous toes, not only in the middle-aged, premature, or otherwise unexpected case, where diabetes could not be blamed, but also, as we now realise, quite wrongly in older people as well. About 1929–30 it is on record [21] as twice as common as all other arterial occlusive conditions put together. Opinion over the next thirty years swung to the opposite extreme: its existence as an entity began to be questioned, and from Harvard Medical School in 1960 [21] came an indictment the content of which repays careful study.

Based on a clinico-pathological appraisal of the case records of men under forty-five years with peripheral arterial insufficiency, amputated limbs from patients of various ages, a few autopsies, and some vein biopsies, the decisive classifying feature was the presence or not of heart disease. Using these criteria, no specific clinical, morbid anatomical, or histological picture could be made out to support the concept of a primarily peripheral occlusive process in young men. Tobacco smoking, a history of phlebitis, and membership of the Jewish faith were equally common in both groups.

The period covered by the study (1928–56) precluded the use of arteriographic evidence. All patients were excluded from the analysis whose 'diagnosis could not be derived from a careful study of the hospital record', a group which might have contained cases of Buerger's disease whose severe ischaemia with large, proximal pulses still present could at that time have clouded the clinical appraisal and confused the record. Objection might also be made to the classification as heart disease, in this context, of valvular or hypertensive disease, and certainly to the inclusion of diabetes and hypercholesterolaemia.

Study of the amputated legs, though it yielded important and useful data which we will later consider, confined the pathological evidence to the lower and smaller vessels; this no doubt perpetuated the chief fault of the whole work, which arteriograms might have set right; an almost total disregard of the state of the main limb artery.

This narrowness in the topographic approach (of which the small attention paid to upper limb occlusions is another example), together with the uncertain relevance of some cases in the 'cardiac' group, should dismiss the indictment. Clinical evidence to be presented in this chapter can leave little doubt that the condition known as Buerger's disease does exist as a definite entity, though perhaps more from the descriptive clinical and angiological viewpoint than as a specific disease: here we may agree that the histological picture of the affected small artery gives no support to the 'absolutely typical and diagnostic' pathology of thromboangiitis obliterans* of Buerger's concept [3]. It seems more likely that cellularity of the arterial wall is a normal reaction to contained thrombus, and later fibrosis is the end result (*see* p. 99).

The Harvard study concluded that lesions in the

---

* The term 'thromboangiitis obliterans' should be avoided, for it contains pathological implications that still remain unfounded. A better name is 'Buerger's disease'. For exactly similar reasons, we in Great Britain have kept to the name 'Crohn's disease' rather than 'regional ileitis'.

vessels in these young men were indistinguishable from those in small arterial occlusions from 'atherosclerosis, systemic embolisation or peripheral thrombosis singly or in combination'. This is an important observation: small arterial lesions, typical in severe ischaemia (*see* Chapter 3, p. 38) *may be* either thrombotic, embolic, or both. Another origin, it is now believed, is from unstable inner deposits of occlusive material that form the lining of the stenosing main artery lesion, the consequent double or multiple blocks then determining the onset of gangrene.

Modern practice in clinical examination of peripheral arterial cases, and the confirmatory evidence of arteriography, have made familiar the association of large irregularities in the main limb artery with distal secondary occlusions beyond. Nevertheless, cases do present in young and middle-aged subjects in which distal blocks occur on their own. These we will now consider.

Comparison with Arteriosclerosis Obliterans

Buerger's disease	*Arteriosclerosis obliterans*
Age 20–45	Age 45 and over
Females rarely affected, most cases premenopausal	Females 10% of all cases. Female incidence rises after menopause
Upper limbs often involved	Upper limbs seldom
Superficial veins often indicate disease activity	Deep veins occasionally, mostly secondary to ischaemic stasis
Onset with foot pain, claudication or at rest	Onset with calf claudication
Gangrene common, and often early, limited, and with nearby pulses often present	Gangrene 10%, later, and with widespread loss of limb pulses
Cigarette smoking absolutely related to progress of disease, and abstention to arrest	Cigarette smoking of direct importance in cases developing gangrene but other factors influence outcome, and deterioration may follow abstention
Sympathectomy and anticoagulants effective if tissues viable	Sympathectomy sometimes, anticoagulants questionable
Serum cholesterol norma	Serum cholesterol raised
Diabetes not relevant	Diabetes contributory
No calcification	Calcification common
Normal ECG	ECG often abnormal in approximately 25%
Life prognosis good	Life prognosis reduced

Incidence Relative to Other Causes of Limb Ischaemia

In Western countries this appears to be in the region of 1 per cent. Most large clinics have records of many cases. Among approximately 4,000 patients with peripheral arterial disease seen by the writer between 1950–1971, there were 54 probable cases of Buerger's disease, most of which were subsequently confirmed at arteriography. In an analysis of 1,000 femoral arteriograms at St Mary's Hospital, London, there were forty cases of Buerger's disease. The remaining 96 per cent were obviously 'atheromatous' [18]. This can, therefore, hardly be called a rare disease.

In the Middle and Far East, a much higher proportion of patients with limb ischaemia show the peripheral, four-limb, youthful type of picture than in Europe and the United States, and the Jewish race was thought by Buerger to be particularly prone to it. The ancient migrations of the Jewish people divided the race into the Ashkenazim (Eastern European communities) and several other groups mostly living in the Middle East, including the Yemenites (*see also* Chapter 1, p. 6). Recent clinical, epidemiological and shown ethnological studies from Israel [7, 11A] have a highly significant preponderance of Ashkenazim, especially from Eastern Poland. These were the people who made up the bulk of the cases first described by Buerger in New York in 1909 [3]. A familial incidence was also found, and a relationship to earlier frostbite.

In Ceylon, China, Korea, and Japan [9, 11B, 12] this is a form peripheral occlusive arterial disease very often takes; these are also the countries in which

'young female arteritis' is seen (see Chapter 7), and though the anatomical distribution and the sex incidence of the two conditions are completely opposite the geographical and pathological features show striking resemblances.

Women are seldom affected by Buerger's disease (see Fig. 4.3); by 1960 there were only sixty cases in the literature [10].

Aetiology and Pathology

The cause of Buerger's disease is cigarette smoking. A few cases have been described in non-smokers but, in a disease such as this, in which the diagnosis depends upon precise clinical and arteriographic evidence, exceptions to the smoking rule will usually be better explained by making another diagnosis; either arteriosclerosis of the peripheral-type if there are any clinical or radiological signs of proximal plaques and diffuse irregularity of larger arteries, or entrapment, or cystic adventitial disease of the popliteal (see Chapter 3, p. 45).

How cigarette smoking causes arterial occlusion in Buerger's disease is not yet known. In normal subjects, inhalation of the smoke at a normal aver-

age rate of once a minute produced no fall in measured blood flow in the extremities, although if frequency was increased to every twenty seconds a sharp fall in hand blood flow occurred, also when the number of cigarettes smoked was increased [17].

The vasoconstrictor action of nicotine, while appropriate to this disease, hardly explains its striking effects when the habit is only moderate, or when serious relapse occurs immediately after resuming cigarette smoking, nor the fact that while sympathetic denervation prevents nicotine vasoconstriction [17] it gives no protection against the damaging effects of smoking in Buerger's disease; neither does the administration of reserpine, one of whose actions is

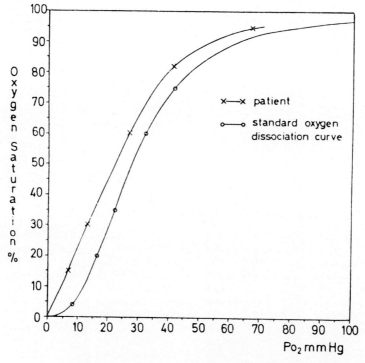

Fig. 4.1. Oxygen dissociation curve for normal subjects and for patient with Buerger's disease. (By permission of the author and *Lancet*.)

the dissipation of catecholamines held in the vessel wall [4].

A tendency to Raynaud's phenomenon, and to excessive sweatiness of the hands [8, 19], could be regarded as evidence of excessive sympathetic activity, which might increase the action of nicotine on the peripheral blood flow. Previous frostbite or other cold exposure injury was obtained in 35 per cent of the Israel cases [7], most of whom had suffered these conditions in the concentration camps. The findings were similar in the Korean study [12].

Tobacco extracts have been injected intradermally to determine whether there might be a sensitivity in subjects with Buerger's disease, but results were conflicting and no recent reports exist.

Antibodies against an antigen prepared from normal artery have been demonstrated in patients during the acute phase and are reduced by giving steroids [15]. While such a process might be part of the cause, it could, like the cellular response in the occluded small artery, be an effect of inflammatory reaction.

An increase in carboxyhaemoglobin has been found in the blood of patients with this disease [1, 2,

6, 11A], which might explain the common occurrence of ischaemic pain and necrosis in digits in which the skin colour is still reasonably good and the capillary return appears normal. The oxygen dissociation curve is moved to the left (Fig. 4.1), which means that at low oxygen tensions the haemoglobin holds on to its oxygen instead of yielding it to the tissues. This could aggravate the ischaemia caused by the occlusive lesions and might be concerned also in the production of these lesions. The effect, however, seems not to be exclusive to Buerger's disease subjects. Healthy male smokers, especially those over forty years of age, show increased oxygen affinity and in these the cause was shown to be a rise in carboxy-haemoglobin [2].

A familial incidence has been suggested by enquiries in the USA and in Israel [7]. A constitutional tendency, perhaps genetically determined, to small arteries has been recognised in a group of thirty patients in France [20]. In two large series the incidence was lower in the professional classes and higher in the lower socio-economic groups, though the effects of differences in cigarette consumption were not distinguished [7, 12].

Histological Features

From the numerous descriptions in the literature, no conclusions as to the nature of the morbid process can at present be drawn except that it differs radically from the common, main arterial lesion of arteriosclerosis, and that at its various stages there is an inflammatory response in the smaller arteries and veins which, later, become fibrous.

Very little is known of the morbid processes of this condition except that they differ sharply from arteriosclerosis obliterans both in body distribution of the lesions and in their gross and microscopic appearances (Fig. 4.2). It is now believed that cellular patterns in and around the occluded small arteries and superficial veins represent the effects of thrombosis, and not its cause. Yet, portions of artery or vein not yet thrombosed do also show cellular infiltration (Fig. 4.2a and c). Two characteristic later features in occluded segments are:

(a) Marked periarterial fibrosis with adherence to surrounding structures (Fig. 4.2b).

(b) Recanalisation of the cellular thrombus (Fig. 4.2b).

These are probably nothing more than a natural sequel to acute occlusion: a vigorous early inflammatory reaction (Fig. 4.2c) in response to the irritant thrombus is followed by healing and organisation. In arteriosclerosis the initial slow process of laminar deposition of occluding material probably provides less stimulus to cellular activity, which might also be prevented by the dense, amorphous composition of the plaque or plug from extending much beyond the internal elastic lamina, although adventitial cellular reaction to advanced arteriosclerotic lesions is common (see p. 12).

The advance of the disease, as in chronic ischaemia from arteriosclerosis, is centripetal, by successive further thromboses in remaining normal tibial or forearm arteries, and probably also, in the territory of the fine, rich screen of collaterals in the ischaemic distal segment of the lesion.

Clinical Features

Pain is the dominant symptom. The following types are listed in the order of their frequency:

1. Claudication in the foot muscles.
2. Rest pain in the toes and forefoot.
3. Painful digital gangrene.

4. Fulminating acute ischaemia of the foot with distal pulses still present.

The onset is sub-acute, though the later course may last many years. The patient presents himself after having endured a few weeks' pain of one of the

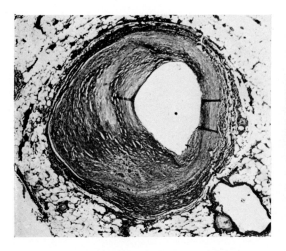 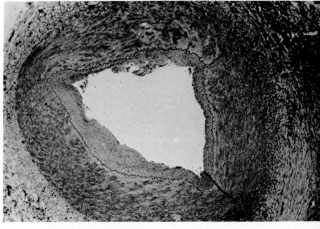

(a)

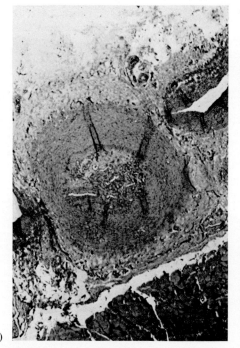 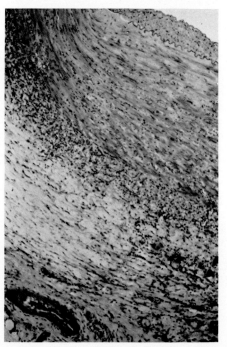

(b) (c)

Fig. 4.2. Contrasting appearances of arteriosclerosis and Buerger's disease. (Photomicrographs by Dr E. A. Wright.)

(a) Left: a partly occluded main coronary artery with typical eccentric narrowing of the lumen with laminated amorphous material containing numerous cholesterol clefts. The media is thin where the plug is thick (× 40).

Right: the posterior tibial artery of a doctor aged thirty-two, showing the preocclusive stage of Buerger's disease. Most of the thickening is in the wall of the artery (× 40).

(b) Buerger's disease: the late lesion. The posterior tibial artery from an amputation specimen showing organised, recanalising thrombus and still, considerable medial thickening. From a ship's officer aged thirty-six who also had a gangrenous little finger (× 40).

(c) The doctor's posterior tibial artery at higher magnification (× 100). There is marked cellular infiltration of all coats and the intimal thickening is also of an organised cellular pattern.

first three types, or with a longer history progressing through these same three stages. He is exhausted from lack of sleep, and from the use of hypnotics and analgesics that have failed to give relief.

Pain is at first confined to one foot or, less often, one hand; and very occasionally a hand and foot both give symptoms at the same time.

In late or relapsed cases, although both feet are obviously affected the pain is mainly confined to one side, the story again, being that of a recent sub-acute relapse, often following a return to smoking. The patient may also mention that a discharge has appeared from between the two most painful toes.

Such a patient sits miserably on his bed holding his worse foot, the knee flexed up; dependency gives less relief from rest pain than in arteriosclerosis.

A HISTORY OF SUPERFICIAL PHLEBITIS

Superficial thrombophlebitis occurs in a high proportion of cases; between 40 per cent [16] and, perhaps, 100 per cent [13] at some time have had it so that, although it should represent a very common cause of symptoms, the discomforts are slight, with only minor pain and tenderness, the redness and localised swelling are often all that is remembered; trivial in the patient's view, and tending to be forgotten in the distress of the serious arterial effects that follow.

PHYSICAL SIGNS

In a mild, early case (Fig. 4.3) there is slight *swelling*

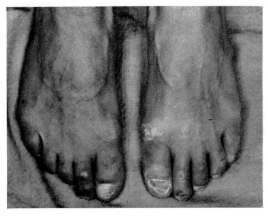

Fig. 4.4. A more advanced case in a merchant seaman aged twenty-six. All toes were swollen and discoloured with deformed nails. Early necrosis over head of first left metatarsal. This patient's arteriograms and subsequent clinical course are shown in Fig. 4.12.

and redness of all the toes, one or more of which are obviously worse affected; the patient confirms that these are the painful ones. Later they become cyanotic, though the capillary return still remains brisk. The nails are thickened and deformed (Fig. 4.4) and there may be signs of infection beneath one or more of them. Fungal infections are common here, and

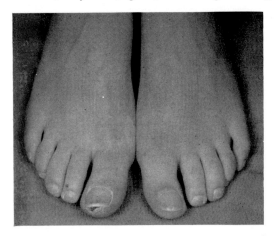

Fig. 4.3. A mild early case, unusual in that it occurred in a thirty-two-year-old woman. The right hallux was swollen, congested and painful, with early subungual necrosis and thickening of the nail. The next toe also had a painful necrotic patch near the nailfold. There had been superficial phlebitis in recent months. Complete relief and regression occurred on cessation of cigarette smoking.

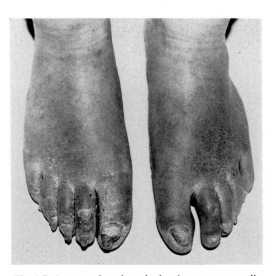

Fig. 4.5. A severe chronic and relapsing case personally observed over twenty years in a man now aged fifty-six. There was clear correlation of relapse with resumption of cigarette smoking. This patient was greatly helped by heparin and LMDX infusion during acute phases, and with low dosage prednisone in the intervals.

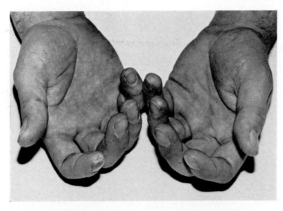

Fig. 4.6. Secondary Raynaud's phenomenon with painful necrosis of right index finger-tip, occurring in the same patient as Fig. 4.5. He had long before undergone bilateral lumbar sympathectomy, but has not yet required sympathectomy for his hands.

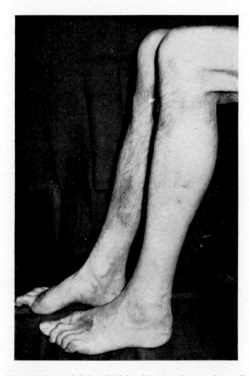

Fig. 4.7. Superficial phlebitis of both calves and a well-healed amputation of the right hallux in a man of thirty-four with a history of symptoms for three years, and who stated that he had not been told to stop smoking. On doing so, the condition abated.

in the webs, and were once thought to be the underlying cause of the 'angiitis'. There is little to support this view, but the presence of penetrating infected lesions must aggravate ischaemia, and such toes are always the worst affected.

In the chronic phase (Fig. 4.5), the feet and toes are generally slightly swollen, with a cylindrical appearance and loss of anatomical contours, the skin is obviously thin and atrophic, and the toes cool, and bluish, with tapered, hard pulps as in advanced Raynaud's disease and scleroderma. By now the hands may also be involved (Fig. 4.6).

Superficial phlebitis, though a common part of the history, does not often show itself during the acute phases of the foot condition. The lesions are typical, occurring most often over the front of the tibia (Fig. 4.7), unlike the acute thrombosis on the inner aspect of the calf, which sometimes complicates varicose veins: in Buerger's disease the main saphenous trunk is usually spared and, instead, short segments of the narrow subcutaneous tributaries become raised, with reddened skin over them. Such veins are tender, though not noticeably hot. Cord-like thrombosis may also occur in the subcutaneous veins of the fingers.

Raynaud's phenomenon and hyperhidrosis have already been mentioned (p. 99). The *skin temperature* of the ischaemic areas is reduced, but less than would be expected, perhaps because with loss of the principal peripheral arteries much of the fine system of collaterals runs close beneath the skin, and possibly also, because the tissue anoxia in Buerger's disease may be partly a humoral phenomenon not entirely determined by reduced blood flow [1].

Pulse deficiencies are diagnostic; the disease can be recognised by their distribution:

1. Severe ischaemia of the feet or hand is associated with loss of ankle or wrist pulses only. Exceptionally, even these are still present.
2. Pulses may be absent in an extremity that is free from symptoms.
3. Wrist pulses are often missing, typically the ulnars [7], (*see* Fig. 4.13).
4. Pulses are usually normal at the knee and elbow.
5. Arterial murmurs are rare.
6. Palpable collateral pulses are seldom present.

Oscillometry in the upper calf typically shows normal readings equal on the two sides. Further down they are sharply reduced, and so is the pressure gradient between the ankle and toes [4A].

Diagnosis

If the features described are present, diagnosis should present little difficulty, though some of them also occur in other conditions; these include:

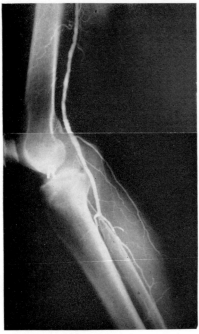

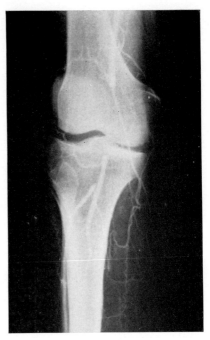

Fig. 4.8. Arteriosclerotic irregularity of the femoro-popliteal artery in a man of fifty with foot claudication and early rest pain. Occluded tibial arteries are here presumably due to embolic migration of intimal thrombus from lesions of the kind shown in the irregular proximal artery. (*See also* [21])

Fig. 4.9. Recent acute thrombosis of the popliteal artery in a woman aged forty-nine. Exploration revealed the cause to be thrombosis within a narrowed segment of cystic adventitial disease.

Secondary Raynaud's phenomenon from other causes in the upper or lower limbs, for example thoracic outlet syndrome, a previous brachial embolism, popliteal aneurysm with embolism, disseminated lupus erythematosus, temporal arteritis, rheumatoid arteritis, ergotism and old frostbite.

Diabetic distal arterial occlusive disease. Glycosuria, neuropathy and small artery calcification are usually present; if not, the case may be misdiagnosed as Buerger's disease, until investigation shows a raised blood sugar or serum insulin abnormality (*see* p. 114).

Arteriosclerosis in the middle-aged should be recognisable from the several ways in which it differs from Buerger's disease (p. 95), though in this age group cases do occur in which the diagnosis may be wrongly made, for example:

1. Peripheral ischaemia with proximal arterial disease and murmurs that have been missed (Fig. 4.8).
2. Popliteal occlusion with abrupt clinical onset (Fig. 4.9).

3. Embolic gangrene of the toes from detachment of proximal thrombus in diffuse arteriosclerosis. (Another form of secondary Raynaud's phenomenon (*see* Fig. 3.11, p. 38)).
4. Arteriosclerotic occlusion of the brachial artery (Fig. 4.10).

A thorough clinical examination should yield supporting evidence for the diagnosis of arteriosclerosis, but cases of doubt do occur at this age; in these the problem is usually solved by arteriography.

Murmurs are the surest clinical evidence; the groin and the adductor opening being auscultated as a routine. Any irregularity in the proximal artery should at once exclude Buerger's disease.

Arteriographic Appearances (Figs 4.11, 4.12, 4.13, and 4.14)

1. The main artery is usually perfectly smooth and normal-looking, usually as far as the knee or elbow region, though there may be 'corrugation' (*see* p. 54).
2. The point of occlusion is clear and sharp, without proximal irregularity.

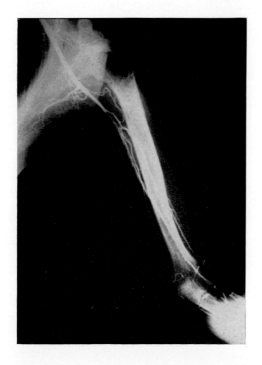
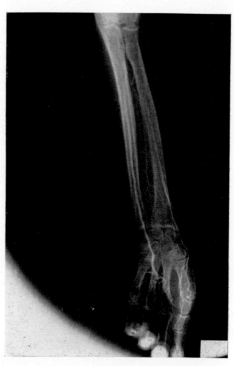

Fig. 4.10. Arteriosclerotic occlusion of the brachial and radial arteries and of the palmar arch in a middle-aged woman with severe, painful secondary Raynaud's phenomenon. (Good response to sympathectomy.)

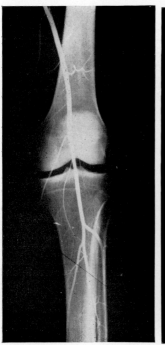
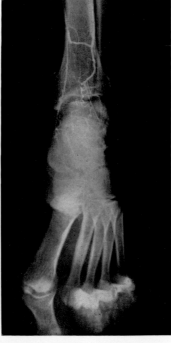

Fig. 4.11. A typical arteriogram in Buerger's disease carried out in 1952 on a man of forty-six.

LEFT. Normal femoro-popliteal and upper calf arteries.

RIGHT. Occluded lower tibial arteries with fine, root-like collaterals insufficient to maintain foot circulation. Major amputation was required.

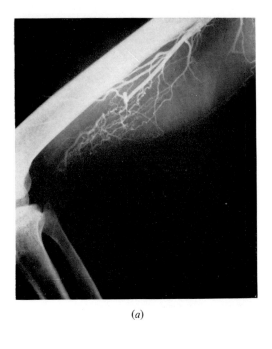

(a)

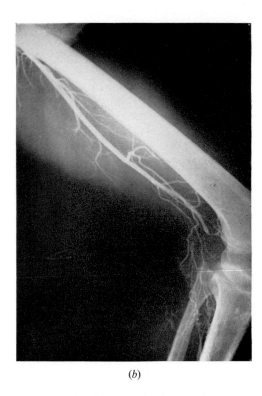

(b)

(a, b) Femoral arteriograms of the seaman whose feet are shown in Fig. 4.4, and taken at the same stage of the disease. There was dependent rubor of the foot on the worse-affected right side.

Fig. 4.12.

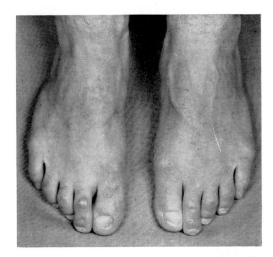

(c) Bilateral sympathectomy was contra-indicated in this young man, but he made a striking improvement on stopping smoking, and when seen again two years later was free from symptoms and had regained a normal appearance of the feet and toes.

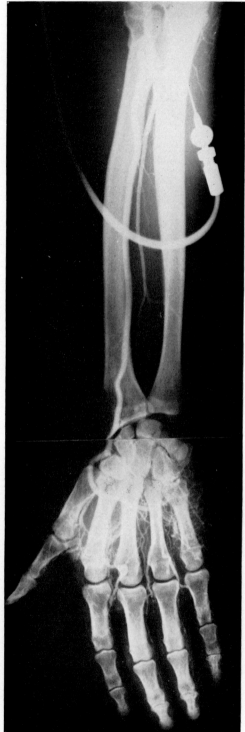

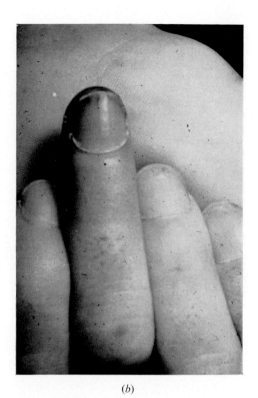

(b)

Fig. 4.13. Buerger's disease of the upper limb.

(a) Occlusion of almost the whole length of the left ulnar artery.

(b) Painful secondary Raynaud's phenomenon with commencing pulp gangrene.

Patient was a thirty-two-year-old lorry driver first seen in 1959 who had smoked forty cigarettes a day for some years. Early improvement following continuous intravenous heparin for one week, followed by sympathectomy. Symptomless ten years later. He has not resumed smoking.

(a)

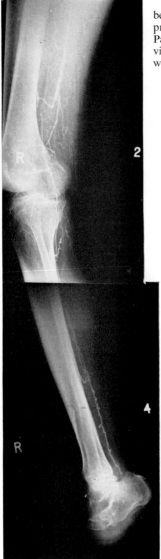

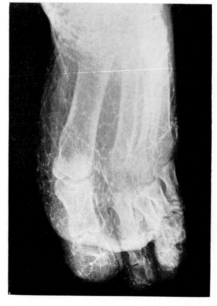

(*a*) Occlusion of popliteal and all main arteries beyond, root-like collaterals, insufficient to support previously stable right through-foot amputation. Patient had been smoking when away from supervision at home in Iraq. Below-knee amputation healed well.

(*b*) The phenomenon of early venous filling strikingly shown in the ischaemic left foot of this patient. Following left lumbar sympathectomy there was an acute deterioration, thought to be due to further arterial thrombosis (*See* Chapter 10, p. 198). Below-knee amputation was required on this side also.

Fig. 4.14. A severe progressive case in a middle-aged Arab patient.

3. There is no patent segment of the main artery beyond the block.

4. One or both tibial or forearm arteries are lost, the process being centripetal.

5. A fine complex of root-like collaterals springs from the lower end of the patent part of the main artery but does not re-enter it below.

6. Early venous filling (Fig. 4.14): rich contrast values are sometimes shown unexpectedly, though the extremity may be obviously ischaemic (*see also* Chapter 3, p. 56). Arteriovenous shunting may be responsible: it has been blamed for worsening of ischaemia after sympathectomy (*see* Chapter 10, p. 198).

Prognosis

Smoking is the crucial factor. If it is continued, the disease will inevitably progress, but the rate of deterioration is not necessarily related to the number of cigarettes smoked. The compulsive smoker may be in no way deterred by loss of one leg or even two.

which time the patient feels he has lost a good deal and gained nothing. Even so, arrest is certain, and improvement highly probable (Figs 4.15 and 4.16), the exception being those cases whom ischaemic damage and secondary infection have gone beyond

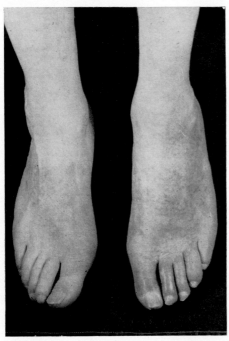

Fig. 4.15. Arrest of Buerger's disease over twenty-two years. This patient now aged fifty-five underwent left lumbar sympathectomy by the late Mr Gwynne Williams, in 1945, and stopped smoking. Appearances of chronic ischaemia persisted, but the patient is completely symptomless.

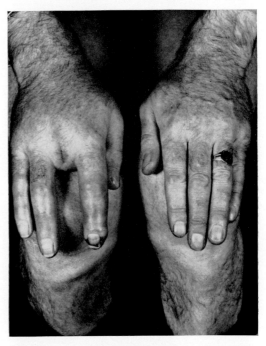

Fig. 4.16. This man of forty-four had a five-year history of multiple-limb ischaemia for which he had undergone bilateral lumbar sympathectomy, double below-knee amputation, and of the right middle finger. Good response to 'bridging treatment' (*see* p. 109), then transaxillary sympathectomy (to avoid shoulder strap of leg prosthesis).

Warning to the patient should be frank and firm; it seldom needs to be repeated, and seldom should, even in the patient who is deteriorating, for he has made his decision and is prepared to abide by the consequences.

Yet, in almost every case, no matter how advanced, provided the extremity is still viable, abstinence from all forms of tobacco will bring an improvement. This may take several weeks to show itself, during

the point at which the restricted blood supply can overcome them.

The Life Prognosis. This is now believed to be almost as good as that of the normal population, of the same age group [13] (Fig. 4.17). Arteriosclerosis, though less often causing the loss of a limb is much more likely to lead to the death of the patient. Coronary deaths predominate in both groups, and may relate to continued use of tobacco.

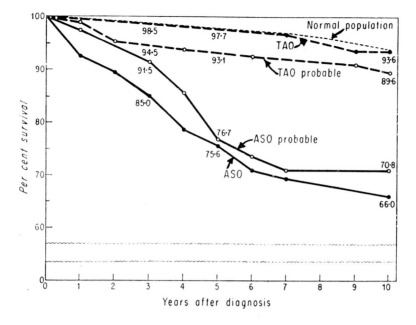

Fig. 4.17. Widely differing ten-year survival rates in Buerger's disease (TAO) and arteriosclerosis (ASO). Confirmed cases of Buerger's disease show no significant difference from the normal population (from McPherson *et al.* [13], by permission of the publishers of the *Annals of Internal Medicine*).

TREATMENT: GENERAL AND SURGICAL

The first step is to warn the patient about the effects of smoking. While the physician and family doctor may already have done this, the patient and his relatives may still not realise the imperative significance of what has been said, for the ultimate and strongest move on the doctor's side, the threat to discontinue the professional relationship, cannot be justified in those who are responsible for the patient's continued care. The surgeon, however, and particularly the vascular surgeon, may be right to use this method for the patient's own good. In fact, it is not often necessary.

Conservative Treatment

It is essential that something active shall be done to try to help the patient over the difficult time between the establishment of the diagnosis and the onset of clinical improvement. Tobacco withdrawal effects are then at their worst. Sedatives and non-vasoactive tranquillisers are necessary. Most cases are best dealt with in hospital at this stage.

Other forms of 'bridging' treatment can then be given and include:

(*a*) Body heating
(*b*) Heparinisation for a week or more
(*c*) Intravenous infusion of low molecular weight dextran (LMDX)
(*d*) Induced hypertension (*see* p. 57)
(*e*) Steroids.

The aim of these is to reduce stasis, sludging, and thrombosis in the small vessels, and to improve tissue perfusion.

Sepsis must be dealt with, using the appropriate antibiotic, according to the results of sensitivity testing of organisms grown from discharge from the line of separation if gangrene is already present, or from moisture from the sodden interdigital skin or the fissure which is found, on separating, in the toe cleft. Oedema and lymphangitis of the nearby area of the dorsum of the foot should soon resolve, the painful swollen parts become wrinkled and less tender, and rest pain is eased. Incising for pus usually

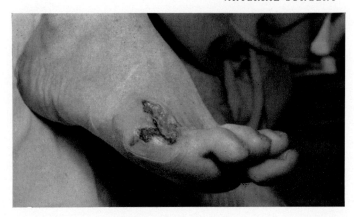

Fig. 4.18. The result of conservative toe amputation in Buerger's disease. A dorsal racquet incision had been used. Below-knee amputation was necessary. Patient now a non-smoker, and remains well fourteen years later.

does more harm than good, for there is no tense collection, because of the lack of blood supply.

Debridement and local amputation require careful judgement. Conservatism is the best policy in this kind of local surgery. The aim is to remove only dead tissue and, thus, to improve drying, drainage and separation of the necrotic part. To open up underlying tissues of low vitality is to spread the gangrene (Fig. 4.18).

Local applications cannot help much on their own. The obvious choice, a topical antibiotic spray containing neomycin, bacitracin, and polymyxin B is badly tolerated as a rule, because of the chilling produced by the propellant and the irritant effects of the agents themselves. Astringent lotions or pastes are better; lotio rubra BPC, zinc oxide or peroxide, and bismuth iodoform paste are worth trying. Otherwise, it is best to keep to gentle interdigital cleansing and drying, leaving small sterile gauze pledgets between the toes so as to separate their skin surfaces without forcing them apart. The same methods and principles apply to the upper limb.

Improvement occurs within the first one or two weeks or not at all. After this time plans must be made for elective operation.

Operative Treatment

In order of usefulness these are: 1. Sympathectomy; 2. Amputation; 3. Arterial reconstruction; 4. Adrenalectomy has been suggested.

Sympathectomy

This is indicated in most cases, for it provides permanent freedom from vasoconstrictor activity in the distal part of the limb, which is the part usually affected by the disease. A strong flow and pressure head are available from the nearby, normal main artery. Anhidrosis of the skin is of positive value in reducing bacterial and fungal activity, which may be

a potent aggravating factor in these patients who so often show a hyperhidrosis (*see* p. 102).

The techniques and results of sympathectomy are discussed in Chapter 10. Some special points concerning Buerger's disease include:

1. Bilateral lumbar sympathectomy, though desirable when both feet are affected, seriously may impair sexual function in these young subjects (*see* Chapter 10, p. 197). This should cause the surgeon to operate first upon the worst side. Milder ischaemia on the other may later improve the removal of the cigarette factor.

2. There is a risk that the patient may find himself worse as a result of the operation (*see* Chapter 10, p. 197). Hypotension during or after operation should be prevented by careful anaesthetic and operative technique. Undue retraction upon the aorta or the vena cava is particularly undesirable.

3. When an upper and a lower limb are severely affected at the same time it is better to deal with the leg first. As with the second foot, an improvement may establish itself in the hand during the time in hospital, and further sympathectomy may not then be necessary. Also, conservative amputations heal better in the upper limb.

Amputations

A conservative approach is often successful in Buerger's disease with its normal proximal arteries and good power of recovery in the affected distal circulation. With a positive programme of medical treatment and timely sympathectomy no major amputation should be necessary, though in the neglected case some ablative surgery will be required after a short trial of conservative treatment in hospital.

Digital, transmetatarsal, Syme's, and below-knee amputations should each do well in the appropriate case according to previous clinical and arteriographic assessment. With normotensive anaesthesia, trial skin incision confirms the suitability of the chosen

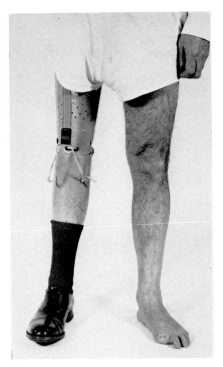

Fig. 4.19. An Austrian Jewish patient first seen by the author in 1947 with painful advanced gangrene of the right foot for which major amputation was undertaken according to the practice of that period. Occlusion extended up to the mid-thigh. This patient had, in 1945, undergone left lumbar sympathectomy and amputation of the left hallux by Sir James Paterson Ross, and this limb remains healthy with a strong popliteal pulse.

site. If lumbar sympathectomy has not already been performed it should immediately precede the amputation.

Operative methods and management after amputation are discussed in Chapter 6.

Arterial Reconstruction

In a few cases, a localised obstruction in a proximal artery may be restored. The lesion is densely adherent to surrounding structures, and within the artery the plane of cleavage between the obstructing tissue and the wall is difficult to define. Endarterectomy is unlikely to succeed, but a by-pass graft may be more suitable. Good results can be obtained in this minority of patients with reconstructable lesions in Buerger's disease, particularly if the symptoms are early [5]. Patients with gangrene have additional occlusions in the smaller arteries and do less well. (Most of these patients are wrongly diagnosed and more probably have early-appearing arteriosclerosis.)

Adrenalectomy

Hyperplasia of the zona fasciculata with increased lipoid content and atrophy or even disappearance of the zona glomerulosa [14], and alteration in urinary catecholamine excretion pattern [11] are both described in Buerger's disease, and may correlate with the common clinical finding of hyperhidrosis and Raynaud's phenomenon seen in early cases. An abnormal activity of the adrenals might, through disturbances in the interrelated cortical and medullary functions, in time lead to such widespread peripheral vasoconstriction of the extremities that vascular occlusion would be made more likely.

On the continent of Europe, surgeons have been interested for some years in the possibility of controlling the disease by sub-total adrenalectomy, and when combined with extensive sympathectomy the clinical course appears to have been arrested in an impressive number of cases [14, 20]. Experience among surgeons in the English-speaking nations is small, and most would point out the regularity with which the disease can be checked by the patient ceasing to smoke. Failing this, in an advancing case this strategy might be tried.

On the other hand, Japanese experience of steroid administration in a large series has been favourable; both clinically and by histological confirmation that collagenolysis of the perithrombotic lesion had been brought about [11]. The author has found steroids effective as a last resort (Fig. 4.5).

Results of Treatment (Table 4.1)

Contrary to general belief, Buerger's disease can be controlled, pain relieved, and gangrene arrested. Among 54 probable cases observed by the author between 1950–71, major amputation was required in only 13, and in most of these the presentation was that of a persistently smoking amputee when first referred. Some had never been warned, or stated so. Figure 4.15 shows the feet of a patient who underwent left lumbar sympathectomy in 1945, and

stopped smoking. The disease was checked, and though the appearance of chronic ischaemia persisted, pain and necrosis stopped, and he has remained well for the twenty years that have followed. The patient shown in Fig. 4.19 was first seen in 1947, and an above-knee amputation was required at once. He stopped smoking and has remained well under regular personal observation ever since. A recent arteriogram confirmed the diagnosis.

Table 4.1. 62 Patients with Suspected Buerger's Disease
All had severe digital ischaemia or foot claudication. Average age at onset 34 years.

Accepted as Buerger's disease	54	Sympathectomy		25
clinical 25		previous	8	
arteriogram 29		subsequent	17	
Diabetic	4	Amputation		24
Peripheral A.S.O.	4	previous	11	(minor 4, major 7)
Superficial phlebitis	16	subsequent*	13	(minor 6, major 7)
Upper limbs involved	16			

* All during first hospital admission on joining this series, except for one persistent smoker. No further amputations during follow-up.

REFERENCES

1. Astrup, P. (1964) An abnormality in the oxygen-dissociation curve of blood from patients with Buerger's disease and patients with non-specific myocarditis. *Lancet*, **ii**, 1152.
2. Birnstingl, M., Cole, P. and Hawkins, L. (1967) Variations in oxyhaemoglobin dissociation with age, smoking, and Buerger's disease. *Brit. J. Surg.*, **54**, 615.
3. Buerger, L. (1908) Thrombo-angiitis obliterans: a study of the vascular lesions leading to presenile spontaneous gangrene. *Amer. J. med. Sci.*, **136**, 567.
4. Burn, J. H. and Rand, M. J. (1958) Effect of reserpine on vasoconstriction caused by sympathomimetic amines. *Lancet*, **i**, 673.
4A. Carter, S. A. and Lezack, J. D. (1971) Digital systolic pressures in the lower limb in arterial disease. *Circulation*, **43**, 905.
5. De Bakey, M. E., Crawford, E. S., Garrett, H. E., Cooley, D. A., Morris, G. C. and Abbott, J. P. (1964) Occlusive disease of the lower extremities in patients 16 to 37 years of age. *Ann. Surg.*, **159**, 873.
6. Dormandy, T. L. (1965) Abnormal oxygen-dissociation curves. *Lancet*, **ii**, 80.
7. Goodman, R. M., Elian, B., Mozes, M. and Deutsch, V. (1965) Buerger's disease in Israel. *Amer. J. med.*, **39**, 601.
8. Hershey, F. B., Pareira, M. D. and Ahlvin, R. C. (1962) Quadrilateral peripheral vascular disease in the young adult. *Circulation*, **26**, 1261.
9. Inada, K., Hayashi, M. and Okatani, T. (1964) Chronic occlusive arterial disease of lower extremity in Japan, with special reference to Buerger's disease. *Arch. Surg.*, **88**, 454.
10. Kaiser, G. C., Musser, A. W. and Shumacker, H. B. (1960) Thromboangiitis obliterans in women; report of two cases. *Surgery*, **48**, 733.
11. Kamiya, K. (1964) Buerger's disease. *Vasc. Dis.*, **1**, 186.
11A. Kjeldsen, K. and Mozes, M. (1969) Buerger's disease in Israel. *Acta chir. Scand.*, **135**, 495.
11B. Kradjian, R., Bowles, L. T. and Edwards, W. S. (1971) Peripheral arterial disease in Ceylon. *Surgery*, **69**, 523.
12. McKusick, V. A., Harris, W. S., Ottesen, O. E., Goodman, R. M., Shelley, W. M. and Bloodwell, R. D. (1962) Buerger's disease: a distinct clinical and pathologic entity. *J. Amer. Med. Assoc.*, **181**, 5.
13. McPherson, J. R., Juergens, J. L. and Gifford, R. W. (1963) Thromboangiitis obliterans and arteriosclerosis obliterans clinical and prognostic differences. *Ann. Int. med.*, **59**, 288.
14. Orban, F. (1961) New trends in the treatment of thromboangeiosis (Buerger's disease). *Ann. Roy. Coll. Surg. Eng.*, **28**, 69; also Personal communication (1966).
15. Pokorny, J. and Jezkova, Z. (1962) Significance of immunological studies in peripheral obliterating vascular diseases. *Circ. Res.*, **11**, 961.
16. Richards, R. L. (1953) Thrombo-angiitis obliterans. Clinical diagnosis and classification of cases. *Brit. med. J.*, **i**, 478.
17. Shepherd, J. T. (1963) In *Physiology of the Circulation in Human Limbs in Health and Disease*. Philadelphia and London: W. B. Saunders Company, pp. 384, 387.
18. Sutton, D. (1966) Personal communication.
19. Szilagyi, D. E., DeRusso, F. J. and Elliott, J. P. (1964) Thromboangiitis obliterans. Clinico-angiographic correlations. *Arch. Surg.*, **88**, 824.
20. Wertheimer, P., Perrin, M. and Minassian, J. (1964) La place de la surrénalectomie bilatérale dans le traitement de la thromboangiose. *Lyon Chir.*, **60**, 801.
21. Wessler, S., Ming, S-C., Gurewich, V. and Freiman, D. G. (1960) A critical evaluation of thromboangiitis obliterans. The case against Buerger's disease. *New Eng. J. med.*, **262**, 1149.

5 Diabetic Gangrene

General Effects of Diabetes upon the Circulation

The circulatory effects of diabetes are complex, widespread, often clinically silent and, like the glycosuria which precedes them, they may be missed. Since extensive arteriosclerosis may also remain undetected until a complication develops, it has been difficult to establish the relationship between the two processes in the development of peripheral ischaemia, though it is now nearly certain that they are closely linked.

BLOOD CHANGES

Hypercholesterolaemia, though often associated with vascular disease, is also a feature of several other medical disorders besides diabetes, not all of which show any striking predisposition to vascular disease.

It is commonest in elderly female diabetics, who compose a large proportion of those attending most diabetic clinics, yet among diabetics these are the least affected by severe arterial disease.

Reduced fibrinolytic activity, seen in thromboembolic disease of many kinds is also present in diabetes [9]. A relationship between arterial obliteration and diabetes would suggest that this factor might be significant. Fibrinolysis has been shown to exert an effect on platelet function (*see* Chapter 1, p. 9) tending to disperse aggregation in the early stages. It is increased by some oral antidiabetic drugs.

Platelet adhesiveness has been found to be raised in diabetic patients [6], as well as after oral and intravenous glucose administration in both normal and diabetic subjects, and by the addition of glucose to blood *in vitro*.

Blood viscosity increases during alimentary lipacmia [7, 25]. Measurements in diabetes have been few. Whole venous blood from patients of various ages was found to show a 20 per cent higher viscosity in diabetes compared with a similar sample of normal subjects [24]. This may be of some haemodynamic significance through aggravation of turbulence, thus favouring an increase in platelet accumulation (*see* Chapter 1, p. 9) at sites of arterial irregularity. Capillary permeability may be reduced in diabetes: radio-iodinated albumin is lost more slowly from three-hour blood samples in them than in normal subjects [12].

The *microcirculation* is distributed in organs such as the eye and the kidney whose structure and function can be readily studied for lesions during life. Lesions in these finely differentiated tissues exert obvious clinical effects. The same processes in limb muscles and the skin, though widespread [14, 17], might not be so conspicuous but their total effect could be to enhance the effects of major arterial disease, already known from study of amputation specimens to be more widely disseminated, and affecting branches of intermediate size more than in non-diabetic cases. This may be part of the reason for the poorer prognosis of established arterial disease in diabetes. Small-vessel lesions might also, on their own, account for some cases of gangrene in which pulses are still present yet without much neuropathy. A parallel with Buerger's disease has been suggested [5].

Nervous control of the peripheral circulation is affected in neuritis of several kinds, with low blood pressure, warm hands, and prominent veins as clinical evidence of loss of circulatory reflexes, proved experimentally by failure to respond to tipping or to the Valsalva manoeuvre [3]. This was present in 17 out of 337 diabetic patients. An afferent block to the baroceptor response was thought responsible [26]. Such patients may be poor operative risks from their failure to compensate for loss of blood volume or barbiturate administered in normal anaesthetic dosage.

One unexplained feature of this study was the presence of impotence in most of the men. An autonomic neuropathy would account for this, and also for the bladder disturbance in diabetes [16]. There is now support for the long-held clinical impression that diabetic patients often show loss of sympathetic function, with warm, dry extremities, even when there is accompanying peripheral vascular occlusive disease. 16 out of 29 diabetics with neurological signs, and 3 of 14 without them were found to have complete sympathetic denervation, as shown by their total failure to alter their foot circulation (digital skin temperatures) in response to body heating and cool-

ing [18]. Moreover, a local form of cold and adrenaline sensitivity was demonstrated (resembling that of a recurrent primary Raynaud condition after sympathectomy) which might aggravate the tendency to local physical damage in these neuropathic extremities.

The clinical importance of such changes is thus considerable. For example, an operative sympathectomy may be superfluous and undesirable in some patients who might at first sight seem to qualify for it on the grounds of local digital ischaemia. Results in these patients are often disappointing [10]. In cerebral ischaemia the 'diabetic auto-sympathectomy' or loss of the afferent baroceptors might aggravate postural hypotension.

Arterial Disease and Diabetes

The common clinical association of these two diseases is a matter of everyday experience, and the limb prognosis is known to be more than twice as bad when ischaemia is complicated by diabetes [24]. As many as 20 per cent of a series of 520 patients attending the Mayo Clinic with peripheral arteriosclerosis proved to be diabetic [13], but in another series of 44 patients with Buerger's disease there were none [19]. On the other hand, among 3,788 diabetic patients seen at King's College Hospital, [20] there were only 146 with obvious peripheral arterial disease, an incidence of 3·9 per cent. If, however, we exclude 2,422 women and 408 men younger than forty years of age the 958 remaining older men included 82 with arterial disease, or 8·3 per cent, which is approximately the same figure as in the prospective studies of normal populations in Basle, Switzerland, and Framingham, USA, as well as in a study of normal old people in Great Britain (see Chapter 1, p. 2). The duration of the diabetes appeared to bear no relationship to the incidence of arterial disease in the King's College Hospital series, and in a large group of young diabetics with severe and unstable disease there were no cases, suggesting that advancing age is more important than close control of the diabetes.

We have already referred (Chapter 1, p. 6) to the finding in a large population study in Bedford, England, of a relationship between symptomless impairment of glucose tolerance and the occurrence of arteriosclerotic disease. The same was found in

Michigan, USA, where arterial disease was about twice as common in people whose blood sugar level was in the top 20 per cent of the range [22]. In Oslo [28], too, the glucose tolerance test results were abnormal in nearly half of a group of patients with arteriosclerosis but without clinical diabetes, compared with only 10 per cent of a comparable normal series. Later studies from the same clinic [28A] showed that such patients also have a decreased hypoglycaemic response to insulin. Moreover, in insulin-dependent diabetics of long standing the same reduction in this effect was significantly associated with both microangiopathy and with arteriosclerosis [15A]. Fredrickson's Type III hyperlipidaemia (see Chapter 1, p. 5), in which both coronary and peripheral arteriosclerosis are a special risk, is also associated with a family history of diabetes; patients with this lipid defect usually have an abnormal glucose tolerance [9A]. In some patients with small vessel disease a glucose load fails to produce any rise in serum insulin [11].

Arterial disease may be aggravated during periods of weight reduction in diabetes, possibly from some products of the mobilisation of the fat stores [4].

The inference from all these studies is that impaired sugar tolerance and other prediabetic states may promote the development of arteriosclerosis and that once both conditions are clinically manifest the course of the disease is worse than in those with normal glucose metabolism.

Diabetic Neuropathy

This is the most important single factor in the development of diabetic gangrene, and the one most often overlooked, though easy to recognise even in its early stages. The onset may be insidious or fairly

rapid. Burning discomfort at night may suggest ischaemia [16]. The skin does not sweat.

Loss of deep reflexes and vibration sense are first present up to the ankles, later reaching the knees,

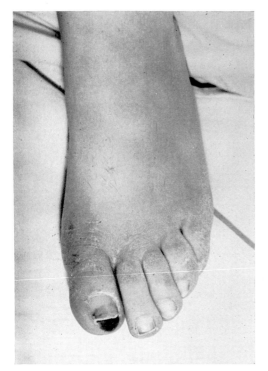

Fig. 5.1. Early diabetic gangrene from pressure in a patient with neuropathic sensory impairment over the fore-foot.

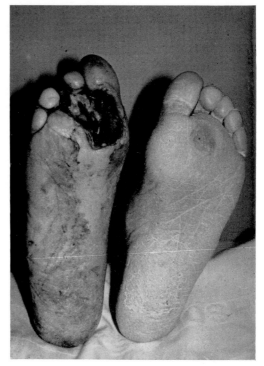

Fig. 5.2. Typical infected diabetic gangrene beneath the anterior metatarsal arch. Tendons exposed, also plantar vessels causing secondary haemorrhage. Note the characteristic dry, finely wrinkled skin of the intact left foot with early pressure lesion already present.

and usually with normal neurological signs over the remainder of the body. Sporadic and unexpected involvement of cranial and other nerves may confuse the diagnosis. Later pin prick and other pain sensations are lost from the forefoot.

Motor, sensory, asymmetrical, and amyotrophic cases are now thought to share a common basis. Lesions in the vasa nervorum, to suggest a vascular basis for neuropathy, have not been confirmed [1].

Local necrosis at pressure points is typical. The tips of the toes (Fig. 5.1) and the undersurface of the middle metatarsal heads (Fig. 5.2) are most often affected, though the heel may also slough (Fig. 5.3), particularly in bedridden patients, such as those who have recently undergone a major amputation of the opposite lower limb.

The neuropathic foot is highly vulnerable to develop progressive infection within painless cracks or blisters at points of normal or unusual pressure, the patient not being aware that a series of spreading infection may be beginning.

A diagnostic sign is the finding of a Charcot's joint. Any of the distal joints of the lower limb may become

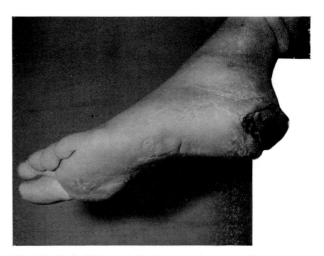

Fig. 5.3. Full thickness infective pressure sore with osteomyelitis of the underlying calcaneus. Later developed spreading gas infection in the calf (*see* Fig. 5.8).

115

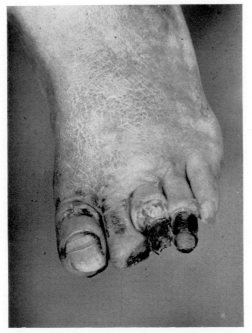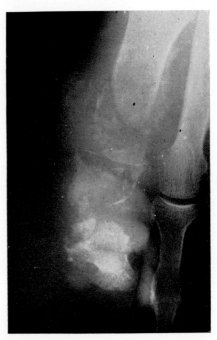

Fig. 5.4. Neuropathic joints of great toe in a neglected diabetic.

painlessly disorganised and grossly deformed in this way (Fig. 5.4). Abscess formation may lead to the formation of sinuses. When these appear in the region of a swollen ankle, a wrong interpretation of peripheral vascular insufficiency may be made in a case in which the main fault is the neuropathy.

The Role of Infection

Although diabetics are specially liable to infection, many other factors exist that foster its establishment and spread. Old age, stiffness, and inability to care for the feet, also social and medical neglect, are at times as much responsible as the diabetes. When infection develops in such a patient who also has ischaemia of his lower limbs, the situation is serious and the best of treatment may fail. Prevention is much easier than cure: good supervision of the diabetes, and at the same clinic visits a careful watch on the condition of the feet, with chiropody and special shoe-fitting, should ensure that diabetic gangrene will be a rarity in the co-operative type of diabetic clinic patient.

Clinical Presentation—Three Varieties

Ischaemia

1. Senile arteriosclerotic gangrene (in a diabetic)
2. Infective gangrene with added ischaemia
3. Infective neuropathic diabetic gangrene (with no ischaemia).

Neuropathy

Senile Arteriosclerotic Gangrene in a Diabetic

Pain is the dominant feature when severe ischaemia develops in an elderly subject who happens also to be diabetic, and so he will be seen early, often with only minor necrosis. The foot is cool, often with dependent rubor and slow venous refilling, and unless the circulation can be improved and infection and the diabetic condition brought under control, the limb prognosis will be bad, tending indeed to be worse than in a non-diabetic.

Infective-neuropathic Gangrene with Added Ischaemia

The patient with neuropathic damage and early spreading infection may not possess a blood supply sufficient to meet and overcome the infection. This

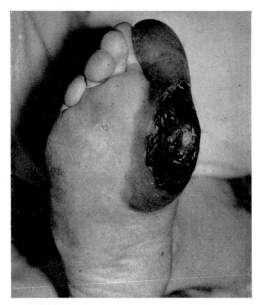

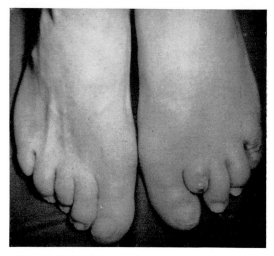

Fig. 5.6. Digital lesions in a middle-aged diabetic patient with bilateral, symmetrical femoro-popliteal occlusive disease. Loss of pain and vibration sense in the left foot and absent tendon reflexes in the left lower limb.

Fig. 5.5. Spreading diabetic gangrene arising from an infected pressure sore beneath the head of the first metatarsal in a patient with arterial insufficiency and neuropathy.

is a difficult condition to assess, for the cause is uncertain, the foot is not cold, sepsis is indolent, and there is less pain and tenderness than would be

expected (Fig. 5.5). It may be difficult to decide how much of the damage is due to lack of blood supply, possibly micro-vascular [17], and how much is the result of neuropathy. Signs of both may be present, with absent ankle pulses (though commonly on both sides, so, therefore, less significant; more important clinically is absence of the popliteal or superficial femoral pulses); loss of vibration sense and diminution of tendon reflexes (also, usually, bilateral, but a useful guide if more marked on the affected side (*see* Fig. 5.6)). Skin temperature is sometimes misleading, for the affected foot may be warmer, either from the presence of numerous subcutaneous arterial collaterals in a case of chronic ischaemia with multiple,

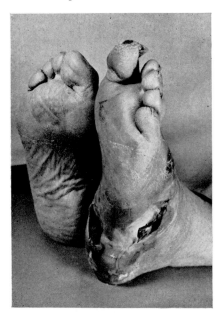

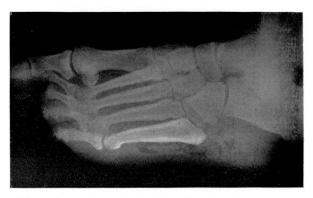

Fig. 5.7. Spreading infection in the sole of a diabetic foot, with gas formation. Healed well with local drainage and strict diabetic regime.

small distal blocks, or from loss of sympathetic tone where neuropathy is the main cause of the local lesion. Inflammation also contributes warmth. With a marginal blood supply, the wide, free incisions necessary to drain extensive infection within such a foot may fail to heal.

Infective Gangrene without Evidence of Ischaemia — Neuropathic Gangrene

Once recognised, this condition is easier to assess and to treat than when ischaemia is present as well. It occurs in careless, alcoholic, neglected or derelict patients who, on the average, are ten years younger than those with pure ischaemia [15]. It is more related to lack of control of the diabetes than to the length of its history. Motor neuropathy leads to deformities, and abnormal pressure points are developed with callosities which insidiously or quite rapidly break down; painlessly as a rule because of the sensory loss. A clean defect soon becomes infected. With a free blood supply, a large amount of pus, which tracks backwards along the tendons and fascial planes of the sole of the foot (Fig. 5.7) may soon form; in other cases the heel is first affected (*see* Fig. 5.3). Extensive infective sloughing of the skin is accompanied by osteomyelitis of the calcaneum. Tracking up into the calf muscles may occur, with gas formation due to coliform infection [6A] (Fig. 5.8), yet still the skin of the foot is pink, warm, and dry up to the line of demarcation. The condition remains painless, without distress except for the general malaise and discomforts of fever, often minor out of all proportion to the danger of the illness, and the patient or his family may need positive persuasion to agree to the necessary major amputation. Characteristically, the smell of the infection may prove decisive.

Principles of Treatment

Each of the factors responsible is assessed and treated. Rest is essential whichever features are presented. The diabetic condition is reviewed, although full control may not yet be possible. Cultures are taken, and the correct antibiotic is given as soon as possible.

Pus is released, in ischaemic patients by softening and lifting the margin of the gangrene, in spreading or neuropathic patients by free incision along the line of tenderness; or inflammation in the soft tissues (Fig. 5.9). The diabetes should now become controllable.

When ischaemia is the dominant factor, it should be treated energetically (*see* Chapters 2 and 3). Sympathectomy, arterial reconstruction, or both, will sometimes enable a conservative amputation to

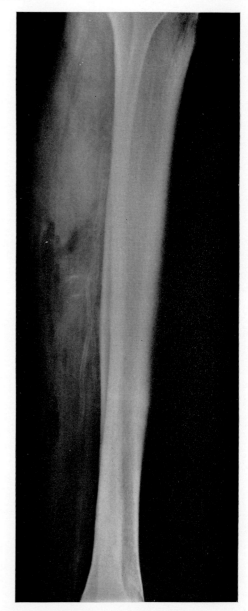

Fig. 5.8. Gas formation in the calf muscles in an elderly diabetic subject, as a complication of the infective gangrenous lesion of the heel shown in Fig. 5.3. Note calcified tibial arteries.

succeed in patients who otherwise would have needed a major ablation [30]. Good care and the passage of time may be sufficient in a patient recovering from acute ischaemia, when the re-establishment blood flow may reach the line of demarcation on the

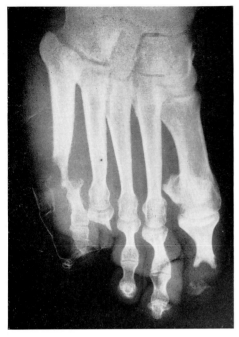 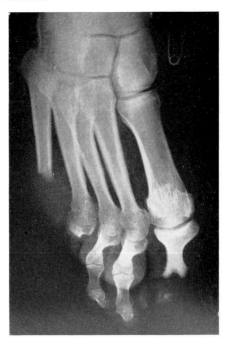

Fig. 5.9. Chronic osteomyelitis of the 5th metatarsal and of neuropathic 4th and 5th toe joints. Primary healing with excision and debridement.

forefoot. Arteriography may help to decide the line of section [2]. Amputations through the toe often do well in these improved ischaemia patients, as well as transmetatarsal or mid-tarsal removal of the whole forefoot, though among 366 such patients the failure rate was one-third [29].

In non-ischaemic patients, local surgery need not be so cautious, and free incision and excision are permissible in the drainage of pus, or the removal *en bloc* of gangrenous areas. Delayed closure by suture or skin grafting usually succeeds [8A]. With an intractable neuropathic ulcer, the whole of the skin area in which sensation is lost may be excised [15]. Toes may be excised at the metatarsal joint: it is sometimes best to remove all rather than one [21]. The transmetatarsal amputation gives excellent results in this type of diabetic gangrene, for which it was first introduced [15]. Great care must be taken after amputation or arterial surgery to prevent a pressure sore developing on the opposite heel or malleoli. The whole limb should be suspended from a beam in well-padded slings [21].

Prognosis and the Results of Treatment

Limb-prognosis in chronic ischaemia is worse when diabetes is present. At Mayo Clinic, a ten-year follow up of 500 patients with lower limb ischaemia showed a 10 per cent amputation rate overall, but among the diabetics the figure was 27 per cent [19]. A repetition of events on the opposite side, leading to a second leg amputation, often within a year or two, is characteristic of diabetic ischaemia, occurring in as many as 25 per cent [8, 27]. The average survival time for one group of patients was five and a half years [8]. The same prognostic significance attaches to diabetes as regards the mortality and end-results of direct arterial surgery, both of which have been found to be several times worse in diabetes than in non-diabetic arteriosclerotics [10]. Yet the results of active, modern treatment are encouraging. The following cases show what is now possible in a condition that only ten years ago so often led to a mid-thigh amputation.

Three Typical Cases

CASE 1: *Severe ischaemia. A 'rescue operation'*
A well-controlled diabetic man of seventy with severe left hemiparesis, developed acute ischaemia of the

119

right lower limb, upon which he depended for his mobility. The limb was cold, pale, weak, and pulseless below the groin. Arteriography (Fig. 5.10)

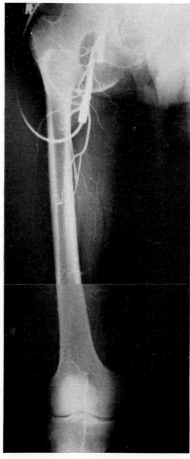

Fig. 5.10. Severe acute ischaemia in a frail elderly diabetic subject. Poor filling of narrowed distal arteries. Good result from emergency femoro-popliteal bypass graft with a knitted dacron prosthesis.

showed a long femoro-popliteal occlusion. A by-pass graft of knitted dacron was inserted, with full restoration of the circulation, which remained so in the four years that followed.

Comment: An unfavourable case in which an early operation saved an important limb. Diabetes was incidental, and in no way contra-indicated the operation.

CASE 2: *Ischaemic gangrene with neuropathy*
An obese, hypertensive woman aged seventy de-

veloped intermittent claudication in the right calf. Six weeks later she noticed discoloration of the forefoot and some pain. Glycosuria was discovered

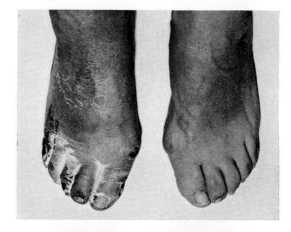

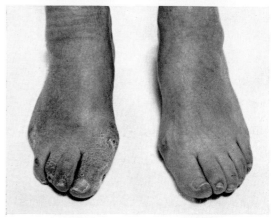

Fig. 5.11. Ischaemic neuropathic gangrene in a recently diagnosed diabetic. Good response to grafting a short popliteal block.

at this stage, also reduction of the lower limb reflexes. Frank gangrene soon affected the hallux, middle and little toes (Fig. 5.11, *upper*) and led to arteriography which showed an upper popliteal occlusion with much tibial disease also. A short femoro-popliteal vein by-pass graft was inserted. At once the foot became hot and pain ceased. Good result at two years (Fig. 5.11, *lower*).

Comment: Neuropathy often shows itself in recently diagnosed patients. In this one the spread of gangrene was quickly checked by combined and concentrated attack on infection, neuropathy, and the arterial block.

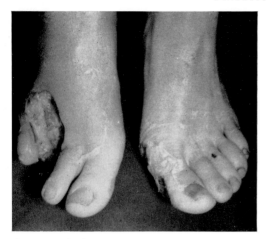

Fig. 5.12. Infective neuropathic gangrene in a middle-aged diabetic, all of whose peripheral pulses were strongly present.

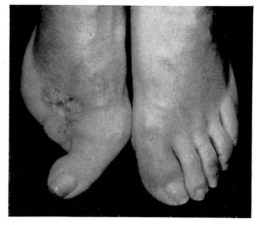

Fig. 5.13. The feet of the same patient as Fig. 5.12 following in-patient local care and minor skin grafting.

CASE 3

A long-distance lorry driver aged fifty-four was forgetful about his insulin injections and neglected to report the painless, spreading ulceration of both forefeet and the right heel (Fig. 5.12). Strong pulses were present in all four tibial arteries at the ankle level, and the feet were warm and dry. Gross sensory and reflex signs of neuropathy were present. With rest in hospital, antibiotics by systemic and local administration, close supervision of his diabetes, and the provision of some split skin cover, full healing took place (Fig. 5.13).

Comment: This patient suffered minor recurrences of his foot condition until he changed his job to local driving; the work is lighter, and he could cope with his diabetic life, with regular visits to the outpatient clinic.

Conclusion

The warm, dry, and painless foot, showing necrosis only at pressure areas, is usually neuropathic and should improve with local and diabetic care. The cold, discoloured painful foot requires treatment of the ischaemia, which is the principal cause of symptoms. In both forms the control of infection may be decisive. Diabetic gangrene is a complex condition in which major occlusive arterial disease, lesions in small vessels, and sensory neuropathy may each play an important part. To be successful, treatment must take all these possibilities into account.

REFERENCES

1. Annotation (1964) Diabetic neuropathy. *Lancet*, **ii**, 1002.
2. Baddeley, R. M. and Fulford, J. C. (1964) The use of arteriography in conservative amputations for lesions of the feet in diabetes mellitus. *Brit. J. Surg.*, **51**, 658.
3. Barraclough, M. A. and Sharpey-Schafer, E. P. (1963) Hypotension from absent circulatory reflexes. *Lancet*, **i**, 1121.
4. Beckett, A. G. and Lewis, J. G. (1960) Mobilisation and utilisation of body-fat as an aetiological factor in occlusive vascular disease in diabetes mellitus. *Lancet*, **ii**, 14.
5. Blumenthal, H. T., Berns, A. W., Goldenberg, S. and Lowenstein, P. W. (1966) Etiologic considerations in peripheral vascular diseases of the lower extremity, with special reference to diabetes mellitus. *Circulation*, **33**, 98.
6. Bridges, J. M., Dalby, A. M., Millar, J. H. D. and Weaver, J. A. (1965) An effect of d-glucose on platelet stickiness. *Lancet*, **i**, 75.
6A. Brightmore, T. (1971) Non-clostridial gas infection. *Proc. Roy. Soc. Med.*, **64**, 1084.
7. Bronte-Stewart, B. (1965) Epidemiology and dietary factors in occlusive vascular disease. *Ann. Roy. Coll. Surg. Eng.*, **36**, 206.
8. Cameron, H. C., Lennard-Jones, J. E. and Robinson, M. P. (1964) Amputations in the diabetic. Outcome and survival. *Lancet*, **ii**, 605.
8A. Catterall, R. F. C. (1968) Vascular disease and diabetes. The surgeon's viewpoint. *Postgrad. med. J. Suppl.*, p. 969.
9. Fearnley, G. R., Chakrabarti, R. and Avis, P. R. D. (1963) Blood fibrinolytic activity in diabetes mellitus and its bearing on ischaemic heart disease and obesity. *Brit. med. J.*, **i**, 921.

9A. Fredrickson, D. S. (1967) Mutations and hyperlipid-aemia. In *Arteriosclerotic Vascular Disease*. (Ed.: Brest, A. N. and Moyer, J. H.) New York: Appleton-Century-Crofts, p. 158.

10. Gensler, S. W., Haimovici, H., Hoffert, P., Steinman, C. and Beneventano, T. C. (1965) Study of vascular lesions in diabetic, nondiabetic patients. *Arch. Surg.*, **91**, 617.

11. Ghilchik, M. W. and Morris, A. S. (1971) Abnormal insulin response in patients with small-vessel disease. *Lancet*, **ii**, 1227.

12. Ismail, A. A., Khalifa, K. and Madwar, K. R. (1965) Capillary loss of radio-iodinated serum albumen in diabetics. *Lancet*, **ii**, 810.

13. Juergens, J. L., Barker, N. W. and Hines, E. A. (1960) Arteriosclerosis obliterans: review of 520 cases with special reference to pathogenic and prognostic factors. *Circulation*, **21**, 188.

14. Lundbaek, K. (1954) Diabetic angiopathy, a specific vascular disease. *Lancet*, **i**, 377.

15. McKittrick, L. S., McKittrick, J. B. and Risley, T. S. (1949) Transmetatarsal amputation for infection or gangrene in patients with diabetes mellitus. *Ann. Surg.*, **130**, 826.

15A. Martin, F. I. R. and Stocks, A. E. (1968) Insulin sensitivity and vascular disease in insulin-dependent diabetics. *Brit. med. J.*, **2**, 81.

16. Miller, H. (1966) Polyneuritis. *Brit. med. J.*, **ii**, 1219.

17. Moore, J. M. and Frew, I. D. O. (1965) Peripheral vascular lesion in diabetes mellitus. *Brit. med. J.*, **ii**, 19.

18. Moorhouse, J. A., Carter, S. A. and Doupe, J. (1966) Vascular responses in diabetic peripheral neuropathy. *Brit. med. J.*, **i**, 883.

19. McPherson, J. R., Juergens, J. L. and Gifford, R. W. (1963) Thrombo-angiitis obliterans and arteriosclerosis obliterans. Clinical and prognostic differences. *Ann. Int. Med.*, **59**, 288.

20. Oakley, W. (1954). Diabetes in surgery. *Ann. Roy. Coll. Surg. Eng.*, **15**, 108.

21. Oakley, W., Catterall, R. C. F. and Martin, M. M. (1956) Aetiology and management of lesions of the feet in diabetes. *Brit. med. J.*, **ii**, 953.

22. Ostrander, L. D., Francis, T., Hayner, N. S., Kjelsberg, M. O. and Epstein, F. H. (1965) The relationship of cardiovascular disease to hyperglycemia. *Ann. Int. Med.*, **62**, 1188.

23. Schadt, D. C., Hines, E. A., Juergens, J. L. and Barker, N. W. (1961) Chronic atherosclerotic occlusion of the femoral artery. *J. Amer. Med. Assoc.*, **175**, 937.

24. Skovborg, F., Neilsen, Aa. V., Schlichtkrull, J. and Ditzel, J. (1966) Blood-viscosity in diabetic patients. *Lancet*, **i**, 129.

25. Swank, R. L. and Cullen, C. F. (1953) Circulatory changes in the hamster's cheek pouch associated with alimentary lipemia. *Proc. Soc. Exp. Biol. Med.*, **82**, 381.

26. Sharpey-Schafer, E. P. and Taylor, P. J. (1960) Absent circulatory reflexes in diabetic neuritis. *Lancet*, **i**, 559.

27. Smith, B. C. (1956) A twenty-year follow-up in fifty below knee amputations for gangrene in diabetics. *Surg. Gynec. Obstet.*, **103**, 625.

28. Wahlberg, F. (1962) The intravenous glucose tolerance test in atherosclerotic disease with special reference to obesity, hypertension, diabetic heredity and cholesterol values. *Acta med. Scand.*, **171**, 1.

28A. Wahlberg, F. (1966) Intravenous glucose tolerance in myocardial infarction, angina pectoris and intermittent claudication. *Acta med. Scand. Suppl.*, **453**, 51.

29. Wheelock, F. C., McKittrick, J. B. and Root, H. F. (1957) Evaluation of the transmetatarsal amputation in patients with diabetes mellitus. *Surgery*, **41**, 184.

30. Wheelock, F. C. and Filtzer, H. S. (1969) Femoral grafts in diabetics. Resulting conservative amputations. *Arch. Surg.*, **99**, 776.

6 Amputations

Indications for Amputation in Vascular Patients

Ablation of a limb is the antithesis of all that the arterial surgeon hopes to achieve for his patient, yet it must often be done to save life. Whenever an extremity is hopelessly damaged by ischaemia, injury, or infection the appropriate type of amputation must be undertaken without delay. Lesser degrees of damage justify early amputation when recovery and rehabilitation depend upon it. *Pain* may hasten the decision or, in severe ischaemia, the absorption of *toxic products* of soft tissue damage with obvious general deterioration and the possibility of renal damage. *Infection* may spread quickly in diabetes, and after injury, when anerobes may be responsible.

Massive ischaemia occurs in ill patients with high-level arterial thrombosis or embolism, or after ligation at the limb-root; nowadays a failed arterial reconstruction is sometimes the cause (Fig. 15.10, p. 283). Unless the ischaemia can be positively corrected, amputation should not be delayed once the extent of irreversible change can be seen.

The same is true of extensive damage to tissues and their blood supply resulting from *injuries* or from the explosive *rupture of a large peripheral arterial aneurysm.* Other vascular diseases incurable except by amputation include some massive *arterio-venous fistulae,* especially those which develop, or recur in an amputation stump, and some extensive congenital cases with unmanageable complications. Venous insufficiency from fistula, or following massive venous occlusion may be so severe as to be treatable only in this way. The same is true of some late cases of *lymphoedema* when ulceration or verruca are extensive and pain is unbearable. *Primary malignancy* may be present, as in the upper limb in some longstanding cases of post-mastectomy oedema.

Choosing the Level of Section

Only in recent years have alternatives to the mid-thigh operation come to be considered correct practice in the treatment of the gangrenous lower limb. Previously, even minor neerosis in the foot was sufficient to justify this major ablation.

We know now, that almost always the site of amputation is clearly indicated by factors that can be accurately assessed before operation. These are as follows:

1. The level of the main arterial occlusion.
2. The extent of ischaemic damage and the rate at which it develops.
3. Whether infection is present.
4. The general condition of the patient.

The first two generally go together, but not always, for secondary distal occlusions often augment the main vessel ischaemia locally (*see* Chapter 3, p. 38) and may compromise one of the proposed flaps. Figure 6.1 shows some common main arterial occlusions and the amputations they may require. Acute aorto-iliac closure, and sometimes also the loss of common femoral, may require mid-thigh section, although both these sites are favourable for reconstruction of the artery, which should almost always be attempted unless the artery is hopelessly diseased

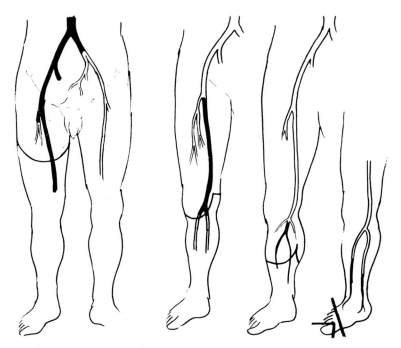

Fig. 6.1. Level of amputation required for severe ischaemia, with corresponding extent of arterial occlusion shown in black.

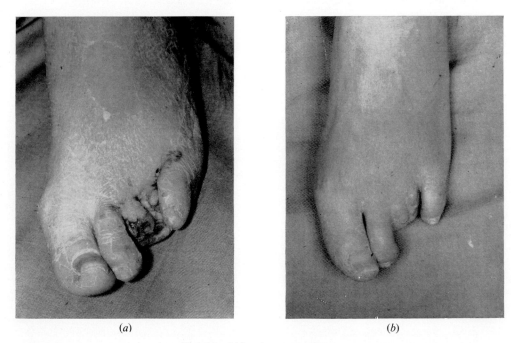

(a)　　　　　　　　　　　　　　　　　　(b)

Fig. 6.2. *Ad hoc* toe amputation.

(a) At time of first dressing. Note irregular flaps loosely opposed by a single stainless-steel wire suture. The skin changes over the rest of the foot are those of recently recovered severe ischaemia following popliteal endarterectomy.

(b) This good result has been maintained for nine years.

or there is extensive secondary thrombosis, with tissue damage of corresponding severity. Mid-thigh operation should not often be called for today, except in some aged patients with thrombosis, and after failed arterial surgery, or massive embolism seen too late or in which delay is to blame. This operation now begins to assume the character of a surgical reproach.

When the common and deep femoral arteries are spared, a through-knee amputation will nearly always be successful. Here the line of section consists of little more than skin, tendons, ligaments, and the neurovascular bundle; the procedure is therefore much less traumatic than when the large muscles of the thigh are cut across at their widest point.

Whenever possible the knee should be spared; this is possible in most femoro-popliteal cases. The anterior flap is usually more ischaemic, so a long posterior muscle-based flap [1B, 5B] should be remembered as a useful solution when the shin is cool or of a poor colour. Failure occurs in 20–30 per cent [1E, 1F, 5B], though less often in diabetic patients, who often retain their popliteal pulse [1F].

Gangrene of the toes, when due to plantar or tibial occlusion without any more proximal obstruction, should prove suitable for digital or transmetatarsal amputation, as in Buerger's disease, frostbite, or arteriosclerotic gangrene after successful restoration of the main arterial occlusion, or digital arterial occlusion from athero-embolism (*see* Chapter 3, p. 38). With good timing and a meticulous technique, toe amputations should succeed in most cases of this type, also in diabetic gangrene of the milder kind (Figs. 6.2 and 5.11, p. 120).

Finger amputations for ischaemia are somewhat rare, though the causes are similar to those mentioned for the toes. Slow separation of a lateral digital slough is more often seen, for though, locally, the blood supply may be seriously reduced, the remarkable collateral circulation of which the upper limb is capable usually ensures localisation and repair. Elective finger amputations heal well, for the same reason.

Conservative amputations for ischaemia are attractive in principle, and frequently succeed in correctly selected patients. No incision, however, should be made near any area of skin rubor, or ulceration with resistant infection, or, as a general rule, far from a palpable pulse, though arteriography may give more accurate information as a basis for planned conservative ablation with good prospects of healing (Fig. 6.3). Arterial reconstruction should ensure a more satisfactory outcome after a distal amputation than if the main artery remains occluded (Fig. 6.4). Special indications for conservative amputations in diabetic gangrene are discussed in Chapter 5.

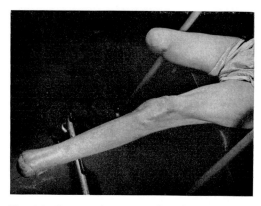

Fig. 6.3. Conservative amputations for symmetrical painful gangrene of both forefeet. Right: Stokes-Gritti, Left: Syme's.

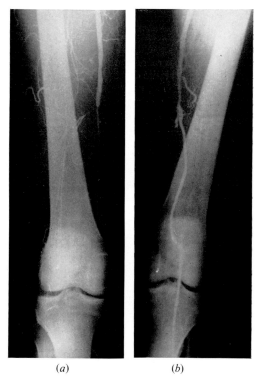

(a)   (b)

Fig. 6.4. Arteriograms of the patient shown in Fig. 6.3.

(*a*) Femoro-popliteal occlusion extending throughout calf though with good collateral branches to the skin of the knee. A good case for through-knee amputation.

(*b*) The left femoro-popliteal occlusion spared the lower popliteal, and a vein graft could be inserted. Syme's amputation healed well in consequence, and vein graft remained patent for seven years.

Infection near the intended flap or in the lymphatics entering the wound from distal parts should contra-indicate any elective amputation in the region. Treating the infection and leaving open flaps with an excess of skin and underlying tissue may be successful, and are useful, in infective diabetic gangrene.

The general condition of the patient is usually decisive. Poor cardiorespiratory reserve, 'brittle' diabetes, postoperative depletion or shock mean that the simplest course must be chosen. Venous insufficiency may cause swelling and necrosis of the skin flaps whose arterial supply is inadequate. Healing of such a stump may be helped by elevating it.

Chilling or freezing the extremity [1, 6, 13A], when once a major amputation becomes inevitable, may provide valuable time during which the patient's general condition may improve, and the collateral circulation to the proposed amputation flaps. Normally, ice cubes are applied, in a plastic bag. Using solid CO_2, amputation can be postponed almost indefinitely, as putrefaction cannot take place at these very low temperatures. This method of deliberate, vigorous chilling or freezing of mortally damaged tissues is quite different from the common practice of air cooling, using an electric fan, which aims, quite wrongly in the author's view, at conserving vitality in a hand or foot in severe but not hopeless ischaemia. Such cold exposure can hardly be less damaging to a critically ischaemic limb than it is known to be when applied to healthy subjects such as sea survivors or mountaineers. The fact that freezing temperatures are not reached is no safeguard in either circumstance.

Exploration for Reconstruction or Amputation

If arteriography should show medium entering part of the main artery (usually the popliteal) below the occlusion (Fig. 6.4), and the patient is ready to accept the amputation he will probably need, it may be worth while to explore the occluded artery,

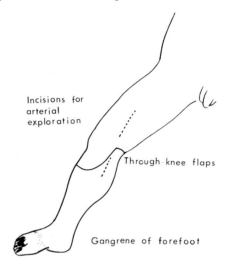

Incisions for arterial exploration

Through-knee flaps

Gangrene of forefoot

Fig. 6.5. Exploration of the femoral or popliteal artery in severe ischaemia should avoid skin likely to be required for amputation flaps.

limiting this first incision and placing it so that it will not interfere with the positioning of amputation flaps should the artery prove to be unsuitable for reconstruction (Fig. 6.5).

General Points in Technique

Meticulous, deliberate operating, with clean sharp incision of the layers and the minimum possible handling and retraction of the tissues should give the best chance of primary healing. Penicillin should be given in full systemic dosage to cover the operative period, and at least a week afterwards. This will minimise the otherwise real danger of gas gangrene as a complication of major amputation for limb ischaemia.

No tourniquet is ever necessary in ischaemia, except rarely when gangrene is due to injury, arteriovenous fistula, or ruptured peripheral aneurysm. A second assistant holds the limb, and an extra, horizontal spotlight should be ready to focus upon the open end of the stump. Judgement and experience are required in planning the flaps. It is wise to base these a little proximal to the proposed line of bone section so that, later, they will fold back well clear of the saw. The skin is never undercut; nor must it be gripped with dissecting forceps. The deep fascia is cut in the same line as the skin, and the muscles are then boldly bevelled in to the bone. In this way, the remaining circulation to the flaps is left undisturbed. At this stage the flaps should be moulded between the hands of the operator so as to lie comfortably around the bone, whose correct point of section can then be chosen (Fig. 6.6).

A few muscular arteries may bleed, particularly in the thigh—from the profunda femoris branches, also from the artery of the sciatic nerve. These should be ligated finely (not diathermised). The main artery does not bleed, but its accompanying vein usually does, and so must be securely ligated. Catgut should be used for all buried ligatures and sutures. After

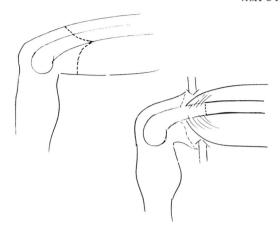

Fig. 6.6. To ensure good apposition of musculo-cutaneous flaps in thigh and calf amputations, these are held in against the bone whose correct line of section can then be selected.

spraying with antibiotic, the deep fascia beneath the flaps is approximated so that these lie together accurately. There is a trend towards myoplastic repair of opposing muscles [2]. Catgut sutures are used, of adequate strength, placing all knots deep to the fascia. A vacuum drainage tube is passed beneath the flaps, and its end is brought out at the lateral extremity of the wound. The skin is now closed, using vertical mattress sutures of 36 gauge stainless steel wire, or adhesive strips of polymer, either of which can be left in place indefinitely without causing any reaction in the skin. The vacuum drain is secured with an encircling stitch of black silk that can easily be seen and cut without taking down the whole dressing when the tube is removed on the second day; it should not be delayed beyond the fifth day otherwise there will be discomfort and possible damage from the pressure of the hardened clot in the gauze.

STANDARD AMPUTATIONS THROUGH THE LOWER LIMB

The general procedure is as already described; some special points apply to each site:

1. Toes

For stable, dry gangrene it is often sufficient to snip off the toe through its dead portion, using bone forceps. In diabetic gangrene, unorthodox flaps, their shape determined by the line of separation, if loosely sutured after filleting the toe, will generally heal well (Fig. 6.2).

If the blood supply to the foot is considered sufficient, a formal amputation is preferable. The flaps must clear the head of the metatarsal without tension: usually they should encircle the skin at the base of the toe, joining the adjacent webs. The dorsal 'racquet' extension is quite unsuitable for ischaemic cases. The fifth toe is difficult: the metatarsal head tends to project between the flaps and may have to be removed, though this may harm the flaps.

2. Transmetatarsal (Fig. 6.7) [18]

This is an exacting operation requiring experience and attention to detail, but it is so useful that its technique should be mastered. The essentials are: a healthy dorsum to the foot, and the cutting of a long, thick plantar flap (Fig. 6.8).

The dorsal cut is made straight across and down to periosteum, a little proximal to the metatarsal heads, without dissection or mobilisation of any of the structures or layers. The plantar flap is curved along near the toe webs and is bevelled obliquely and cleanly with a sharp scalpel upwards towards the metatarsal necks, and then on into the deep hollow

formed by the transverse arch of the anterior ends of the metatarsal shafts (Fig. 6.9), now directing the cut deeply inwards, almost at right angles to the bones.

Unless at this stage fresh bleeding can be seen coming from the soft tissues of both flaps, it is better to abandon the procedure. Pale ischaemic flaps, oozing slightly from stagnant veins, can never survive. If there is doubt, the next step may decide: the metatarsals are divided with a small saw or large bone forceps at, or slightly proximal to, the dorsal skin cut, using rongeurs to shorten the bones if the flaps seem at all tight. They must be carefully protected during the bone section. At this point, fresh bleeding from the divided interosseous structures confirms that the deep blood supply is maintained; perfusion of the flaps should soon improve.

Closure is meticulous, and in two layers, the inverted catgut sutures help to secure the long plantar flap over the end of the stump, and take most of the strain from the fine wire used for the skin (Fig. 6.10). No suture should be tight. Drainage is often necessary.

3. Syme's amputation [1, 4] (Figs. 6.3, 6.11)

This amputation has a restricted place in ischaemia, for if the blood supply will not support healing of a transmetatarsal operation, neither, as a rule, can the extensively dissected heel flap of the Syme operation be hoped to survive. Healing may take place in some cases of distal occlusion or after a proximal block has been restored. In such patients the good prospects for this useful weight-bearing amputation

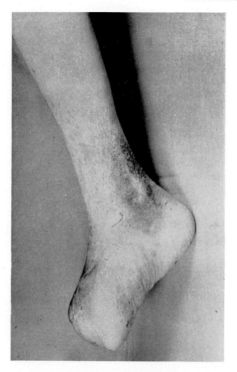

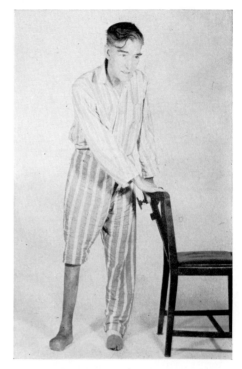

Fig. 6.7. Early weight-bearing by an elderly subject after transmetatarsal amputation made possible by recent femoro-popliteal vein graft (Mr J. R. Kenyon's case). (*See also* Fig. 3.7, p. 37.)

should always be kept in mind. A lumbar sympathectomy may help.

4. Below Knee (Fig. 6.12) [1E, 1F]
Except in infected diabetic cases it is seldom necessary to leave long, open flaps. Primary closure is preferable, and usually possible. Antero-posterior flaps give the best cover to the bone ends, which can be shorter than the classical 7 inches; as little as 4

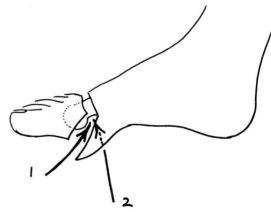

Fig. 6.9. Deeper dissection of flaps; dorsal by guillotine cut; plantar by: (1) sharp bevelling a good thickness of muscles and ligaments of the sole within the flap; (2) a vertical scalpel cut deeply into the transverse metatarsal arch, down to bone.

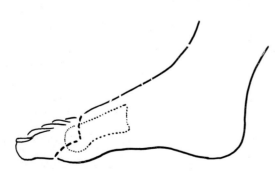

Fig. 6.8. Long plantar, and transverse dorsal flaps for transmetatarsal amputation.

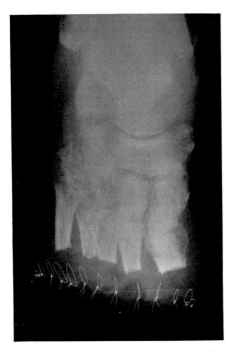

Fig. 6.10. A proximal transmetatarsal amputation for Buerger's disease. Healing, though slow, was much assisted by the retention of stainless-steel wire skin sutures for over a month.

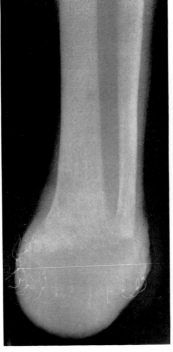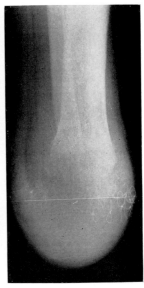

Fig. 6.11. Syme's amputation; retaining maximum area of transected tibial medial malleolus and cartilage surface. Good healing in an elderly subject with severe ischaemia following femoral artery reconstruction.

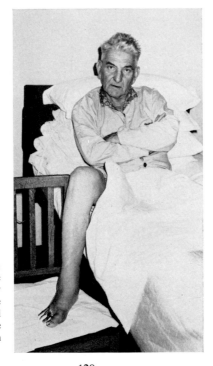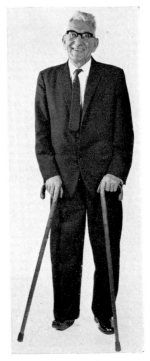

Fig. 6.12. Gangrene of right toes with severe ischaemia of foot due to extensive femoro-popliteal occlusion. Mobility regained on temporary below-knee prosthesis. On the day of the second picture, six weeks after operation, the patient had hung a door in his room single-handed.

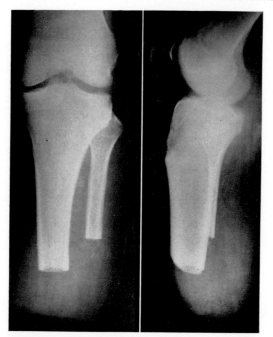

Fig. 6.13. Correct bone and soft tissue shaping for below-knee amputation.

inches is satisfactory [3]. Lateral flaps may conserve the blood supply of the anterior part of the stump because they can be cut much thicker [3, 9], but a longer posterior flap probably does this better [1B, 1F, 5B]. With any method the fibula is cut first, and higher (Fig. 6.13); in a very short stump it may be excised. The tibia must be bevelled, and all edges of its cut end must be filed smooth and round, including the posterior border. Healing should take place in 80 per cent of non-diabetic patients (1F, 1G). In diabetes, as with most other conservative amputations, results are surprisingly good, as many as 98 per cent of below-knee sections healing well [1G]. The advent of the patellar tendon bearing prosthesis has improved results [10].

5. Through Knee

Both the standard amputations at this level use a long anterior flap whose blood supply is usually good, and a straight transverse cut above the knee posteriorly. End weight-bearing is now allowed [4].

The *Stokes-Gritti* operation (Figs. 6.2, 6.14) [7] is preferable in many cases, as the long anterior flap maintains the important connection with the patella with its sizeable collaterals, and fits well over the end of the stump. Drilling and wiring give better fixation to the bones than suturing with catgut: non-union

of the freshened patello-femoral surfaces should never happen, but it is a common and painful complication of this amputation unless secure wire fixation is used. Bone ischaemia may be responsible [9].

This amputation gives good control and muscular leverage, and retains a useful amount of proprioception so that mobility with or without prosthesis is much better than after mid-thigh section which destroys most of the natural use of the thigh muscles. (Bedsores, already present before the amputation will heal, with the relief of painful immobility, once the patient can move about in bed.)

The transarticular operation has its advocates [3, 4, 5A, 7B] and offers simplicity and the advantage, in infected cases, that there is no bone cut. The flaps are somewhat difficult to plan to fit well over the large bulbous end of the femoral condyles, whether equal antero-posterior (Fig. 6.15), or with a long anterior flap (Fig. 6.16) with good weight-bearing potential, as in the Stokes-Gritti operation. Skin necrosis is common. Between 50 per cent [1C] and 80 per cent [5A, 7B] heal well; the difference no doubt reflects case selection.

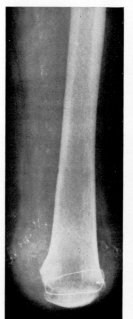
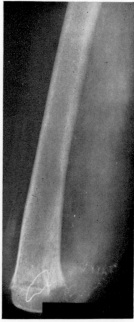

Fig. 6.14. The Stokes-Gritti amputation, with wire fixation of the cut bony surfaces of the patella and femur, conserves the action of most of the long muscles of the thigh. The long anterior flap containing the patella and covered with special skin form a natural weight-bearing surface, and healing of the posterior suture line is usually good.

130

6. Mid-thigh and Above

These are technically simple and heal well [3A]. Shock may be considerable, and disability much greater than with the more distal amputations. Phantom pain is commoner and more distressing.

Causes of Failure

Necrosis of one or both skin flaps may take place during the days between removal of the drain and removal of the sutures. It is usually accompanied by pain. The causes are:

1. *Technical Errors.* Cutting the flaps too short or the bone too long, so that the stitches must be too tight if they are to close the wound; some tissue strangulation must occur as a result. Oedema of the stump may aggravate the condition.
2. *Insufficient Blood Supply.* Although the flaps may be well-fashioned, there may be insufficient blood flow within them to ensure good healing. This should not happen if the patient has been carefully assessed before operation, though it may be due to further arterial thrombosis following it. Venous insufficiency, shock and heart failure may impair the micro-circulation as severely as arterial ischaemia.
3. *Haematoma* due to lack of haemostasis or to inefficient drainage causes tension under the flaps and leads to necrosis, centred over the haematoma. If the first dressing is unduly delayed the hard coagulum on the gauze may cause local pressure necrosis.
4. *Infection* usually follows when one or more of these three factors damages the flaps and should, therefore, be avoidable, though in some cases of conservative amputation, with a line of section not far from the line of demarcation, infection may be present from the time of operation.

Most serious of all is the development of *gas gangrene.* This is a real risk after major amputation, e.g. through the thigh, where a large ischaemic muscle mass may have been enclosed beneath over-tightly sutured skin with clostridial contamination from the nearby anus, either at the time of operation, or shortly afterwards via a drainage tube. Pressure from an early ambulation plaster cast may also contribute to this disaster, but the omission of penicillin from the scheme of treatment is the most usual finding [8A]. It is probably true that, as with haemolytic streptococcal infection, penicillin in high

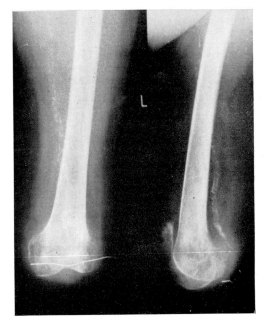

Fig. 6.15. Through-knee amputation with nearly equal antero-posterior flaps, the line of the incision being marked by the opaque wire.

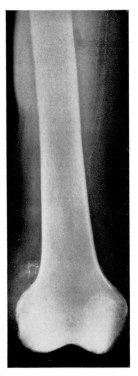
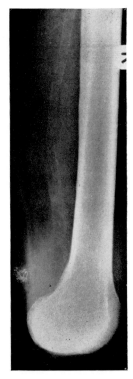

Fig. 6.16. Through-knee amputation with long anterior flap. Removal of the patella may damage the blood supply to this.

dosage is also the most effective preventive measure against gas gangrene, yet these infections still occur, either from omission of antibiotics altogether [3A] or because broad-spectrum agents are used instead of penicillin. Hyperbaric oxygen has reduced the mortality of established gas gangrene from over 50 per cent to less than 15 per cent [7A].

Other Complications

Lack of progress, with general depression and decline, poor stump movements, and progressive flexion contracture may be due to senility or other constitutional causes, but pain is the usual reason, and the fault most often lies in the surgery, from faulty case-selection or mistakes in technique.

Nevertheless, there is a fairly high general morbidity and mortality after peripheral vascular amputations [12], with death in 10 to 18 per cent of cases, many of which are due to pulmonary embolism or other vascular complications [9, 15] often associated with failure of the operation as well, a catastrophe that may happen in almost a third of a large series at a first-class centre [8].

Good medical care, better choice of operation, and perhaps the use of preventive anticoagulant treatment after drainage has ceased, may help to reduce the danger and suffering in these patients.

Upper-limb Amputations

These are not often required for arterial disease. Conservatism should be the deciding factor in all cases in order to preserve function. Secondary operations are often justifiable, for they do not immobilise the patient. Cooperation with a plastic surgeon may prove the means for remarkable function: e.g. using skin tunnels for loops to moving parts, or to dispense with a prosthesis by fashioning the forearm into the split lobster claw or Krukenberg-shape which offers good grip and sensation [3]. In some patients the hand prosthesis is fitted with interchangeable tools.

Rehabilitation and Limb-fitting [2A, 3, 3A, 5, 14, 16, 17]

No patient is too old to use a prosthesis. In an otherwise fit subject, whatever the age, a healthy painless stump should be anticipated for limb fitting as soon as possible after the operation, or even before it [1E, 2A]. A temporary pylon may be constructed in the hospital, using plaster of Paris and other light materials [17]. Physiotherapy is directed towards developing movements important in the subsequent use of the new limb. (Adduction and extension of the mid-thigh stump; and strong, full extension below the knee.) Limb-fitting techniques are changing [10]: surgeons no longer need always excise the knee; long femoral stumps with total weight-bearing are now favoured, likewise the patellar tendon bearing below-knee socket, both recent advances in simplification and improvement of limb design. Early mobility and weight-bearing are now commonplace (Figs. 6.7, 6.12).

Phantom Pain. Vivid sensations from the lost extremity occur from time to time in most patients. In some, they cause mental distress, though seldom from persistence of pre-operative pain. Explanation and reassurance are usually sufficient. Active treatment is needed in only the worst cases. In such, there may be feelings of distortion of size or position, together with intervals of pain that are described as very severe. Analgesics should be used only with great caution for this condition. Percussion of an amputation neuroma is sometimes helpful, and so is periarterial sympathectomy. Re-amputation should not be advised. Recent reports on the topical use of dimethyl sulphoxide (DMSO) show promise [13].*

Limb Fitting [14]

In Great Britain, high standards have been set by the Ministry of Health limb-fitting centres. It is the important duty of surgeons and physiotherapists to help the special centres by good preparation of the patient and his stump and by supporting the policies and recommendations of the centre throughout the patient's hospital treatment. Nevertheless, it is a distressing fact that 30 to 50 per cent of lower limb amputees die within two years [1A, 2A, 3B] and that, of the survivors, a half subsequently lose the other limb. Age, diabetes and widespread arterial disease are responsible. Fewer than half of a followed-up group were actively ambulant [3B].

---

* 15 ml of 90 per cent DMSO are applied morning and evening.

REFERENCES

1. Baker, C. W. and Stableforth, P. G. (1969) Syme's amputation. A review of 67 cases. *J. Bone Jt. Surg.*, **51B**, 482.

1A. Brodie, I. A. D. (1970) Lower limb amputation. *Brit. J. hosp. Med.*, **4**, 596.

1B. Burgess, E. M., Romano, R. L., Zettl, J. H. and Schrock, R. D. (1970) Amputations of the leg for peripheral vascular insufficiency. *J. Bone Jt. Surg.*, **53A**, 874.

1C. Chilvers, A. S., Briggs, J., Browse, N. L. and Kinmonth, J. B. (1971) Below- and through-knee amputations in ischaemic disease. *Brit. J. Surg.*, **58**, 824.

1D. Cohen, S. M. (1944) Amputation under ice anaesthesia. *Proc. Roy. Soc. Med.*, **37**, 232.

1E. Condon, R. E. and Jordan, P. H. (1969) Immediate postoperative prosthesis in vascular amputation. *Ann. Surg.*, **170**, 435.

1F. Condon, R. E. and Jordan, P. H. (1970) Below-knee amputation for arterial insufficiency. *Surg. Gynec. Obstet.*, **130**, 641.

1G. Cranley, J. J., Krause, R. J., Strasser, E. S. and Hafner, C. D. (1969) Below-the-knee amputation for arteriosclerosis obliterans with and without diabetes. *Arch. Surg.*, **98**, 77.

2. Dederich, R. (1967) Technique of myoplastic amputations. *Ann. Roy. Coll. Surg. Eng.*, **40**, 222.

2A. Devas, M. B. (1971) Early walking of geriatric amputees. *Brit. med. J.*, **1**, 394.

3. Gillis, L. (1954) *Amputations.* London: Heinemann, pp. 60 (disarticulation at the knee); 154 (the short below-knee stump); 304 (lateral flaps below the knee); 243 (Kineplastic forearm stumps); 251 (the Krukenberg forearm operation).

3A. Hall, H. R. and Shucksmith, H. S. (1971) The above-knee amputation for ischaemia. *Brit. J. Surg.*, **58**, 656.

3B. Hamilton, E. A. and Nichols, P. J. R. (1972) Rehabilitation of the elderly lower-limb amputee. *Brit. med. J.*, **2**, 95.

4. Harding, H. E. (1967) Knee disarticulation and Syme's amputation. *Ann. Roy. Coll. Surg. Eng.*, **40**, 235.

5. Harris, E. E. (1967) Early prosthetic rehabilitation. *Ann. Roy. Coll. Surg. Eng.*, **40**, 266.

5A. Howard, R. R. S., Chamberlain, J. and Macpherson, A. I. S. (1969) Through-knee amputation in peripheral vascular disease. *Lancet*, **ii**, 240.

5B. Hunter-Craig, I., Vitali, M. and Robinson, K. P. (1970) Long posterior-flap amputation in peripheral vascular disease. *Brit. J. Surg.*, **57**, 62.

6. Johnstone, F. R. C. (1964) The use of dry ice in the refrigeration of gangrenous extremities. *Amer. Surg.*, **30**, 830.

7. Martin, P. and Wickham, J. E. A. (1962) Gritti-Stokes amputation for atherosclerotic gangrene. *Lancet*, **ii**, 16.

7A. Maudsley, R. and Arden, G. P. (1959) Postoperative gas gangrene. *Brit. med. J.*, **4**, 301.

7B. Newcombe, J. F. and Marcuson, R. W. (1972) Through-knee amputation. *Brit. med. J.*, **2**, 95.

8. Otteman, M. G. and Stahlgren, L. H. (1965) Evaluation of factors which influence mortality and morbidity following major lower extremity amputations for arteriosclerosis. *Surg. Gynec. Obstet.*, **120**, 1217.

8A. Parker, M. T. (1969) Postoperative clostridial infections in Britain. *Brit. med. J.*, **3**, 671.

9. Perlow, S. (1962) Amputation for gangrene because of occlusive arterial disease. Results in 312 amputations. *Amer. J. Surg.*, **103**, 569.

10. Redhead, R. G. (1966) Recent developments in prosthetics. *Proc. Roy. Med.*, **59**, 3.

11. Robb, H. J., Jacobson, L. F. and Jordan, P. (1965) Midcalf amputation in the ischemic extremity. (Use of lateral and medial flap). *Arch. Surg.*, **91**, 506.

12. Schlitt, R. J. and Serlin, O. (1960) Lower extremity amputations in peripheral vascular disease. *Amer. J. Surg.*, **100**, 682.

13. Stewart, G. and Jacob, S. W. (1965) Use of dimethyl sulfoxide (DMSO) in the treatment of post-amputation pain. *Amer. Surg.*, **31**, 460.

13A. Still, J. M., Wray, C. H. and Moretz, W. H. (1970) Selective physiological amputation. A valuable adjunct in preparation for surgical amputation. *Ann. Surg.*, **171**, 143.

14. Symposium on limb ablation and limb replacement (1967) *Ann. Roy. Coll. Surg. Eng.*, **40**, 203–288.

15. Thompson, R. C., Delblanco, T. L. and McAllister, F. F. (1965) Complications following lower extremity amputation. *Surg. Gynec. Obstet.*, **120**, 301.

16. Vitali, M. (1966) Rehabilitation of the amputee. *Proc. Roy. Soc. Med.*, **59**, 1.

17. Vitali, M. and Redhead, R. G. (1967) The modern concept of the general management of amputee rehabilitation including immediate post-operative fitting. *Ann. Roy. Coll. Surg. Eng.*, **40**, 251.

18. Wheelock, F. C., McKittrick, J. B. and Root, H. F. (1957) Evaluation of the transmetatarsal amputation in patients with diabetes mellitus. *Surgery*, **41**, 184.

7 Arteritis

Definition. Arteritis is an inflammatory or proliferative cellular response in arteries of all sizes, from damaging factors, local or general, known, and unknown.

Mechanical Stress

A necrotising arteritis of the mesentery sometimes follows resection of an aortic coarctation. By 1963 [60] there were eighty-two cases in the literature of this condition which has become familiar in most cardiac surgical units [28A]. It occurs most often in boys of about ten. The gut arteries are stretched, and their medial coat is damaged [46]. Abdominal pain from about the third day, with a rising blood pressure and striking leucocytosis, if accompanied by peritoneal signs, will require operation, at which the bowel is found to be grossly hyperaemic. Later intervention in missed cases who fail to improve may show arterial thrombosis, ulceration, and gangrene, adhesions, and fistulae. If the diagnosis is made, and the need for operation is not evident from the local signs, the condition responds well to reserpine, and to phenoxybenzamine [28A].

Irradiation Damage

Arterial involvement in neoplastic disease of the neck or limb-root can lead to haemorrhage, thrombosis or aneurysm and the role of previous irradiation may be uncertain. In some cases the blame can be more definitely laid for such complications [30A], which follow three to seven years after treatment for a benign or early malignant condition (*see* Fig. 8.12, p. 154).

Infective Arteritis

Of all forms of arterial disease this is one of the most serious and difficult to treat.

Pyogenic Arteritis

This is most often due to direct spread from local sepsis, as in a compound fracture of a long bone; also from postoperative wound infection with a special risk in arterial surgery. Weakening of the wall of the artery is due to a spread of infection into its substance, and not to the mechanical effects of undrained pus, which is not usually present when the wound is explored. Secondary carcinomatous breakdown in cervical or inguinal lymph nodes, or a local malignant recurrence near an artery may erode the vessel wall in the same way. Massive secondary haemorrhage occurs when the softened media gives way, having usually been heralded by minor bleeding. Often, by this time, the organism can be grown from the blood stream, and clinical evidence of septicaemia may precede the haemorrhage, with high swinging fever, rigors, and great prostration. The spleen may be palpably enlarged, and red cells appear in the urine. Arterial blood culture is more often positive than venous [32].

Sepsis and Arterial Surgery

A *Staphyloccocus aureus* is usually responsible, of an antibiotic-resistant, 'hospital' strain often from organisms carried in the nose or skin flexures, or contamination in the implanted material, particularly an arterial homograft. Potential sources of infection should always be cultured before operation. Even highly resistant strains can usually be cleared away in a few days if the patient is given neomycin-bacitracin ointment to the nares, and hexachlorophene soap for use in the bath, also hibitane-spirit lotion to the skin flexures [64]. Prophylactic antibiotic treatment should be given only when a known infection or contamination persists after these measures and the effectiveness of the proposed therapeutic agent has been confirmed in the laboratory. Local antibiotic spray after simple cleansing of an infected lesion may eliminate a dangerous bacterial strain without danger of setting up resistance.

Sustained fever is the first warning. Patients to whom postoperative anticoagulant treatment has been commonly develop a large haematoma that may, at first, be correctly blamed for the pyrexia. The point at which sepsis takes its full place is uncertain, for there may be no local signs of infection, the swelling of the soft tissues being mainly from oedema and blood clot. Haemorrhage may be the first sign. The management of this catastrophe is discussed in Chapter 3.

Infection may show itself long after surgery as a cause of graft failure, with leakage from anastomosis or, in less acute cases, a mycotic type of false aneurysm may form. There may be multiple emboli to the lower limbs [35].

Infected Arteriosclerosis

'Atheromatous' ulceration into the media of a large artery may provide a breach and a foothold for the invasion of circulating bacteria, at first into the thrombus and debris of the surface layers, and then spreading into the unhealthy tissues of the sclerotic media. Sepsis outside the artery, for example a paravertebral abscess or peritoneal abscess near the aorta or iliac artery, may penetrate the outer layers of the diseased artery. Whichever path is taken by the infection, it ends by causing a mycotic aneurysm of the erosive type, or, worse still, a sudden fatal secondary haemorrhage, for example:

CASE REPORT
A man aged fifty-two underwent right hemicolectomy for recurrent starch granuloma. Six weeks later he died suddenly from intraperitoneal bleeding from just above the aortic bifurcation. The cause was found to be a perforated arteriosclerotic ulcer close to an abscess. The bowel anastomosis was intact.

A localised infective arteritis can be set up without apparent local cause, probably most often from blood-borne infection although, as in some cases of subacute bacterial endocarditis, the blood cultures may have been repeatedly negative. Usually in such patients the artery is already diseased or has been submitted to undue local wear and tear, as for example near a large arterio-venous fistula that becomes infected (*see* Chapter 16). This complication of mechanical stress and strain may explain why some synthetic cloth prostheses fail from late rupture at the anastomosis, with evidence of a low-grade infection around the separated suture line. An infected heart valve prosthesis may work itself loose, with fatal haemorrhage or aortic dissection; a Salmonella infection, long after surgery, was responsible in one patient [63].

Specific Bacterial Infections of Large Arteries

In recent years, a new pattern of disease has emerged, in which an arteriosclerotic lesion becomes infected with a more or less virulent, antibiotic-resistant organism, often one of the following:

1. *Salmonella cholerasuis* [59]
2. *Salmonella typhimurium* [35A, 66]
3. *Staphylococcus aureus* [6]

Destructive changes are accelerated which end in massive haemorrhage, either from a mycotic aneurysm or from acute arterial rupture, as in the patient described above.

Sometimes the persistent blood infection and arterial embolic manifestations [45] may follow a long course of the wrong antibiotic, as in the following:

CASE REPORT
A woman of thirty-five, living in the Middle East, became ill over several weeks and was thought to have developed subacute bacterial endocarditis. Chlortetracycline had been given during the latter part of her illness but she deteriorated and was transferred to St Mary's Hospital, where a blood culture

grew *Streptococcus viridans.* Massive continuous intravenous penicillin treatment was begun, and her general condition began to improve. During the journey she had noticed something wrong with her right lower limb, and on arrival was found to have a tender, thickened, and swollen common femoral artery with absent pulsation at and beyond this point. The limb, however, was only mildly ischaemic, having partly recovered a circulation by this time.

Exploration at the groin showed the artery to be inflamed, oedematous, and adherent to its surroundings. When opened, the lumen contained a pale, friable accumulation of supposedly embolic material which, later, grew the same streptococcus on culture. Though the local infection was advanced, the organism was known to be sensitive to penicillin, and the arteriotomy was closed in the normal way using silk sutures. With continued penicillin, healing and revascularisation of the limb were uneventful.

A few days later the patient experienced severe pain in the right side of her neck, and petechae appeared over that half of the face, particularly in the conjunctiva. There was swelling and exquisite tenderness of the bifurcation of the common carotid artery. No cerebral or retinal effects could be detected. Another infected embolus was found and removed from the inflamed carotid. Again the arterial repair healed uneventfully and remained patent.

Without penicillin treatment such a patient would almost certainly have died, either of the bloodstream infection or its embolic complications. We may expect to see more late arterial infective lesions in future, and a renewed incidence of mycotic aneurysm is likely [39], including some due to resistant organisms.

Mycotic Aneurysm

Like the infections which cause it, this is a changing disease. As first described by Sir William Osler [40] it was due to blood spread of organisms, usually streptococci, from an infected heart valve, as in the patient reported above. Today most cases are iatrogenic, from resistant organisms and opportunistic invasions in patients receiving antibiotics, steroids or immunosuppressive drugs [10A, 15A].

Three types are recognised: embolomycotic, cryptogenic and erosive. Most resemble false aneurysms in that they are rounded, with a small opening into an otherwise relatively healthy main artery, the defect being due to septic destruction of that portion of the arterial wall, commonly at a bifurcation (Fig. 7.1), where an infected embolus may have lodged.

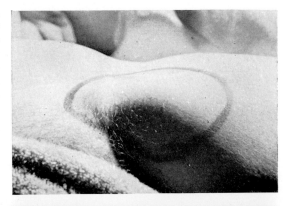

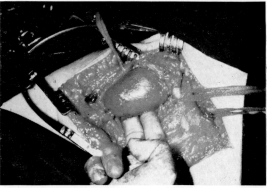

Fig. 7.1. Mycotic aneurysm of the left common femoral artery in a woman aged fifty previously treated for bacterial endocarditis due to streptococcus viridans. Note: typical rounded form and situation at a bifurcation.

1. *Embolomycotic type*

This is a quiet infection, often without suppuration, yet containing micrococci on histological section. Host-resistance to the infection may have been partly developed. In a series of cases of bacterial endocarditis examined for the Medical Research Council in 1951 [11A], ten per cent of the deaths were the result of rupture of a mycotic aneurysm. Figure 7.1 shows the presentation of a typical case in a woman who had noticed a gradually increasing swelling in her groin for about five years. She had suffered from chorea as a child, and at the age of forty developed subacute bacterial endocarditis which was treated for several months with penicillin. This type may be multiple.

2. *Cryptogenic Type*

Nowadays the classical condition is less often seen. Rheumatic fever has declined and penicillin has not only helped to control both its incidence and its complications but has led to the emergence of organisms such as the salmonellae and the 'hospital' staphylococci with greater antibiotic resistance, and the infected cardiovascular lesion is seen less often in the heart of a young subject than in the diseased artery of an older one [6]. Yet salmonella infection may lead to fatal rupture of the heart when it invades damaged tissue from some already established lesion [52]. The invasive and septicaemic tendency of such infections in the elderly patient may persist in spite of adequate dosage of an antibiotic such as chloramphenicol, shown to be effective against the infecting organism *in vitro* [28]. Osteomyelitis of the lumbar spine has been found to be present in several published cases of suppurative aortitis or infected aneurysm [59] and nearly half of one case series had either diarrhoea or faecal incontinence [66].

The management of mycotic aneurysm (or arteritis) demands effective antibiotic control of infection during and after any necessary surgical procedure [38A]. This is often difficult to arrange, for diagnosis may not be possible until the condition reaches the acute stage of imminent rupture. Yet cases are reported in which patients were saved by excision, with repair either by simple suture [49] or by grafting with autogenous vein (Fig. 7.1) or with a by-pass prosthesis through a completely clear field [12B, 22A, 39, 45A], though there is the risk that the fabric may form a nidus for persistent systemic infection as also happens with an infected prosthetic heart valve [45, 63].

3. *Erosive Type* (Fig. 7.2)

Local sepsis is the cause, e.g. from a soft tissue abscess, such as occurs at the groin in drug addicts [22A], or from osteomyelitis or infected malignant lymph nodes. A massive ligature may be responsible, perhaps one that was placed there to control an earlier erosive aneurysm that had bled.

CASE REPORT

A woman aged sixty-three was X-rayed for backache and found to have a large, rounded paravertebral shadow in the left mid-thoracic region, diagnosed radiologically as a tuberculous abscess from her sharply-wedged spine at the level (Fig. 7.2). It did not pulsate on screening. Exploration via a costo-transversectomy led to a violent aortic haemorrhage, which was controlled by passing a Foley catheter into the hole and pulling back on the inflated balloon. The chest wall was closed with wire. Seven weeks later, using atrio-femoral shunt, the aorta was transected above and below the sac and a by-pass dacron prosthesis was inserted. Shortly afterwards the Foley catheter was removed and the cavity

drained; it soon healed up. She remains well two years later.

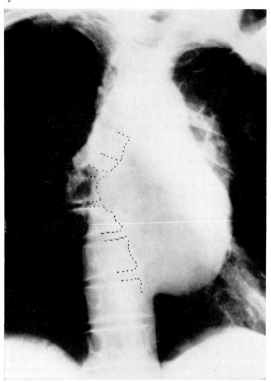

Fig. 7.2. Mycotic aneurysm of the thoracic aorta, suspected to have been tuberculous (*see* text). (Patient treated with Mr Nigel Harris and Mr L. L. Bromley.)

Tuberculous Arteritis and Aneurysm

This uncommon, lethal disease can now be cured by operation, as Rob and the author showed in 1954 [48] by using a prosthetic graft and giving specific antituberculous drug treatment.

Of the 100 cases in the literature up to 1963 [61], most were situated in the aorta and were due to direct local erosive spread from an adjacent tuberculous lesion, either caseating lymph nodes, carious vertebrae, tuberculous empyema or lung focus with cavitation.

Serious local complications can occur without actual aneurysm formation; for example, the ureter may be obstructed by a tuberculous lesion in the iliac artery, which may rupture [33], or vice versa. Dissection within the vessel wall is also described [61].

In the neck there have been cases in which tuberculous nodes had been treated by irradiation [25]. The author has had such a patient, treated by resection and end-to-end anastomosis. Other cases have had prosthetic grafts [27, 43, 48].

Infected Aortic Aneurysm

A significant proportion of abdominal aortic aneurysms become infected. At the Mayo Clinic [58], evidence in the form of inflammation, abscesses and necrosis of the wall of the sac was found in 6 patients among 172 abdominal aneurysms encountered at post-mortem. Gram positive cocci were seen in 5 of these in the stained sections; 4 had ruptured.

Gram negative bacilli are equally serious in their effects upon such aneurysms [45A]. Patients with *Salmonella typhi* [65] and *S. cholerasuis* [28] developed secondary bleeding in spite of chloramphenicol treatment to which the organism had been shown to be sensitive. Infection seems to be a cause of premature rupture of aneurysms of small or moderate size.

CASE REPORT

A man aged sixty-two underwent prostatectomy, following which he developed a continuous fever, and a persistent urinary infection with a coliform organism. During the third week he deteriorated, with renewed abdominal pain and heightened pyrexia, culminating in a general collapse with severe abdominal and back pain, and a tender pulsating swelling in the central abdomen. At operation this was confirmed to be an abdominal aortic aneurysm, $2\frac{1}{2}$ inches in diameter, whose softened, inflamed wall had given way posteriorly. A graft was inserted in its place, but the sutures held badly in the oedematous, friable arterial wall. He remained acutely ill and died two days later, after further high fever, from haemorrhage from the graft.

Syphilitic Arteritis

By tradition, syphilitic arteritis has been blamed for peripheral occlusive disease and popliteal aneurysms, but today such effects are so rare that for practical purposes the lesion can be safely omitted from the differential diagnosis of causes of these common clinical conditions, the vast majority of which are the result of degenerative arteriosclerosis. Apart from cerebrovascular lesions and small arterial narrowing by endarteritis around a gumma, the only remaining syphilitic arterial lesion in the practice of today is aortitis, usually of the thoracic aorta, and often associated with saccular or fusiform aneurysm of part or whole of the arch or descending portion (*see* Chapter 15, p. 314).

The intimal lesion is much less striking than that of arteriosclerosis, but there are destructive effects upon the elastic fibre system of the media, with replacement by fibrous scar tissue which stretches to become aneurysmal. As a result, the aortic valve often becomes incompetent, as in dilatation due to dissecting aneurysm, but also by infection in the valve itself.

Treatment with penicillin should precede operation, preferably by several weeks.

Candida Arteritis and Mycotic Aneurysm [53]

Cardiovascular operations, diagnostic catheterisation, prolonged intravenous infusions, and, above all, the administration to ill patients of broad spectrum antibiotics have been followed by candida infection in the blood stream with true mycotic endocarditis. Sometimes this leads to aortic aneurysm, at the aortic suture line, as well as to smaller multiple mycotic aneurysms elsewhere.

Non-infective Arteritis

Though primarily presenting the features of a general medical disease with fever, anaemia, joint pains, and a raised ESR, this group of conditions should be familiar to the surgeon who may be called in because of Raynaud's phenomenon, abdominal pain, or involvement of the larger limb arteries. Clinically, the general effects of the disease may be hidden, though not as a rule on investigation. Drugs may be the cause, e.g., chlorthiazide in necrotising vasculitis of the skin [15], hydrallazine in systemic lupus erythematosus [2], methysergide, causing retroperitoneal fibrosis which may obstruct the aorta and its branches [15]; also drug abuse by addicts [12A, 16A].

The following will be considered:

1. Disseminated lupus erythematosus
2. Polyarteritis nodosa
3. Rheumatoid arteritis
4. Giant-celled (temporal) arteritis
5. Pulseless (Takayasu's) disease

Disseminated Lupus Erythematosus (DLE) [20, 26]

This occurs mainly in young and middle-aged women, in some of whom poor general health is complicated by the development of secondary Raynaud's phenomenon; in others it may be the earliest symptom. It is present in at least 4 per cent of all cases of this common condition. The digital effects may be acute and severe, with several gangrenous finger tips (Fig. 11.9, p. 208), also the toes, heels and elbows may be affected. There may be a link with the presence of cryoglobulins, which are present in 15 per cent of cases, but not all these suffer such serious results. Fever, chest and joint pains, and the appearance of a discoid rash on the shins and elsewhere should lead to a search for LE cells which, though not specific to this condition, are usually present. The ESR is usually raised. Major pulse deficiencies and aneurysms are rare, though one patient of the author's, a woman of thirty-five, presented with a disabling aorto-iliac occlusion and failed to improve after a by-pass operation which restored all her distal pulses (*see* Fig. 3.64, p. 72). She had continued fever, weakness and some joint pains, which led to biopsy of a small rounded skin lesion on the calf, which, with the finding of LE cells in the blood, confirmed the diagnosis of DLE. There was a striking and well-maintained improvement on steroid treatment.

This regime should control the general and vascular symptoms for some time. Gangrenous tips of digits should separate cleanly, and heal. Eventually, however, there is a fatal decline, with renal, hepatic or cardiac complications or steroid difficulties.

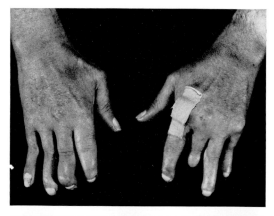

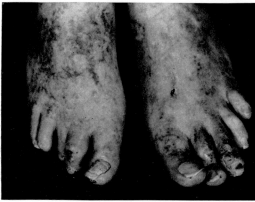

Fig. 7.3. Ischaemic digital lesions of rheumatoid arteritis in a man aged forty-five. Condition relatively painless.

Polyarteritis Nodosa

Three times commoner in men, with polyarteritis nodosa there may be the complaint of pain, tenderness, numbness, and weakness, usually in one lower limb, due to nerve involvement in the vascular disease; cutaneous gangrene is also seen. Pulse deficiencies are sometimes present but are not necessarily related to gangrene. They may coincide with the mononeuritis areas. Raynaud's phenomenon may occur as in DLE, and for the same reason. The abdominal viscera are usually affected, causing pain and gastrointestinal or intraperitoneal haemorrhage. There may be ileal obstruction with or without gangrene [14] (Fig. 17.14, p. 372). Fever, hypertension, albuminuria, haematuria, and renal failure are common; also chest symptoms and signs including haemoptysis. Nodules may be palpable along the testicular artery in the spermatic cord. Muscle biopsy should show the typical lesions in the outer coats of small arteries with small false aneurysms, which can be demonstrated at aortography [9] (Fig. 7.7, p. 143). After an operation for acute abdominal pain, the lesion may be noticed in the histology of the artery to the appendix or gall bladder [46A]. The ESR is consistently raised, and eosinophilia is sometimes present, also Australia antigen [23A].

Many resemblances are shown by these two diseases and their response to treatment with steroids, which at present offer the most effective method of controlling symptoms and prolonging life. Failure seems to be commoner in polyarteritis nodosa, possibly because of the greater severity of visceral involvement, which is the chief determining factor in prognosis. Many patients die within three months of the onset, especially those without lung involvement, which tends to be associated with a better prognosis [50].

Rheumatoid Arteritis

Secondary Raynaud phenomenon developing in the hands and feet of some patients with late or advanced rheumatoid arthritis is usually due to specific occlusive lesions of the digital arteries [56]. The familiar deformity of the fingers and toes plus the added changes of stagnation, congestion, and local ulceration should identify this interesting condition whose appearance is quite typical (Fig. 7.3). Symptoms are usually less severe than this would suggest, but the course is not always slow: tips, phalanges, or even the whole hand may be lost [10]. Neuropathic features are often present [41] and may explain the mildness of symptoms with such striking local signs. Sometimes the onset is more abrupt;

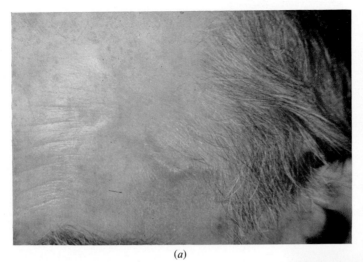

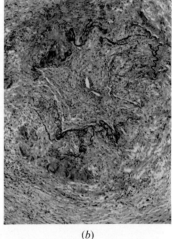

(a)

(b)

Fig. 7.4. Temporal arteritis.

(a) Typical scalp lesion.
(b) Biopsy from this patient showing giant-cell reaction in media and fragmentation of internal elastic coat with organising thrombus within the lumen. (Photomicrograph by Dr J. Guthrie.)
(c) Another case, under higher power showing giant cells. (Photomicrograph by Dr E. A. Wright.)

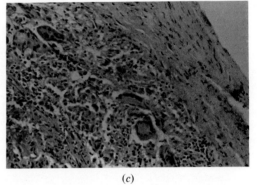

(c)

this may follow the start of steroid treatment [10]. The Rose-Waaler test for rheumatoid factor is invariably positive [13].

Two pathological lesions may be seen:

1. The digital artery may be narrowed and, later, occluded by a concentric fibrous intimal thickening.
2. An inflammatory cellular infiltration is irregularly disposed, with interruption of the elastic laminae, also in the digital arteries, but like polyarteritis, which it resembles histologically, affecting the abdominal and other systemic arteries [10] and relatively more common in men (*see* Chapter 17, p. 382).

Arteriography in early cases of rheumatoid arthritis tends to show normal digital arteries. Later studies, and those carried out on cadavers, show segmental digital arterial occlusive lesions irregularly disposed as in other conditions with secondary Raynaud's phenomenon.

In most patients the course is slow and benign. Some with a more acute illness, and severe neuropathy, have a much worse prognosis [13].

Giant-celled (temporal) Arteritis [36]

Another uncommon inflammatory disease of arteries, though becoming less so [11], temporal arteritis also has certain similarities with systemic lupus and polyarteritis, for its clinical features are varied and wide-ranging, and its natural course and prognosis are much influenced by steroid treatment. It is chiefly a disease of the over-sixties and predominantly affects the carotids and their branches, particularly the temporals as they run in the scalp (Fig. 7.4), causing severe headache with local tenderness, redness and swelling, amounting on occasion to actual gangrene. The tongue may be affected likewise [7]; more often it and the jaw muscles may claudicate [23B, 23D, 26A]. In the Mayo Clinic series [25A] this was the second commonest presenting symptom. Though the average age was seventy-four years, there were no deaths; all patients lived at least four years after diagnosis. Some cases are silent, except for the scalp nodules, until blindness suddenly descends [23C]. Giant-celled arteritis is sometimes found in excised aorto-iliac specimens. Aneurysm formation is rare [23]. As in the other two forms of arteritis, there is often a low fever, anaemia and a raised ESR and alteration in the plasma globulin fraction. There are no LE cells and antinuclear factor is not present.

Arterial Lesions in Polymyalgia Rheumatica

A commoner, milder condition probably related to giant-celled arteritis is polymyalgia rheumatica. The incidence is higher in females, and most patients are elderly. Morning pain and stiffness in the muscles of the limb girdles is associated with a raised ESR, and accompanying disturbances of plasma globulins and increased fibrinogen. Biopsy of the affected muscles shows no specific vascular lesion, though when the temporal arteries have been studied a giant-celled arteritis has often been found [3]. More striking is the finding of widespread arterial murmurs in 30 out of 52 Swedish patients compared with 6 out of an equal number of matched control subjects [24]. Arteriography in 5 cases showed that there was narrowing of the artery at the point where the murmur was heard. Unlike arteriosclerosis, lesions appear to be much commoner in the upper part of the body. Aortic arch syndrome is a recognised complication [3, 24] though it would be incorrect to imply any close relationship with Takayasu's (pulseless) disease, which affects a much younger age group.

Amyloid Disease affecting Small Arteries

Muscle pain is common in systemic amyloidosis, and may cause intermittent claudication. The smaller vessels to the limb muscles are found on biopsy to be extensively involved, and later at autopsy these changes are found to be very generalised [67]. (*See also* p. 373.)

Obliterative Arteritis of Kidney Homograft Rejection [44]

Fever, oliguria, hypertension, and leucocytosis in a patient with a renal homograft are signs of rejection. There are marked arterial changes in the graft as early as thirteen days [21], with intimal proliferation and thrombosis, which resemble the arterial lesions of polyarteritis nodosa, scleroderma and malignant hypertension. The fact that thrombosis is so important in kidney rejection may suggest that it is also part of the microvascular response in these other angiopathies. Rejection changes can be prevented by anticoagulants and dipyridamole [31A].

Pulseless Disease (aortic arch syndrome, Takayasu's disease, young oriental female arteritis, constrictive arteritis)

Sir William Broadbent, in 1875, [8] described a St Mary's Hospital patient with absent radial pulsations, yet these arteries were palpably full of blood, except when the arms were raised. Post mortem showed the cause to be stenosis of the innominate and left subclavian at their origin.

In 1908, Takayasu, a Japanese ophthalmologist, saw a young woman for attacks of blindness and syncope and found that her carotid pulses were absent.

Since then, many cases have been reported from Far Eastern countries, most of which conformed to this classical pattern with absent pulses in the upper half of the body, and cerebrovascular and retinal insufficiency. Some of these patients may have had hypertension: lack of brachial pulsations would mask this feature in a routine examination. Coldness and paraesthesiae of the arms, and a tendency to hold the head forward were noticed by McKusick [34] who saw many cases in Japan and Korea, and who reviewed the world literature up to 1962, drawing attention to the hypertensive complications. Other Japanese [51], Chinese [62], Malayan [18] and Indian [57] series at about this time mentioned the lower aortic and lower limb involvement, which had tended to be classified as 'atypical coarctation', also the renal arterial involvement with the aortic lesion. Further oriental cases were published in Siamese children [42], and in Japanese women living in Hawaii [12].

Arterial disease in Africans [55] has many similar features, mostly occurring in young women with aortic narrowing sufficient to produce murmurs, and with peripheral arterial occlusions, cerebrovascular insufficiency and, occasionally, aneurysms [1, 29, 30]. Some were first seen in pregnancy [22].

Diagnosis of pulseless disease should be given first place in any young woman, whatever her race, who presents with unexplained peripheral pulse deficiencies (Figs. 7.5, 7.6), hypertension, or cranio-brachial arterial insufficiency. There is usually a low fever. Investigations should include ESR and plasma protein estimations, both of which are almost invariably abnormal. Aortography, like blood pressure measurements, may be hampered by the lack of available peripheral arteries. LE cells may be found [37].

A special form occurs in very young children, with severe involvement of the thoraco-abdominal segment of the aorta and hypertensive renal arterial narrowing (Fig. 17.13), perhaps part of the rubella syndrome (Chapter 17, p. 357, [105]).

No sure pathological basis yet exists for this mysterious disease. Surgical material is scarce, because resection and endarterectomy are so difficult. Autopsy reports are few, but the vessel walls have been seen to be thickened, with a wrinkled intima and necrotic damage to the elastic tissue in

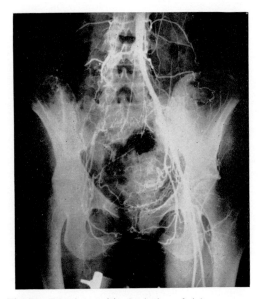

Fig. 7.5. Female arteritis. Occlusion of right common iliac artery in a woman aged thirty-two presenting with claudication in 1951. This patient subsequent thrombosed both subclavian arteries, the right renal artery, and twelve years later died of a coronary occlusion.

all layers. Round-celled infiltration of the adventitia is described [55]. It is believed that auto-immune processes are responsible [47], probably with genetic predisposition.

Prognosis is poor, and surgery difficult [28B], but the course of the disease is often slow (Fig. 7.5). Renal-hypertensive or cardiac death is to be expected. Reports of benefit from steroid administration have been made in Japan. Pulseless disease is probably an entity which differs with the age and sex of the patient. Among 299 patients with aortic arch syndromes reported from Houston, Texas [17], all those under 35 years of age were women, at middle age the sex incidence was about equal, and after fifty-five most were men; the lesions in these older cases were those of obliterative arteriosclerosis rather than of arteritis.

Further reference to the diagnosis and treatment of aortic arch syndrome will be made in Chapter 8.

Summary

Infective arteritis is caused by the invasion of an artery, locally or from the blood stream, at a point where it is already diseased or injured, including during healing after operation. Pathogens such as resistant staphylococci, anaerobic streptococci, salmonella, and *M. tuberculosis* are responsible. Treatment is directed against the cause, and in resistant infections, reconstruction of the artery through a fresh, uninfected region.

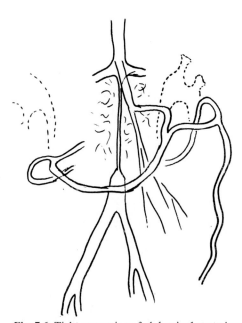

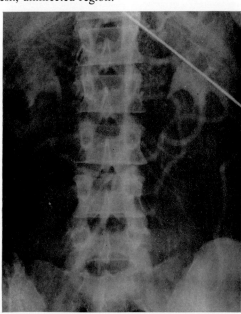

Fig. 7.6. Tight narrowing of abdominal aorta in a Greek Cypriot woman aged thirty-two. Renals and iliacs were spared. Grossly dilated marginal artery is acting as an aortic collateral, for superior mesenteric branches fill well. Around the stenosed aorta are numerous fine branches, making it impossible to mobilise the aorta.

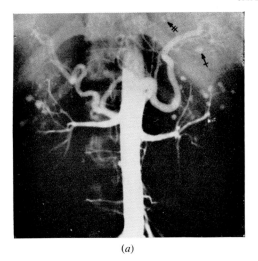 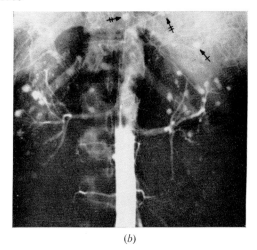

(a)   (b)

Fig. 7.7. Polyarteritis nodosa. Small false aneurysms demonstrated by aortography.

(a) Early phase showing normal main branches.
(b) Late phase showing many renal aneurysms and two hepatic (-‖→) and one splenic (+→).
(By courtesy of Bron *et al.* [9], and the publishers of the *Annals of Internal Medicine.*)

Non-infective arteritis is thought to be due to a sensitivity or auto-immunity process with arteries as the target organ. A febrile illness with raised ESR is followed by chronic inflammatory infiltration with destruction of connective tissues in the artery wall. Mostly young women are affected. The prognosis in general is bad, but steroid treatment may give great relief, and prolong life.

REFERENCES

1. Abrahams, D. G. and Cockshott, W. P. (1962) Multiple non-luetic aneurysms in young Nigerians. *Brit. Heart J.*, **24**, 83.
2. Alarćon-Segovia, D., Worthington, J. W., Ward, L. E. and Wakim, K. G. (1965) Lupus diathesis and the hydralazine syndrome. *New Eng. J. Med.*, **272**, 462.
3. Alestig, K. and Barr, J. (1963) Giant-cell arteritis. A biopsy study of polymyalgia rheumatica, including one case of Takayasu's disease. *Lancet*, **i**, 1228.
4. Ask-Upmark, E. (1954) On 'the pulseless disease' outside of Japan. *Acta med. Scand.*, **149**, 161.
5. Björnberg, A. and Gisslén, H. (1965) Thiazides: a cause of necrotising vasculitis? *Lancet*, **ii**, 982.
6. Blum, L. and Keefer, E. B. C. (1964) Clinical entity of cryptogenic mycotic aneurysm. *J. Amer. Med. Assoc.*, **188**, 505.
7. Brearley, B. F. and MacDonald, J. G. (1961) Temporal arteritis resulting in infected gangrene of tongue. *Brit. med. J.*, **i**, 1151.
8. Broadbent, W. H. (1875) Absence of pulsation in both radial arteries, the vessels being full of blood. *Trans. Clin. Soc.*, **8**, 165.
9. Bron, K. M. Strott, C. A. and Shapiro, A. P. (1965) The diagnostic value of angiographic observations in polyarteritis nodosa. A case of multiple aneurysms in the visceral organs. *Arch. Int. Med.*, **116**, 450.
10. Bywaters, E. G. L. (1957) Peripheral vascular obstruction in rheumatoid arthritis and its relationship to other vascular lesions. *Ann. rheum. Dis.*, **16**, 84.
10A.Callard, G. M., Wright, C. B., Wray, C. and Minor, G. R. (1971) False aneurysm due to Mucor following repair of coarctation with a dacron prosthesis. *J. Thorac. Cardiovasc. Surg.*, **61**, 181.
11. Cameron, A. (1959) Temporal arteritis in general practice. *Brit. med. J.*, **ii**, 1291.
11A.Cates, J. E. and Christie, R. V. (1951) Subacute bacterial endocarditis. A review of 442 patients treated in 14 centres approved by the Penicillin Trials Committee of the Medical Research Council. *Quart. J. Med.*, **20**, 93.
12. Cheitlin, M. D. and Carter, P. B. (1965) Takayashu's disease. *Arch. Int. med.*, **116**, 283.
12A.Citron, B. P., Halpern, M. and McCarron, M. (1970) Necrotising angiitis associated with drug abuse. *New Eng. J. Med.*, **283**, 1003.
12B.Cliff, M. M., Soulen, R. L. and Finestone, A. J. (1970) Mycotic aneurysms—a challenge and a clue. *Arch. int. Med.*, **126**, 977.
13. Clinicopathological Conference (1966) A case of rheumatoid arthritis with polyarteritis. Demonstrated at the Post-graduate Medical School of London. *Brit. med. J.*, **i**, 1027.
14. Colton, C. L. and Butler, T. J. (1967) The surgical

problem of polyarteritis nodosa. *Brit. J. Surg.*, **54**, 393.

15. Conley, J. E., Boulanger, W. J. and Mendeloff, G. L. (1966) Aortic obstruction associated with methysergide maleate therapy for headaches. *J. Amer. Med. Assoc.*, **198**, 808.

15A. Conn, J. H., Hardy, J. D., Chavez, C. M. and Fain, W. R. (1970) Infected arterial grafts: experience in 22 cases with emphasis on unusual bacteria and techniques. *Ann. Surg.*, **171**, 704.

16. Cooke, W. T., Cloake, P. C. P., Govan, A. D. T. and Colbeck, J. C. (1946) Temporal arteritis: a generalised vascular disease. *Quart. J. med.*, **15**, 47.

16A. Correspondence: (1971) Angiitis in drug abuse. *New Eng. J. Med.*, **284**, 111.

17. Crawford, E. S., De Bakey, M. E., Morris, G. C. and Howells, J. F. (1969) Surgical treatment of occlusion of the innominate, common carotid and subclavian arteries: a 10-year experience. *Surgery*, **65**, 17.

18. Danaraj, T. J., Wong, H. O. and Thomas, M. A. (1963) Primary arteritis of aorta causing renal artery stenosis and hypertension. *Brit. Heart J.*, **25**, 153.

19. Donnelly, G. H. and Campbell, R. E. (1954) Surgical aspects of periarteritis nodosa. *Arch. Surg.*, **69**, 533.

20. Dubois, E. L. and Arterberry, J. D. (1962) Gangrene as a manifestation of systemic lupus erythematosus. *J. Amer. Med. Assoc.*, **181**, 366.

21. Dunea, G., Nakamoto, S., Straffon, R. A., Figueroa, J. E., Versaci, A. A., Shibagaki, M. and Kolff, W. J. (1965) Renal homotransplantation in 24 patients. *Brit. med. J.*, **i**, 7.

22. Emanuel, L. A., Ikomi, E. A. and Nwokedi, C. (1966) Takayashu's or pulseless disease in pregnancy. *J. Obstet. Gynaec. Brit. Commonwealth*, **73**, 119.

22A. Fromin, S. H. and Lucas, C. E. (1970) Obturator bypass for mycotic aneurysm in a drug addict. *Arch. Surg.*, **100**, 83.

23. Garret, R. (1962) Chronic diffuse giant cell mesaortitis, with dissecting aneurysm and rupture. *Amer. J. Clin. Path.*, **38**, 406.

23A. Gocke, D. J., Hsu, K., Morgan, C., Bombardieri, S., Lockshin, M. and Christian, C. L. (1970) Vasculitis in association with Australia antigen. *J. exp. Med.*, **134**, 330s.

23B. Graham, R., Bluestone, R. and Holt, P. J. L. (1968) Recurrent blanching of the tongue due to giant-cell arteritis. *Ann. Int. Med.*, **69**, 781,

23C. Gutrecht, J. A. (1970) Occult temporal arteritis. *J. Amer. med. Ass.*, **213**, 1188.

23D. Hamilton, C. R., Shelley, W. M. and Tumulty, P. A. (1971) Giant-cell arteritis: including temporal arteritis and polymyalgia rheumatica. *Medicine*, **50**, 1.

24. Hamrin, B., Jonsson, N. and Landberg, T. (1965) Involvement of large vessels in polymyalgia arteritica. *Lancet*, **i**, 1193.

25. Hara, M. and Bransford, R. M. (1963) Aneurysm of the subclavian artery associated with contiguous pulmonary tuberculosis. *J. Thorac. Cardiovasc. Surg.*, **46**, 256.

25A. Hauser, W. A., Ferguson, R. H., Holley, K. E. and Kurland, L. T. (1971) Temporal arteritis in Rochester, Minnesota, 1951 to 1967. *Mayo Clin. Proc.*, **46**, 597.

26. Hejtmancik, M. R., Wright, J. C., Quint, R. and Jennings, F. L. (1964) The cardiovascular manifestations of systemic lupus erythematosus. *Amer. Heart J.*, **68**, 119.

26A. Henderson, A. H. (1967) Tongue pain with giant-cell arteritis. *Brit. med. J.*, **4**, 337.

27. Hsien-min, M., Yü-ch'üan, T., Chieh, W. and Tse-lin, C. (1963) Tuberculous abdominal aortic aneurysm —report of a case treated with resection and artificial graft. *Chinese med. J.*, **82**, 452.

28. Hyde, R. D. and Davis, P. K. B. (1962) Infection of an aortic aneurysm with Salmonella choleraesuis. *Brit. med. J.*, **i**, 30.

28A. Ibarra-Perez, C. and Lillehei, C. W. (1969) Treatment of mesenteric arteritis following resection of coarctation of the aorta. *J. Thorac. Cardiovasc. Surg.*, **58**, 135.

28B. Inada, K., Katsumura, T., Hirai, J. and Sunada, T. (1970) Surgical treatment in the aortitis syndrome. *Arch. Surg.*, **100**, 220.

29. Isaacson, C. (1961) An idiopathic aortitis in young Africans. *J. Path. Bact.*, **81**, 69.

30. Joffe, N. (1965) Idiopathic panarteritis with aneurysm formation. *Clin. Radiol.*, **16**, 251.

30A. Johnson, A. G., Lane, B., Rains, A. J. H., O'Donnell, D. and Ramsay, N. W. (1969) Large artery damage after X-irradiation. *Brit. J. Radiol.*, **42**, 937.

31. Kalmasohn, R. B. and R. W. (1957) Thrombotic obliteration of the branches of the aortic arch. *Circulation*, **15**, 237.

31A. Kincaid-Smith, P. (1969) Modification of the vascular lesions of rejection in cadaveric renal allografts by dipyramidole and anticoagulants. *Lancet*, **ii**, 920.

32. Krøll, J. (1965) Arterial blood culture. *Danish med. Bull.*, **12**, 131.

33. McCune, W. R., Galleher, E. P. and Oster, W. (1965) Ureteral obstruction following rupture of an iliac artery secondary to tuberculous arteritis. *J. Urol.*, **94**, 391.

34. McKusick, V. A. (1962) A form of vascular disease relatively frequent in the Orient. *Amer. Heart J.*, **63**, 57.

35. Martin, A. and Copeman, P. W. M. (1967) Aortojejunal fistula from rupture of teflon graft, with septic emboli in the skin. *Brit. med. J.*, **ii**, 155.

35A. Meade, R. H. and Moran, J. M. (1969) Salmonella arteritis. Preoperative diagnosis and cure of S. typhimurium aortic aneurysm. *New Eng. J. Med.*, **281**, 310.

36. Meadows, S. P. (1966) Temporal or giant cell arteritis. *Proc. Roy. Soc. Med.*, **59**, 329.

37. Miller, G. A. H., Thomas, M. L. and Medd, W. E. (1962) Aortic arch syndrome and polymyositis with LE cells in peripheral blood. *Brit. med. J.*, **i**, 771.

38. Miller, H. G. and Daley, R. (1946) Clinical aspects of polyarteritis nodosa. *Quart. J. med.*, **15**, 255.

38A. Mundth, E. D., Darling, R. C., Alvarado, R. H., Buckley, M. J., Linton, R. R. and Austen, W. G. (1969) Surgical management of mycotic aneurysms and the complications of infection in vascular reconstructive surgery. *Amer. J. Surg.*, **117**, 460.

39. Nabseth, D. C. and Deterling, R. A. (1961) Surgical management of mycotic aneurysms. *Surgery*, **50**, 347.

40. Osler, W. (1885) The Gulstonian lectures on malignant endocarditis. *Brit. med. J.*, **i**, 467.

41. Pallis, C. A. and Scott, J. T. (1965) Peripheral neuropathy in rheumatoid arthritis. *Brit. med. J.*, **i**, 1141.

42. Paton, B. C., Chartikavanij, K., Buri, P., Prachuabmoh, K. and Jumbala, M. R. B. (1965) Obliterative aortic disease in children in the tropics. *Circulation. Supp. I.*, **31**, and **32**, 197.

43. Peyton, R. W. (1965) Surgical correction of tuberculous pseudoaneurysm of upper abdominal aorta. *Ann. Surg.*, **162**, 1069.

44. Porter, K. A., Thomson, W. B., Owen, K., Kenyon, J. R., Mowbray, J. F. and Peart, W. S. (1963) Obliterative vascular changes in four human kidney homotransplants. *Brit. med. J.*, **ii**, 639.

45. Rabinovich, S., Evans, J., Smith, I. M. and January, L. E. (1965) A long-term view of bacterial endocarditis. 337 cases 1924–1963. *Ann. Int. Med.*, **63**, 185.

45A. Reichle, F. A., Tyson, R. R., Soloff, L. A., Lautsch, E. V. and Rosemond, G. P. (1970) Salmonellosis and aneurysm of the distal aorta. *Ann. Surg.*, **171**, 219.

46. Reid, H. C. and Dallachy, R. (1958) Infarction of ileum following resection of coarctation of the aorta. *Brit. J. Surg.*, **45**, 625.

46A. Remigio, P. and Zaino, E. (1970) Polyarteritis of the gall bladder. *Surgery*, **67**, 427.

47. Riehl, J.-L. and Brown, W. J. (1965) Takayasu's arteritis. An autoimmune disease. *Arch. Neurol.*, **12**, 92.

48. Rob, C. G. and Eastcott, H. H. G. (1955) Aortic aneurysm due to tuberculous lymphadenitis. *Brit. med. J.*, **i**, 378.

49. Robb, D. (1962) Surgical treatment of mycotic aneurysm. *Surgery*, **52**, 847.

50. Rose, G. A. and Spencer, H. (1957) Polyarteritis nodosa. *Quart. J. med.*, **26**, 43.

51. Ross, R. S. and McKusick, V. A. (1953) Aortic arch syndromes. *Arch. Int. Med.*, **92**, 701.

52. Sanders, V. and Misanik, L. F. (1964) Salmonella myocarditis: report of a case with ventricular rupture. *Amer. Heart J.*, **68**, 682.

53. Sanger, P. W., Taylor, F. H., Robicsek, F., Germuth, F., Senterfit, L. and McKinnon, G. (1962) Candida infection as a complication of heart surgery. Review of literature and report of two cases. *J. Amer. Med. Assoc.*, **181**, 88.

54. Saphra, I. and Winter, J. W. (1957) Clinical manifestations of Salmonellosis in man. *New Eng. J. Med.*, **256**, 1128.

55. Schrire, V. and Asherson, R. A. (1964) Arteritis of the aorta and its major branches. *Quart. J. med.*, **33**, 439.

56. Scott, J. T., Hourihane, D. O., Doyle, F. H., Steiner, R. E., Laws, J. W., Dixon, A. St. J. and Bywaters, E. G. L. (1961) Digital arteritis in rheumatoid disease. *Ann. rheum. Dis.*, **20**, 224.

57. Sen, P. K., Kinare, S. G., Kulkarni, T. P. and Parulkar, G. B. (1962) Stenosing aortitis of unknown etiology. *Surgery*, **51**, 317.

58. Sommerville, R. L., Allen, E. V. and Edwards, J. E. (1959) Bland and infected arteriosclerotic abdominal aortic aneurysms: a clinicopathological study. *Medicine*, Baltimore, **38**, 207.

59. Sower, N. D. and Whelan, T. J. (1962) Suppurative arteritis due to Salmonella. *Surgery*, **52**, 851.

60. Trummer, M. J. and Mannix, E. P. (1963) Abdominal pain and necrotising mesenteric arteritis following resection of coarctation of the aorta. *J. Thorac. Cardiovasc. Surg.*, **45**, 198.

61. Volini, F. I., Olfield, R. C., Thompson, J. R. and Kent, G. (1962) Tuberculosis of the aorta. *J. Amer. med. Assoc.*, **181**, 78.

62. Wan, H. and Li-sheng, L. (1962) Constrictive arteritis of the aorta and its branches. *Chinese med. J.*, **81**, 526.

63. Weinstein, L. and Kaplan, K. (1965) Salmonella aortitis in a patient with a Hufnagel valve. *Circulation*, **31**, 755.

64. Williams, R. E. O., Blowers, R., Garrod, L. P. and Shooter, R. A. (1966) *Hospital Infection, Causes and Prevention*. London: Lloyd-Luke (Medical Books), Second Edition. p. 242.

65. Wright, J. T. and Raeburn, C. (1962) Infection of aortic aneurysm with Salmonellae. *Brit. med. J.*, **i**, 563.

66. Zak, F. G., Strauss, L. and Saphra, I. (1958) Rupture of diseased large arteries in the course of enterobacter (Salmonella) infections. *New Eng. J. Med.*, **258**, 824.

67. Zelis, R., Mason, D. T. and Barth, W. (1969) Abnormal peripheral vascular dynamics in systemic amyloidosis. *Ann. Internal Med.*, **70**, 1167.

8 Carotid-Vertebral Insufficiency

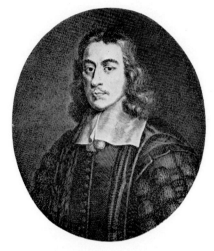

Thomas Willis (1621–1675)

The Cerebral Blood Supply

Thomas Willis, in 1664, clearly grasped the important potential of the arterial circle which now bears his name, when he wrote: 'if the carotid of one side should be obstructed, then the vessels of the other side might provide for either province . . . further, if both the carotids should be stopt, the offices of each might be provided through the vertebrals' [93].

It is a reflection on the importance of the cerebral blood supply that it should reach the brain by four such large arteries.

Factors Affecting Cerebral Blood Flow [53]
Each 100 g of brain requires an average of 50 ml of blood a minute throughout the twenty-four hours, sleeping or waking. Few factors change this rate of flow. It declines with age, cerebral arteriosclerosis, with profound fall in blood pressure, rising intracranial pressure, and, very strikingly, with polycythaemia. By far the most potent substance to stimulate cerebral blood flow is carbon dioxide. A small increase occurs in normal sleep, acute alcoholic intoxication, with administration of 1-nor-

adrenalin, and in anaemia. Sympathetic denervation is without effect, and so are hypotensive drugs in therapeutic dosage.

Measurements are still too complicated for clinical application. Most methods give total cerebral blood flow. Separate values for individual neck arteries are now possible during operation, using the electromagnetic flow meter [36], and regional cerebral flow can be estimated by the intra-arterial injection of isotopes such as ^{133}Xe, ^{85}Kr, and ^{32}P. Even so, it is not yet possible to conduct serial studies of the flow in the four main arteries with sufficient convenience to establish the patterns of the blood supply in health and disease. That there may be wide individual variations would be expected from the variable effects of carotid ligation in the absence of occlusive cerebrovascular disease, as well as from the extraordinary range of disability from nil (Fig. 8.1) to severe (Fig. 8.2) in carotid occlusive disease, whose degree in fact may be inversely proportional to the associated neurological deficit. It has been shown that, in healthy subjects, temporary constriction

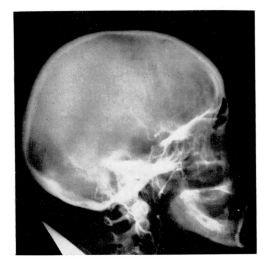
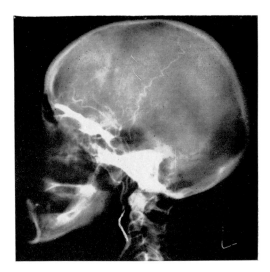

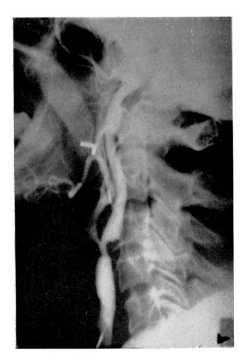

Fig. 8.1. Bilateral complete internal carotid occlusion in a middle-aged woman. History of transient ischaemic attacks but with no residual neurological defect. (Dr Helen Dimsdale's case.)

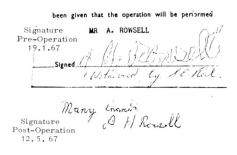

been given that the operation will be performed

Signature
Pre–Operation   MR A. ROWSELL
19.1.67

_____Signed_____

Signature
Post–Operation
12. 5. 67

Fig. 8.2. Severe stenosis of left carotid bifurcation in a man aged fifty-four. After three recent transient ischaemic attacks with right hemiplegia and aphasia, he was left with a moderately severe neurological defect. Left internal carotid endarterectomy was followed by a striking early improvement, and complete neurological recovery was confirmed by his signature four months later.

147

of a carotid artery has no effect upon the blood flow within it unless the cross-sectional area is less than 2 mm², and that this is still true in the presence of stenosis of the other three main afferent arteries, provided the critical area is not reached [12].

Carotid Ligation

In 1805, Astley Cooper performed this, then unique, operation upon a middle-aged woman for rapidly enlarging carotid aneurysm in the middle region of the right side of the neck, and the patient was able to stand up immediately afterwards [13].

Today, either the common or the internal carotid, or both, may require ligation in order to control bleeding from an intracranial aneurysm. In 142 of Jefferson's patients there was no death attributable to the ligation [48, 49]. There were, however, 11 hemiplegias, 7 of which were dense, with some recovery; mean carotid pressure had been reduced by 40 to 60 per cent, the desired effect in this instance [82]. Triple ligation of the carotid bifurcation is more serious. In the past, this was sometimes necessary for uncontrollable bleeding during the removal of a carotid body tumour, or malignant cervical lymph nodes. The mortality was as high as 30 per cent [68], with hypovolaemic hypotension no doubt responsible for aggravating the ischaemic intracranial damage.

The effects of carotid ligation cannot be forecast with any certainty even though trial occlusion of the artery for ten to thirty minutes may have been used as a routine (Matas's test) [8, 74A]. A negative result is no guarantee of safety, but the test should continue to be used because the positive finding of weakness during trial occlusion is strong evidence that hemiplegia will follow permanent ligation. If the ligature can be removed within fifteen minutes, a full recovery is the rule. These data suggest that the location of the intracranial lesion with respect to the circle of Willis might be as important in determining the results of carotid ligation as the point of the carotid ligation. Aneurysms in this situation may impede the cross flow in much the same way as an arteriosclerotic obstruction.

Syndromes of Cerebrovascular Insufficiency

Interfaces of static blood occur in the healthy circle of Willis [58] and boundary zones in corresponding areas of the cerebrum [59]. These frontiers must vary in situation according to the anatomy of the main arteries and the pressure and flow within them and their communicating branches.

The same must be true of the cerebral circulation in disease; it is possible to envisage a state in which at most times a given area of brain has stable blood supply though there may be inequalities in the four main arteries, yet when some alteration of the general circulation occurs to reduce the total available cerebral blood flow via the neck arteries, the haemodynamic effect at the periphery will be uneven, for the equilibrium of collateral flow to the cerebral areas in question may be lost, and transient ischaemia could result [67].

This is thought to occur in patients with arteriosclerotic heart disease, but though the clinical association is familiar it is not easy to prove cause and effect. In rheumatic heart disease, the mechanical fault can be corrected surgically; the cerebrovascular effects are then abolished, and furthermore, recurrence of the mitral stenosis brings renewed neurological symptoms [46].

Episodes (transient ischaemic attacks, *see also* p. 156)

These are of two kinds:

1. *Hemisphere* effects of *carotid* insufficiency.
2. *Hind-brain* effects of *vertebro-basilar* insufficiency.

Motor, sensory and visual features may occur in either type, and the recognition of the location of the disturbance is not usually difficult. Well-lateralised episodes in an arm, leg or half the face are usually a result of ischaemia of the opposite hemisphere. Mixed effects on both sides of the body are more likely to be due to brain-stem ischaemia, particularly if accompanied by vertigo, hemianopia or other field defects. Intermittent complete blindness of one eye from failure of the flow in the ophthalmic artery is a typical feature of carotid obstruction.

We have seen how haemodynamic factors, together with inequalities in the complex circuit of cerebral arteries, may produce a tidal effect during disturbances of the central body circulation. Together with local 'steal' effects (*see* pp. 31, 48 and 170), this process probably accounts for most repetitive episodes of cerebrovascular insufficiency.

Embolism, though it may be less common as the cause of episodal ischaemia can, however, be positively identified by direct observation of the retinal arteries during attacks of transient blindness.

Platelet Emboli. White and red bodies have been observed traversing the vessels [5, 57, 79, 80] at retinoscopy during visual attacks, and similar material has been recovered at autopsy from the retinal arteries and was identified as platelet aggregate [57], which we know to form the inner layer of many obliterative main arterial lesions.

Figures 8.3 and 8.4 show the appearance of the left retina in a man aged fifty-one with a previous

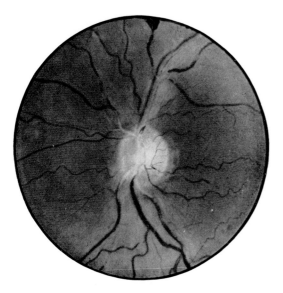

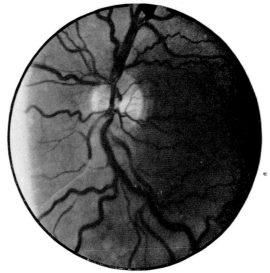

Fig. 8.3. Platelet emboli entering the retinal arteries of a man aged fifty-one, who had transient blindness of that eye in recurrent attacks lasting up to five minutes.

Fig. 8.4. Four and a half minutes later: the emboli have almost passed. Fourteen days after his last attack a left carotid arteriogram showed complete occlusion, and symptoms ceased (Dr Michael Ashby's case [5] and courtesy *British Medical Journal*).

history of right hemiparesis. Over twenty of the visual attacks were recorded, lasting one to five minutes. Fourteen days after attack, which was almost certainly due to a platelet embolus, a left carotid arteriogram showed a complete occlusion, almost certainly recent, of the internal carotid artery beginning at the sinus [5]. Small retinal emboli may be symptomless; such a condition has been seen and photographed during a chance examination [86].

Although such transient retinal changes may not occur at a time when they can be witnessed, this mechanism should be suspected when a patient with transient blindness is shown to have irregular stenosis of the internal carotid sinus on the same side (Fig. 8.5a). At operation, this will be found partly blocked by an accumulation of platelet thrombus (Fig. 8.5b). In many such patients a cure has followed correction of the lesion in the carotid. The incidence of such 'ulcerated' irregularities is cited as between 7 and 54 per cent [50, 102A]. Stasis can be demonstrated (Fig. 8.5c) in the boundary layer of the stream within the carotid sinus: platelets might lodge here even in the absence of ulceration.

Cholesterol emboli are sometimes seen as brightly shining deposits lodged at the bifurcation of a retinal artery, and probably arise from the discharge of a pocket of mural atheroma substance into the carotid lumen; thus their origin as well as their appearance is different from the transient paler

platelet emboli from the surface of the main artery lesion [80].

Aneurysm of the internal carotid artery carries a risk of serious stroke complications when sizeable pieces of contained thrombus become detached [84]. Transient episodes of constant pattern may then precede the major event, with loss of vision on the side of the lesion and hemiparesis of the opposite side (Fig. 8.6) (*see also* Chapter 9).

Smaller emboli, however, could scarcely be the reason for repeated minor localised cerebral episodes; if this were the mechanism the fragments would be required to take exactly the same anatomical course down the branching arterial tree on each occasion. A static lesion with haemodynamic shifts of a more general, systemically determined origin would seem a better explanation of these.

Progressive Cerebral Ischaemia

Patients whose episodes become more frequent, with a neurological defect which increases with the episodes or between them, and often mental deterioration also [4], have progressive ischaemia. It is not yet known how much of this is due to an increase in the main artery obstruction, and how much to further loss, perhaps embolic, of small branches, or to continuing cerebral impairment from previous ischaemia. Neither is it easy to exonerate general

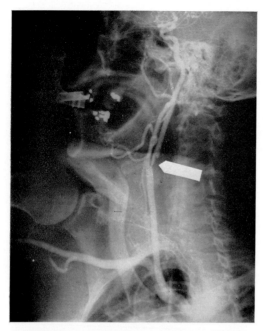

(a) Irregular stenosis of right carotid sinus in an oil-rig driller aged forty-nine, who had been having transient attacks of blindness in the right eye. Relieved after carotid endarterectomy.

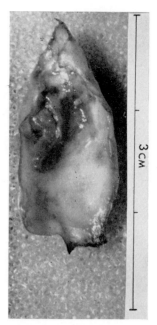

(b) Endarterectomy specimen from right carotid sinus of a man aged sixty-five who, while under observation for intermittent claudication, developed transient paralysis of the left hand on awakening. Soft recent thrombus was loosely adherent to the intima just proximal to the stenosis. Good recovery following endarterectomy. Patency of repair $2\frac{3}{4}$ years later at post-mortem for carcinoma of bronchus.

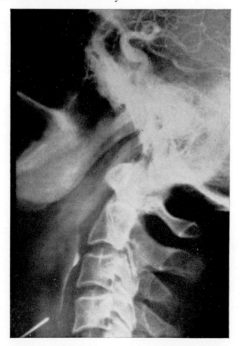

(c) Stasis of marginal blood stream in carotid sinus proximal to a stenosis at its upper end. Contrast medium lingers in this region. Platelet thrombus might build up here.

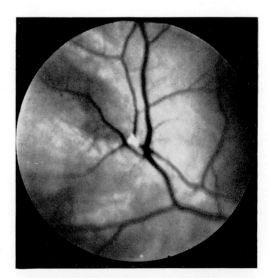

(d) Cholesterol retinal embolus. Transient attacks of blindness, relieved after carotid endarterectomy.

Fig. 8.5.

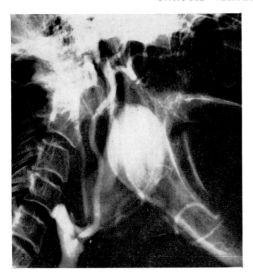

Fig. 8.6. A large retropharyngeal aneurysm of the right internal carotid artery whose removal was complicated by cerebral embolism.

and circulatory factors which would tend to accelerate such local deterioration. Another difficulty concerns the vague and bilateral effects of vertebrobasilar obstruction; there is no healthy side to compare with the ischaemic region. Cases of progressive hind-brain ischaemia are easily missed. Now that some of these are suitable for surgical treatment, for example the lesion known as 'subclavian steal' (*see* p. 171), there is practical value in the recognition of progressive hind-brain ischaemia which might otherwise be mistaken for senility and general decline.

The Completed Stroke: Cerebral Infarction

Once a major and sustained stroke has occurred, with subsequent recovery which is delayed and incomplete, a *cerebral infarction* is considered to be present. Loss of consciousness occurs only when an ischaemic lesion is massive but is more common when the stroke is due to cerebral haemorrhage, a point of immediate importance in management, for if the condition is wrongly considered to be thrombotic, and either anticoagulants are given or a carotid reconstruction is undertaken for a stenosis, which may also be present, further fatal bleeding is probable [104]. The same significance attaches to the finding of blood in the cerebrospinal fluid, also rare in thrombotic stroke. Echo-encephalography has been successfully used in detecting shift of the midline structures caused by cerebral haemorrhage, but seldom present in infarction [1].

The Size and Implications of the Stroke Problem

Figures published by the Registrar General for the years 1942 to 1962 show that stroke deaths, mostly from cerebral infarction [108], have more than doubled in the past twenty years (Fig. 8.7). In Great Britain, the mortality exceeds that of other western countries (*see* Chapter 1, p. 1), and is higher than for any other form of peripheral arterial disease in this country, especially in women.

Survival in 'hard-hit' hemiplegics who recover from their acute illness is not so short as is often supposed. With institutional care, which many of them require, they may live longer than other chronic sick. Unfavourable factors include age over sixty-five [3], diastolic blood pressure above 110 mm, and abnormality of the ECG [63]. A patient free from these may survive for years.

To the vascular surgeon this common tragedy provides an incentive to earlier recognition of the warning stages and the presence of main artery stenosis so often associated with them, for at the present time only surgery can correct this.

The role of stenosis of the extracranial arteries in cerebral infarction was the subject of a Special

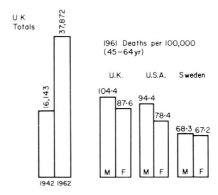

Fig. 8.7. Stroke deaths. (International figures from Burgess *et al.*, *see* Chapter 1 [12].)

Report published by the Medical Research Council in 1961 [107]. The authors, Yates and Hutchinson, examined at autopsy the whole main arterial supply from the aorta to the brain in 100 cases in whom death was thought to be due to cerebral ischaemia. They accept that their series was selected, for other patients with cerebral ischaemia died outside the hospital in which the study was conducted, e.g. those with psychiatric symptoms or transient, remittent neurological episodes, who later died from massive ischaemia. Even so, the group examined was found

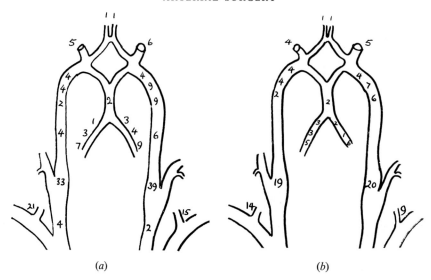

(a)   (b)

Fig. 8.8. Incidence and distribution of severe atheroma and stenosis in the main cerebral supply arteries (*after* Yates and Hutchinson, 1961 [107]).

(*a*) in 100 patients with the clinical diagnosis of cerebral infarct.
(*b*) in 31 patients with proven cerebral infarct.

to contain 28 cases of hæmorrhage, and 26 of circulatory failure, most of them due to postoperative shock or recent myocardial infarction or both.

The following important conclusions arose from the Report (Fig. 8.8):

(*a*) Nearly all infarcts were associated with stenosis or occlusion of extracranial cerebral arteries.

(*b*) Less than one-third of infarcts were associated with stenosis or occlusion of intracranial arteries (*see also* p. 158, radiology of strokes).

(*c*) Severe obstructive disease was present in the carotid arteries in 51 patients and in the vertebrals in 40.

(*d*) General systemic factors such as anaemia, hypotension, coronary arteriosclerosis, and postoperative shock, all contribute to the occurrence of cerebral infarction in the presence of main arterial obstruction. Sludging of blood in the cerebral capillary bed may be an important further cause of continuing stasis.

Morbid Anatomy of Main Artery Lesions

1. *Distribution*

An unselected series of 93 autopsies was subsequently examined in the same way by Schwartz and Mitchell [83], and each of the main arteries in the specimens was graded for area of arterial disease, severity of stenosis, and presence of ulceration or occlusion (Fig. 8.9). Severe arteriosclerosis and stenosis were common, particularly in the carotid sinuses. Stenosis occurred about equally in the proximal parts of the innominate and left subclavian arteries. The right subclavian and vertebral arteries were more often stenosed than the left. The common carotids differed: on the left, the narrowing was greatest proximally (near the aortic origin), while on the right the termination was more often

affected. Innominate and proximal subclavian stenoses were much commoner in men, also vertebral stenosis, probably as a part of the condition of the subclavian. It was unusual for one main artery to be narrowed without similar changes in the others, a fact that should be remembered clinically when considering, for example, an abnormality in a single carotid arteriogram.

Another important practical implication of both these studies is that almost all the sites liable to severe stenosis are accessible to the surgeon, whereas after complete occlusion has occurred and thrombus has spread distally into the bony course of the carotid or vertebral artery, no restoration of flow will be possible (Fig. 8.10).

2. Structure

Study of the narrowed carotid sinus in arteriosclerosis [72] shows that the lining is composed of fibrin-platelet thrombus, beneath which is amorphous fibrin thrombus, then an organised fibrous

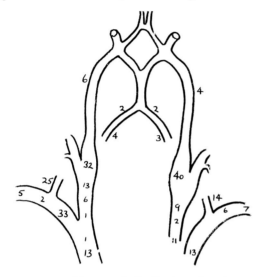

Fig. 8.9. Incidence and distribution of neck-artery stenosis in a series of ninety-three unselected autopsies (*after* Schwartz and Mitchell, 1961).

layer, deep to which appear cholesterol clefts, then comes adherent inner layers of the arterial media. Sometimes, in this type of lesion, here or in other parts of the carotid-vertebral system, the plaque gives way, and blood from the lumen enters the deep clefts of the lesion under considerable pressure and lifts the plaque, thereby further narrowing the artery or even closing it. If, later, such a lesion is explored, it will be found to contain thick, greenish soupy substance, a true atheroma (athere = porridge), which may at any time discharge its contents into the cerebral circulation, with possibly serious results [52].

Causes of Carotid Occlusion Other than Arteriosclerosis

Fibromuscular hyperplasia of the arterial wall, first described in the renal artery (*see* Chapter 17, p. 358) affects the internal carotid next in frequency [20, 53A]. It may be an incidental finding during investigation for cerebral aneurysm or tumour [4A, 6A, 80A]. Cerebral symptoms are more often diffuse than focal. Other arteries can be affected [17].

The proximal carotid is sometimes involved in *pulseless disease* (*see* Chapter 7, p. 141).

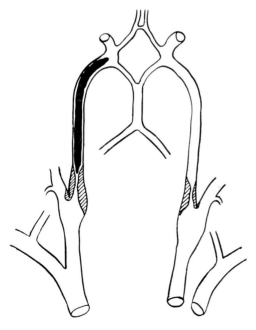

Fig. 8.10. Intracranial extension of distal thrombus beyond stenosis of carotid sinus.

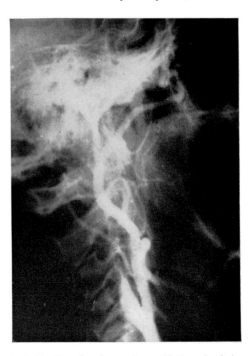

Fig. 8.11. Complete internal carotid thrombosis in a young woman following extraction of an infected molar tooth. Temporarily hemiplegic with full recovery.

Fig. 8.12.

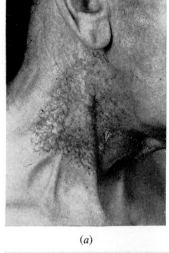

(*a*) Area of previous irradiation for hypopharyngeal carcinoma in an engine driver aged sixty.

(*b*) Complete occlusion of both carotid arteries in irradiated zone.

(*c*) The left internal carotid is also occluded.

(*d*) Collateral supply to cerebrum via left external carotid and ophthalmic arteries. Loud bruit over left eye.

Dementia and decline with further stroke.

(*a*)

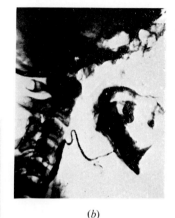

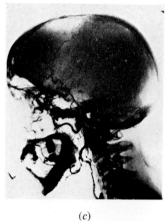

(*b*)

(*c*)

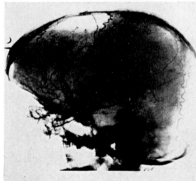

(*d*)

Neck sepsis (Fig. 8.11) [7, 33], irradiation (Fig. 8.12), temporal arteritis (*see* Chapter 7, p. 140), and dissecting aneurysm (*see* Chapter 15, p. 319) are other causes. Injury is considered on page 155.

Tortuosity

When, as a result of hypertensive aortic lengthening, the great vessels become lifted up at their origin, and the neck arteries themselves stretch also, the latter may become much too long for their anatomical course. They then assume a meandering, tortuous appearance, with kinking or even looping. Figure 8.13 shows the *innominate and right common carotid* often affected. It is common for a hypertensive woman in her fifties to seek advice for the pulsatile swelling in the right side of her neck, which these arteries then produce. The condition is quite harmless; it may in fact resolve perceptibly with hypotensive drugs, though in itself no indication for such treatment. Arteriography would be indicated only if there were real doubt over the possibility of a

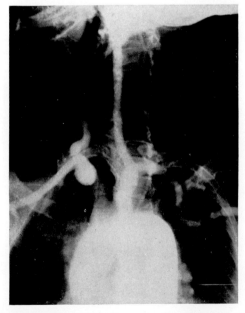

Fig. 8.13. Kinked dilated innominate artery presenting in the suprasternal notch. Right common carotid artery also kinked and laterally displaced. From a woman aged fifty-four.

true aneurysm as the cause of the pulsation, a much rarer lesion in this site, though occasionally seen in connection with female arteritis (*see* Chapter 7).

Kinking of the internal carotid (Fig. 8.14) is common at all ages, and is unrelated to hypertension [66]. It may be congenital, from a cause such as failure of the artery to straighten the long and angulated course it earlier assumed from the joining of the third aortic arch and the dorsal aorta. It has been described clinically as a pulsatile prominence in the lateral pharynx, commoner in females, of whom over a third are under fifteen years of age [51]. Another malformation is the fixation of the carotid bifurcation by a band of fibrous tissue in place of the external carotids [75]; obstruction may be caused, with dilatation of the common carotid, and a looped internal carotid that is narrower than normal, though occasionally the redundancy is associated with aneurysm (Fig. 8.6), *see also* Chapter 9, p. 188, which further suggests some factor localised to the internal carotid itself, for the external carotid is seldom affected in this way.

It is believed that looping of the internal carotid may cause neurological effects from interference with its blood flow [39, 74, 88]. This has been shown to be so in experimental work on dogs [24], in which the haemodynamic effect was proportional to the degree of the deformity (*see also* p. 173).

Kinking of the vertebral artery [39] (*see* Fig. 8.36) may occur with certain head movements, either at the short segment between its origin and entering the bony canal, or where osteoarthritic thickening of the intervertebral sections of the canal may nip the artery higher in its course [37, 43]. Hind-brain ischaemia in the form of drop attacks with neck turning or extension should justify arteriography if the patient is otherwise well.

Injuries and Cerebral Ischaemia

Closed injury to the internal carotid is easily missed; there may not be much local bruising and the neurological complications are almost always delayed. Young people are affected, in whom the neck has been violently extended or twisted, as in athletic or car accidents. Older patients are less liable to such stretching of their carotid for it is longer, even tortuous, and thus will not be 'bow-strung' across the vertebrae. They may, however, sustain a local blunt injury to an already thickened, narrowed and stiff carotid bifurcation which may fracture, dissect or thrombose, and the patient later develops hemiplegia. In all these injuries there should be time to repair the damage to the artery before neurological effects show themselves [40, 55A, 77]. The same applies to the hidden carotid injury that a child sustains when he falls on to an object such as a pencil carried in the mouth [94].

Damage to the neck arteries may occur in *birth injury*. Probably some cases of cerebral palsy are caused in this way [106]. The vertebral artery is most often involved.

In adults, the vertebral artery may be injured during manipulation for painful spondylosis, as well as by accidental violence. The prognosis is grave.

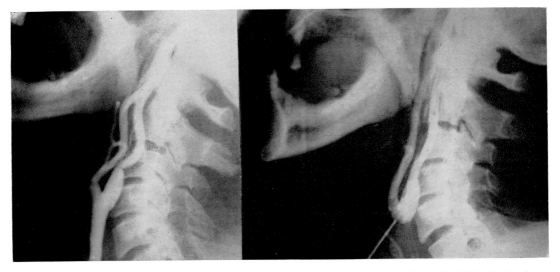

Fig. 8.14. Kinked, angulated left internal carotid artery in a man aged sixty with right-sided TIAs. Relieved after common carotid resection and anastomosis (*see* also Fig. 8.36).

Five out of six recently reported cases died [55]. Infarcts of the cerebellum and occipital lobe were found at autopsy. The occlusion may spread to the vertebral artery from a traumatic thrombosis of the subclavian [29, 55]. Patients who survive may show severe brain stem disability. The spinal artery may also thrombose in fractures of the cervical spine, and aggravate the cord lesion already caused by the injury.

Operative injury to the extracranial cerebral arteries is rare. Some cases have followed thyroidectomy, perhaps from excessive retraction upon the carotid, though the vertebral artery may be damaged also, either in its canal by the extended position of the neck, or by direct damage in the open part of its course, for scar tissue found there, when removed, was followed by full recovery [96].

Clinical Diagnosis [4, 46A] Table 8.1

Table 8.1. Clinical Features in 100 Patients before Carotid Endarterectomy

Transient ischaemic attacks	almost all
Neck bruit	69
Unilateral lesion	65
Motor symptoms	40
(right and left equal)	
Residual neurological defect	36
(mild, 22; severe, 14)	
Visual symptoms	26
Hind brain features	20
Sensory symptoms	12
Ipsilateral retinal ⎫	
Contralateral hemiphenomena ⎭	8
Evidence of arteriosclerosis at other sites	64
(myocardial, 34; limbs, 30)	

The steps are as follows:

1. Recognition in a middle-aged or elderly patient of ischaemic neurological symptoms and signs focal or general.
2. Detection of occlusive arterial disease in the neck or the upper limbs.
3. Radiological confirmation and localisation of obstruction to these arteries.
4. A full general survey of the patient for evidence of any associated, general, neurological or vascular disease.

Although the vascular surgeon may be experienced in this field, he should not normally take it upon himself to make the neurological assessment.* Co-operation with a neurologist is essential, both before and after surgery.

In summary, the table following gives the main clinical features:

---

* Three patients referred to the author for carotid surgery proved on investigation to be suffering from cerebral tumour as well as their carotid lesion.

Neurological

Hemisphere: four types [62]:

1. Attacks of monocular blindness and later hemiplegia.
2. Episodes of hemiparesis or sensory disturbance, by increments leading to hemiplegia.
3. Gradually progressive focal lesion (resembles cerebral tumour).
4. Common stroke, with or without premonitory effects. The common form.

Hind brain: two types:

1. Sudden fatal illness.
2. Episodes with diffuse or varied neurological and visual symptoms. Vertigo commonest.

Cardiovascular and associated

Generalised obliterative arterial disease.
Bruits over carotids or subclavians.
Unequal arm blood pressures.
Coronary heart disease, including heart block.
Hypertension.
Carotid sinus syndrome.
Rheumatic heart disease.
Spondylitis of cervical spine.
Recent injury, hypotension, surgical operation.
Thiazide diuretics [16], the contraceptive pill [95A].
Carbon monoxide poisoning.
Anaemia, or polycythaemia.

TRANSIENT ISCHAEMIC ATTACKS (TIA)

The mechanism of these has been discussed, and we have seen that they may occur in either the carotid or the vertebro-basilar territory, yet not often in both, although occlusion in one area may give rise to symptoms in the other.

They often occur when the patient arises from bed; or with head turning.

Headache may come on with the attacks. The diagnosis will then be from migraine, tumour, and other neurological diseases. The vascular evidence, with the help of the neurologist, should usually resolve this important point. The surgeon should go no further until this has been settled. Transient attacks 'should be repetitive and initially there should be full recovery of function between the attacks, [whose duration] should be less than an hour' [2].

What relationship may exist between TIAs and massive cerebral ischaemia? Three possibilities should be considered [62]:

1. Patients first seen with a major stroke often give a history of recent attacks, some short, some prolonged. These have a higher mean blood pressure, and *haemorrhage* may in fact be the cause of the stroke.
2. About the same number of patients present with the *TIAs only*, which in the vertebro-basilar group tend to be very short, though the total history might be a long one. The typical symptoms occur in wide variety.
3. A smaller number of patients experience *TIAs after a major attack*.

Marshall has emphasised that in the carotid territory the interval between onset and major stroke tends to be short, with only one or two TIAs in 75 per cent of his cases. A sense of urgency is therefore needed in the management of such patients, for in them the condition is truly one of 'impending stroke'.

Residual neurological features, if present, are of the usual upper motor neurone type, and may be quite mild; there may also be clumsiness, speech impairment, poor signature, and mental depression. If in such a patient a bruit is present over the carotid bifurcation on either side, the case for arteriography is strong.

Vertebro-basilar TIAs are about equally common. Neurological features are less clear than in the carotid type. Vertigo, scattered limb pareses, dim vision or bilateral field defects, and facial paraesthesias are common, and may be noticed on head turning. In normal subjects it is possible to demonstrate interference with vertebral artery flow on the side opposite to the movement, a factor likely to be important, also, in patients with vertebral artery narrowing. In cervical spondylosis, obstruction occurs on the side towards which the head is turned, also on looking up, producing a typical form of 'drop attack' [11, 37].

Head turning may also elicit attacks of another kind: e.g. in the carotid sinus syndrome [45, 98, 99] where the effects may be purely syncopal and generalised, or the hypotension may 'pick out' a focal zone so that a more typical TIA is produced.

Yet another form of ischaemic attack occurs in a patient with rheumatic heart disease [46]; 14 per cent of one group of 323 patients had already had cerebral embolism and another 12 per cent had experienced disabling neurological disturbances. Previous subclinical embolic incidents were considered possible cause for the transient attacks in this latter group, with exertion, or tachycardia acting as a trigger mechanism. Surgical correction of mitral stenosis relieved the attacks.

Ischaemic heart disease, a known cause of severe cerebral infarction from embolism [7A], may also cause TIAs. Polycythaemia, which strikingly reduces cerebral blood flow [53], has been associated with TIAs [2]; full stroke led to the diagnosis in three of the author's patients.

INTERPRETATION OF CAROTID BRUITS

A soft, low-pitched murmur is common in healthy subjects [35], especially in childhood when the neck is thin and the cerebral blood flow reaches its highest level [53]. Anaemia also produces arterial murmurs, as it does in the heart; more than half of a group of patients whose haemoglobin was less than 60 per cent had a loud systolic murmur in the neck [97].

Undue pressure upon the stethoscope bell will, as with other peripheral arteries, produce a carotid murmur, though with head turning it should disappear as the bell is displaced by the movement; a true carotid bruit is more often increased with head turning (N.B. Carotid sinus compression may cause cardiac standstill (*see* p. 176)).

The bruit of carotid stenosis is unmistakable. It is localised to the bifurcation, and is usually loud, rough, and often has a curious high-pitched squeaking prolongation like the cry of a seagull. Such a bruit is reliable evidence of carotid stenosis and should weigh heavily in the clinical diagnosis of carotid insufficiency. In perhaps 10 per cent of cases, the sound originates in the external carotid near its origin [101] (Fig. 8.15), or both branches of the common carotid may be sufficiently narrowed to produce it (Fig. 8.16). Reduction in the superficial temporal pulse, or the occurrence of masseteric claudication may help in recognising external carotid stenosis, also thermography of the face.

The quality of the bruit may change during an observation period in which TIAs or retinal platelet emboli take place [85].

SUBCLAVIAN AND INNOMINATE BRUITS

As with the carotid, if these other neck murmurs are truly obstructive, the sound produced is loud and rough, and is confined to the area where they are generated, behind the sternoclavicular joint or manubrium, for there is insufficient blood flow to carry them along the distal course of the artery. (After relief of the obstruction by endarterectomy a softer bruit usually persists which, with the increased blood flow, is well transmitted peripherally.) A bruit confined to the distal part of the subclavian artery is

perfectly operable, and with such severe reduction in blood flow already having developed there is much less risk and uncertainty with carotid surgery than with lesser degrees of obstruction. All that is required is a steady trickle of blood sufficient to maintain distal patency in the carotid.

Arteriography, like the morbid anatomical studies discussed on page 152, has shown that intracerebral occlusion is much less common as a cause of cerebral ischaemia than is generally supposed. Among 80 cases of acute stroke investigated in this way, the clinical diagnosis of middle cerebral occlusion was made 41 times, and arteriography confirmed it in only 3. The commonest abnormal finding was a main neck artery occlusion [14].

Carotid Arteriography or Arch Aortography?

Carotid arteriography gives the clearest view of the carotid bifurcation. It also shows the cerebral vessels, an important consideration when the diagnosis is at all in doubt, and a useful means of assessing the cross-flow between the hemispheres in patients with bilateral disease (Fig. 8.17(*b*)). It is, however, not entirely without risk. The necessary manipulations of the carotid, both with digital compression and during the actual needle puncture, may either dislodge thrombus or atheromatous material into the brain, or cause carotid sinus reflex effects. Bilateral studies are essential, and the needle must always appear in the picture. 'Trickle' injection (Fig. 8.5(*c*)) confirms local stasis and the probability of embolism [41A].

Arch aortography [91] is finding an increasing place in routine practice, for it gives information on all four neck arteries at once, providing a full anatomical study, and comparing flow rates in the two cranio-brachial areas, an essential need when there is suspicion of proximal stenosis of the great arteries, as in subclavian steal. It is also valuable in the investigation of hind-brain ischaemia of all kinds, including intrinsic vertebral artery lesions, and those secondary to compression, as in cervical

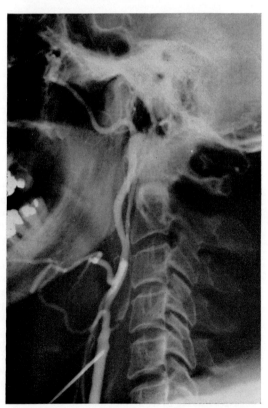

(*a*) Tight localised stenosis within carotid sinus with grossly reduced flow into patent distal internal carotid.

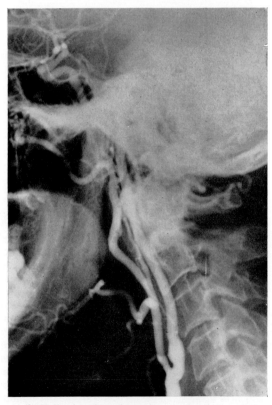

(*b*) Following thrombo-endarterectomy, the whole of the internal carotid and its branches are seen to be patent.

Fig. 8.18. The final stage of carotid stenosis.

spondylosis [11, 37]. In pulseless disease or in generalised arteriosclerosis of the central type there may be difficulty in obtaining an aortic injection from the limbs. *Intravenous aortography* may give a useful indication of the extent of aortic arch disease in such patients.

Vertebral arteriography via an axillary catheter gives excellent pictures (Fig. 8.19), but is not free from risk of overdosage to the hind brain.

Thermal scanning of the face [14A, 102] usually shows decreased heat elimination in the supra-orbital region in patients whose ophthalmic perfusion is reduced by internal carotid occlusion or stenosis (Fig. 8.20).

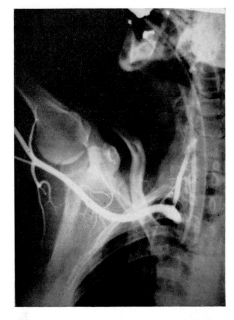

Fig. 8.19. Stenosis of right vertebral origin. Good contrast values obtained via axillary catheterisation.

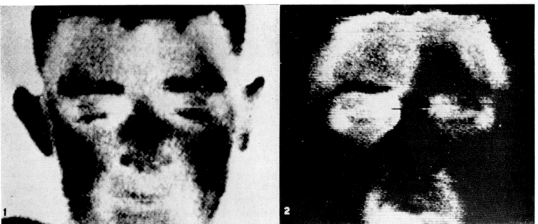

Fig. 8.20. The thermographic pattern of heat elimination from the head.

(*a*) A normal subject; the dark areas representing cold skin, e.g. ears, cheeks, and nose.

(*b*) In a patient with left internal carotid obstruction: the area of the frontal branch of the left ophthalmic artery is dark. This effect can sometimes be recognised on simple palpation with the back of the finger. (Courtesy of the publishers of *Radiology* [102].)

Course and Prognosis

The severity of the neurological features [2], and the age at which they first appear [3], both influence the mortality, although, as we have seen [3], once the patient has survived a major stroke he may have five years or so of more or less severely limited existence before a further cerebral or cardiovascular attack brings this to an end.

In 153 patients with radiologically proved internal carotid occlusion [38], the highest mortality was in those with sudden onset; the majority of patients with TIAs as the first feature went on to a full stroke. Of 11 patients with bilateral occlusion 5 succumbed in an average of just over six months. The overall mortality in this series was 46 per cent over 3·7 years.

In a prospective study of 177 stroke patients over three years [63], the chief factors affecting the outcome were the presence of a diastolic blood pressure above 110 mm Hg or an abnormal pattern in the ECG. Patients with features of brain-stem ischaemia did worse than those with hemisphere effects. The opposite applies to those with only TIAs [62].

Medical Treatment [10, 30B]

As with arteriosclerosis elsewhere in the body, there is as yet no certain effective medical treatment, and no ready way of assessing those that are in use. Anticoagulants must not be used if there is any possibility that the stroke may be haemorrhagic [15]. The probability of this mistake in diagnosis is high [107]. Opinion is divided on the possible benefits of anticoagulants in non-haemorrhagic cerebral ischaemia, whether it has caused infarction or only TIAs [54]. Controlled study has not established its value [39A]. One danger is that of 'rebound thrombosis' on stopping the anticoagulant [61].

SURGICAL TREATMENT

In the fifteen years that have passed since the first successful carotid reconstruction for hemiparesis [28], nothing has diminished the confidence of the writer in the value of the well-timed operation for cerebral ischaemia. Our first patient, operated upon in 1954 for repeated and worsening episodes, remains free from cerebrovascular symptoms after fifteen years. This experience has been repeatedly confirmed since (Table 8.4, p. 168).

There now exists an established case for surgery in cerebral ischaemia, when the following conditions can be satisfied:

1. Where reconstruction of a main artery should increase the total cerebral blood supply, without the necessity for proof that the arterial obstruction concerned is directly related to the region of the brain thought, clinically, to be ischaemic.
2. Where repeated ischaemic attacks are related to the narrowed main artery to the region of the brain in question, or to one eye, whether or not the evidence suggests that embolism is responsible.
3. As a preventive measure where tight stenosis is discovered in a patient with a previous history suggesting cerebrovascular disease, or before major surgery for some other condition such as an abdominal aneurysm.

Contra-indications: the Irreversible Lesion

There are two such lesions and both are extremely common:

1. Complete occlusion of the internal carotid.*

2. A cerebral infarct, with dense persisting hemiplegia.

Commonly the two occur together. Nothing that surgery can offer will overcome the direct and completed effects of these two lesions, but there may be a place for supplementary operation for incomplete arterial or cerebral lesions occurring in the same patient, as for example:

(a) where there is stenosis of the opposite carotid artery;
(b) where there is a residual defect (not massive) with delayed recovery.

A third important contra-indication to carotid surgery is a deterioration in the general condition of the patient. Confusion, senility, or heart failure are severe impediments, and a good result is unlikely in such patients who usually also show minor residual neurological defects, due to previous infarction. Old age alone is no contra-indication if the general condition is good and the neurological picture suggests the need for operation. Acute, severe recent deterioration is a warning that surgery may be dangerous, particularly in fresh strokes with loss of consciousness, in which oedema or haemorrhage may be more important than the ischaemia that caused them (see p. 168).

Preventive Operation [26, 47A, 94B]

In a sense, most of the indications for operation come under this heading, for though transient attacks may be alarming, they do not, in themselves, disable. It is in the expectation that complete occlusion may be postponed or prevented altogether that localised obstruction in the carotid, vertebral, and subclavian arteries now require serious consideration for surgical correction whenever they are recognised, for, as yet, there is no means of knowing whether or not the obstructed artery is dispensable until it is too late.

---

* A minority view among surgeons favours an attempt at clearance of a recent total occlusion, hoping to remove consecutive thrombus by suction, or using balloon catheters [32, 94A] as in embolectomy (see Chapter 14, p. 271). Only time will show which of such cases, if any, should be explored.

Carotid Endarterectomy

Technique

Choice of anaesthetic. Special measures must be taken to protect the brain from further ischaemia during carotid clamping. Each of the following methods has been adopted in its turn (Table 8.2); all were found satisfactory in the majority of cases.

(*a*) General anaesthesia with induced hypothermia.

(*b*) Local analgesia by cervical plexus block.

(*c*) General anaesthesia with routine use of an indwelling carotid shunt.

Fresh neurological sequelae were encountered in seven per cent.

Table 8.2. Anaesthesia and Cerebral Protection

Method	Total	Fresh neurological defect
Hypothermia	30	3
Local	18	2
Shunt	26	3
G.A. only	36	0†
	100	7*

* One patient had shunt and hypothermia.
† Eight operations under total body heparin (3 mg per kg body wt.) [52].

Induced hypothermia with general anaesthesia was used for the first time in 1954 [28], and remained routine until 1962. Surface cooling, originally with ice bags, wet sheets, and fans, took one and a half hours or more in an obese patient. Later, a collapsible canvas bath was introduced (Fig. 8.21) which, with the advent of halothane, shortened the cooling time to about thirty minutes. It is a cumbersome and time-consuming technique, and we now only use it in:

1. Patients who show a residual neurological deficit before operation, and in whom temporary shunting, which may involve several minutes' total clamping during setting up and removal, could be considered an extra risk.

2. In those with such an extensive or high-placed lesion of the internal carotid that a shunt cannot be conveniently placed. The maximum time we allow under hypothermia is twenty minutes. In the sinus region this is ample unless a patch graft is to be used.

These and other lesions requiring a longer period of clamping will require the setting up of a temporary shunt.

3. For the patient with multiple occlusions in whom there would be less safety margin in manipulating the remaining artery at normal body temperature.

4. When multiple reconstructions are contemplated.

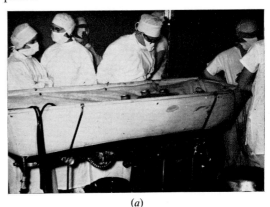

(*a*)

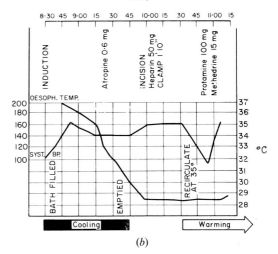

(*b*)

Fig. 8.21. Induced hypothermia by surface cooling.

(*a*) Waiting for the body temperature to fall. Patient is almost completely immersed with ice bags on the trunk, and ice cold water is being circulated through the bath by means of a mechanical pump.

(*b*) Cooling record: the systolic pressure rises sharply in the early cooling phase before the body temperature has fallen. Likewise, it falls again during early rewarming.

An oesophageal thermistor registers the temperature of the deep tissues and of the circulating blood in the great vessels. Gentle surface warming with a water-filled blanket and pump circuit may be necessary to prevent a further fall in body temperature after the emptying of the bath. Rewarming takes about five hours and, like cooling, is slower in fat subjects.

Local anaesthesia was extensively used before 1967, in the hope of detecting ischaemic cerebral damage from the operation in its earliest stages, with the patient conscious during the clamping. In fact this test proved unreliable, with postoperative strokes in patients who had tolerated both the trial and the actual clamping well. Others had a stroke even before the clamp was applied, and were thought to have sustained embolism from dislodgement of obstructing material in the carotid sinus [7c]. Exposure and apprehension might lower the patient's resistance to temporary ischaemia. In the author's experience there was little difference between this and other methods of cerebral protection.

General anaesthesia is obviously preferable, but on its own gives no protection against operative cerebral ischaemia. To guard against this, various suggestions have been made, including:

(*a*) The use of cyclopropane, with which can be given a high proportion of oxygen [19], though cyclopropane has been found to influence the function of the carotid baroceptors [73].

(*b*) Hypoventilation at 6 to 8 respirations per minute [100] produces a rise in PCO_2, considered useful because of its potent cerebral vasodilator action.

(*c*) Vasopressors have been given with the object of increasing cerebral blood flow [100], but there is little evidence that induced hypertension does this, though it is important to maintain the normal blood pressure; any fall, whether induced by the anaesthetic agent or by foot-down tilting, can cause a sharp reduction in cerebral flow.

(*d*) With a short-acting barbiturate such as intravenous 1 per cent methohexitone, the patient may be roused from time to time to assess the neurological state [19]. Not all subjects will be able to co-operate effectively under such circumstances, as is found after drowsing during cervical plexus block with heavy basal narcosis.

More important is the virtually certain protection provided by an *indwelling carotid shunt* which provides for the flow of blood through the affected carotid during almost the whole of the arterial procedure. Setting up and removing the shunt takes only two or three minutes. This is now the writer's routine practice. No difficulties have been encountered, and the technique is simple and involves almost no blood loss. It is described on page 167.

SURGICAL EXPOSURE

The carotid bifurcation is exposed by a short incision along the upper half of the anterior border of the sterno-mastoid (Fig. 8.22). Oblique skin crease

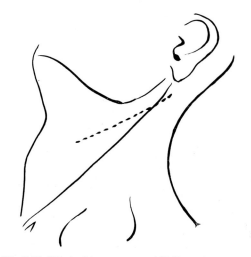

Fig. 8.22. Skin incision over carotid bifurcation should not be too oblique.

incisions are not well suited to vascular surgery in the neck, for they cannot be extended along the artery.

With a self-retaining retractor in the left hand, the superficial and deep fasciae are divided with the scalpel. The retractor is then re-inserted to include these layers and is lifted up, while further sharp dissection with the scalpel exposes the common facial vein. The retractor is then laid down while the vein is ligated and divided (Fig. 8.24), close to the internal jugular so as to leave a portion for possible use as a patch graft.

The carotid bifurcation can now be felt pulsating close beneath. The external carotid is identified first by means of its superior thyroid branch (Fig. 8.25). Two per cent xylocaine (without adrenalin) is now injected between the internal and external carotids and, after allowing a few moments for this to take effect, the mobilisation of the three carotids can be completed (Fig. 8.26), and a tape sling placed under each. The hypoglossal nerve must be carefully protected. Any fall in blood pressure or cardiac arrhythmia should be treated with atropine 0·6 mg

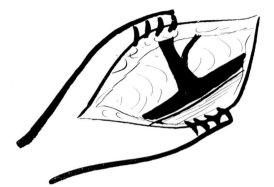

Fig. 8.23. Superficial exposure.

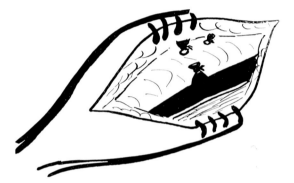

Fig. 8.24. Division of the common facial vein.

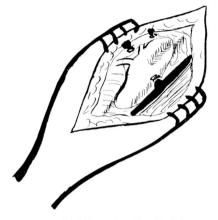

Fig. 8.25. Carotid bifurcation identified by superior thyroid branch.

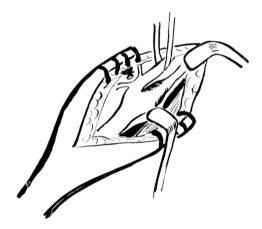

Fig. 8.26. Bifurcation mobilised and branches are taped.

intravenously, and more local anaesthetic is injected between the carotid bifurcation.

If bilateral surgery is required, care should be taken to preserve the carotid sinus nerve and the carotid body, otherwise physiological disturbances of blood pressure and gases may result (*see* Chapter 9, pp. 181 and 185).

Preparations should be made for an internal shunt.

CLAMPING (Fig. 8.27)
A Craaford clamp is applied to the common carotid well down in the lower end of the wound, in order to lift the vessel up into good view, and the internal and external carotids are closed off with bulldog clamps, heparin 50 mg having been injected into the lumen of the bifurcation just beforehand. The time is noted, and a stop watch started.

Acknowledgement
Figures 8.22 to 8.30, the 'technique of internal carotid thrombo-endarterectomy', are from Martin's *Indications and Techniques in Arterial Surgery* by courtesy of the publishers, E. and S. Livingstone.

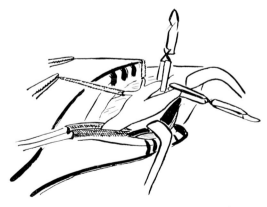

Fig. 8.27. The three carotids are clamped.

165

ENDARTERECTOMY (Fig. 8.28)

A short longitudinal incision is made over the hardest part of the atheromatous plaque, using a No. 15 blade, and entering the plane of cleavage the roll of obstructing material is readily freed from the healthy plane of the media, using a Watson-Cheyne dissector. The thin fringe of sclerosed intima at the distal limit of the block is usually well attached to the artery wall and can be trimmed carefully away so as not to lift it free. The proximal end takes less time to deal with, for it can be neatly avulsed close to the position of the Craaford clamp, using short, curved artery forceps.

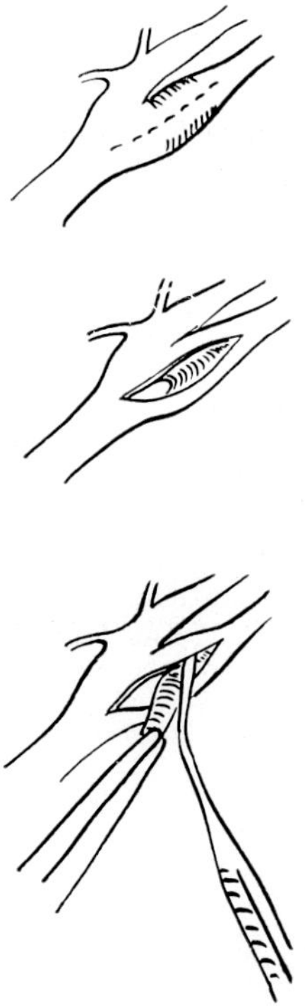

Internal carotid stenosis is usually short, and though it may sometimes extend up into the less accessible higher course of the artery, much more often the lesion is part of the more proximal thick plaque in the terminal common carotid and with the same lesion running into the external carotid opening (Fig. 8.16).

Sometimes the stenosis may lie at a little distance beyond the carotid sinus. When it does, there is often redundant artery that may account for the situation of the lesion; this slack portion can be pulled down to improve the access of this otherwise high-lying lesion to reconstructive surgery.

Occasionally, the common carotid bifurcates low in the neck; sometimes higher, but rarely higher than the angle of the jaw, for it must supply structures at and below this level. The internal carotid artery may lie anterior to the external at the bifurcation. In both these anatomical abnormalities internal carotid stenosis that in no way differs from that of the normally placed artery has been seen.

REPAIR

After brief release of all three clamps, in turn, and a final inspection of the lumen for any loose material remaining, the arteriotomy is closed from above downwards (Fig. 8.29), using 5 or 6/0 arterial silk, with very fine bites at the upper end; the size and interval can be increased as the sinus and the common carotid portions of the opening are reached.

The heparin is reversed, using protamine 100 mg, and the clamps are released, noting the total occlusion time, which should not normally exceed

Fig. 8.28. Stages in open thrombo-endarterectomy of carotid sinus.

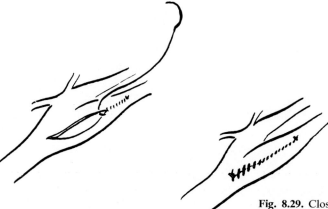

Fig. 8.29. Closure of arteriotomy; very fine stitches distally becoming larger proximally.

166

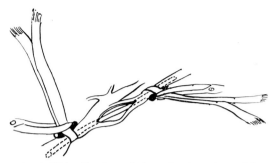

Fig. 8.30(*a*). Simple technique for insertion of indwelling polythene carotid shunt.

nine to ten minutes, an acceptable time for an uncomplicated, short lesion and an operation under local analgesia.

Technique for Internal Shunt

Many cases are likely to require more detailed work, taking longer to complete, e.g. securing stitches to the distal edge of intima, or the placing of a patch graft in the arteriotomy; for these, a temporary shunt should always be set up. It is also highly advisable if the internal carotid backflow is poor, or the measured distal carotid pressure is low [30c, 68a].

A firm polythene tube of at least 2 to 3 mm internal diameter is cut to length to fit the dissected portions of the carotid and internal carotids. The latter artery is intubated first. It may be necessary to dilate it, using either a Watson-Cheyne probe pointed dissector or a small Bakes dilator.* If back flow through the tube is brisk, its lower end should be clipped in an artery forceps. A simple way of inserting the proximal end of the shunt is for the operator to hold the common carotid between the finger and thumb, having removed the Craaford clamp from its lower end. It is then easy to slip the proximal end of the shunt tube into the finger-gripped portions having first snipped off the portion flattened by the artery forceps. Once the tube is lying well down into the artery, the proximal tape can be tightened and held (Fig. 8.30(*a*)). Provided the patient has been heparinised, the shunt will continue to function for as long as may be needed.

Javid's shunt is shown in Fig. 8.30(*b*); it has a tapering form with bulbous ends, which fit the common and internal carotid well, and are secured there by the special ring clamps.

Removal of the shunt is usually through the lower part of the arteriotomy, which can then be sutured

---

* This is also the recommended, definitive operative manoeuvre for the correction of narrowing due to fibromuscular hyperplasia [68b].

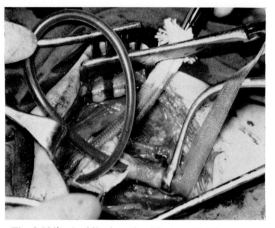

Fig. 8.30(*b*). Javid's shunt in right carotid bifurcation.

quickly during a further short period of complete clamping, the whole process taking only 1–2 minutes.

This method has been found completely satisfactory over periods of up to one and threequarter hours at normal body temperature.

WOUND CLOSURE

After a final check for wound haemostasis, the deep fascia is closed with catgut, having placed a perforated polythene vacuum tube drain (REDIVAC) along the line of the vessels, and brought it out below the main wound. The skin is clipped or sutured with 36 gauge stainless-steel wire.

Results of Carotid Endarterectomy (Fig. 8.31)

Several large surgical series have now been reported [7c, 8, 23, 26, 30, 30b, 30c, 94c, 104a, 105, 109]. The chief lesson concerns the danger of operation in patients with acute recent stroke or severe defect. Table 8.3 shows the findings of the Joint Study of Extracranial Arterial Occlusion in the three common kinds of patient that are referred to surgeons. Haemorrhage into a recent infarct was first recognised as a real risk in 1964 [104], and most papers admit this. Operative mortality has in fact been almost entirely cerebrovascular. Table 8.4 gives the figures for six of the largest series. In general, mortality is declining, no doubt a reflection of more stringent case selection, and also perhaps from improved methods of cerebral protection during operation. The author's own experience agrees with these findings: among ninety-one patients operated upon for TIAs there were three operative deaths, all cerebrovascular. Five other patients were made worse by operation, with probable cerebral infarction. Bilateral carotid disease, ECG

**Table 8.3. Carotid Reconstruction:
Operative Mortality and Neurological
State**

(Joint Study IV [7B])

	No deficit	Deficit present	Acute stroke	All cases
No. of cases	494	1673	50	2217
Operative mortality (%)	2	5	42	5*

* Carotid bifurcation 4, proximal common carotid 8·5, vertebral 4·2, subclavian 5. These figures closely corresponded with the incidence of new strokes after operation at each site.

changes, polycythaemia and severe hypertension were associated preoperative findings in this group.

One good risk patient received no heparin at operation and sustained a massive stroke the same day.

There were two *brain-stem infarcts*. Both had previously shown clinical and radiological evidence of hind-brain ischaemia and both had bilateral carotid stenosis. One had already made a good immediate recovery from operation, but with a period of hypotension due to a 'heparin haematoma'. This episode may have caused the fatal thrombosis. The other patient never regained consciousness; as in the aneurysm patient described above, his was an emergency operation for stroke and coma.

Late mortality in the follow-up period was mainly from coronary thrombosis, with one cerebral infarct in a patient with stenosis in the carotid siphon, and in another patient from a general decline with diffuse cerebrovascular features. All the late deaths were in patients with either known heart disease or hypertension before operation.

Table 8.4. Carotid Endarterectomy: Mortality and Morbidity

Authors	Total patients	Operative mortality (%)	Fresh or worsened defect (%)
Bloodwell *et al.* (1968) [8] (G.A. with hypoventilation)	374	5·6	4·8
Young *et al.* (1969) [109] (G.A. with hypoventilation)	137	4·4	2·9
Thompson *et al.* (1970) [94c] (G.A. with shunt)	358	1·5	2·0
Bland *et al.* (1970) (7c) (Local anaesthesia G.A. with hypercarbia and mild hypertension)	488	3·6	11·4
Joint Study V (1970) (30B) (Various methods)	150	3·5	7·7
DeWeese *et al.* (1971) [26] (Mostly G.A. with B.P. maintenance)	313	3·0	5·5
Firt *et al.* (1971) [30c] (Back pressure measurement re need for shunt)	287	3·0	1·0

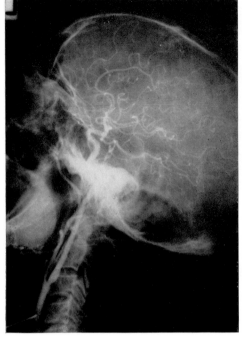

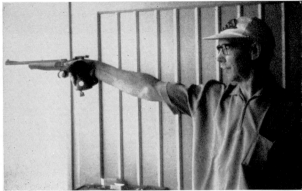

Fig. 8.31. Left internal carotid stenosis diagnosed in 1960 producing transient ischaemic attacks, probably of embolic origin. This patient was recently placed among the winners at a world pistol shooting contest. The scar over his left carotid bifurcation can be clearly seen.

The late results of carotid endarterectomy show the same variability as the early outcome, and depend on closely similar factors, such as case selection (degree of defect, number of arteries involved), experience of the surgical team and much besides [30B]. From a single, highly-specialised centre at which 247 patients were followed for an average of four years, the proportion remaining neurologically symptom-free was 70 per cent for those initially presenting with multiple lesions and hind-brain symptoms. Where only one carotid had been affected, and with pure hemisphere symptoms, the figure was over 90 per cent [104A]. The Joint Study [30B], as would be expected, found results that fell far short of this. Transient attacks were present equally at 42 months in about a third of both the surgical and non-surgical groups. Here there had been random selection of the type of treatment. There was agreement, however, that patients did better after unilateral carotid operation than bilateral, not only in terms of post-operative defect (*see* Table 8.4), but also as far as late, serious strokes were concerned. At St Mary's Hospital, London, Mr. Kenyon and I followed up our complete series of carotid reconstructions for stroke of varying severity. Of 200 patients, mostly with transient attacks, and unilaterally affected in 129 instances, just over 60 per cent of the operative survivors remained neurologically intact after an average follow-up of five years. This figure was weighted by the inclusion of 27 who had developed fresh defects of varying severity immediately after operation.

Vertebral Endarterectomy and Widening

Direct operation upon the stenosed vertebral origin has not yet become accepted as routine; it is technically more difficult and, perhaps, less justifiable because the symptoms and prognosis of hind-brain ischaemia are much less serious than those of the carotid territory.

Indirect operations have been successful, however, including:

(*a*) Carotid endarterectomy with the object of improving hind-brain collateral circulation through the circle of Willis. Twenty-five per cent of one large series of patients surgically treated for carotid occlusive disease had vertigo, and all were relieved following operation [42].

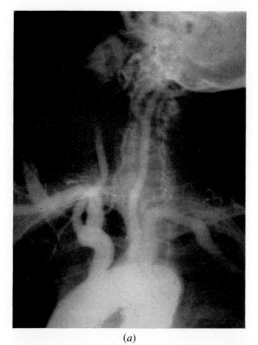
(a)

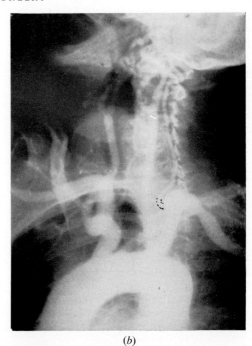
(b)

Fig. 8.32(a). Severe stenosis of the left vertebral artery at its origin in a hypertensive woman of sixty who had been troubled by repeated hind-brain ischaemic attacks.

(b) Good patency following vertebral endarterectomy and patch grafting. Relief from attacks.

(b) Correction of vertebral kinking (see p. 175).

(c) Relief of subclavian steal (see p. 171–3).

(d) Decompression of the vertebral canal [37].

Yet there is a place for vertebral arterial reconstruction which, in selected cases and experienced hands, is safe and satisfactory. Where it appears certain that a narrowed vertebral orifice is contributing to a total cerebrovascular insufficiency, as when one or both carotids are already occluded (Fig. 8.32), the progressive trend of the disease may be checked for a while by vertebral surgery. As with reconstruction of the solitary, 'inappropriate' carotid stenosis (see p. 162), the preventive value of a vertebral widening operation would seem to justify it where experience and facilities are good.

Technique

The standard supraclavicular exposure of the subclavian artery (see Chapter 13) is made under hypothermia if more than one other neck artery is known to be occluded.

The portion of the artery proximal to the internal mammary artery is fully mobilised with the aid of tape traction; the thyro-cervical trunk may require division; the subclavian can then be drawn downwards and laterally to show up its large and unmistakable vertebral branch at its origin.

Remaining branches are controlled with loops or bulldog forceps, and a good length of the open course of the vertebral is now available for exploration, once the proximal Craaford clamp has been applied well down on the first part of the subclavian. The arteriotomy should be one-third over the vertebral and two thirds over the adjacent subclavian.

A shunt must be inserted if the patient also has occluded internal carotids. Technically, this is little more difficult than at the carotid bifurcation, and the sequence of movements is similar. With the distal, vertebral tape loosened, the tube is very gently inserted into the vertebral end of the arteriotomy, checking the backflow before the tape is re-tightened. The proximal end is passed back into the subclavian between the finger and thumb with the Craaford clamp removed, and the tape is then tightened. Heparin is given systemically.

Vertebral endarterectomy tends to be marred by difficulty with tearing during suturing of the thin, remaining layers of the artery. Unless there is gross local irregularity, it is better to leave the plaque and simply to widen the vertebral origin and the subclavian portion of the arteriotomy with a flat dacron patch graft. Fine suturing is essential at the distal part of the patch.

Subclavian Steal [81]

The union of the two vertebral arteries to form the basilar is an efficient arrangement only as long as the pressure within both is fully maintained. If, as a result of a proximal obstruction, the pressure falls in one subclavian, the flow may be reversed in its vertebral branch, which then constitutes a large collateral to the deprived upper limb. This takes place at the expense of the flow into the basilar, so affecting the supply to the hind brain and, sometimes, the general cerebral circulation also.

This is one site in which intermittent neurological changes can be quite definitely related to haemodynamic shifts within the arterial system. Exercise or reactive hyperaemia of the affected upper limb 'milks' the cerebral circulation, and the patient may notice that the neurological episodes are associated with claudication and cooling of the limb.

In the patient with subclavian steal there is always an obvious difference between the arterial status of the two upper limbs. The pulses on the side affected are usually reduced or absent, or if not, there must be a significant difference between the two brachial blood pressures.

AETIOLOGY

Most patients with subclavian steal are men in their fifties with well localised arteriosclerotic narrowing or obstruction of the first part of the left subclavian artery. In a collected series, the left side was affected in 54, and the right in only 17 [81]. A bilateral case has been reported [81]. Other causes of the syndrome include 'young female arteritis' (see Chapter 7), surgical diversion of the proximal subclavian by a Blalock operation, usually some years earlier [31], traumatic injury [78], congenital abnormalities of the origins of the left subclavian and common carotid arteries, embolism [22] and vertebral arteriovenous fistula.

THE CLINICAL PICTURE

Symptomless cases are probably fairly common, and these are sometimes detected when the upper limb pulses are compared during the routine examination for other ischaemic difficulties, such as intermittent claudication of the lower limbs [47]. Dizziness and visual disturbances are the commonest presenting symptoms. The history tends, as with other types of hind-brain ischaemia, to be fairly long: two years on the average for the neurological features and slightly less for the upper limb effects [81], though about a half of the patients do not complain of these.

A bruit is present near the stenosis in about a half of all patients [81] and may be present only in certain positions [95].

Unequal upper limb circulation is always present, the average difference between the brachial blood pressures being 55 mm Hg, and with innominate occlusion the right carotid pulsations are also reduced. Neurological and electroencephalographic examinations are not often helpful.

Arteriography

Most cases show up well with arch aortography [91], as that in Fig. 8.33. Not only are the left vertebral and subclavian usually late in filling, but other collaterals can be seen running down from the head to the shoulder. Care should be taken to exclude a separate aortic origin of the left vertebral, which would be unaffected by proximal subclavian obstruction. Right vertebral steal is less common and not always so easy to recognise (Fig. 8.35) though the delayed filling of the right subclavian should attract attention to the vertebral.

Innominate obstruction seems to produce a similar picture. In this case the right common carotid also 'steals' blood which may produce recurrent right-sided monocular blindness [47]. The writer also had one such patient whose symptoms were reversed by innominate endarterectomy.

The effects of proximal obstruction of the great vessels are made worse if distal carotid or vertebral narrowing is also present. An important anatomical anomaly that may affect this syndrome, present in 16 per cent of all subjects, and over twice as often in negroes is the brachiocephalic trunk, from which the innominate and the left carotid both arise [60, 91]. Another common variation is the separate origin of the left vertebral from the aortic arch [91]. Both these arrangements may be of clinical importance in individual cases of suspected steal, when they may support or preclude the diagnosis.

Technique for Surgical Correction (Fig. 8.34) [21]

The object of operations for subclavian steal is to check the reversed flow in the affected vertebral artery. This is usually ensured if the proximal obstruction to the subclavian is removed or by-passed. It may, however, be sufficient simply to prevent the passage of vertebral blood into the subclavian, as when the vertebral is ligated [76, 110] or its subclavian opening becomes thrombosed [47].

1. Innominate and First and Part of Right Subclavian

Good exposure is obtained by extending the normal supraclavicular dissection of the subclavian medially and downwards beneath the left innominate vein, by means of a vertical split in the sternum, which

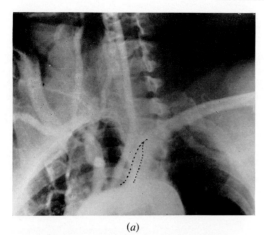

(a)

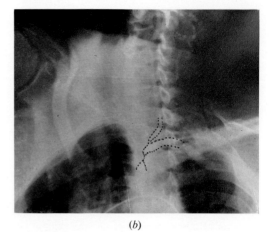

(b)

Fig. 8.33. Subclavian steal. The patient was a man of fifty-five who had transient ischaemic attacks affecting the right arm with some residual defect.

(*a*) Early phase arch aortogram good filling of all proximal vessels including right vertebral. Narrowing of left subclavian just proximal to vertebral, which is only faintly outlined.

(*b*) Late phase, showing well-filled left vertebral and other head vessels flowing down towards the shoulder. Left subclavian now filling well beyond the stenosis.

(*c*) Patient's signature before and after operation. A grossly reduced blood pressure in the left arm was restored to normal following thrombo endarterectomy of the proximal subclavian.

(c)

provides limited access to the aortic origin (Fig. 8.34*a*), sufficient for the application of a lateral clamp.

2. *First Part of Left Subclavian*

The following methods are applicable:

(*a*) For obstruction nearer to the vertebral than to the aortic origin in a thin subject, a medial extension of the standard *supraclavicular exposure* may be tried with the pleura wall mobilised laterally away from the upper medistinal course of the subclavian and left common carotid, provided good control of the subclavian can be secured with a Craaford clamp, well proximal to the stenosis (Fig. 8.34*c*); then with the vertebral and second part of the subclavian lightly clamped an endarterectomy can then be completed.

(*b*) If the lesion is near the aorta, endarterectomy may be carried out through a *thoracic exposure* via the fourth rib bed (Fig. 8.34*d*). There may be difficulty with the repair of the thin-walled remnant, especially at the distal end of the suture line; also,

separation of the subclavian origin from the aorta has been known to occur.

(*c*) For these reasons it may be preferable to by-pass the left subclavian origin, by inserting a knitted dacron graft between the ascending aorta and the supraclavicular part of the artery (Fig. 8.34*e*). A long sternum split with a lateral extension into the right third rib line will allow a safe lateral clamping of the aorta. This anterior approach cannot be used for the proximal left subclavian; therefore, the decision between endarterectomy and by-pass must be made before the operation has begun.

3. *First Part of Either Subclavian*

The morbidity and pain inevitable with either a thoractomy or sternum split can be avoided, provided the carotids are fully patent and reasonably free from disease, by the simpler shunt shown in Fig. 3.44*f*. The standard left or right supraclavicular exposure is extended a little medially to mobilise the

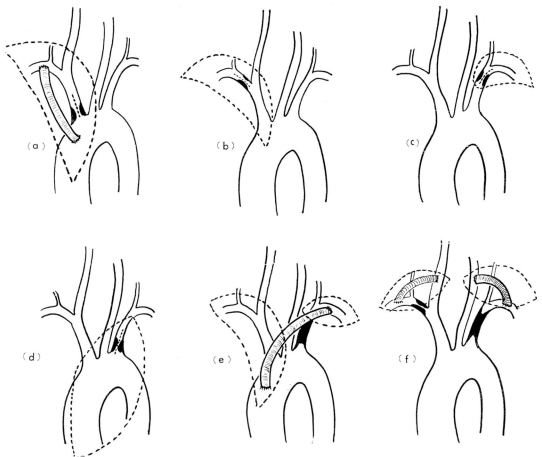

Fig. 8.34. Methods for the surgical correction of subclavian steal. (The dotted ellipses show the operative exposure required.)

(*a*) Innominate endarterectomy or by-pass. Right supraclavicular and sternum split.
(*b*) Right subclavian endarterectomy. Right supraclavicular and manubrium split.
(*c*) Left subclavian endarterectomy—first part, distal. Left supraclavicular.
(*d*) Left subclavian endarterectomy—first part, proximal. Left 4th rib thoractomy.
(*e*) Left subclavian by-pass: a combination of (*a*) and (*c*).
(*f*) Left or right carotid-subclavian shunt, a simple method for any obstruction in the first part of the subclavian.

Experience is proving methods (*b*) and (*f*) to be the most effective. A branching graft can be used in some cases of of aortic arch syndrome. A cross-over graft between the two subclavians is useful to overcome an innominate block.

nearby common carotid, which is then joined to the second or third part of the subclavian with a dacron or saphenous vein graft. This relatively easy operation has largely taken the place of those that require thoracotomy, which have proved to carry a mortality as high as twenty per cent [21]. With the change to the neck approach this figure fell to five per cent or less. Good end results are reported in 90 per cent of survivors [21, 104A].

In all shunt procedures involving clamping of the common carotid it is essential to use heparin and either an indwelling plastic tube in the taped carotid, or hypothermia, or both if there are multiple occlusions present.

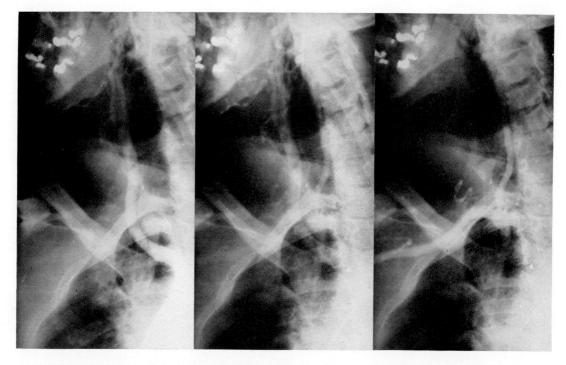

Fig. 8.35. Right-sided subclavian steal. Failure to fill right subclavian or vertebral when right carotid fully shown. Late, retrograde, filling of right vertebral, then subclavian. From a professional singer, aged fifty-eight, with intermittent basilar ischaemia and absent pulses in the right upper limb. Relieved by endarterectomy; recurrent laryngeal nerve preserved as it passed over the stenosed proximal subclavian. (Case referred by Dr Barham Carter.)

Correction of Carotid and Vertebral Kinking

If, in considering the causes of cerebral ischaemia, uncertainty must still be admitted over the role of main artery stenosis [6], though the obstructive possibilities of the lesion are manifest, there will naturally be greater doubt that kinking of the arteries can exert any cerebral haemodynamic effects. Yet, after a survey of 1,000 carotid arteriograms at the Institute of Neurology, London [66], it was concluded that:

(a) Kinking was present in 16 per cent.

(b) It occurred in every age decade.

(c) It was unrelated to hypertension.

(d) There was a strong suggestion that cerebrovascular episodes were commoner in this group of patients than in normal subjects.

(e) In such patients the question of surgical correction should be carefully considered.

Operative correction either by arteriopexy [39], or by resection [39, 74, 88] (Fig. 8.36), gave good initial results; more recent experience confirms this. Among 240 patients having arteriography for cerebrovascular symptoms, 46 showed tortuosity and buckling [39]. Most of these were explored, and fibrous bands were found, often dense and blending with the arterial wall. Good results were obtained, particularly in patients with progressive symptoms. A suitable length of the common carotid should be resected, and re-anastomosed, with division of the external carotid if necessary, thus straightening the internal carotid (Fig. 8.14).

Kinking of the first part of the vertebral artery is corrected by mobilising the whole cervical course of the subclavian artery, dividing the thyrocervical trunk and suturing its stump to the scalene tubercle on the first rib (Fig. 8.37).

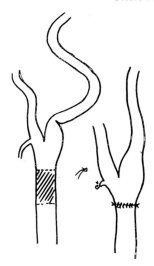

Fig. 8.36. Correction of internal carotid kinking with encroachment of the lumen by a fold. Resection of the common carotid with division of the external carotid or its superior thyroid branch should straighten the kink. No shunt was used in the author's cases unless there was a residual neurological defect. (*See also* Fig. 8.14.)

Fig. 8.37. Kinking of the vertebral artery before (*left*) and after subclavian arteriopexy (*right*). Relief of recurrent transient hind brain attacks during seven years follow up. (Patient referred by Dr John Marshall.)

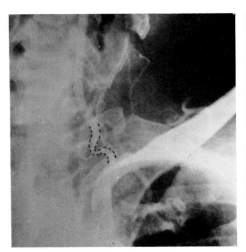
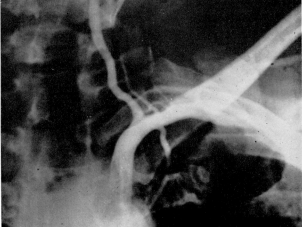

Carotid Sinus Syndrome [98, 99]

The cardiovascular effects of carotid sinus stimulation are directly important to surgeons, in three ways:

1. Cardiac slowing and a fall in blood pressure occur in many normal subjects on local stimulation of the sinus, e.g. from the pressure of the stethoscope bell. A heightened reflex may cause cardiac standstill in response to quite gentle pressure. This is the most important type of carotid sinus syndrome (Fig 8.38).

2. Dissection in the region of the carotid bifurcation often has the same effect; sometimes a profound fall in blood pressure also occurs, which with cardiac slowing might aggravate the effects of carotid occlusion.

3. Patients with incipient or partial heart block may develop complete ventricular asystole during manipulation of the carotid (Fig. 8.39).

Spontaneous attacks of carotid sinus syndrome are often produced by neck movements—another form of 'drop attack'—or from tying the tie, as well as by quite gentle pressure on one or both sinuses.

Cerebrovascular symptoms are common [45] and include vertigo, syncope, focal episodes, and mental changes which may be due, as in Stokes Adams

175

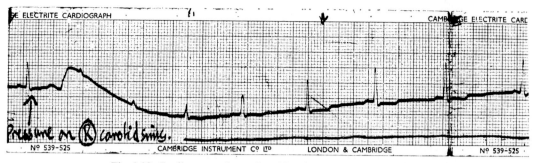

Fig. 8.38. Cardiac asystole produced by gentle pressure on carotid sinus.

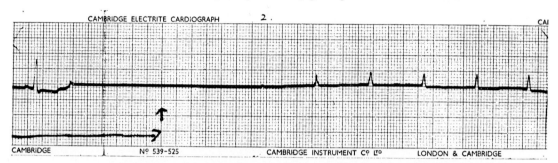

Fig. 8.39. Cardiac arrest occurring during dissection between the carotids.

disease, to repeated ischaemic cerebral insult. The first attack is usually the worst, for patients learn to fear and to avoid them.

In the management of this syndrome, atropine and adrenalin are useful for they control, respectively, the vagal, or cardioinhibitory, and the depressor responses; in the cerebral type neither drug is effective [99].

Surgery is the treatment of choice for the severe examples of this condition, and may need to be bilateral.

The carotid bifurcation is approached as described and with the utmost caution, and then only after generous infiltration with 2 per cent xylocaine without adrenalin; in fact, it is advisable to use a weaker solution first, to block the initial stimulatory phase of the 2 per cent injection.

Carotid denervation is best carried out by means of a complete stripping of the bifurcation of its adventitial and all local connections; the carotid body is clearly seen as a rounded structure, 2 to 3 mm in diameter, closely applied to the back of the bifurcation, and it usually comes away with the adventitia; the nerve is also seen and should be divided at least 2 cm above the point where it joins the artery.

Bilateral carotid surgery, which often involves this type of dissection and mobilisation, may leave the patient in a changed physiological state. This was discovered when studying the response of asthmatic patients to bilateral excision of the carotid body (involving also a complete sinus denervation) [103]. These patients showed two striking effects:

1. They failed to develop hyperpnoea in response to partial anoxia.
2. They became hypertensive and no longer showed the normal fall in blood pressure on foot down tilting.

Although the unilateral operation has been advocated and widely practiced, there should be grave restrictions as to the place of the bilateral procedure in any patient, asthmatic or otherwise [103] (*see also* Chapter 9). Loss of 'hypoxic drive' and a rise in resting arterial PCO_2 have been confirmed in seven patients after bilateral endarterectomy [95B].

Carotid Sinus Nerve Stimulation for Reduction of Hypertension

Experimental work on hypertensive dogs has shown that their blood pressure can be depressed for short periods by passing a low-frequency current to the sinus nerve at 30 to 50 cycles per second, for 0·1 to 0·3 milliseconds [69, 71]. The same effect can be achieved by widening the carotid sinus with a patch graft, which increases the tension in the carotid wall for the same arterial pressure [30A].

REFERENCES

1. Achar, V. S., Coe, R. P. K. and Marshall, J. (1966) Echoencephalography in the differential diagnosis of cerebral haemorrhage and infarction. *Lancet*, **i**, 161.

2. Acheson, J. and Hutchinson, E. C. (1964) Observations on the natural history of transient cerebral ischaemia. *Lancet*, **ii**, 871.

3. Adams, G. F. and Merrett, J. D. (1961) Prognosis and survival in the aftermath of hemiplegia. *Brit. med. J.*, **i**, 309.

4. Alvarez, W. C. (1966) *Little Strokes*. Philadelphia and Toronto: J. B. Lippincott Co.

4A.Andersen, P. E. (1970) Fibromuscular dysplasia of the carotid arteries. *Acta radiol.*, **10**, 90.

5. Ashby, M., Oakley, N., Lorentz, I. and Scott, D. (1963) Recurrent transient monocular blindness. *Brit. med. J.*, **ii**, 894.

6. Battacharji, S. K., Hutchinson, E. C. and McCall, A. J. (1967) Stenosis and occlusion of vessels in cerebral infarction. *Brit. med. J.*, **iii**, 270.

6A.Bergan, J. J. and MacDonald, J. R. (1969) Recognition of fibromuscular hyperplasia. *Arch. Surg.*, **98**, 332.

7. Bickerstaff, E. R. (1964) Aetiology of acute hemiplegia in childhood. *Brit. med. J.*, **ii**, 82.

7A.Blackwood, W., Hallpike, J. F., Kocen, R. S. and Mair, W. G. (1969) Atheromatous disease of the carotid arterial system and embolism from the heart in cerebral infarction: a morbid anatomical study. *Brain*, **92**, 897.

7B.Blaisdell, W. F., Clauss, R. H., Galbraith, J. G., Imparato, A. M. and Wylie, E. J. (1969) Joint Study of Extracranial Arterial Occlusion. IV. A review of surgical considerations. *J. Amer. med. Ass.*, **209**, 1889.

7C.Bland, J. E., Chapman, R. D. and Wylie, E. J. (1970) Neurological complications of carotid artery surgery. *Ann. Surg.*, **171**, 459.

8. Bloodwell, R. D., Haleman, G. D., Keats, A. S. and Cooley, D. A. (1968) Carotid endarterectomy without a shunt. Results using hypercarbic general anaesthesia to prevent cerebral ischemia. *Arch. Surg.*, **96**, 344.

9. Brackett, C. E. (1953) Complications of carotid artery ligation in the neck. *J. Neurosurg.*, **10**, 91.

10. Bradshaw, P. and Casey, E. (1967) Outcome of medically treated stroke associated with stenosis or occlusion of the internal carotid artery. *Brit. med. J.*, **i**, 201.

11. Brain, R. (1963) Some unsolved problems of cervical spondylosis. *Brit. med. J.*, **i**, 771.

12. Brice, J. G., Dowsett, D. J. and Lowe, R. D. (1964) Haemodynamic effects of carotid artery stenosis. *Brit. med. J.*, **ii**, 1363.

13. Brock, R. C. (1952) *The Life and Work of Astley Cooper*. Edinburgh and London: Livingstone, p. 51.

14. Bull, J. W. D. (1960) 'Radiological investigation of acute stroke.' In *Pathogenesis and Treatment of Occlusive Arterial Disease*. The Proceedings of a Conference at the Royal College of Physicians of London. (Ed. McDonald, L.) London: Pitman Medical Publishing Co., p. 73.

14A.Capistrani, T. D. (1971) Thermographic facial patterns in carotid occlusive disease. *Radiology*, **100**, 85.

15. Carter, A. B. (1961) Anticoagulant treatment in progressing stroke. *Brit. med. J.*, **ii**, 70.

16. Carter, A. B. (1965) Thiazides and cerebral ischaemia. *Lancet*, **ii**, 1127.

17. Claiborne, T. S. (1970) Fibromuscular hyperplasia. Report of a case with involvement of multiple arteries. *Amer. J. Med.*, **49**, 103.

19. Coleman, D. J. and Gillespie, J. A. (1963) Management of carotid endarterectomy with special reference to anaesthesia. *Brit. J. Surg.*, **50**, 856.

20. Connett, M. C. and Lansche, J. M. (1965) Fibromuscular hyperplasia of the internal carotid artery. Report of a case. *Ann. Surg.*, **162**, 59.

21. Crawford, E. S., DeBakey, M. E., Morris, G. C. and Howell, J. P. (1969) Surgical treatment of occlusion of the innominate, common carotid and subclavian arteries: a 10-year experience. *Surgery*, **65**, 17.

22. Dardik, H., Gensler, S., Stern, W. Z. and Glotzer, P. (1966) Subclavian steal syndrome secondary to embolism; first reported case. *Ann. Surg.*, **164**, 171.

23. DeBakey, M. E., Crawford, E. S., Cooley, D. A., Morris, G. C., Garrett, H. E. and Fields, W. S. (1965) Cerebral arterial insufficiency; one to 11 year results following arterial reconstructive operation. *Ann. Surg.*, **161**, 921.

24. Derrick, J. R., Estess, M. and Williams, D. (1965) Circulatory dynamics in kinking of the carotid artery. *Surgery*, **58**, 381.

25. De Villiers, J. C. (1966) A brachiocephalic vascular syndrome associated with cervical. *Brit. med. J.*, **ii**, 140.

26. DeWeese, J. A., Rob, C. G., Safran, R., Marsh, D. O., Joynt, R. J., Lipchik, E. O. and Zehl, D. N. (1971) Endarterectomy for athero-sclerotic lesions of the internal carotid artery. *J. Cardiovasc. Surg.*, **66**, 299.

27. Dillon, M. L., Reeves, J. W. and Postlethwait, R. W. (1965) Carotid artery flows and pressures in twenty-two patients with cerebral vascular insufficiency. *Surgery*, **58**, 951.

28. Eastcott, H. H. G., Pickering, G. W. and Rob, C. G. (1954) Reconstruction of internal carotid artery in a patient with intermittent attacks of hemiplegia. *Lancet*, **ii**, 994.

29. Edgar, M. A. and Joyce, M. (1969) Cerebral embolus after traction injury to the arm. *Brit. med. J.*, **2**, 805.

30. Edwards, C. H., Gordon, N. S. and Rob, C. (1960) The surgical treatment of internal carotid artery occlusion. *Quart. J. Med.*, **29**, 67.

30A.Fadali, A. M., Ramos, M. D., Johnson, J. R. and Gott, V. C. (1969) Enlarging the lumen of the carotid sinus. An experimental treatment of systemic arterial hypertension. *Arch. Surg.*, **99**, 624.

30B.Fields, W. S., Maslenikov, V., Meyer, J. S., Hass, W. K., Remington, R. D. and Macdonald, M. (1970) Joint Study of Extracranial Arterial Occlusion. V. Progress report of prognosis following surgery or non-surgical treatment for transient cerebral ischemic attacks and carotid artery lesions. *J. Amer. Med. Ass.*, **211**, 1993.

30C.Firt, P., Hejhal, L. and Weiss, K. (1971) Remarks on the reconstruction of obliterating atherosclerosis of the internal carotid artery. *J. Cardiovasc. Surg.*, **12**, 447.

31. Folger, G. M. and Shah, K. D. (1965) Subclavian steal in patients with Blalock-Taussig anastomosis. *Circulation*, **31**, 241.

32. Garamella, J. J., Lynch, M. F., Jensen, N. K., Sterns, L. P. and Schmidt, W. R. (1966) Endarterectomy and thrombectomy for the totally occluded extracranial internal carotid artery. Use of Fogarty balloon catheters. *Ann. Surg.*, **164**, 325.

33. Garland, H. and Pearce, J. (1965) Carotid arteritis as a cause of cerebral ischaemia in the adult. *Lancet*, **i**, 993.

34. Gilroy, J. and Meyer, J. S. (1963) Compression of the subclavian artery as a cause of ischaemic brachial neuropathy. *Brain*, **86**, 733.

35. Hammond, J. H. and Eisinger, R. P. (1962) Carotid bruits in 1,000 normal subjects. *Arch. Int. Med.*, **109**, 563.

36. Hardesty, W. H., Roberts, B., Toole, J. F. and Royster, H. P. (1961) Studies on carotid artery flow. *Surgery*, **49**, 251.

37. Hardin, C. A. (1965) Vertebral artery insufficiency produced by cervical osteoarthritic spurs. *Arch. Surg.*, **90**, 629.

38. Hardy, W. G., Lindner, D. W., Thomas, L. M. and Gurdjian, E. S. (1962) Anticipated clinical course in carotid artery occlusion. *Arch. Neurol.*, **6**, 138.

39. Harrison, J. H. and Davalos, P. A. (1962) Cerebral ischemia: surgical procedure in cases due to tortuosity and buckling of the cervical vessels. *Arch. Surg.*, **84**, 85.

39A.Hill, A. B., Marshall, J. and Shaw, D. A. (1962) Cerebrovascular disease: trial of long term anticoagulant therapy. *Brit. med. J.*, **ii**, 1003.

40. Hockaday, T. D. R. (1959) Traumatic thrombosis of the internal carotid artery. *J. Neurol. Neurosurg. and Psychiat.*, **22**, 229.

41. Holton, P. and Wood, J. B. (1965) The effects of bilateral removal of the carotid bodies and denervation of the carotid sinuses in two human subjects. *J. Physiol.*, **181**, 365.

41A.Hugh, A. E. (1970) Trickle arteriography: demonstration of thrombi in the origin of the internal carotid artery. *Brit. med. J.*, **2**, 574.

42. Humphries, A. W., Young, J. R., Beven, E. G., LeFevre, F. A. and DeWolfe, V. G. (1965) Relief of vertebrobasilar symptoms by carotid endarterectomy. *Surgery*, **57**, 48.

43. Hutchinson, E. C. and Yates, P. O. (1956) The cervical portion of the vertebral artery: a clinico-pathological study. *Brain*, **79**, 319.

44. Hutchinson, E. C. and Yates, P. O. (1957) Caroticovertebral stenosis. *Lancet*, **i**, 2.

45. Hutchinson, E. C. and Stock, J. P. P. (1960) The carotid sinus syndrome. *Lancet*, ii. 445.

46. Hutchinson, E. C. and Stock, J. P. P. (1963) Paroxysmal cerebral ischaemia in rheumatic heart-disease. *Lancet*, **ii**, 653.

46A.Hutchinson, E. C. (1969) Little strokes. *Brit. med. J.*, **3**, 32.

47. Irvine, W. T., Luck, R. J. and Jacobey, J. A. (1965) Reversed blood-flow in the vertebral arteries causing recurrent brain-stem ischaemia. *Lancet*, **i**, 994.

47A.Javid, H., Ostermiller, W. E., Hengesh, J. W., Hunter, J. A., Najafi, H. and Julian, O. C. (1971) Carotid endarterectomy for asymptomatic patients. *Arch. Surg.*, **102**, 389.

48. Jefferson, G. (1952) The pathology, diagnosis and treatment of intracranial saccular aneurysms. *Proc. Roy. Soc. Med.*, **45**, 300.

49. Johnson, R. (1952) The pathology, diagnosis and treatment of intracranial saccular aneurysms. *Proc. Roy. Soc. Med.*, **45**, 301.

50. Julian, O. C., Dye, W. S., Javid, H. and Hunter, J. A. (1963) Ulcerative lesions of the carotid artery bifurcation. *Arch. Surg.*, **86**, 803.

51. Kelly, A. B. (1924) Tortuosity of the internal carotid in relation to the pharynx. *Proc. Roy. Soc. Med.*, **17**, Section Laryngology and Otology, 1.

52. Kenyon, J. R., Thomas, A. B. W. and Goodwin D. P. (1972) Heparin protection for the brain during carotid-artery reconstruction. *Lancet*, **ii**, 153.

53. Kety, S. S. (1958) 'The physiology of the cerebral circulation in man.' In *Circulation*, Proceedings of the Harvey Tercentary Congress held at Royal College of Surgeons of England. (Ed. McMichael, J.). Oxford: Blackwell Scientific Publications, p. 324.

53A.Lamis, P. A., Carson, W. P., Wilson, J. P. and Letton, A. H. (1971) Recognition and treatment of fibromuscular hyperplasia of the internal carotid artery. *Surgery*, **69**, 498.

54. Leading Article (1965) Anticoagulants for cerebral arteriosclerosis. *Lancet*, **i**, 34.

55. Lewin, W. (1965) Cerebral effects of injury to the vertebral artery. *Brit. J. Surg.*, **52**, 223.

55A.Little, J. M., May, J., Vanderfield, G. K. and Lamond, S. (1969) Traumatic thrombosis of the internal carotid artery. *Lancet*, **ii**, 926.

56. Lowe, R. D. and Stephens, N. L. (1961) Carotid occlusion; its diagnosis by ophthalmodynamometry during carotid compression. *Lancet*, **i**, 1241.

57. McBrien, D. J., Bradley, R. D. and Ashton, N. (1963) The nature of retinal emboli in stenosis of the internal carotid artery. *Lancet*, **i**, 697.

58. McDonald, D. A. and Potter, J. M. (1949) Blood flow in the circle of Willis. *J. Physiol.*, **108**, 34p.

59. McDonald, D. A. and Potter, J. H. (1951) The distribution of blood to the brain. *J. Physiol.*, **114**, 356.

60. McDonald, J. J. and Ason, B. J. (1940) Variations in the origin of arteries derived from the aortic arch

in American whites and negroes. *Amer. J. Phys. Anthrop.*, **27**, 91.

61. Marshall, J. (1963) Rebound phenomenon after anticoagulant therapy in cerebrovascular disease. *Circulation*, **28**, 329.

62. Marshall, J. (1964) The natural history of transient ischaemic cerebro-vascular attacks. *Quart. J. Med.*, **33**, 309.

63. Marshall, J. and Kaeser, A. C. (1961) Survival after non-haemorrhagic cerebrovascular accidents: a prospective study. *Brit. med. J.*, **ii**, 73.

63A. Marshall, J. (1971) Angiography in the investigation of ischaemic episodes in the territory of the internal carotid artery. *Lancet*, **i**, 719.

64. Martin, M. J., Whisnant, J. P. and Sayre, G. P. (1960) Occlusive vascular disease in the extracranial cerebral circulation. *Arch. Neurol.*, **3**, 530.

65. Meadows, S. P. (1966) Temporal or giant cell arteritis. *Proc. Roy. Soc. Med.*, **59**, 329.

66. Metz, H., Murray-Leslie, R. M., Bannister, R. G., Bull, J. W. D. and Marshall, J. (1961) Kinking of the internal carotid artery in relation to cerebro-vascular disease. *Lancet*, **i**, 424.

67. Meyer, J. S. and Denny-Brown, D. (1957) The cerebral collateral circulation. I. Factors influencing collateral blood flow. *Neurol.*, **7**, 447.

68. Monro, R. S. (1950) The natural history of carotid body tumours and their diagnosis and treatment. *Brit. J. Surg.*, **37**, 445.

68A. Moore, W. S. and Hall, A. D. (1970) Carotid artery back pressure. A test of cerebral tolerance to temporary carotid occlusion. *J. Cardiovasc. Surg.*, **11**, 72.

68B. Morris, G. C., Lechter, A. and DeBakey, M. E. (1968) Surgical treatment of fibromuscular disease of the carotid arteries. *Arch. Surg.*, **96**, 636.

69. Neistadt, A. and Schwartz, S. I. (1966) Implantable carotid sinus nerve stimulator for reversal of hypertension. *Surg. Forum*, **17**, 123.

70. Osler, W. (1911) Transient attacks of aphasia and paralysis in states of high blood pressure and arteriosclerosis. *Canad. Med. Assoc. J.*, **1.**, 919.

71. Parsonnet, V., Myers, G. H., Holcomb, W. G. and Zucker, I. R. (1966) Radio-frequency stimulation of the carotid baroreceptors in the treatment of hypertension. *Surg. Forum*, **17**, 125.

72. Pickering, G. (1964) Pathogenesis of myocardial and cerebral infarction: nodular arteriosclerosis. *Brit. med. J.*, **i**, 517.

73. Price, H. L. and Widdicombe, J. (1962) Actions of cyclopropane on carotid sinus baroreceptors and carotid body chemoreceptors. *J. Pharm. Exp. Therap.*, **135**, 233.

74. Quattlebaum, J. K., Upson, E. T. and Neville, R. L. (1959) Stroke associated with elongation and kinking of the internal carotid artery. Report of 3 cases treated by segmental resection of the carotid artery. *Ann. Surg.*, **150**, 824.

74A. Raja, I. A., Marshall, M. and Hankinson, J. (1970) Effects of low-molecular-weight dextran and other factors in common carotid ligation. *Angiology*, **21**, 151.

75. Riser, M., Geraud, J., Ducoudray, J. and Ribaut, L. (1951) Dolicho-carotide interne avec syndrome vertigineux. *Rev. Neurol. (Par.)*, **85**, 145.

76. Rob, C. (1965) 'Subclavian occlusive disease and reversal of flow in the ipsilateral vertebral artery: treatment.' In: *Cerebral Vascular Diseases.* Transactions of the Fourth Conference. (Ed. Millikan, C. H., Siekert, R. G. and Whisnant, J. P.). New York and London: Grune and Stratton, p. 122.

77. Robinson, R. (1961) Restitution of the internal carotid artery. *Lancet*, **ii**, 52.

78. Rojas, R. H., Levitsky, S. and Stansel, H. C. (1966) Acute traumatic subclavian steal syndrome. *J. Thorac. Cardiovasc. Surg.*, **51**, 113.

79. Russell, R. W. R. (1961) Observations on the retinal blood-vessels in monocular blindness. *Lancet*, **ii**, 1422.

80. Russell, R. W. R. (1965) Retinal disease in neurology. *Proc. Roy. Soc. Med.*, **58**, 1045.

80A. Sandok, B. A., Houser, O. W., Baker, H. L. and Holley, K. E. (1971) Fibromuscular dysplasia. Neurologic disorders associated with disease of the great vessels of the neck. *Arch. Surg.*, **24**, 462.

81. Santschi, D. R., Frahm, C. J., Pascale, L. R. and Dumanian, A. V. (1966) The subclavian steal syndrome: clinical and angiographic considerations in 74 cases in adults. *J. Thorac. Cardiovasc. Surg.*, **51**, 103.

82. Schorstein, J. (1940) Carotid ligation in saccular intracranial aneurysms. *Brit. J. Surg.*, **28**, 50.

83. Schwartz, C. J. and Mitchell, J. R. A. (1961) Atheroma of the carotid and vertebral arterial systems. *Brit. med. J.*, **ii**, 1057.

84. Schwartz, C. J., Mitchell, J. R. A. and Hughes, J. T. (1962) Transient recurrent cerebral episodes and aneurysm of carotid sinus. *Brit. med. J.*, **i**, 770.

85. Siekert, R. G. and Millikan, C. H. (1966) Changing carotid bruit in transient cerebral ischemic attacks. *Arch. Neurol.*, **14**, 302.

86. Skovborg, F. and Lauritzen, E. (1965) Symptomless retinal embolism. *Lancet*, **ii**, 361.

87. Solomon, S. (1966) Evaluation of carotid artery compression in cerebrovascular disease. An electroencephalographic clinical correlation. *Arch. Neurol.*, **14**, 165.

88. Spence, W. T. (1963) Pseudostroke. Acute cerebrovascular insufficiency with congenital carotid kinking. *J. Amer. Med. Assoc.*, **186**, 76.

89. Spencer, F. C. and Eiseman, B. (1962) Technique of carotid endarterectomy. *Surg. Gynec. Obstet.*, **115**, 115.

90. Stern, W. E. and Good, R. G. (1960) Studies of the effects of hypothermia upon cerebrospinal fluid oxygen tension and carotid blood flow. *Surgery*, **48.**, 13.

91. Sutton, D. and Davies, E. R. (1966) Arch aortography and cerebrovascular insufficiency. *Clin. Radiol.*, **17**, 330; *Proc. Roy. Soc. Med.*, **59**, 759.

92. Symonds, C. P. (1927) Two cases of thrombosis of subclavian artery, with contralateral hemiplegia of sudden onset, probably embolic. *Brain*, **50**, 259.

93. Symonds, C. (1955) The circle of Willis. *Brit. med. J.*, **i**, 119.

94. Therkelsen, J. and Hornnes, N. (1963) Traumatic occlusion of the internal carotid artery in a child. Restored circulation by means of thrombectomy. *Circulation*, **28**, 101.

94A. Thompson, J. E., Austin, D. J. and Patman, R. D. (1967) Endarterectomy of the totally occluded carotid artery for stroke. *Arch. Surg.*, **95**, 791.

94B. Thompson, J. E. and Patman, R. D. (1970) Endarterectomy for asymptomatic carotid bruits. *Heart Bull.*, **19**, 116.

94C. Thompson, J. E., Austin, D. J. and Patman, R. D. (1970) Carotid endarterectomy for cerebrovascular insufficiency. Long-term results in 592 patients followed up to 13 years. *Ann. Surg.*, **172**, 663.

95. Toole, J. F. and Tucker, S. H. (1960) Influence of head position upon cerebral circulation. *Arch. Neurol.*, **2**, 616.

95A. Vessey, M. P. and Doll, R. (1969) Investigation of relation between use of oral contraceptives and thromboembolic disease. A further report. *Brit. med. J.*, **2**, 651.

95B. Wade, J. G., Larson, C. P. and Hickley, R. F. (1969) Effects of carotid endarterectomy on carotid chemoreceptor and baroceptor function in man. *New Eng. J. Med.*, **282**, 823.

96. Wagner, M., Kitzerow, E. and Taitel, A. (1963) Vertebral artery insufficiency. *Arch. Surg.*, **87**, 885.

97. Wales, R. T. and Martin, E. A. (1963) Arterial bruits in anaemia. *Brit. med. J.*, **ii**, 1444.

98. Waller, A. (1862) Experimental researches on the functions of the vagus and the cervical sympathetic nerves in man. *Proc. Roy. Soc.*, **11**, 302.

99. Weiss, S. and Baker, J. P. (1933) The carotid sinus reflex in health and disease. Its role in the causation of fainting and convulsions. *Medicine, Baltimore*, **12**, 297.

100. Wells, B. A., Keats, A. S. and Cooley, D. A. (1963) Increased tolerance to cerebral ischemia produced by general anesthesia during temporary carotid occlusion. *Surgery*, **54**, 216.

101. Wetzel, N., Tuncbay, E., Kaupp, H. A. and Trippel, O. H. (1964) Stenotic lesions of the external carotid artery (Cause of bruit in the neck). *Arch. Surg.*, **88**, 842.

102. Wood, E. H. (1965) Thermography in the diagnosis of cerebrovascular disease. *Radiology*, **85**, 270.

102A. Wood, E. H. and Correll, J. W. (1969) Atheromatous ulceration in major neck vessels as a cause of cerebral embolism. *Acta radiol. Scand.*, **9**, 520.

103. Wood, J. B., Frankland, A. W. and Eastcott, H. H. G. (1965) Bilateral removal of carotid bodies for asthma. *Thorax*, **20**, 570.

104. Wylie, E. J., Hein, M. F. and Adams, J. E. (1964) Intracranial hemorrhage following surgical revascularisation for treatment of acute strokes. *J. Neurosurg.*, **21**, 212.

104A. Wylie, E. J. and Ehrenfeld, W. K. (1970) *Extracranial Occlusive Cerebrovascular Disease*. Philadelphia: Saunders, p. 221.

105. Yashon, D., Jane, J. A. and Javid, H. (1966) Long-term results of carotid bifurcation endarterectomy. *Surg. Gynec. Obstet.*, **122**, 517.

106. Yates, P. O. (1959) Birth trauma to the vertebral arteries. *Arch. Dis. Child.*, **34**, 436.

107. Yates, P. O. and Hutchinson, E. C. (1961) *Cerebral Infarction: the role of stenosis of the extracranial cerebral arteries*. Med. Res. Counc. Spec. Rep. Series No. 300. London: H.M.S.O.

108. Yates, P. O. (1964) A change in the pattern of cerebrovascular disease. *Lancet*, **i**, 65.

109. Young, J. R., Humphries, A. W., Beven, E. G. and de Wolfe, V. G. (1969) Carotid endarterectomy without a shunt. *Arch. Surg.*, **99**, 293.

110. Yum, K. Y. and Myers, R. N. (1969) Vertebral artery ligation in management of subclavian steal syndrome. *Arch. Surg.*, **98**, 199.

9 Carotid Body Tumours

The normal carotid body is composed of chemo-receptor tissues which are markedly sensitive to changes in O_2 tension, much less so to CO_2, and still less to pH. Bilateral carotid body extirpation, in man, may result in serious disturbances of respiration, principally from failure of hypoxia to increase ventilation [13]. This condition tends to correct itself in time, presumably because other chemoreceptor tissues take over carotid body function. Many sites other than the carotid bifurcation are known to contain this tissue; apart from the aortic bodies [9] most of these are in the head and neck, particularly in the region of the jugular foramen (Fig. 9.1) where the vagal ganglia and branches of this nerve and the glossopharyngeal are also common situations. Tumours of the carotid body type (chemodectoma) occur in all these places, as well as in the retroperitoneal tissues [6A, 29] and along the femoral arteries [31]. Their histology is the same as that of the normal carotid body (Fig. 9.2 and 9.3).

Types of Chemodectoma

The *carotid body tumour* (Fig. 9.4) is the least rare. Of 900 published cases of chemodectoma reviewed in 1969 [27A], 600 were of this, the type most familiar to general surgeons, at least from their academic training if not in practical experience. The remainder, situated in or about the ear, are of a similar interest to ear, nose, and throat surgeons.

Those arising from the undersurface of the carotid bifurcation remain closely adherent to it as they expand and extend, mostly growing upwards as a rounded encapsulated tumour which surrounds the internal and external carotid, replacing their adventitia but seldom involving surrounding structures. The tumour is very richly vascular from an abnormal supply by a multitude of small branches from the carotids, but it does not, as a rule, pulsate.

Local invasion occurs only in the largest examples and in some variant forms; though the vagus or hypoglossal nerves are sometimes enveloped (Fig. 9.5), and the jugular vein may be closely adherent, not, however, because of abnormal venous connections, for in contrast to the close, diffuse arterial adherence of the tumour to the carotids, its venous drainage is more superficial, through dilated tributaries of the common facial.

Extension into the tissues at the base of the skull, when it occurs, signifies that the tumour has lost its encapsulated form, and though not necessarily malignant it so closely involves the deepest layers of the neck and the vessels and nerves of the skull base that operative separation is impossible (Figs 9.7 and 9.10).

Non-arterial sites [1, 6A, 7, 18, 29, 31] must be recognised but are not the main concern of the vascular surgeon. They present with aural symptoms or nerve palsies or both, according to whether the origin is from the tympanic body or the glomus jugulare (*see* Fig. 9.1), and the stage reached by the tumour [1].

The Natural Course of the Carotid Body Tumour

The fact that most of these tumours are first seen in middle adult life, and often with a long history, suggests that the tumour may have been there longer still before being recognised by the patient, so that progress is usually slow. It is the same when a diagnosed tumour is treated expectantly, though here the evidence is scanty, for most patients request operations eventually, and the end stages are therefore seldom seen. A few patients followed up during ten to twenty years after biopsy showed no serious effects of the tumour [22].

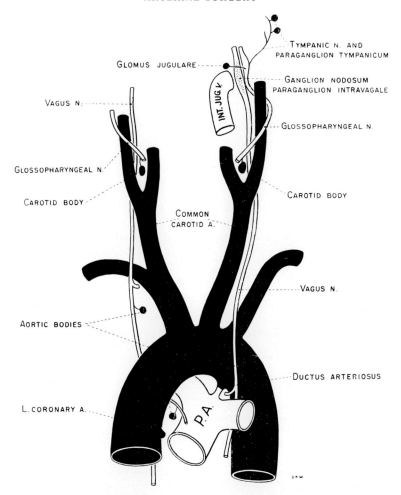

TYMPANIC N. AND
PARAGANGLION TYMPANICUM

GLOMUS JUGULARE

GANGLION NODOSUM
PARAGANGLION INTRAVAGALE

VAGUS N.

INT. JUG. V.

GLOSSOPHARYNGEAL N.

GLOSSOPHARYNGEAL N.

CAROTID BODY

CAROTID BODY

COMMON
CAROTID A.

VAGUS N.

AORTIC BODIES

DUCTUS ARTERIOSUS

L. CORONARY A.

P.A.

Fig. 9.1. The anatomy of chemoreceptor organs. (By permission of Drs R. Lattes and P. M. LeCompte and the Director of the U.S. Armed Forces Institute of Pathology. *See also* [18].)

The Question of Malignancy

Metastasis undoubtedly occurs either in local lymph nodes, viscera or bone [19, 24, 25, 26, 28, 31], but most of the reports in the literature concern cases other than the typical carotid body tumour, either with local invasive features [25] or from the first extending to the skull base. The other cases are those arising from the glomus jugulare or other nearby chemodectoma tissue [29, 32]. Histological appearances of malignancy are commoner. Some have placed it as high as 50 per cent [11]. It may be that more tumours would develop metastasis if they were left untreated, for it has been shown that a perfectly benign-appearing example may spread to bone after many years, and still show much the same histological pattern [8]. Other tumours have shown a more pleomorphic appearance in late-appearing bone secondaries, yet growth continued to be slow; pathological fracture occurred as an incident without affecting the rate or, apparently, causing further spread [24]. It seems that the histological pattern is a poor guide to malignancy [21, 27].

Some of these cases may have been thyroid carcinoma; their behaviour would suggest this.

Diagnosis

When a patient in middle adult life complains of a long-standing, symptomless swelling situated in the

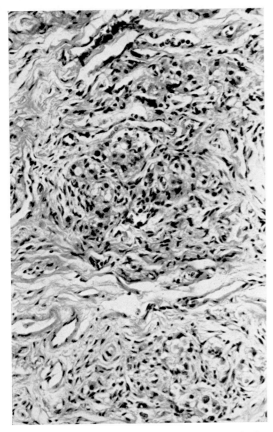

Fig. 9.2. Histological section of a normal carotid body (× 40) removed as a treatment for asthma [13]. (Photomicrograph by Dr E. A. Wright.)

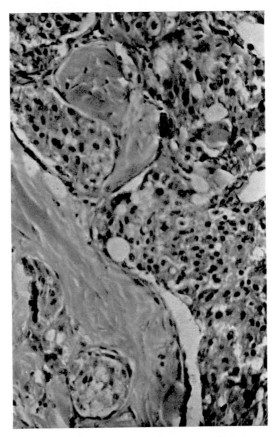

Fig. 9.3. Histological section of a carotid body tumour (× 40), containing more than usual amount of fibrous tissue. (Photomicrograph by Dr E. A. Wright.)

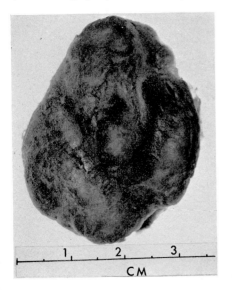

Fig. 9.4. Excised carotid body tumour; well encapsulated and grooved on its undersurface by the carotid bifurcation.

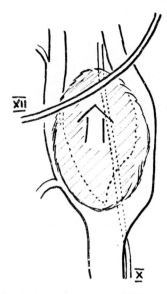

Fig. 9.5. Local expansion of a benign carotid body tumour opens up the bifurcation and may envelop the vagus or hypoglossal nerves.

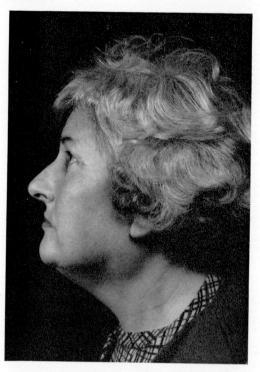

Fig. 9.7. Chemodectoma of the higher type, extending from the carotid bifurcation deep to the jaw and parotid gland. Figure 9.10 shows the arteriographic appearance in this case, confirming the clinical impression of vascular invasion at the base of the skull. An excellent response was obtained with high-voltage radiotherapy. (Miss Irene Cade's and the author's case.)

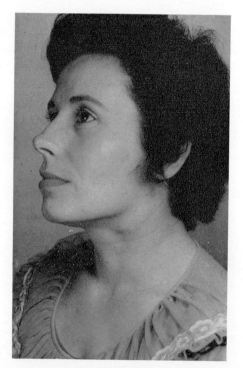

Fig. 9.6. A typical carotid body tumour in a woman aged thirty-two.

carotid triangle, which has not varied in size, though it may have slowly increased, a carotid body tumour should be considered (Fig. 9.6).

A transmitted arterial impulse is usual, and occasionally an arterial bruit; expansile pulsation is unusual. The external carotid may be felt as it crosses the tumour. Mobility is slight and only across the line of the carotid.

The upper limit of the tumour is usually at the angle of the jaw, or deep to the lower part of the carotid, but sometimes it extends upwards much higher, where its own outline is lost; the swelling below the ear is deep and diffuse (Fig. 9.7). In some patients the swelling is first noticed in the throat (Fig. 9.8). Bilateral cases are not exceptionally rare [26, 37A, 38]. Families may be affected [37A].

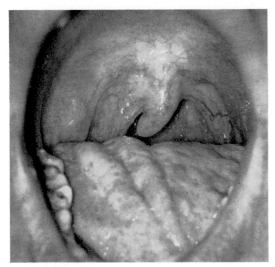

Fig. 9.8. Another chemodectoma of the high carotid type presenting as a pharyngeal swelling. (Mr A. W. Morrison's case.)

In some series the incidence of vocal cord paralysis is as high as 25 per cent [22], although major cranial nerve palsies should suggest locally invasive malignancy, which will later be proved at operation and histological section [25].

Chemoreceptor or carotid sinus symptoms have been reported [10, 29, 34], with blackouts, hypotension, nystagmus, and vertigo often related to exertion or over-ventilation.

The clinical diagnosis of carotid body tumour is by exclusion. The common causes of a hard swelling in the carotid region, secondary carcinoma and tuberculous lymphadenitis show their own progressive and familiar features, and doubt remains in only a few cases. If carotid body tumour is seriously considered, it is better that biopsy should not be undertaken; carotid arteriography is safer and more informative.

Arteriographic Appearance of Carotid Body Tumour (Fig. 9.9)

The characteristic 'goblet' displacement of the carotids is almost always present, with abnormal vessels richly filling the tumour zone in the later films. This is an essential finding, for spreading of the carotid bifurcation is produced by enlargement of lymph nodes. If the extent of abnormal vascularity is not clearly demarcated, and particularly if it extends upwards towards the base of the skull (Fig. 9.10), the lesion is not a true carotid body tumour, and surgical exploration may be contra-indicated.

SURGICAL TREATMENT

This is indicated whenever the diagnosis is made and confirmed, but with the provision that the facilities for arterial reconstruction should be ready, the patient fit for prolonged anaesthesia, perhaps involving hypothermia, and the surgeon must be experienced in the field.

Operative hazards are mainly those of uncontrollable haemorrhage and that to which it could lead, a multiple ligation of the carotids with the probability of hemiplegia. This fearful combination of accidents has in the past carried a mortality of about 30 per cent [10, 21, 22], so that the cure might be worse than the disease. To this must be added the risks of operative damage to surrounding structures, particularly cranial nerves [29A]. Bilateral operation may deprive the patient of the normal function of the carotid sinus.

Nevertheless, the results of excision today are good, with the provisions stated; our experience at St Mary's Hospital, London [26] has been satisfactory: a total of twenty-nine tumours excised between 1956 and 1964 without mortality or hemiplegia. No internal or common carotid was ligated, though an arterial graft was required in one case.

Technique

The principles of the operation are those of Gordon-Taylor [10], who stressed the importance of meticulous and painstaking dissection within a subadventitial line of cleavage, which, if maintained, ensures the complete removal of the tumour without the need for carotid clamping or ligation.

Anaesthesia should aim at minimising unnecessary oozing without lowering the blood pressure sufficiently to reduce cerebral blood flow. Slight foot-down tilt may reduce venous congestion in the early stages of the dissection but carries the risk of an exaggerated fall in cerebral flow in the event of an unexpected fall in carotid perfusion such as may occur with brisk blood loss, or during temporary carotid clamping.

Hypothermia has been recommended [36] for its protective effect should carotid interruption be needed. In the writer's experience it is probably unnecessary, and has the disadvantage (in this operation) that bleeding is increased.

The approach to the carotid bifurcation has been described in Chapter 8, p. 164, the only special feature of the early phase being the greater extent

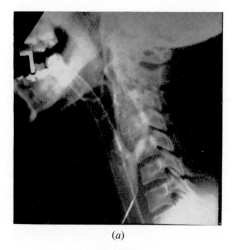

(a)

Fig. 9.9.

Arteriography and carotid body tumour.

(a) 'Goblet' displacement of carotids with abnormal tumour vessels in the expanded intercarotid area.

(b) Six years after excision of the tumour the carotids now lie parallel and close together. This is the normal postoperative appearance, excluding recurrence of the tumour.

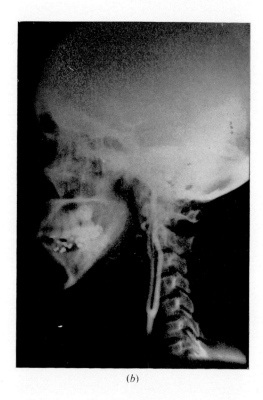

(b)

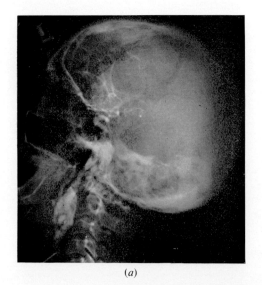

(a)

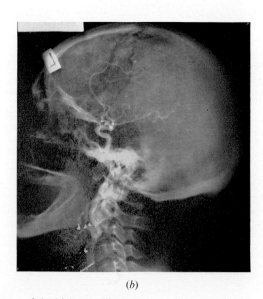

(b)

Fig. 9.10. Inoperable chemodectoma of the high carotid type.

(a) The low component, highly vascular with coiled external carotid.

(b) In the later contrast phase, the same appearance is seen extending into the tissues at the base of the skull. (From the patient whose swelling is shown in Fig. 9.7.)

of the venous plane of dissection in carotid body tumour. After the division of the common facial vein a large number of abnormal tributaries are encountered; these are draining the tumour, and if patiently ligated and divided, the surface of the tumour or of the normal common carotid will be reached without difficulty.

The dissection aims at finding the 'white line' of Gordon-Taylor, and is best begun on the common carotid at the lower limit of the tumour. If this plane is patiently developed, with minute attention to the numerous small vessels that cross it, using diathermy through fine non-toothed dissecting forceps (Mac-Indoe's), the tumour will eventually be freed. Some larger arteries of supply may come from the external carotid, or from the back of the bifurcation itself whence arises the normal arterial origin of the carotid body. Such vessels require fine silk ligation and division. Carotid clamping should be avoided unless absolutely necessary. It is much easier to injure the artery when it is clamped. The operation closely resembles the removal of a meningioma. The external carotid may be tied if access to a deep lying tumour would thus be improved (Figs 9.11 and 9.4). The dissection becomes easier as it proceeds, for the upper connections should be less vascular provided the case has been correctly assessed from the arteriograms. Injury to the hypoglossal nerve must be avoided (Fig. 9.5). If it should run deeply through the tumour it must be divided and resutured at the end of the operation. In removing a very large,

producing respiratory difficulties and trouble with swallowing.

The wound should be drained for two days. Recovery is uneventful, provided the carotids have been kept intact.

In summary, this is an exacting operation which may involve a vascular procedure other than dissection, so that experience and facilities of this special kind must be available, yet in such circumstances the need for them will be small.

As we have noted, carotid clamping tends to lead the dissection further still into the lumen, and ligation may then be forced upon the operator, for there will seldom be sufficient normal carotid above the tumour to which a graft could be attached.

An exception to these rules is the management of the *rare malignant tumour*. Here, nothing less than a radical resection will suffice, with removal not only of the length of carotid bearing the tumour but also any adherent structures, including nerves. Simple ligation-excision may be safe, as with ligation in the treatment of bleeding intracranial aneurysm, if the cross flow within the circle of Willis is sufficient (*see* Chapter 8, p. 148). Carotid reconstruction by grafting may be possible [20]. In any of these difficult circumstances a tube shunt into the carotid may help to control and remedy the situation.

Results of Excision

Local recurrence after complete excision is rare, except where invasive morbid anatomical features

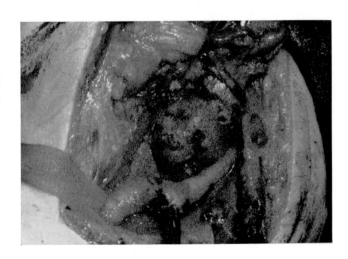

Fig. 9.11. Final stages of removal of tumour from the patient whose clinical appearance is shown in Fig. 9.6. Division of the external carotid, though not often necessary, has here facilitated the separation and preservation of the lower deeper aspect of the internal carotid seen running along the back of the tumour.

deeply placed tumour care should be taken not to injure the vagus, for otherwise not only would recurrent laryngeal palsy result, but also there may be loss of upper laryngeal and pharyngeal sensation, were noted at the operation. Nerve palsies are common after removal of the larger tumours, particularly of the hypoglossal, recurrent laryngeal, and cervical facial nerves; while still more disabling is the loss of pharyngeal sensation and severe, drooling dysphagia which follows damage to the glosso-pharyngeal and sensory vagal fibres. Because of these complications, incomplete excision may be preferable, with radiotherapy to follow.

Radiotherapy for Chemodectomata

Fortunately, although these tumours are well differentiated and slow growing they are often radiosensitive, particularly the glomus tumours. Shrinkage of the tumour (Fig. 9.7) and recovery of nerve palsies should follow treatment. Megavoltage therapy is preferable because of its greater precision of application in depth and lower incidence of bone necrosis compared with standard source rays (250 kV). A tumour dose of 5,000 to 5,500 rads over five weeks is recommended for glomus jugulare tumours [37]. Good results followed in 85 per cent, after this treatment, though surgery remains the treatment of choice for limited tympanic tumours, and for glomus jugulare tumours without local invasion. It has also been recommended in the after-treatment of incompletely excised carotid body tumours [15].

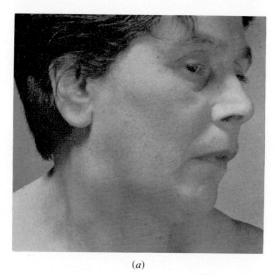
(a)

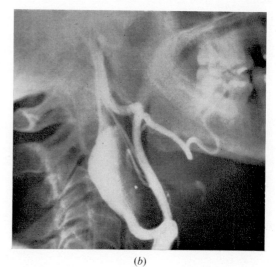
(b)

Fig. 9.12. Internal carotid aneurysm.
(a) Presenting in the neck.
(b) Arteriogram of this patient showing elongation and kinking in association with the aneurysm. Treated by excision and end-to-end anastomosis.

Carotid Aneurysm

The common intracranial aneurysm of the internal carotid is the concern of the neurosurgeon, who has to deal with bleeding and local pressure effects upon nerves, and upon the venous return in the cavernous sinus, presenting as unilateral ocular palsy or proptosis. Extracranial carotid aneurysm is rare [6B, 22A], though the diagnosis is often made in error in hypertensive females, in whom the common carotid has become elongated and widened to form a prominent kink or curl, thought to be aneurysmal [4]. Arteriography shows the true state (Fig. 8.12, p. 154).

Internal carotid aneurysm occurs either as:

(a) a dilatation of the carotid sinus [28] from which thrombus may become detached, producing transient cerebral ischaemia; or

(b) a more distal dilatation, usually in association with elongation and kinking of the artery, presenting either as a lump in the neck (Fig. 9.12a, b) or in the pharynx (Fig. 8.6), and like the carotid body tumour it may involve the hypoglossal or vagus, causing difficulties with speech and with swallowing [39]. The pulsatile nature of the swelling may be missed, and there is a risk that incision or exploration may lead to serious haemorrhage.

The common carotid artery, like the innominate and aorta near the left subclavian, may be torn by deceleration injury, and in the confined space of the retrosternal tissues a false aneurysm may form later, developing pain and pressure effects. This is much

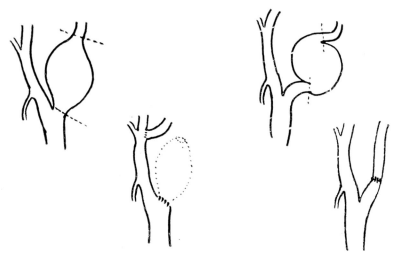

Fig. 9.13. Techniques for excision of internal carotid aneurysm and restoration of the artery.

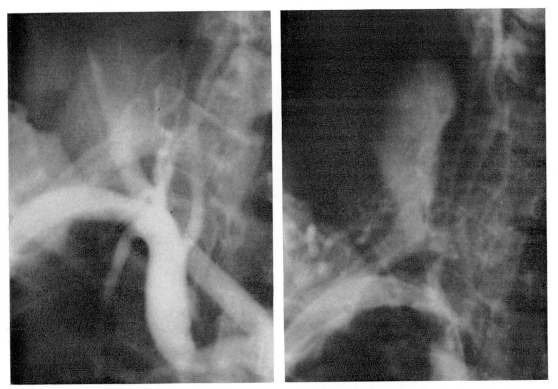

Fig. 9.14. A large false aneurysm of the right common carotid artery, excised and homografted under hypothermia in 1957. Patient remains well. (*From* Sutton's *Arteriography*, by courtesy of the author and publishers.)

the commonest type of cervical carotid anenrysm (Fig. 9.14) (*see also* Chapter 13, p. 248).

Surgical Treatment

The possibility of spontaneous thrombosis was considered by Matthew Baillie in 1789 [2], and he cited the view of John Hunter that carotid ligation on one or both sides might be possible. Astley Cooper successfully performed this operation in 1805 [6]. Little further advance was made until the late 1950s, when reports of reconstructive operation for carotid aneurysm began to appear [5, 30, 33, 39], though the number of such operations is still small [16].

Technique. A favourable feature in most cases is the associated redundancy of the internal carotid (Fig. 9.12). This may allow an end-to-end anastomosis, or the distal stump of the carotid to be drawn down into the operative field sufficiently to be anastomosed to the external carotid in its wider proximal portion, either end to side, or end to end after division of the external carotid (Fig. 9.13).

One important precaution must be observed: the distal carotid is secured as gently and as soon as possible, and the aneurysm is manipulated very cautiously, for otherwise it is possible to dislodge thrombus of sufficient size to cause a massive cerebral embolism.

Like the various non-arteriosclerotic occlusive lesions of the popliteal, renal and carotid arteries that have become better known since arteriography became routine, the rarity of internal carotid aneurysm may not last much longer. Though by 1968 only 20 cases had been reported [22A], the writer has already operated upon six: four in the internal carotid of older women, one erosive-mycotic from a quinsy in a child of $2\frac{1}{2}$ years, and one false aneurysm from failure of a patch graft. All but the first patient, in 1956 (Fig. 8.6) did well.

A Note on Nerve Tumours of the Carotid Sheath

Patients are sometimes referred to the vascular surgeon with a hard pulsatile swelling in the upper carotid region. Arteriography excludes aneurysm or

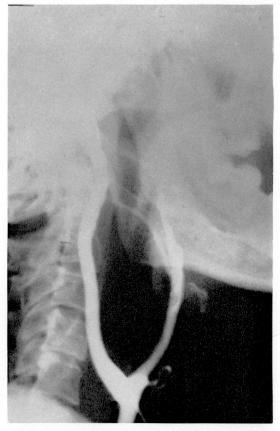

Fig. 9.15. Neurilemmoma of the cervical sympathetic chain in a woman aged fifty-one. No vessels between carotids.

chemodectoma, from the fact that the carotids are splayed, without any abnormal vessel filling (Fig. 9.15). When exposed, the mass is found to be easily separable from the arteries, though much involved with a nerve, which is usually the vagus or the sympathetic trunk. Not all cases can retain the nerve intact; in these the voice and swallowing may be much impaired.

REFERENCES

1. Alford, B. R. and Guilford, F. R. (1962) A comprehensive study of tumors of the glomus jugulare. *Laryngoscope, St Louis,* **72,** 765.
2. Baillie, M. (1844) In *Observations on Aneurism* (Ed. Erichsen, J. E.). London: Sydenham Society, p. 175.
3. Benvenuto, R., Despres, J. P., Pribram, H. F. W. and Callaghan, J. C. (1961) Excision of an extracranial aneurysm of the internal carotid artery employing hypothermia. *J. Cardiovasc. Surg.,* **2,** 165.
4. Bergan, J. J. and Hoehn, J. G. (1965) Evanescent cervical pseudoaneurysms. *Ann. Surg.,* **162,** 213.

5. Boatman, K. K. and Bradford, V. A. (1958) Excision of an internal carotid aneurysm during pregnancy employing hypothermia and a vascular shunt. *Ann. Surg.,* **148,** 271.
6. Brock, R. C. (1952) *The Life and Work of Astley Cooper.* Edinburgh and London: E. & S. Livingstone.
6A.Carmichael, J. D., Daniel, W. A. and Lamon, E. W. (1970) Mesenteric chemodectoma. *Arch. Surg.,* **101,** 630.
6B.Cifarelli, F. and Sadig, S. (1971) Bilateral carotid

aneurysms treated by resection and replacement grafts. *Arch. Surg.*, **102**, 74.

7. Dallachy, R. and Simpson, I. C. (1960) Chemoreceptor tumours in the neck, arising away from the carotid body, with report of a case presenting as a swelling in the pharynx. *J. Laryngol. Otol.*, **74**, 217.

8. Donald, R. A. and Crile, G. (1948) Tumors of the carotid body. *Amer. J. Surg.*, **75**, 435.

9. Gillis, D. A., Reynolds, D. P. and Merritt, J. W. (1956) Chemodectoma of an aortic body. *Brit. J. Surg.*, **43**, 585.

10. Gordon-Taylor, G. (1940) On carotid tumours. *Brit. J. Surg.*, **28**, 163.

11. Harrington, S. W., Clagett, O. T. and Dockerty, M. B. (1941) Tumors of the carotid body. Clinical and pathologic considerations of twenty tumours affecting nineteen patients. *Ann. Surg.*, **114**, 820.

12. Harrison, E. G., Soule, E. H. and Judd, E. S. (1957) Chemodectoma of the glomus intravagale (vagal-body tumor). *Cancer*, **10**, 1226.

13. Holton, P. and Wood, J. B. (1965) The effects of bilateral removal of the carotid bodies and denervation of the carotid sinuses in two human subjects. *J. Physiol.*, **181**, 365.

14. Huppler, E. G., McBean, J. B. and Parkhill, E. M. (1955) Chemodectoma of the glomus jugulare: report of a case with vocal cord paralysis as a presenting finding. *Proc. Mayo Clin.*, **30**, 53.

15. Jepson, R. P. and Opit, L. J. (1961) Carotid body tumours. *Austral. N.Z. J. Surg.*, **30**, 175.

16. Kianouri, M. (1967) Extracranial carotid aneurysms: treatment by excision and end-to-end anastomosis. *Ann. Surg.*, **165**, 152.

17 Killian, H. (1951) Aneurysmen des brachiocephalen Stromgebietes und weitere Erfahrungen mit der Mediastinotomia sterno-clavicularis. *Arch. klin. Chir.*, **269**, 200.

18. LeCompte, P. M. (1951) Tumours of the carotid body and related structures. In: *Atlas of Tumor Pathology*. Sect. IV, Fasc. 16, Armed Forces Institute of Pathology, Washington D.C.

19. Morfit, H. M., Swan, H. and Taylor, E. R. (1953) Carotid body tumors. Report of twelve cases, including one case with proved visceral dissemination. *Arch. Surg.*, **67**, 194.

20. Morris, G. C., Balas, P. E., Cooley, D. A., Crawford, E. S. and DeBakey, M. E. (1963) Surgical treatment of benign and malignant carotid body tumors: clinical experience with sixteen tumours in twelve patients. *Amer. Surg.*, **29**, 429.

21. Monro, R. S. (1950) The natural history of carotid body tumours and their diagnosis and treatment, with a report of five cases. *Brit. J. Surg.*, **37**, 445.

22. Nelson, W. R. (1962) Carotid body tumours. *Surgery*, **51**, 326.

22A. Ohara, I., Utsumi, N. and Ouchi, H. (1968) Resection of extracranial internal carotid aneurysms. *J. Cardiovasc. Surg.*, **9**, 365.

23. Pettet, J. R., Woolner, L. B. and Judd, E. S. (1953) Carotid body tumors (chemodectomas). *Ann. Surg.*, **137**, 465.

24. Pendergrass, E. P. and Kirsh, D. (1947) Röentgen manifestations in the skull of metastatic carotid body tumor (paraganglioma), of meningioma, and of mucocele. *Amer. J. Röent.*, **57**, 417.

25. Reese, H. E., Lucas, R. N. and Bergman, P. A. (1963) Malignant carotid body tumors. Report of a case. *Ann. Surg.*, **157**, 232.

26. Rob, C. G., Owen, K. and Eastcott, H. H. G. (1966) Surgical treatment of carotid body tumours. Unpublished data.

27. Romanski, R. (1954) Chemodectoma (non-chromaffinic paraganglioma) of the carotid body with distant metastases. *Amer. J. Path.*, **30**, 1.

27A. Salyer, K. E., Ketchum, L. D., Robinson, D. W. and Marten, F. W. (1969) Surgical management of cervical paragangliomata. *Arch. Surg.*, **98**, 572.

28. Schwartz, C. J., Mitchell, J. R. A. and Hughes, J. T. (1962) Transient recurrent cerebral episodes and aneurysm of carotid sinus. *Brit. med. J.*, **i**, 770.

29. Sessions, R. T., McSwain, B., Carlson, R. I. and Scott, H. W. (1959) Surgical experiences with tumors of the carotid body, glomus jugulare and retroperitoneal nonchromaffin paraganglia. *Ann. Surg.*, **150**, 808.

29A. Shamblin, W. R., ReMine, W. H., Sheps, S. G. and Harrison, E. G. (1971) Carotid body tumour (chemodectoma). Clinicopathologic analysis of 90 cases. *Amer. J. Surg.*, **122**, 732.

30. Shea, P. C., Glass, L. F., Reid, W. A. and Harland, A. (1955) Anastomosis of common and internal carotid arteries following excision of mycotic aneurysm. *Surgery*, **37**, 829.

31. Smetana, H. F. and Scott, W. F. (1951) Malignant tumors of nonchromaffin paraganglia. *Mil. Surg.*, **109**, 330.

32. Taylor, D. M., Alford, B. R. and Greenberg, S. D. (1965) Metastases of glomus jugulare tumors. *Arch. Otolaryngol.*, **82**, 5.

33. Thompson, J. E. and Austin, D. J. (1957) Surgical management of cervical carotid aneurysms. *Arch. Surg.*, **74**, 80.

34. Tuckman, J., Slater, S. R. and Medlowitz, M. (1965) The carotid sinus reflexes. *Amer. Heart J.*, **70**, 119.

35. Van Miert, P. J. (1964) The treatment of chemodectomas by radiotherapy. *Proc. Roy. Soc. Med.*, **57**, 946.

36. Westbury, G. (1960) The management of carotid body tumours, with a report of seven cases. *Brit. J. Surg.*, **47**, 605.

37. Williams, I. G. (1957) Radiotherapy of tumours of the glomus jugulare. *J. Facult. Radiol. Lond.*, **8**, 335.

37A. Wilson, H. (1970) Carotid body tumours: familial and bilateral. *Ann. Surg.*, **171**, 843.

38. Wychulis, A. R. and Beahrs, O. H. (1965) Bilateral chemodectomas. *Arch. Surg.*, **91**, 690.

39. Zakrzewski, A. (1963) Spontaneous extracranial aneurysms of the internal carotid artery. *J. Laryngol. Otol.*, **77**. 342.

10 Sympathectomy

History [15, 17]. Most of the early observations on sympathectomy were made in France. Claude Bernard, in 1852, and Jaboulay, in 1899, both showed that vasodilatation follows removal of sympathetic nerves, respectively, in the ear of the rabbit, and the human lower limb. These were postganglionic sections, and consequently their effects were transient. Later it was found by Royle and Hunter in Sydney, Australia, that ganglionectomy produced more lasting changes of the same kind in patients with spastic paralysis, and from the late 1920s this type of denervation, after early successes at the Mayo Clinic, found an increasing place in the treatment of limb ischaemia.

Anatomy of Sympathetic Nerves to the Limbs

Although centralised, and deeply placed in its paravertebral course, the sympathetic ganglionic chain is accessible to surgical manipulations, and much has been learned from clinical experience about the topography and neurology of sympathetic innervation. Figure 10.1 shows the segmental upper limb distribution by ganglia, and by preganglionic rami. Variations occur mainly in the position of the ganglia, so that at operation it may not be possible to be sure of the extent of the denervation. The chain is deeply placed at all its levels and is often crossed by segmental arteries and veins. Most of the white rami to the upper limb arise from the second to the sixth anterior spinal nerve roots, often with extra preganglionic fibres from two segments above and below. The lower limb is supplied from the tenth thoracic to the second lumbar roots, relaying segmentally in the lumbar ganglionic chain, as shown in Fig. 10.2. Considerable overlap exists because of branching within the chain, and many postganglionic fibres may arise from a single relay of a single afferent fibre. This may be relevant to the problem of recurrent vasoconstrictor tone after cervical sympathectomy.

Early and Late Effects of Sympathectomy

The distribution of postganglionic fibres within the limbs is to plain muscle of vessel walls, sweat glands, and pilomotors. Effective sympathetic denervation is confirmed if, in comparison with the patient's unoperated limbs, there is *increased warmth and redness, lack of perspiration, and failure to raise goose flesh*, the last named with a test stimulus such as pinching, pricking or exposure to cold sufficient to do this in regions outside the denervated area.

These effects may not be locally distinctive at the end of the operation, either from a general interference with sympathetic tone by anaesthetic agents or inhibitors (e.g. tubocurarine, hexamethonium), or locally because of transient stimulation of the cut end of the postganglionic fibre, or an axon reflex within it. In any of these circumstances a more or less striking degree of goose flesh may be noticed in the recently sympathectomised skin area.

The highest rate of blood flow after sympathectomy occurs early, but not necessarily immediately after the operation [2] (Fig. 10.3). Whether the section is preganglionic or by ganglionectomy seems to make no difference to the level of the early hyperaemia, which is more related to the resting preoperative level, from factors such as intrinsic tone [17] or structural disease. During the first week, as tone returns, the blood flow falls to near normal levels but the digital skin temperature remains raised, and cold vasoconstriction is abolished.

The extent to which these effects are maintained depends upon the part of the body concerned and the disease for which the operation was performed. Nearly all lumbar sympathectomy patients show permanent effects [7]. In the upper limb, vasoconstrictor response tends gradually to return in a much larger proportion. If the patient has Raynaud's disease, the rate of recurrence is as high as 50 per cent in the first six months (*see* Chapter 14). Sudomotor effects are more lasting in all areas but less so in the upper limb.

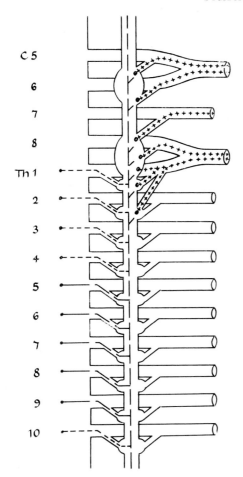

Fig. 10.1. Sympathetic innervation of the upper limb. Broken line = preganglionic fibres; crosses = postganglionic fibres. (Adapted from Ross's *Surgery of the Sympathetic Nervous System* by courtesy of the author and publishers [15].)

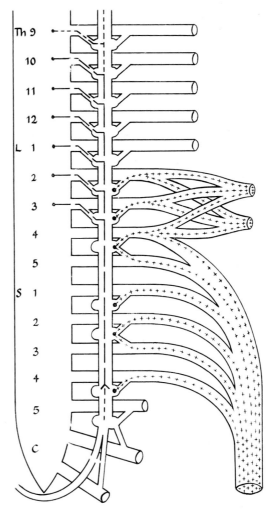

Fig. 10.2. Sympathetic innervation of the lower limb. Broken line = preganglionic fibres; crosses = postganglionic fibres. (Adapted from Ross's *Surgery of the Sympathetic Nervous System* by courtesy of the author and publishers [15].)

Indications for Sympathectomy

NON-ARTERIAL DISEASE

These include hyperhidrosis; primary acrocyanosis; secondary acrocyanosis, e.g. in spastic paralysis as originally introduced by Hunter and Royle, and in old poliomyelitis; post-traumatic dystrophy; traumatic neuroma, phantom limb and causalgia. Some cases of erythromelalgia are helped (*see* p. 213). Frost-bite damage can be ameliorated by early sympathectomy [8]. Relief of angina pectoris is reported in over 50 per cent of cases [4].

ARTERIAL DISEASE

These are discussed in detail in the chapters on chronic ischaemia, Raynaud's syndromes, and upper limb occlusion. The object of the operation in these conditions is:

1. To remove vasoconstrictor tone tending to reduce limb blood flow for long periods in each day, and many days each year. Sustained higher flow rates should mean a lower rate of thrombosis and an improvement in the development of a collateral circulation.

2. By drying the skin to discourage infection.

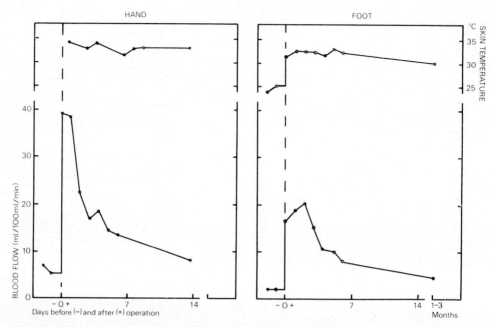

Fig. 10.3. Effect of sympathectomy on blood flow and skin temperature in hand and foot. Blood flow soon subsides, but skin temperature is maintained. (Adapted from Barcroft and Swan, *Sympathetic Control of Human Blood Vessels* by permission of the authors and publishers, [2].)

These merits of so simple a procedure should ensure its continued use in the treatment of limb ischaemia, either as a support to the existing circulation, or as a useful addition to an arterial reconstruction. Another good use of sympathectomy is to assist the early healing of a doubtful amputation through the foot, taking advantage of the maximal flow during the first few days by performing both operations at the same time. Where a main artery must be ligated, as in some cases of peripheral aneurysm, though the limb may survive the acute phase of the subsequent ischaemia, the residual circulation may be marginal, and chronic ischaemic difficulties may be averted or minimised by coincident sympathectomy.

Contra-indications

Too much is sometimes expected of this operation. It cannot be hoped to have any good effect in *acute, massive ischaemia* (*see* Chapter 2); neither can it help the patient with chronic ischaemia due mainly to proximal occlusion of the main limb artery at or above the level of the groin or first rib.

The ideal case is one in which the occluded arteries are mainly in the distal segment of the limb, once the acute ischaemia has been overcome.

OPERATIVE TECHNIQUE

Cervical Sympathectomy (*see* Chapter 12, p. 227).

Lumbar Sympathectomy

As the most important single operation in the treatment of arterial disease, it will be described in full. By modern methods it is no longer a major procedure; the older technique using a long posterolateral lumbar exposure should now be abandoned. The lumbar sympathetic chain is much more easily approached from the front, for the vertebral bodies upon which it lies are projected forwards into the mid-abdomen.

A short transverse incision is made with its medial third over the rectus sheath (Fig. 10.4), and its outer two-thirds over the oblique muscles well clear of the costal margin, to reduce postoperative pain. The key step in this operation is the *division of the linea semilunaris* (Fig. 10.5). The upper and lower cut edges are picked up with the artery forceps and are held up into the wound by the assistant. Each of the

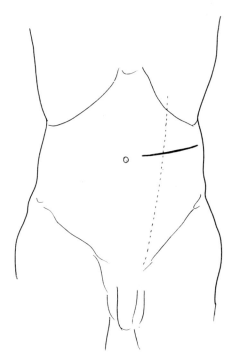

Fig. 10.4. Skin incision for antero-lateral approach to left lumbar sympathetic chain.

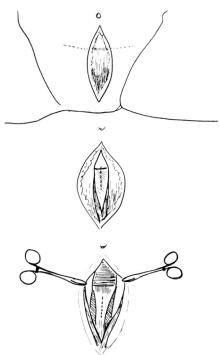

Fig. 10.5. Stages in the approach to the extra-peritoneal plane as viewed by the surgeon standing on the patient's left side.

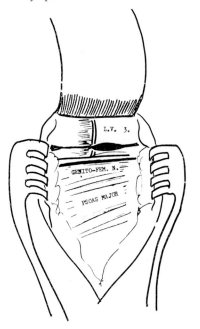

Fig. 10.6. The lumbar sympathetic chain widely exposed; the peritoneum being retracted by the lateral packs and central Deaver's retractor.

oblique muscles can then be cut separately and haemostasis is easily secured, keeping the muscles lifted up on the stretch. The transversus abdominis aponeurosis is carefully divided *in situ* along the line of its fibres, using a scalpel: it must not be picked up and divided, otherwise the peritoneum may be opened. Once the transversus fibres are separated *the peritoneum is pushed away* from its inner surface, using mounted dental cotton swabs, until a sufficient extraperitoneal working space has been obtained to complete the division of the posterior part of the transversus muscle. Then, the process of lifting the peritoneum off the parietes can be completed with little risk of opening the cavity, for the posterior part of the membrane is strong and well supported.

The *psoas major muscle is felt*, and the fatty tissue over it is lifted up with the peritoneum; the fingers of the right hand are then advanced until the vertebral bodies are reached.

A gentle lengthwise stroking of the *tissues over the vertebrae* will clear the way for the sympathectomy; often the chain can now be clearly felt, tight and distinct as it runs down over the vertebral aponeurosis.

195

Two, large, folded abdominal packs are then inserted, one under each side of the wound, firmly tucked beneath the mobilised peritoneum, as near the midline as possible. The medial part of the peritoneal sac is then drawn back and up from the vertebral column, using a Deaver's retractor. The abdominal wound is opened up, to admit more light, by inserting a Harvey Jackson's self-retaining laminectomy retractor between the muscle layers and as far as the packs.

This gives a perfect exposure of the middle portion of the sympathetic chain (Fig. 10.6), which can be picked up with a long nerve hook and freed by dissection with long, curved scissors. It may be necessary to divide the lower end first, in order to pass the chain under a large lumbar vein. The ganglia are freed by dividing their deep connections. They vary in number from one thick fusiform aggregation to three or four distinct swellings; the chain between is often thin and delicate. A second, narrower Deaver's retractor may help to expose the upper end of the chain, and the light should be redirected from below. Bleeding is negligible unless a lumbar vessel has been injured. Diathermy is usually sufficient for its control: the nearby genito-femoral nerve must be avoided. More brisk bleeding can be checked by applying McKenzie silver clips, or absorbable cellulose gauze.

After removing the retractors and packs the muscles are closed; an accurate three-layer apposition is ensured by replacing the two pairs of artery forceps on the cut linea semilunaris and holding them up and apart as before. Continuous catgut is satisfactory.

If the opposite chain is to be removed as well, the superficial fascia closure of the first side is left until the end of the operation so as to make full use of the period of anaesthetic relaxation without the need for further dosage.

The membranous layer of the superficial fascia is closed with fine catgut, and the skin with interrupted 36 gauge stainless-steel wire, or with clips.

No special after care is required for this relatively minor operation; a light normal diet can be resumed as soon as the patient wishes.

Complications and Undesirable Sequelae

Surgical accidents are rare, and should be recognised and dealt with at once. The most important of these is due to heavy traction upon the great vessels.

Haemorrhage from the lumbar arteries or veins has already been discussed. It may occur after wound closure if the patient has been on large dosage of oral anticoagulants, heavy salicylate medication for pain, or when heparin has been given during a combined procedure with an arterial reconstruction as is often the case in the lower limb, when the sympathectomy will have been completed first and its wound closed. If there has been any warning of this possible complication during the sympathectomy it is advisable to insert a temporary drain down to the vertebral column before closing the wound. It may then be removed before the patient goes back to the ward. The inferior vena cava may be injured by retraction or by cutting into one of the lumbar veins near its entry into the cava. This can give rise to a severe haemorrhage at the deepest point of the wound, though local pressure should control it at once. It is usually possible to secure the small opening in the great vein with a sponge forceps used as a clamp, though it is preferable, if ready on the trolley, to use a Satinsky or other lateral vascular clamp. Fine catgut on a small atraumatic round-bodied needle is often easier to place and tie than a fine silk vascular suture.

Embolism

Figure 10.7 shows how, at a left lumbar sympathectomy, aortic retraction may displace thrombus or atheromatous material, which then passes down the *right iliac artery*, since the left tends to be obstructed by the retractor. At the completion of the operation the right lower limb is seen to be ischaemic, with an absent femoral pulse indicating an embolus at this point or just above, in the external iliac. An immediate embolectomy is usually successful unless the obstructed artery is heavily atheromatous (Fig. 10.8).

Exceptionally, a thrombus present in the inferior vena cava in a bedridden patient may be pushed free and give rise to a pulmonary embolism.

Injury to the Ureter

This is unlikely, for the normal tissue mobility allows the ureter to slip medially and upwards under the central retractor, which then protects it. In patients with retroperitoneal fibrosis or spinal disease, for example an old psoas abscess, the ureter is densely fixed, and injury is likely to occur during the search for the sympathetic chain.

Postsympathectomy Neuralgia [19]

This is a common complication, occurring in a mild form in about 20 per cent of patients; severe pain is

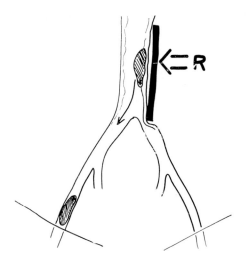

Fig. 10.7. Retraction upon the aorta during left lumbar sympathectomy may cause an embolus to dislodge, it then enters the right iliac artery, the left being occluded by the retractor.

The same retraction may injure the left iliac artery, causing worsening of the limb condition on the operated side, or the occlusion may predispose to thrombosis in the narrowed parts of the artery beyond.

less common. It is seldom bilateral. The onset, often at night, tends to be during the first week, or later, and the pain is described as a dull ache extending over the antero-lateral aspect of the thigh. Usually, there are no abnormal neurological signs, so that the somatic nerve injury is an unlikely explanation. It may be due to reference to this somatic area from the damaged sympathetic fibres which are of the same segmental level. Though some patients state that it is very severe, it is never permanent, in most cases passing off within one to six weeks. Sometimes it occurs after chemical sympathectomy using 10 per cent phenol.

Interference with Sexual Function

In the male, bilateral lumbar sympathectomy is often followed by loss of ejaculation (dry orgasm). It is believed that this complication is less likely to happen if the first lumbar ganglion is preserved on one side, though the writer had a case in which the symptom followed a unilateral sympathectomy.

It is important to warn the patient about this possible complication which, in the younger man with bilateral disease (e.g. Buerger's disease), may afford a serious drawback to a highly necessary operation.

Other Unusual Effects of Sympathectomy

A wide, bilateral sympathectomy may lead to postural hypotension. Reduction in the area of the outflow may also lead to overactivity in the intact remaining fibres, with the development of Raynaud's phenomenon (*see* Chapter 11). For similar reasons, hyperhidrosis may be set up in non-sympathectomised areas.

Unilateral upper limb sympathectomy is reported to prevent digital osteoarthritis [12].

Worsening of Ischaemia After Lumbar Sympathectomy [3]

When a patient with reduced circulation in one or both lower limbs undergoes lumbar sympathectomy the ischaemia is sometimes made worse. Either limb may be affected. Transient changes are common in the early hours and the common 'cold phase' on the operated side will usually be assumed to be responsible, though often more marked than normal. By the next day it will be clear that the patient is worse as a result of the operation. Three possible reasons should be considered:

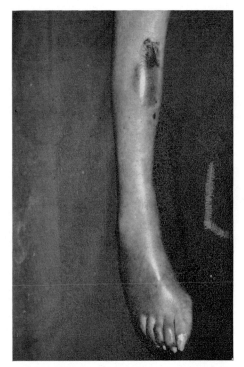

Fig. 10.8. Results of unrecognised right common femoral embolism occurring during left lumbar sympathectomy. Severe ischaemia with muscle contracture of the calf and anterior tibial infarction. High amputation was necessary.

197

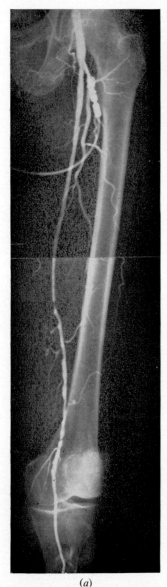

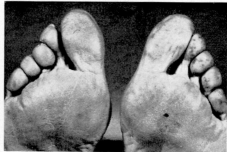

(b)

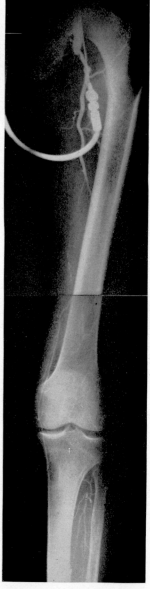

(c)

(a)

Fig. 10.9. Acute worsening of left lower limb ischaemia following left lumbar sympathectomy.

    (a) Diffusely narrowed femoro-popliteal artery before operation.

    (b) Acute ischaemia of left toes with with patchy lividity and pallor at their worst severity on the second postoperative day.

    (c) Postoperative femoral arteriogram showing occlusion of the whole of the femoro-popliteal segment.

A good recovery followed the infusion of heparin in low molecular weight dextran for five days.

1. Thrombo-embolic complications of the operation, the anaesthetic, or a period of postoperative hypotension.
2. Haemodynamic shifts within the balanced system of resistances, serial in one limb, and parallel in bilateral cases.
3. Arterio-venous shunting, already perhaps contributing to the ischaemia (*see* Chapters 3, p. 56, and 4, p. 107).

We have already examined the serious problem of contralateral iliofemoral arterial *embolism* from operative retraction on the aorta. Here the advent of the new pulse deficiencies of major degree should lead to prompt diagnosis and treatment, before irreversible changes take place (Fig. 10.8).

On the operated side, an *acute thrombosis* within a diffusely narrowed and sclerotic artery may take place during the early hours (Fig. 10.9). The iliac artery may have been damaged or unduly compressed during surgery (Fig. 10.7) [3]. A 'thrombophilic' phase in the underlying disease might be blamed, or a general response to operative injury, or the recent withdrawal of long-term anticoagulant treatment for the purposes of the operation.

Haemometakinesia, or the 'borrowing-lending syndrome' [6] from sections of greater to lower resistance, so important a concept in vascular disease, has been applied to the present problem [13] with its various possible combinations of circumstances under which sharp changes of peripheral resistance might follow arterial reconstruction or sympathectomy or both, with worsening of the opposite side, or possibly even parts of the revascularised limb.

Fortunately, this serious and unexpected complication is sufficiently unusual for sympathectomy to continue in its important role as a safe and valuable 'insurance operation' for lower limb ischaemia.

Mortality

For a deep abdominal operation in subjects of questionable cardiovascular status the mortality rate is low. Not all published series give this figure, but an average of 1 per cent should represent an acceptable risk for the real benefits of the procedure. In the author's experience of 204 lumbar sympathectomies in 179 patients (excluding a similar number combined with various arterial reconstructions) there was one death, from myocardial infarction.

Note on Chemical Sympathectomy [10, 14]

Lumbar paravertebral injection of one in fifteen phenol in water (not oil, which inactivates it) is often followed by a striking and lasting release of sympathetic tone in the lower limb on the injected side, with dryness of the skin and good relief of rest pain. Minor gangrene may be induced to heal. For the aged or otherwise unsuitable patient requiring sympathectomy this method is valuable. 3 ml are injected through each of two long splanchnic block needles, four fingers' breadth lateral to the midline, and thence inwards and slightly upwards between the lumbar transverse processes so as to strike the side of the vertebral body near its anterior surface. After aspirating, to avoid the large blood vessels close by this point, the operator should wait for 20 seconds before injecting the phenol, to ensure that C.S.F. has not been reached. Within a few minutes of the injections, if the placing is correct, the skin of the knee and calf show increased warmth.

Reid, of Glasgow, the principal exponent of this method, has had over 7,000 patients who showed similar benefits to those that follow operative sympathectomy, and only one death, cause not found at post-mortem [14].

Results of Lumbar Sympathectomy in Occlusive Arterial Disease

Over 50 per cent of patients with severe ischaemia are helped by this simple operation. There is good agreement in the literature, as the following large case series show:

Gillespie [7] (1960) 100 patients; 41 with rest pain or ischaemic lesions. 55 per cent healing and no amputation. 13 per cent of those with claudication improved.

Taylor and Calo [18] (1962) 113 patients, all with early nutritional disturbance. 60 per cent improved. (Untreated 28 per cent.) 41 per cent of those with claudication improved. (Untreated 39 per cent.)

Blain et al. [5] (1963) 196 patients, most of whom had rest pain or gangrene. 64 per cent excellent or good results.

King et al. [11] (1964) 407 patients, most of whom had rest pain or gangrene. 57 per cent of those with rest pain improved.

45 per cent of those with gangrene improved.

Haimovici et al. [9] (1964) 171 patients, 55 per cent with gangrene, 25 per cent with severe rest pain. More than half diabetic. Rest pain improved in 71 per cent. Ulceration and gangrene improved in 55·4 per cent. Claudication improved in 20 per cent.

Strand [17A] (1969) 167 patients. 56 per cent improved. Rest pain better than gangrene.

The solid advantages of this safe procedure are now being overshadowed by the more spectacular success that often follows arterial reconstruction. Yet failure is common with both operations, the important difference being that after sympathectomy there may still be the prospect of relief with direct arterial surgery, whereas a failed arterial operation in such a case usually determines the need for an early amputation.

REFERENCES

1. Baffes, T. G., Norberg, C. and Katopodis, S. (1959) Some problems encountered in treatment of peripheral arterial disease. *Arch. Surg.*, **79**, 52.

2. Barcroft, H. and Swan, H. J. C. (1953) *Sympathetic Control of Human Blood Vessels*. London: Edward Arnold & Co., p. 6, 58 *et seq.*

3. Bergan, J. J. and Trippel, O. H. (1962) Arteriograms in ischemic limbs worsened after lumbar sympathectomy. *Arch. Surg.*, **85**, 643.

4. Birkett, D. A., Apthorp, G. H., Chamberlain, D. A., Hayward, G. W. and Tuckwell, E. G. (1965) Bilateral upper thoracic sympathectomy in angina pectoris: results in 52 cases. *Brit. med. J.*, **ii**, 187.

5. Blain, A., Zadeh, A. T., Teves, M. L. and Bing, R. J. (1963) Lumbar sympathectomy for arteriosclerosis obliterans. *Surgery*, **53**, 164.

6. De Bakey, M. E., Burch, G., Ray, T. and Ochsner, A. (1947) The 'borrowing-lending' hemodynamic phenomenon (hemometakinesia) and its therapeutic application in peripheral vascular disturbances. *Ann. Surg.*, **126**, 850.

7. Gillespie, J. A. (1960) Late effects of lumbar sympathectomy on blood-flow in the foot in obliterative vascular disease. *Lancet*, **i**, 891.

8. Golding, M. R., Mendoza, M. F., Hennigar, G. R., Fries, C. C. and Wesolowski, S. A. (1964) On settling the controversy on the benefit of sympathectomy for frostbite. *Surgery*, **56**, 221.

9. Haimovici, H., Steinman, C. and Karson, I. H. (1964) Evaluation of lumbar sympathectomy: advanced occlusive arterial disease. *Arch. Surg.*, **89**, 1089.

10. Haxton, H. A. (1949) Chemical sympathectomy. *Brit. med. J.*, **i**, 1026.

11. King, R. D., Kaiser, G. C., Lempke, R. E. and Shumacker, H. B. (1964) Evaluation of lumbar sympathetic denervation. *Arch. Surg.*, **88**, 36.

12. Lilly, G. D. (1966) Effect of sympathectomy on development of chronic osteoarthritis. *Ann. Surg.*, **163**, 856.

13. Murphy, T. O. and Piper C. A. (1965) Hemato-metakinesia effects upon the sympathectomised extremity. *Amer. Surg.*, **31**, 437.

14. Reid, W., Watt, J. K. and Gray, T. G. (1970) Phenol injection of the sympathetic chain. *Brit. J. Surg.*, **57**, 45, and Personal Communication (1972).

15. Ross, J. P. (1958) *Surgery of the Sympathetic Nervous System*. London: Ballière, Tindall and Cox. Third edition.

16. Shumacker, H. B. (1960) Comments on the distribution of blood flow. *Surgery*, **47**, 1.

17. Simeone, F. A. (1963) Intravascular pressure, vascular tone, and sympathectomy. *Surgery*, **53**, 1.

17A.Strand, L. (1969) Lumbar sympathectomy in the treatment of peripheral obliterative arterial disease. *Acta chir. Scand.*, **135**, 597.

18. Taylor, G. W. and Calo, A. R. (1962) Atherosclerosis of arteries of lower limbs. *Brit. med. J.*, **i**, 507.

19. Tracy, G. D. and Cockett, F. B. (1957) Pain in the lower limb after sympathectomy. *Lancet*, **i**, 12.

11 The Raynaud Syndromes

Definition. The Raynaud syndrome is an intermittent cold-induced digital ischaemia progressing to become chronic, with eventual loss of tissue, featuring vascular disease either as cause or effect.

Historical Contributions
Maurice Raynaud published his original thesis, entitled *On Local Asphyxia and Symmetrical Gangrene of the Extremities*, in 1862 [49]. Although his view was that sympathetic over-activity was the cause of the condition, his observations included cases of other kinds which we now recognise as secondary to known disease conditions and only 'spasmodic' in a subsidiary way; for example, he likened some cases to the condition of ergotism; others had peripheral neuritis, but he clearly distinguished diabetic gangrene apart. Several of his patients were fatally ill when they developed digital gangrene at an unnaturally early age.

It was in 1934 that Lewis and Pickering [41] showed that, apart from cases with a 'local fault' there is a large group of diseases, many of them generalised, yet showing the digital vascular features that Raynaud described, and this state they called 'the Raynaud phenomenon', a distinction of the utmost importance, for though the early appearances are much the same in the two types, the treatment and prognosis differ very considerably.

The relative incidence of the two types is not yet established. It may vary in different parts of the world, or it may be changing with an increase in the prevalence of collagen diseases, or with clearer recognition of the effects of vascular occlusion. A related problem is that the digital features of collagen diseases may be the presenting, and indeed the only feature, for a considerable period of time, during which the patient may be thought to have true primary Raynaud's disease. A two-year limit [2] may not be long enough to exclude the possibility of secondary disease [35].

The Two Types

Primary Raynaud's Disease	Secondary Raynaud Phenomenon
Cause not fully known	Many causes recognised
Cool, damp climate	Climate unrelated
Heredity	Some hereditary causes
Mainly females	Both sexes
A 'local fault' in the digital vessels, which over-react to cold	Known causes include: Structural arterial disease Connective tissue disorders Blood diseases
Two or more extremities affected	One alone is diagnostic, but may be multiple

Acrocyanosis (=blue ends) commonly occurs with disuse of a limb. Lewis observed [40e] that in a normal subject resting one hand completely for thirty minutes while using the other normally would result in a marked fall in finger temperature in the resting hand. Moreover, if then the hand were laid at rest on a table, and the hypothenar muscles were exercised, the temperature of this part of the cool hand would then rise above that of the remainder. This type of circulatory depression is seen in longstanding, paralytic states of all kinds, especially with late hemiplegia, birth palsy, poliomyelitis, and traumatic lower motor neurone loss after the early stage of sympathetic release. Such patients tend to improve with sympathectomy, the likely effects of which can be established before the operation by body warming. If, however, the extremity is completely denervated, it will not, Lewis showed, respond to body warming, here resembling a sympathectomised limb.

Four-limb acrocyanosis is quite different, for body activity is normal and general health unimpaired. It is often associated with hyperhidrosis, and therefore suggests sympathetic overactivity, yet local warming of a small area of the affected skin improves its colour and raises its temperature so that a local fault, as in primary Raynaud's disease, seems to be more to blame [40c]. Young women with this condition tend to have fat legs, which when thinly covered in winter time become very blue and puffy, and may ulcerate in places, probably from small foci of fat necrosis. Cases of this severity, unaffected by wearing warmer clothing or other general measures, usually respond well to lumbar sympathectomy.

Three-Phase Cycle of the Raynaud Phenomenon

The following are the typical colour changes shown by the affected digits on exposure to cold:

1. Waxy pallor (due to acute ischaemia as the digital arteries shut down).
2. Cyanosis, often with swelling (as the returning blood becomes quickly deprived of its oxygen, and stagnates, before the venous capillaries recover sufficiently to carry it away).
3. Burning, red reactive hyperaemia, as the circulation is fully restored.

Not all patients show the three stages, often only the first two are described. In the more chronic examples there is persistent cyanosis throughout the cold season, and sometimes in the summer as well. No doubt the persistent features are due to the development of permanent narrowing or obstruction to the arteries of the affected digit, for body heating or sympathetic block produce a markedly unequal rise in skin temperature comparing the 'good' with the 'bad' digits or with other nearby parts of the extremity [14]. Such evidence of structural damage to the arteries can be confirmed by arteriography, which also shows much earlier lesions not yet causing inequalities of skin temperature.

Primary Raynaud's Disease (Fig. 11.1)

Minor degrees of digital ischaemia are common in the young [40a], and in a cool, damp climate such as that of western Norway where the reported incidence of mild forms of Raynaud's disease is high [23]. A hereditary tendency would also be likely in a closed community of this kind. Lewis and Pickering drew attention to this possibility [41]. Other associated factors include a history of emotional instability, hypertension, hyperhidrosis or migraine.

Sympathetic overactivity as the main cause of primary Raynaud's disease is now out of favour, though it may explain attacks with emotion in patients who possess the 'local fault' [51a]. There is one type of case in which it appears to be fully responsible; patients who develop intermittent digital ischaemia after extensive bilateral thoraco-lumbar sympathectomy for hypertension. In these, it is thought, more of the sympathetic outflow from

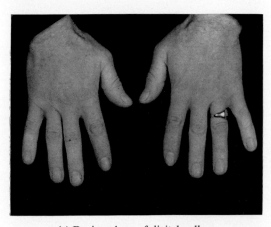

(*a*) During phase of digital pallor.

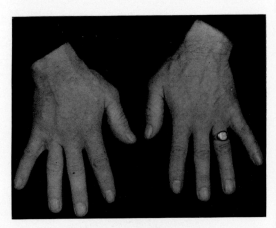

(*b*) During congestive cyanosis.

Fig. 11.1. Primary Raynaud's disease. (Note typically pointed index finger tips.)

the hypothalamus is canalised into the intact neurotomes of upper limbs. A parallel condition is the hyperhidrosis of the trunk sometimes seen after two- or four-limb sympathectomy [51b].

The haemodynamics of affected hands and fingers have been examined. Hand blood flow increased less than normal with local heating and fell more sharply with local cooling [43, 46]. Digital blood pressure at the summit of the capillary loop was grossly reduced during attacks but returned to normal or above [37].

Increased blood viscosity and a raised plasma fibrinogen level have been demonstrated [48], both factors that could bring about stasis in the digital circulation in response to cold, which is known to increase blood viscosity [39], while the presence of more than normal amounts of fibrinogen does increase red cell sludging [16].

Other physiological studies have indicated that there may be a constitutional defect in the response to cold in terms of a *limited heat production* [44] and *excess of catecholamines* detectable in the peripheral veins [45].

Very high levels have been found to be associated with Raynaud phenomenon in some patients with phaeochromocytoma, particularly those with paroxysms. Although bilateral, the condition may be asymmetrical. It is fully relieved by excision of the adrenalin secreting tumour, even if digital changes have been established [29].

As well as the anxious, obsessional personality so common in primary Raynaud's disease, there is

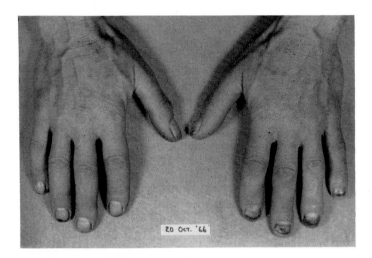

Fig. 11.2. A more advanced case of primary Raynaud's disease with chronically swollen fingers, thickened and discoloured nails, but no necrosis. The digital arteries are often still patent in such cases.

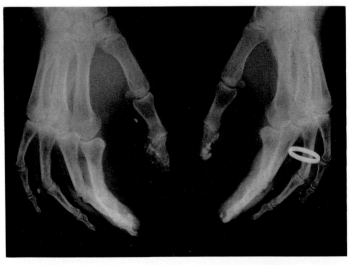

Fig. 11.3. Calcified deposits in finger and thumb pulps occurring in a woman aged sixty with hardened finger tips; yet her Raynaud symptoms were mild.

more evidence of a central neurological factor in the finding of abnormal electroencephalographic patterns suggesting a diencephalic discharge or 'psychomotor seizure' [15].

In simpler terms, a clinical definition of true primary Raynaud's disease was given by Allen and Brown in 1932 [2] and, with qualification, still serves:

(a) The vasomotor phenomenon should be bilateral and paroxysmal.
(b) There should be no more than minimal necrosis of the tips of the digits.
(c) There should be no evidence of any primary disease of the blood vessels or nervous system.
(d) These features should have been present for at least two years.

Today, however, we should re-examine this last condition. If all the milder forms are included, then the definition is true for most cases. If attention is confined to the more severely afflicted, then there is a serious risk of including a fairly high proportion of patients of secondary type in the early, local phase of their disease, which it is now thought may last much longer than two years; collagen disease may develop in an apparently typical primary patient as long as twelve to sixteen years or more after the onset of digital symptoms [14, 35].

Permanent nutritional changes in primary Raynaud's disease are troublesome, but seldom grave. A patient with actual gangrene of the pulp is probably suffering from one of the causes of secondary Raynaud phenomenon. Atrophy and hardening of the tips, particularly of the index finger, are common, apart from scleroderma, and the nails suffer damage (Fig. 11.2) from the impaired circulation in the nail plate, a fact that has been established arteriographically [52]. Paronychia, repeated, indolent, and very painful may prove to be decisive for sympathectomy in patients on conservative treatment.

Calcinosis of the finger pulps is sometimes seen in longstanding cases (Fig. 11.3), though not necessarily with severe symptoms. It is common in systemic scleroderma however [57].

Taking into account the climate, the severity of the symptoms and signs, and the results of a thorough investigation for possible underlying causal disease, a diagnosis of primary Raynaud's disease may be made with some caution in most patients whose symptoms fit these criteria, and treatment may be planned accordingly.

Secondary Raynaud Phenomenon (Fig. 11.4)

Concepts of cause and mechanism in primary Raynaud's disease remain hypothetical, but in the secondary condition known causes are many, mostly well defined and generally accepted in this role. The following list will introduce the subject:

Structural arterial disease
  Peripheral arteriosclerosis
  Thromboangiitis obliterans
  Embolism
  Cervical rib and other mechanical arterial damage
  Vibrating tools
  Frost bite
  Ergot and heavy metal poisoning

Systemic diseases affecting smaller vessels
  Scleroderma
  Disseminated lupus erythematosus
  Polyarteritis nodosa
  Rheumatoid arteritis
  Malignant disease
  Diabetes

Blood abnormalities causing impaired red cell suspension stability
  Cold agglutinins
  Cryoglobulins
  Abnormal globulins on the red cell in rheumatoid disease
  Sickle-celled anaemia
  Polycythaemia
  Pulmonary hypertension
  Congestive heart failure and shock
  The contraceptive pill

Occlusion of the small arteries of the extremity is the essential feature common to all types, whether caused by changes in the intermediate-sized proximal arteries, in the digital arteries, or by accumulating blockage of the lumen of smaller vessels by aggregated red cells from a haematological disturbance or peripheral circulatory depression. It seems that embolism may be a common feature, whatever the underlying cause; shift of small portions of obstructing material onward into the isolated peripheral territory of the small digital arteries may be the ultimate lesion in many patients. This would explain the progressive severity of the disability in striking contrast to the good level of blood flow to adjacent proximal regions of the extremity, and other digits that appear almost normal.

An essential feature of all types of Raynaud's phenomenon is intermittency; the common state of severe progressive chronic ischaemia, with incipient

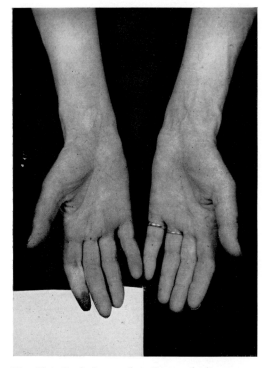

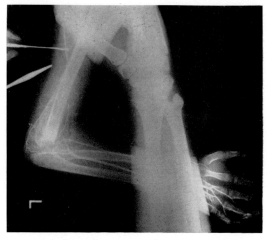

Fig. 11.5. Secondary Raynaud phenomenon of the thumb, index, and middle fingers in a young child who had sustained a brachial artery injury as a result of a supracondular fracture at the elbow. (Mr A. V. Pollock's case.)

1. An absent major pulse.
2. Stenosis as indicated by a localised systolic bruit.
3. Aneurysm at a point of mechanical wear and tear, as at the thoracic outlet or behind the knee.
4. Pallor of the affected extremity after exercising the limb (*see* Chapter 12, Case 6, p. 231, *also* Fig. 3.27).

Fig. 11.4. Typical secondary Raynaud phenomenon in a fifty-nine-year-old woman with thoracic outlet compression of the subclavian artery on the right side. Reduced upper limb pulsations, occluded digital arteries and gangrene of index finger pulp. Photograph taken during phase of pallor after immersion of hands in cold water.

Repeated embolism is now accepted as an important factor, with lesions of the last two types in the pre-occlusive stages of main vessel disease, though even after this has gone on to complete thrombosis, an instability of the collateral circulation may for the first time set up the balanced type of peripheral circulation manifested by the Raynaud phenomenon.

Arteriosclerosis and Buerger's disease* are important causes of intermittent digital ischaemia from digital arterial thrombosis, in which vigorous treatment is often successful. Occasionally, the digital lesion may be severe, yet with the wrist or ankle pulses still present at rest (*see* Fig. 4.13, p. 106). The same applies to cervical rib with arterial damage (*see* Chapter 13), a serious and progressive condition with a bad natural prognosis from repeated embolism which, unless the cause is removed, eventually fills the arteries of the limb with thrombus.

digital gangrene, is a later development in some patients, but before this stage there should have been an equilibrium in the collateral circulation, adversely affected by cold exposure or by emotion, giving rise to the attacks. There may come a time in both the primary and the secondary diseases when progressive occlusive changes in the digital arteries disturb the earlier balance of pressure and resistance so that attacks give place to a steady state of chronic congestive ischaemia. Conversely, favourable factors such as a warm climate, a successful sympathectomy, or removal of a proximal arterial obstruction may swing the balance back towards the normal.

Structural disease of the major arteries includes many important and common causes of secondary Raynaud's phenomenon, most of which are easy to recognise clinically. Usually, only one extremity is affected; examination of its main artery should account for the changes in the hand or foot. Important clinical signs include:

Other arterial damage of a mechanical kind may be followed by Raynaud episodes, for example injury to the brachial at the elbow in *supracondylar fracture* (Fig. 11.5), traumatic thrombosis of the forearm

---

* 57 per cent of one series of patients with Buerger's disease had Raynaud phenomenon at the onset [28].

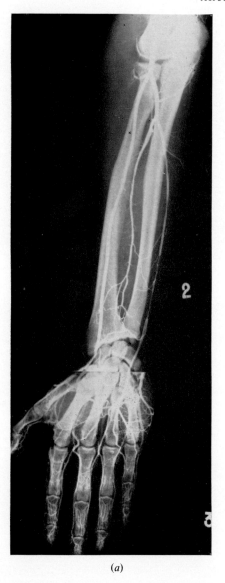

(a)

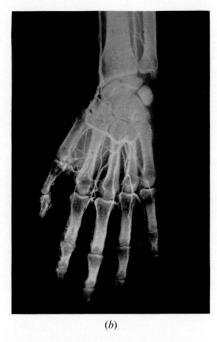

(b)

(a) Occlusive changes in right ulnar and interossous arteries in forearm and radial at wrist in a championship tennis player presenting with Raynaud phenomenon when playing in cold conditions.

(b) Occlusion of the palmar course of the ulnar artery from occupational heavy striking—the 'hypothenar hammer syndrome' [11B].

Fig. 11.6

arteries from over-use (Fig. 11.6a), and of the *palmar arch* from repeated blows to the hand at work [11B] (Fig. 11.6b), and the digital arterial disturbance that follows the long-continued *use of vibrating tools* [1] with a working frequency of between 40–125 cycles per second [34]. Chain-saw workers under cold conditions, both in Norway [32A], and in Scotland [55A], also, in Wales, pedestal grinders, copper swagers and propeller shapers [55A], were particularly liable to Raynaud spasms of blanching and numbness. Smoking also appears to aggravate the condition. Mostly the condition is non-progressive,

and structural changes either in the digital arteries or the skin that they supply are unusual [34]. More severe cases can occur, however, with digital thrombosis and loss of skin [55A].

Frost Bite [20, 27, 54, 57B] (Fig. 11.7)

The thermal injury caused by exposure to below-freezing temperatures produces lesions of interest to the vascular surgeon, whose methods may prove effective in treatment, for it is probable that the degree of vascular damage during freezing of the skin and superficial tissues is what determines their

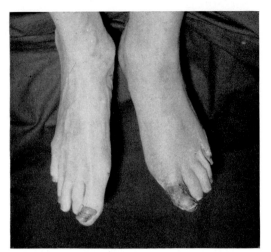

Fig. 11.7. Gangrene of outermost toes and swelling of the left foot during late recovery stage of frost bite. All peripheral pulses were normally present in this elderly subject. Earlier, blistering is typical.

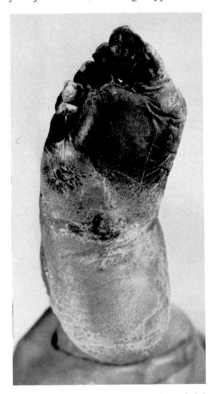

Fig. 11.8. Dry gangrene of distal portion of right foot from ergot poisoning. Appearance at fourteen days, by which time the sole up to the line of demarcation was pink and hot. All pulses had returned. (Mr P. P. McGarry's case.)

survival or necrosis. Skin tolerates extremes of temperature better than any other tissue; super-cooling or unprotected freezing need not kill it. The subcutaneous vessels, however, are more seriously affected, becoming packed with sludged and agglutinated red cells which occlude them and produce a secondary ischaemia of the part. Early arteriography shows spasm of the distal arteries, and arterio-venous shunting [42]. In amputation specimens from frost-bitten extremities, the larger arteries and veins may be seen to be thrombosed and surrounded by perivascular cellular infiltration like that present in Buerger's disease. In extensive damage no large-scale recovery is possible, and gangrene of the distal parts of the hands and feet is likely. The toes are usually affected in the 'ground-type' (in soldiers, farmers, and others exposed to snow or freezing water), and the fingers in 'high altitude' frost bite as occurs in mountaineers and air crews. When seen early, and perhaps even still frozen, rapid warming or thawing, with heparin and low molecular weight dextran infusion are indicated, aiming thus to reduce the occlusive effects of the vascular injury and lessen the extent of probable necrosis. Sympathetic block, or operative sympathectomy are advisable, and hyperbaric oxygen has proved effective [57B].

Large blisters develop during the recovery phase: these patients often do well.

Apart from complete necrosis, with inevitable separation or amputation, the digits may be chronically damaged in other ways, and bear a close resemblance to Raynaud's disease and to scleroderma. The skin is atrophic, and the nails are altered or absent, no doubt from loss of capillary blood supply, and there are nerve lesions with perineural fibrosis and demyelinisation, which are the causes of late sensory symptoms that aggravate the Raynaud diability. Sympathectomy helps this type of patient.

Ergot poisoning [8, 12] is sometimes seen after overdosage with ergotamine in migraine (Fig. 11.8), or when an ergot preparation has been used to procure an abortion. Paraesthesiae and sensory impairment precede the peripheral ischaemic signs in most patients, though those with varicose veins who take ergotamine may notice pain along the course of the affected region, followed, if the drug is continued, by constriction of the veins, leaving grooves in the fat of the subcutaneous tissues to mark their former position. Whatever the degree of vasospasm, improvement is slow even after the drug is stopped. Large arteries may go into spasm with intermittent claudication at first [60]. Deterioration may continue, and the whole limb is then threatened. Treatment is as for frost bite, except that the extremity should not be warmed.

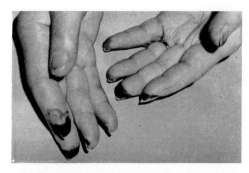 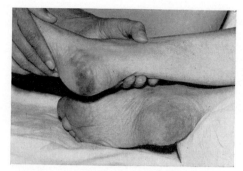

Fig. 11.9. Patchy severe ischaemia of all four extremities of acute onset in an elderly woman who also showed acute polyarthritis and a raised ESR. A suspected case of collagen disease. Acute heart failure may also have played a part.

Collagen Diseases (Fig. 11.9, also Fig. 7.3, p. 139)

This group of conditions appears to be on the increase (Chapter 7). As a cause of the Raynaud phenomenon they are becoming important, in some series outnumbering the primary cases [15]. Age and sex distribution are similar and so the question arises, how long must a patient with apparent primary Raynaud's disease be followed before it can be certain that she is not an early case of disseminated lupus or scleroderma systemica? The peripheral circulatory effects of collagen diseases are the presenting feature in a substantial minority. In such patients acrocyanosis usually affects all four limbs, and in most of them other evidence of the underlying disease can be elicited. General ill health is accompanied by anaemia with low fever and joint pains. The LE cells or other positive laboratory findings may be present. The prognostic and therapeutic significance of such evidence is important, particularly now that steroid treatment alleviates the effects of these diseases for long periods in many cases. Sympathectomy is contra-indicated, for the results are poor.

Malignant disease may be associated with digital ischaemia, particularly in women [30].

Disturbances of the blood and micro-circulation can cause Raynaud phenomenon by altering the red cell suspension stability, or, as in primary Raynaud's disease, the blood viscosity (*see* p. 203), so that there is sludging in the small peripheral vessels which become partly obstructed as a result, when thrombosis may follow. The following conditions may be responsible singly or in combination: congestive heart failure, pulmonary hypertension, polycythaemia, protein abnormalities including cold agglutinins [15], cryoglobulins [19], Waldenström's macroglobulinaemia [17], and other abnormal red cell protein coating, for example in rheumatoid

disease [22]. Any of these may be aggravated by trauma, operative shock or haemorrhage, or by haemoconcentration from fluid losses.

Sickle-celled anaemia may lead to digital artery occlusion (Fig. 11.10) due to repeated application of compression of the arm in taking successive blood-pressure readings, temporary peripheral stagnation

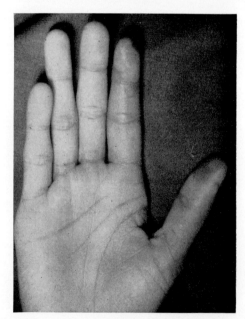

Fig. 11.10. Severe secondary Raynaud phenomenon affecting thumb and index finger of a young negress following repeated blood pressure measurements during a complicated labour.

Note extra flexor creases distal to normal folds—a useful clinical sign in many cases of sickle-cell disease [13].

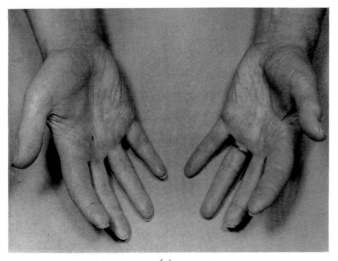

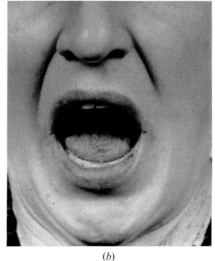

(a)

(b)

Fig. 11.11. Clinical features of scleroderma. Hard, tight contracted skin over (a) fingers, (b) lips and corners of mouth, (c) pretibial skin. Telangiectases were also present in all three situations.

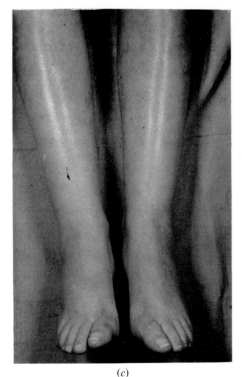

(c)

and anoxia apparently being sufficient to change the haemoglobin and red cells into the pathological form, causing obstruction by sludging. Transient and permanent occlusive effects have been described in patients with sickle-cell haemoglobin—C disease [9].

Investigation of a Case of Raynaud Phenomenon [6A] The history and clinical examination are directed towards the possibility of an underlying general or cardiovascular disease. Inspection may show obvious scleroderma (Fig. 11.11), central or peripheral, or the purple face and extremities of primary or secondary polycythaemia. Mild rheumatoid swelling of the joints is common, and the pulse rate is often raised with the low fever. Digital pulses may be missing in the worse-affected fingers (Fig. 11.12). A raised ESR is characteristic. Except in polycythaemia, the haemoglobin level is below normal. An LE cell test must be carried out as a routine, together with a search for cold agglutinins and cryoglobulins in the serum. The urine may contain free haemoglobin after cold agglutination has occurred. Barium-meal studies may show the visceral type of scleroderma, particularly in the oesophagus (Fig. 11.13). Chest films may show the pulmonary and cardiac changes of polyarteritis nodosa, for confirmation of which muscle biopsy may also be needed. Punch biopsy of the skin may reveal the same abnormalities or those of scleroderma, even away from clinically affected areas.

Arteriography, by brachial puncture under general anaesthesia, gives good pictures which confirm the

209

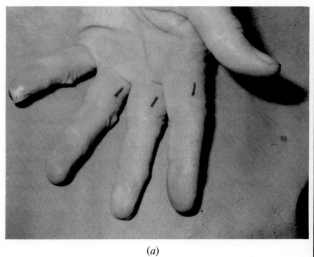

(a)

Fig. 11.12. Secondary Raynaud phenomenon due to arteriosclerotic thrombosis or embolism. (*a*) Sudden onset of painful necrosis of little finger tip in a man aged sixty-four with impalpable ulnar three digital pulses confirmed at arteriography (*b*). (Doppler ultrasound may be sufficient.)

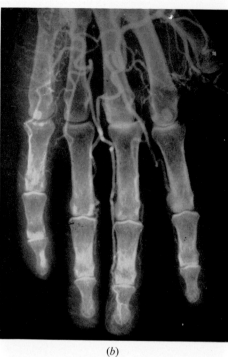

(b)

Fig. 11.13. (*a*) Dilated, atonic oesophagus, and (*b*) Finger tip necrosis in a woman aged sixty with scleroderma.

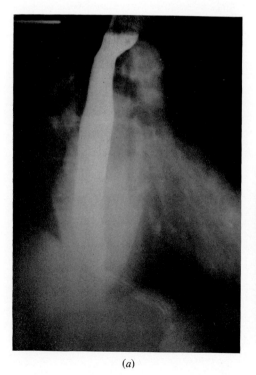

(a)

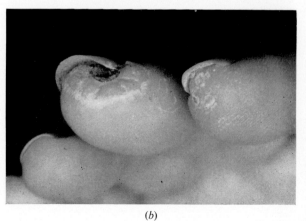

(b)

clinical evidence of digital ischaemia and often show multiple occlusions of the arteries of several fingers [6]. These findings, although they may support the case for sympathectomy, help very little towards the diagnosis of the cause, being present in some severe primary and most secondary types, and sometimes in digits that are symptomless [55] (Fig. 11.12*b*). The examination may, however, demonstrate structural disease of the larger, proximal arteries of the forearm and wrist (*see* Figs 11.6*a* and 11.16*b*).

Non-vascular conditions that resemble Raynaud's disease include the carpal (and tarsal) tunnel syndromes, various generalised neuropathies, and glomus tumour [11c], the latter showing vasomotor effects as well as pain.

Treatment: General and Medical

All patients benefit from conservative measures to protect the extremities from cold, damp or rough use. Gloves should be worn at work and out of doors over most of the year, and warm clothing at all cool times and seasons. Slow-burning hand stoves can be held or safely kept in the pockets at other times. Sepsis should be dealt with early while still subcuticular: deep incisions into the finger pulp are seldom necessary. Antibiotics are often helpful for minor indolent infection without evidence of pus.

These measures apply equally to primary and secondary patients, although in the latter, every emphasis should be upon finding and treating the underlying disease.

Intractable primary Raynaud's disease can be fully controlled by constant warm conditions; good advice for such patients is that they should move to a tropical climate, e.g. Northern Queensland.

Drugs that may be tried include the vasodilators, including alcohol, and the regime of Peacock [47], which consists of the following:

1. 10-methoxydeserpidine 5 mg b.d., which is known to reduce the concentration of catecholamines in the vessel walls [10]. Reserpine 0·5 mg into the brachial or radial arteries may help [50A, 59].
2. Tri-iodothyronine (liothyronine) 60–80 μg daily and:
3. Stenediol, 50 mg daily, both of which stimulate metabolism and may, therefore, lessen cold sensitivity.

Other drugs for which claims have been made include griseofulvin [11A, 12A], which has cardio-vascular properties [1A, 51A], methyldopa [57A], from its sympatholytic effect, and low molecular weight dextran [33, 48] which might lower blood viscosity (*see* p. 27).

SURGICAL TREATMENT

Indications for Sympathectomy

Patients in whom acrocyanosis or hyperhidrosis (Fig. 11.14) are most of the disability, or in whom the feet are more affected than the hands, should all do well.

In the large remainder of patients with primary Raynaud's disease, a prolonged and patient trial of conservative measure and medical treatment is good policy, during which time signs of an underlying disease may emerge; meanwhile operation is kept in reserve. Unreasonable delay is an unkindness to the patient with severe symptoms, however, and it is wrong to wait for complications before advising sympathectomy, for the best results are obtained in the earlier stages.

CHOICE OF OPERATION

Most British surgeons prefer the anterior approach for its excellent exposure of the stellate and upper two or three thoracic ganglia; also because it allows full inspection of the neurovascular bundle for com-

pression at the thoracic outlet. Details of this operation are given in Chapter 13.

The posterior approach through the second rib bed is difficult and causes more postoperative pain. It provides no view of the neurovascular bundle, an objection that also applies to the axillary trans-pleural route, but for good exposure, and cosmetically, this method has much to recommend it [3].

Complications are few: injury to the pleura happens often, but without serious consequence; the air is removed through a suction catheter during wound closure. There may be troublesome bleeding from an intercostal vein; control is more difficult when the pleura is open and, very occasionally, a haemopneumothorax may develop. Pain in the shoulder and upper chest segments may be referred from the damaged sympathetic lesion ('post sympathectomy neuritis'), as is thought to explain the pain in the thigh which commonly follows lumbar sympathectomy.

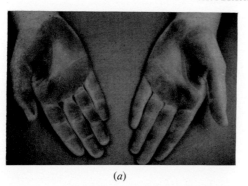
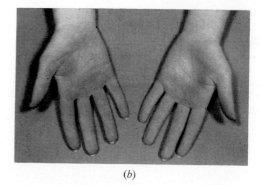

(*a*)   (*b*)

Fig. 11.14. Quinizarin sweat test in a girl aged nineteen with primary acrocyanosis and hyperhidrosis. (*a*) before, (*b*) after cervico-dorsal sympathectomy.

Results of Sympathectomy for Primary Raynaud's Disease

Allowing for varying criteria of severity and revision of the diagnosis during the follow up period, Table 11.1 shows the findings of several papers: it is clear that in the upper limb the late results are not good. Yet, almost all patients show striking early relief, with complete absence of sympathetic tone in the early weeks [31]. In the lower limbs this satisfactory state usually persists [21]. In the common severe form of the disease affecting the upper extremity, the benefits of operation often do not last. Clinical and physiological evidence in one study [21] showed renewed vasomotor activity at six months in 64 per cent of the patients, though this might remain less efficient than before operation [5]. Some patients, however, experienced good results in spite of re-establishment of the vasomotor path [5]. Yet there were few poor results in a group in which persistent denervation could be demonstrated [50]. Whether the section is preganglionic or a ganglionectomy makes little difference according to some [24, 31, 35, 36], though Haxton's modification of the original Telford operation of preganglionic section, in which

Table 11.1. Late Results of Cervico-dorsal Sympathectomy for Primary Raynaud's Disease

Authors	Follow-up years	Total cases	Excellent	Fair	Poor	Remarks
Telford, 1944 [56]	½–several	39	16	8	13	In 19 cases of acrosclerosis: poor.
Haxton, 1947 [31]	1–14	40	14	8	18	Ganglionectomy and preganglionic section: no different.
Barcroft and Hamilton, 1948 [5]	1–6	36	18	14	4	Some good results with recurrent vasomotor tone.
Felder *et al.*, 1949 [21]	½–20	75	36%	28%	36%	Clinical and physiological recurrence in 64% by six months.
Blain *et al.*, 1951 [7]	2–13	24	10	—	—	Untreated, 40% remained the same.
Robertson and Smithwick, 1951 [50]	1–15	86 (limbs)	27	46	13	Fair results with incomplete denervation in 46/86.
Kinmonth and Hadfield, 1952 [36]	1–13	80	56 improved	24 fair or poor		Importance of local fault in recurrence.
Gifford *et al.*, 1958 [24]	1–28	100	54	9	37	Ganglionectomy and preganglionic section no different. Best results in uncomplicated cases.
Johnston *et al.*, 1965 [35]	3–24	31	18 improved			Larger initial series reduced by other diagnoses.
Baddeley, 1965 [4]	6–13	64 (limbs)	13	22	29	T.1–5 ganglionectomy no more effective than T.2–3 or 3–4.

he places the mobilised upper thoracic chain in a tunnel between the ribs and passes it into the posterior muscles, gave better than average late results in its first trials, and is still doing so [32].

Causes of Relapse

With a disease whose nature is so little understood, it is scarcely surprising that its re-emergence after upper limb sympathectomy cannot be explained either. There may not be much difference between treated and untreated patients. In one large series treated conservatively only 25 per cent deteriorated severely; while 40 per cent remained unchanged [7].

Regeneration of upper thoracic sympathetic fibres has been shown histologically in monkeys and in man [32], physiologically by reflex heating [5], and by nerve block with procaine and diodone [32]. The fact that few clinical relapses occur in patients with maintained vasomotor interruption does not prove that regeneration is the cause of relapse, only that it may aggravate it, as Lewis observed [40b] in commenting upon the practical value of the operation in this disease, which he considered to be due to a local fault.

Some have stated that the incidence of relapse is less from re-innervation than from persistence of the local fault [36].

The relapse and the primary disease may, therefore, be much the same, with sympathetic tone, or the lack of it, fulfilling only a secondary role through its action in modifying the prevailing conditions of temperature and heat loss at the extremities.

These differences are not confined to limbs that have been sympathectomised for Raynaud's disease. They also exist when the operation has been performed for other reasons, e.g. arteriosclerosis or hyperhidrosis. Yet, even in untreated Raynaud's disease, there is a marked difference between the degree of vascular tone in the fingers and in the toes, probably better explained without reference to the vasomotor nerves, but more upon the basis of an inequality of the local fault in the two sites.

Results of Sympathectomy in Secondary Raynaud's Phenomenon

1. In patients with arteriosclerosis (Fig. 11.15) or Buerger's disease (see Figs 4.7, 4.14) who have stopped smoking, the outlook is good provided that ischaemic damage is not already advanced. In digital artery thrombosis proven by arteriography, the results are better in men; according to one report 60 per cent were fully cured of all symptoms; women with skin necrosis were helped, but milder symptoms persisted [6].

2. In cervical rib or thoracic outlet syndrome with arterial damage, sympathectomy alone, though useful, may not be sufficient [18] (see Chapter 13).

3. The mild vasospasm produced by vibrating tools may be helped by sympathectomy, but here the local fault within the affected fingers is likely to be the dominant factor [31] in determining response to treatment.

4. In acrosclerosis (scleroderma of the extremities with systemic features of milder degree), some good results are obtainable, but mainly in the early stages of the slowly progressive condition, when the picture may, for several years, be identical with primary Raynaud's disease [14]. Severe digital sclerosis is seldom helped [24].

5. In generalised severe scleroderma, recognised before the sympathectomy, there is little benefit to the hands from the operation; some patients are made worse.

6. In disseminated lupus erythematosus, harm may also be done; with a general deterioration, e.g. from renal failure [14].

Prognosis of Secondary Raynaud Phenomenon with Other Forms of Treatment

Many of the causes can now be treated effectively, e.g. structural disease of a main artery; but in patients with collagen disease the outlook is uncertain even with steroid therapy, the side effects of which, after large or long continued dosage, may constitute a disease in themselves.

NOTE ON ERYTHROMELALGIA, AND ON CAUSALGIA OF THE FINGER FLEXURES

These are two similar, though somewhat obscure, conditions in which the chief complaint is of a burning pain or discomfort in the extremities. Because they are uncommon, and symptoms are intermittent, neurosis may be suspected.

Erythromelalgia

Painful burning episodes, chiefly of the feet, which the patient relieves by cooling, e.g. getting up from bed to walk on a cold floor surface, such as upon tiles, may occur with or without organic disease of the blood or the vessels. Some patients with chronic lower limb ischaemia experience this during rest pain. It also occurs in polycythaemia [58]. In other patients, chilblains are present. Often, there are no abnormal signs. Sympathectomy, as Lewis found [40d] is sometimes highly successful, but it should always be preceded by a trial by paravertebral block. Methysergide (Deseril) is reported to control the symptoms [11], but the risk of retroperitoneal fibrosis might contra-indicate its prolonged use.

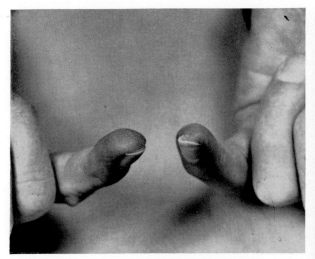

Fig. 11.15. Good result of sympathectomy for digital artery thrombosis (the same patient as in Fig. 11.12).

Causalgia of the Finger Flexures

Not to be confused with causalgia from partial nerve damage, this seems to be a purely vascular condition in which, from time to time, often under conditions of heat or vibration, the patient experiences a sharp needle-like burning pain 'like a bee-sting', usually over the anterolateral part of the proximal interphalangeal finger joint, i.e. along the line of the digital vessels. This is soon followed by a hot bluish tender swelling in the crease, which slowly resolves over the next few days. In the author's view, it is possibly due to some damage to a glomus body beneath this thin area of skin. Reassurance is all that is required, once the diagnosis from Raynaud phenomenon is clear.

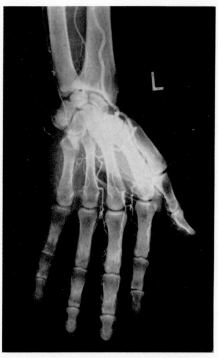

Fig. 11.16. Polycythaemia vera as a cause of digital ischaemia. A man aged sixty developed bilateral ulnar artery thrombosis, with a good response to sympathectomy. Later the blood condition was recognised and relieved by P_{32} treatment.

REFERENCES

1. Agate, J. N. and Druett, H. A. (1947) A study of portable vibrating tools in relation to the clinical effects which they produce. *Brit. J. Indust. med.*, **4**, 141.
1A. Aldinger, E. E. (1968) Cardiovascular effects of griseofulvin. *Circ. Research*, **22**, 589.
2. Allen, E. V. and Brown, G. E. (1932) Raynaud's disease: a critical review of minimal requisites for diagnosis. *Amer. J. Med. Sci.*, **183**, 187.
3. Atkins, H. J. B. (1954) Sympathectomy by the axillary approach. *Lancet*, **i**, 538.
4. Baddeley, R. M. (1965) The place of upper dorsal sympathectomy in the treatment of primary Raynaud's disease. *Brit. J. Surg.*, **52**, 426.
5. Barcroft, H. and Hamilton, G. T. C. (1948) Results of sympathectomy of the upper limb, with special reference to Raynaud's disease. *Lancet*, **i**, 441.
6. Birnstingl, M. (1967) Results of sympathectomy in digital artery disease. *Brit. med. J.*, **ii**, 601.
6A. Birnstingl, M. (1971) The Raynaud syndrome. *Postgrad. med. J.*, **47**, 297.
7. Blain, A. Coller, F. A. and Carver, G. B. (1951) Raynaud's disease. A study of criteria for prognosis. *Surgery*, **29**, 387.
8. Bross, W., Czereda, T., Cisek, T. and Kozminski, S. (1963) Gangrene of the legs after ergotrate by mouth. *Lancet*, **i**, 85.
9. Burchmore, J. W., Buckle, R. M., Lehmann, H. and Jenkins, W. J. (1962) Agglutinating-sickling arterial thrombosis. *Lancet*, **ii**, 1008.

10. Burn, J. H. and Rand, M. J. (1958) Effect of reserpine on vasoconstriction caused by sympathcomimetic amines. *Lancet*, **i**, 673.

11. Catchpole, B. N. (1964) Erythromelalgia. *Lancet*, **i**, 909.

11A.Charles, R. and Carmick, E. S. (1970) Skin temperature changes in Raynaud's disease after griseofulvin. *Arch. Dermatol.*, **101**, 331.

11B.Conn, J., Bergan, J. J. and Bell, J. L. (1970) Hypothenar hammer syndrome. *Surgery*, **68**, 1122.

11C.Cooke, S. A. R. (1971) Misleading features in the clinical diagnosis of the peripheral glomus tumour. *Brit. J. Surg.*, **58**, 602.

12. Cranley, J. J., Krause, R. J., Strasser, E. S. and Hafner, C. D. (1963) Impending gangrene of four extremities secondary to ergotism. *New Eng. J. med.*, **269**, 727.

12A.Creery, R. D. G., Voyce, M. A., Preece, A. W. and Evason, A. R. (1968) Raynaud's disease treated with griseofulvin. *Arch. Dis. Child.*, **43**, 344.

13. DeJong, R. and Platou, R. V. (1967) Sickle cell hemoglobinopathy. An anatomic sign. *Amer. J. Dis. Child.*, **113**, 271.

14. de Takats, G. and Fowler, E. F. (1962) Raynaud phenomenon. *J. Amer. Med. Assoc.*, **179**, 1.

15. de Takats, G. and Fowler, E. F. (1962) The neurogenic factor in Raynaud's phenomenon. *Surgery*, **51**, 9.

16. Ditzel, J. (1959) Relationship of blood protein composition to intravascular erythrocyte aggregation (sludged blood). *Acta med. Scand.*, **164**, Supp. 343, p. 11.

17. Donders, P. C., Imhof, J. W. and Baars, H. (1958) Clinical demonstrations. Ophthalmological phenomena in Waldenström's disease with cryoglobulinaemia. *Ophthalmologica*, **135**, 324.

18. Eastcott, H. H. G. (1962) Reconstruction of the subclavian artery for complications of cervical-rib and thoracic-outlet syndrome. *Lancet*, **ii**, 1243.

19. Ellis, H. A. and Stanworth, D. R. (1961) Physicochemical and immunological observations on the abnormal proteins in three patients with cryoglobulinaemia. *J. Clin. Path.*, **14**, 179.

20. Ervasti, E. (1962) Frostbites of the extremities and their sequelae: a clinical study. *Acta. chir. Scand.*, Supp. 299.

21. Felder, D. A., Simeone, F. A., Linton, R. R. and Welch, C. E. (1949) Evaluation of sympathetic neurectomy in Raynaud's disease. *Surgery*, **26**, 1014.

22. Finkelstein, A. E., Kwok, G., Hall, A. P. and Bayles, T. B. (1961) The erythrocyte in rheumatoid arthritis. I. A method for the detection of an abnormal globulin coating. *New Eng. J. Med.*, **264**, 270.

23. Fretheim, B. (1961) Sympathetic denervation of the upper extremities in Raynaud's disease and secondary Raynaud's phenomenon. *Acta chir. Scand.*, **122**, 361.

24. Gifford, R. W., Hines, E. A. and Craig, W. McK. (1958) Sympathectomy for Raynaud's phenomenon. *Circulation*, **17**, 1.

25. Gillespie, J. A. and Douglas, D. M. (1961) *Some Aspects of Obliterative Vascular Disease of the Lower limb.* Edinburgh and London: E. & S. Livingstone, pp. 57–110.

26. Golding, M. R. Mendoza, M. F., Hennigar, G. R., Fries, C. C. and Wesolowski, S. A. (1964) On settling the controversy on the benefit of sympathectomy for frostbite. *Surgery*, **56**, 221.

27. Goodhead, B. (1966) The comparative value of low molecular weight dextran and sympathectomy in the treatment of experimental frost-bite. *Brit. J. Surg.*, **53**, 1060.

28. Goodman, R. M., Elian, B., Mozes, M. and Deutsch, V. (1965) Buerger's disease in Israel. *Amer. J. Med.*, **39**, 601.

29. Hadfield, J. I. H. (1965) Phaeochromocytoma with unusual presentation. *Proc. Roy. Soc. Med.*, **58**, 262.

30. Hawley, P. R., Johnston, A. W. and Rankin, J. T. (1967) Association between digital ischaemia and malignant disease. *Brit. med. J.*, **iii**, 208.

31. Haxton, H. A. (1947) Regeneration after sympathectomy and its effects on Raynaud's disease. *Brit. J. Surg.*, **35**, 69.

32. Haxton, H. A. (1954) The sympathetic nerve supply of the upper limb in relation to sympathectomy. *Ann. Roy. Coll. Surg. Eng.*, **14**, 247: *also* Personal Communication (1966).

32A.Hellstrøm, B. and Anderson, K. L. (1972) Vibration injuries in Norwegian forest workers. *Brit. J. industr. Med.*, **29**, 255.

33. Holti, G. (1965) The effect of intermittent low molecular dextran upon the digital circulation in systemic sclerosis. *Brit. J. Dermat.*, **77**, 560.

34. Jepson, R. P. (1954) Raynaud's phenomenon in workers with vibratory tools. *Brit. J. Indust. Med.*, **11**, 180.

35. Johnston, E. N. M., Summerly, R. and Birnstingl, M. (1965) Prognosis in Raynaud's phenomenon after sympathectomy. *Brit. med. J.*, **i**, 962.

36. Kinmonth, J. B. and Hadfield, G. J. (1952) Sympathectomy for Raynaud's disease. Results of ganglionectomy and preganglionic section compared. *Brit. med. J.*, **i**, 1377.

37. Landis, E. M. (1930) Micro-injection studies of capillary blood pressure in Raynaud's disease. *Heart*, **15**, 247.

38. Landis, E. M. and Gibbon, J. H. (1933) A simple method of producing vasodilatation in the lower extremities, with reference to its usefulness in studies of peripheral vascular disease. *Arch. int. Med.*, **52**, 785.

39. Langstroth, L. (1919) Blood viscosity. I. Conditions affecting the viscosity of blood after withdrawal from the body. II. Effect of increased venous pressure. *J. exp. Med.*, **30**, 597, 607.

40. Lewis, T. (1949) *Vascular disorders of the Limbs.* London: Macmillan and Co. Second Edition (*a*) p. 66, (*b*) p. 79, (*c*) pp. 95–97, 109, (*d*) p. 102, (*e*) pp. 105–109.

41. Lewis, T. and Pickering, G. W. (1934) Observations on maladies in which the blood supply to digits ceases intermittently or permanently, and upon bilateral gangrene of digits; observations relevant to so-called 'Raynaud's disease'. *Clin. Sci.*, **1**, 327.

42. Martinez, A., Golding, M., Sawyer, P. N. and

Wesolowski, S. A. (1966) The specific arterial lesions in mild and severe frostbite: effect of sympathectomy. *J. Cardiovasc. Surg.*, **7**, 495.

43. Peacock, J. H. (1958) Vasodilatation in the human hand. Observations on primary Raynaud's disease and acrocyanosis of the upper extremities. *Clin. Sci.*, **17**, 575.

44. Peacock, J. H. (1960) The effect of changes in local temperature on the blood flows of the normal hand, primary Raynaud's disease and primary acrocyanosis. *Clin. Sci.*, **19**, 505.

45. Peacock, J. H. (1959) Peripheral venous blood concentrations of epinephrine and norepinephrine in primary Raynaud's disease. *Circulation Res.*, **7**, 821.

46. Peacock, J. H. (1959) A comparative study of the digital cutaneous temperatures and hand blood flows in the normal hand, primary Raynaud's disease and primary acrocyanosis. *Clin. Sci.*, **18**, 25.

47. Peacock, J. H. (1960) The treatment of primary Raynaud's disease of the upper limb. *Lancet*, **ii**, 65.

48. Pringle, R., Walder, D. N. and Weaver, J. P. A. (1965) Blood viscosity and Raynaud's disease. *Lancet*, **i**, 1086.

49. Raynaud, M. (1888) *On Local Asphyxia and Symmetrical Gangrene of the Extremities.* Translated by T. Barlow. Selected monographs. London: New Sydenham Society.

50. Robertson, C. W. and Smithwick, R. H. (1951) The recurrence of vasoconstrictor activity after limb sympathectomy in Raynaud's disease and allied vasomotor states. *New Eng. J. Med.*, **245**, 317.

50A. Romeo, S. G., Whalen, R. E. and Tindall, J. P. (1970) Intra-arterial administration of reserpine. *Arch. int. Med.*, **125**, 825.

51. Ross, J. P. (1958) *Surgery of the Sympathetic Nervous System.* London: Ballière, Tindall and Cox. Third Edition. (*a*) p. 108, (*b*) p. 128.

51A. Rubin, A. A. (1963) Coronary vascular effects of griseofulvin. *J. Amer. Med. Ass.*, **185**, 971.

52. Samman, P. D. and Strickland, B. (1962) Abnormalities of the finger nails associated with impaired peripheral blood supply. *Brit. J. Dermat.*, **74**, 165.

53. Schatz, I. J. (1963) Occlusive arterial disease in the hand due to occupational trauma. *New Eng. J. Med.*, **268**, 281.

54. Schumacker, H. B. and Lempke, R. E. (1951) Recent advances in frostbite, with particular reference to experimental studies concerning functional pathology and treatment. *Surgery*, **30**, 873.

55. Takaro, T. and Hines, E. A. (1967) Digital arteriography in occlusive arterial disease and clubbing of the fingers. *Circulation*, **35**, 682.

55A. Taylor, W. and James, P. B. (1972) Vascular disorders associated with the use of vibrating tools. Personal communication. To be published.

56. Telford, E. D. (1944) Discussion on peripheral vascular lesions. *Proc. Roy. Soc. Med.*, **37**, 621.

57. Tuffanelli, D. L. and Winkelmann, R. K. (1961) Systemic scleroderma. A clinical study of 727 cases. *Arch. Dermat.*, **84**, 49.

57A. Varadi, D. P. and Lawrence, A. M. (1969) Suppression of Raynaud's phenomenon by methyldopa. *Arch. int. Med.*, **124**, 13.

57B. Ward, M. P., Garnham, J. R., Simpson, B. R. J., Morley, G. H. and Winter, J. S. (1968) Frostbite: general observations and report of cases treated with hyperbaric oxygen. *Proc. Roy. Soc. Med.*, **61**, 785.

58. Whitby, L. E. H. and Britton, C. J. C. (1957) *Disorders of the Blood.* London: J. & A. Churchill Ltd., Eighth Edition. p. 498.

59. Willerson, J. T., Thompson, R. H., Hookman, P., Herdt, J. and Decker, J. L. (1970) Reserpine in Raynaud's disease and phenomenon. Short-term response to intra-arterial injection. *Ann. int. Med.*, **72**, 17.

60. Yao, S. T., Goodwin, D. P. and Kenyon, J. R. (1970) Case of ergot poisoning. *Brit. med. J.*, **3**, 86.

12 Cervical Rib and Thoracic Outlet Compression, and Other Causes of Upper Limb Occlusion

Pain in the arm, with numbness or coldness of the hand are common symptoms of neurovascular disease in the upper limb, and many are the possible causes (Table 12.1). As in the lower limb, it is not

Table 12.1. Neurovascular Causes of Pain in the Upper Limb

1. *Nerve Compression:*

Cervico-brachial plexus roots:	Spondylitis, apical lung cancer, secondary deposits.
Brachial plexus trunks:	thoracic outlet syndrome, primary, or from compression by subclavian or axillary aneurysm.
Attrition neuritis at the elbow or wrist.	

2. *Arterial disease:*

Aortic arch syndrome	
Thoracic outlet syndrome:	occlusion, partial or complete. aneurysm embolism
Occlusive arterial disease in the arm and distal vessels:	Arteriosclerosis, and Buerger's disease.
Systemic embolism from heart or great vessels.	
Mechanical damage to artery:	acute injury, irradiation, crutch pressure.
All other causes of secondary Raynaud's phenomenon.	

3. *Axillary or subclavian vein thrombosis.*

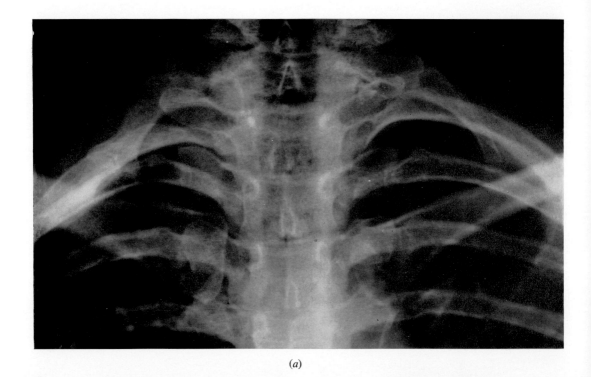

(a)

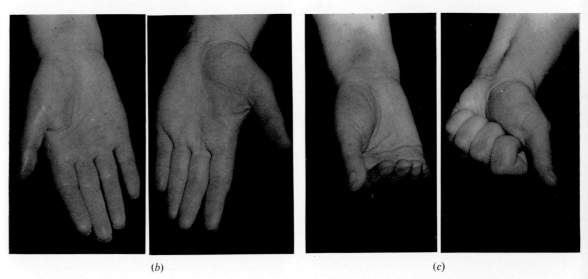

(b)   (c)

Fig. 12.1. (Case 1) The two common types of cervical rib. On the right, a large rib with a broad joint connecting it to the first thoracic rib. On the left, the slender incomplete rib is joined to the first rib by an aponeurotic band.

This patient, a professional musician aged fifty, presented with claudication wasting and stiffness of the right hand. During a spell of cold winter weather, pallor and cyanosis developed with pain at rest. Complete relief following removal of right rib and reconstruction of thrombosed subclavian artery.

Note loss of active flexion and wasting of thenar and hypothenar muscles. A good example of ischaemic brachial neuropathy [11].

always easy to distinguish between the pains of claudication or peripheral ischaemia and pain that is primarily of nerve origin, or that which arises from degenerative disease in the joints.

Other causes will suggest themselves, such as angina pectoris, dissecting or expanding aortic aneurysm, or an old stroke, but our concern here is to recognise only those that are a direct result of arterial disease in the limb or its root, or resemble it closely.

Thorough clinical examination will usually decide the answer, for although the history may be equivocal, there will be the physical signs of arterial narrowing, or dilatation, or thrombo-embolic complications as well as the features of secondary Raynaud's phenomenon. We will first consider the thoracic outlet syndrome, and then the other causes of upper limb ischaemia (p. 233) in the ways in which they differ from it and from one another.

The Anatomy of Thoracic Outlet Compression

Each of the following has been held responsible:

1. A cervical rib, partial or complete.
2. Articulation between a cervical rib and the normal first rib.
3. Fibrous aponeurotic bands joining these, and the scalenus anterior or medius muscles.
4. Nipping between the first rib and the clavicle.
5. The scalenus muscles themselves.
6. The normal first rib.
7. Deformities or tumours of the first rib.
8. Fractures of the clavicle or the first rib with excess of callus or mal-union.
9. The coracoid process.

Common to them all is the relationship of symptoms to exertion and strain, acutely or over long periods, and particularly in cold weather. It may be that these factors by themselves may be sufficient to cause symptoms without any anatomical abnormality. Shoulder sagging and other postural factors, including hyperabduction and the scalenus manoeuvre, regularly produce obliteration or an arterial murmur in the radial pulse in 27 per cent of apparently normal subjects [11], compared with about 50 per cent of those with neurological symptoms from cervical rib [3].

INCIDENCE OF CERVICAL RIB

This has been assessed as 0·4 per cent of the population [16] with a 2:1 preponderance of females. In 70 per cent of patients the condition is bilateral. This takes no account of the other structures thought to be responsible for compression, so that potential thoracic outlet syndrome should be fairly common.

Types of cervical rib are shown in Fig. 12.1 (Case 1). Their relationship to the first thoracic root, the subclavian artery and the vein, from behind forwards is one of decreasing tension (Fig. 12.2), which agrees with the fact that nerve complications are a good deal commoner than arterial effects, and venous compression the rarest of the three. It has also been stated that short ribs produce nerve complications, and long ones, arterial [7].

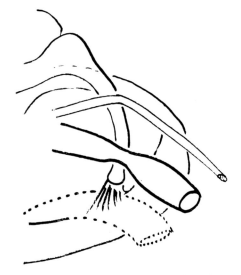

Fig. 12.2. Neurovascular tension at the thoracic outlet is greatest posteriorly where the rib is highest.

The Arterial Lesions of Thoracic Outlet Compression

These are as follows:

1. Narrowing (Fig. 12.3a, b) and eventual thrombosis (Fig. 12.3c) of the subclavian artery; sometimes of a dense and fibrous type with no endarterectomy cleavage plane.
2. Post-stenotic aneurysmal dilatation of the distal subclavian and axillary arteries (Cases 2, 3, 4, 5 and 6).
3. Peripheral embolism to the upper limb (Fig. 12.4) or to the brain (Fig. 12.5).

All may occur in the same patient, but not necessarily in this order; any of the three may open the clinical history. The picture may be complicated by subclavian or axillary venous thrombosis or pulmonary embolism. Peripheral neurological effects are not usually present with vascular compression,

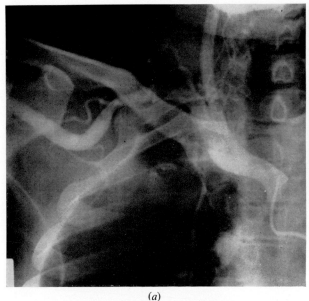

(a)

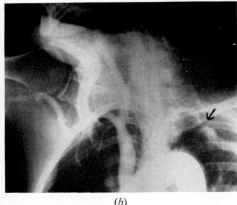

(b)

Fig. 12.3. Narrowing and the thrombotic lesion.

(a) Innominate arteriogram showing compression of right subclavian artery by a deformed first thoracic rib in a man aged thirty-nine with similar early symptoms to Case 1. A few days later, the artery thrombosed and the right hand became severely ischaemic with gangrene of index and middle finger-tips. Full relief and healing followed thrombo-endarterectomy.

(b) Arch aortogram in a woman aged sixty during investigation of cerebrovascular symptoms with low blood pressure readings in left arm. Narrowing at thoracic outlet with marked fusiform post-stenotic dilatation.

(c) Complete arterial thrombosis centring on thoracic outlet—a small right cervical rib being present. Good collateral circulation has developed, and though there is evidence of a previous embolus at the axillary bifurcation, symptoms were mild, though such a patient could develop cerebral embolism via the vertebral artery which is close to the proximal face of the thrombus.

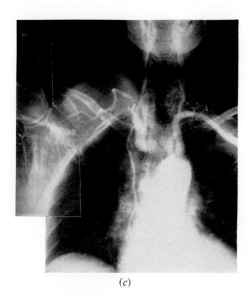

(c)

any weakness or numbness being more likely to be due to peripheral ischaemia (but *see* p. 222 for cerebral embolic effects of subclavian thrombosis). Gangrene of the fingers is more extensive and rapid than with most other forms of the secondary Raynaud phenomenon (*see* Chapter 11). In an elderly arteriosclerotic patient, subclavian artery thrombosis may cause massive ischaemia of the limb with early development of gangrene of most of the hand.

THE CAUSE OF HAND ISCHAEMIA IN PATIENTS WITH CERVICAL RIB

In these younger subjects, local block at the site of arterial compression at the thoracic outlet would not on its own be expected to produce severe ischaemia. The collateral circulation at this region is via the rich supply to the shoulder joint and its muscles (Fig. 12.3c). Only if more peripheral regions in the main artery were already occluded would subclavian thrombosis lead to serious effects in the hand, for in such a patient there is an abnormally high peripheral resistance, exceeding the capacity of the collaterals in the upper arm to supply the more remote parts of the limb. Such a state also explains the effect of cold exposure of such a patient in producing Raynaud phenomenon.

For a long while, digital ischaemia in cervical rib subjects was thought to be explained by spasm, either in the main artery, or peripherally, from irritation of sympathetic fibres in the lowest trunk of the brachial plexus as it passed over the cervical rib. The evidence for this was never completely satisfactory, for the beneficial effects of sympathetic release by body-warming or local nerve block should apply equally, whether the ischaemia were due to a structural block or to a hypothetical state of spasm. Once it became clear that arterial obstruction is usually to be found in patients with vascular effects of cervical rib [17] a new basis was provided for an understanding of this and many other ischaemic states [18]. It is over thirty years since Lewis and Pickering [17] first suggested that the source of the trouble is damage to the artery behind the clavicle, leading not only to local thrombosis but, in some cases, also to emboli affecting the hand. As a logical extension of their work on primary Raynaud's disease (see Chapter 11), in which they found that a local fault in the digital arteries, and not sympathetic overactivity, was the cause of the attacks, they recognised that structural occlusion of the distal arteries in cervical rib would adequately explain the occurrence of Raynaud phenomenon in these patients. Subsequent work [7] confirmed the correctness of the concept of repeated embolism as the cause of progressive, episodal, and incremental ischaemia of the hand in patients with cervical rib, and recent histological studies have shown that there is an accumulation of platelet thrombus over the thickened, oedematous, and infiltrated artery at the point of mechanical drainage [12].

EMBOLISM TO THE UPPER LIMB ARTERIES IN CERVICAL RIB (Fig. 12.4)

At first, only the small arteries of the hand are affected (Case 4, p. 226) with the wrist pulses still present and transient colour changes in response to cold limited to those fingers whose digital arteries are blocked. Later, after another acute episode of unusual severity, the wrist pulses are lost, and subsequently those of the brachial bifurcation. By the time the brachial becomes occluded to the level of the profunda brachii, the hand will have developed chronic ischaemia with wasting, and often with necrosis of those fingers whose arterial supply was

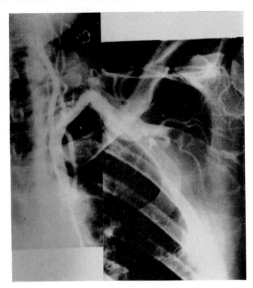

Fig. 12.4. Recent axillary embolism from a subclavian aneurysm from a man aged forty with a left cervical rib. Excision of rib, clavicle, and aneurysm; embolectomy, and reconstruction of the artery by anastomosis. Full functional recovery though with absent wrist pulses, no doubt due to previous smaller emboli.

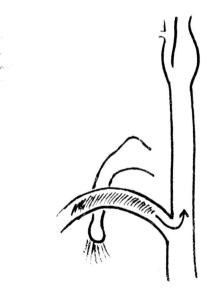

Fig. 12.5. The suspected route of a right carotid embolus from the proximal face of a subclavian thrombus. This can occur only on the right side, though the hind-brain might be affected via the vertebral on either side.

221

blocked early in the disease. At this stage the axillary and upper brachial can still be felt pulsating strongly, although at any time they, too, may become closed off by a further embolus from the subclavian. Arteriography at this critical time may show the thrombus at its source (Cases 2 and 4) and also where portions of it have lodged in the main artery in the upper arm (Fig. 12.4, Cases 2 and 4).

Not only do the cumulative, successive occlusions themselves eventually reduce the upper limb's circulation to danger level, each time with loss of the collateral bed that previously compensated for earlier blocks, but, also, the obstruction offered by the main lesion at the rib margin will steadily increase, both from further narrowing thrombus there, and from rising resistance in the 'run-off'.

The dynamics of flow through the primary lesion can be studied by auscultation. At rest, or perhaps only on head turning or during inspiration, a systolic bruit should be heard [8]. Posture alone may be sufficient cause for temporary aggravation of arterial compression and narrowing; such a state could also favour embolism. Attention should be paid to the effect of exercising the limb: in some patients a soft murmur at rest becomes loud and harsh for a few minutes. During such times there could be detachment of thrombus either from the point of narrowing or into the turbulent stream within the dilated segment beyond it (Case 5, p. 230).

The final closure of the subclavian, and the onset of gangrene, seem often to be determined by the weather. In nearly all the published cases the onset of severe ischaemia occurred during the coldest part of the winter. The end result of the occlusive sequence may be so severe an ischaemia as to require a forearm amputation [6, 14, 10].

Clinical Diagnosis of Upper Limb Ischaemia due to Cervical Rib

Symptoms are usually insidious, but during a spell of cold weather it is noticed that the hand, already colder than the good side, is now also weaker, and clumsy in fine movements such as writing or knitting. These effects are often intermittent and quite mild, with relief after resting and when the weather improves, so that the patient feels reassured and often does not report the trouble.

Even if these early symptoms do bring the patient for advice, if the rib is small or absent it will not be easy to determine whether they are due to thoracic outlet compression or some other more common cause such as brachial root irritation in cervical spondylitis. If thoracic outlet compression is suspected, and the rib is obvious, it still may not be clear whether the effects are nervous or vascular. Changes in colour and temperature are good evidence of an arterial basis for early symptoms; but they can also be caused by disuse when there is neuromuscular weakness. This type of secondary acrocyanosis is never as striking as the true Raynaud phenomenon which complicates the arterial lesion in cervical rib. Later, severe local ischaemia becomes obvious.

Physical Signs

1. The rib may be visible or palpable in the posterior cervical triangle, and the trapezius profile is raised on one, or both sides (Fig. 12.6a, also Cases 3, 4, and 6).
2. Wasting, weakness and stiffness of all the intrinsic muscles and joints of the affected hand without segmental nerve features (Case 1, Fig. 12.1b), and a uniform, centripetal sensory impairment [11].
3. Severe colour changes of Raynaud type on exposure to cold, but confined to one hand or even one finger, commonly the index (Fig. 11.4, p. 205).
4. A systolic bruit over the distal subclavian artery (Case 3 (c)) brought out by inspiration, shoulder movement, and exercise of the affected upper limb, as already described.
5. A low or absent blood pressure reading on the affected side. Pain and pallor in the affected hand after opening and gripping exercises with the hands raised, both sides being tested at once for purposes of comparison (Case 5, p. 231).
6. Pulse deficiencies, developing sequentially, distally at first, sometimes detectable early through loss of the digital arterial pulsations in the fingers most affected by the Raynaud phenomenon. Later, one or both wrist pulses are lost, then the brachial, axillary and, finally, the subclavian itself. Previous removal of the rib does not invariably protect against this sequence of events [23].
7. Visible or palpable prominence of the subclavian arterial pulsation, or obvious aneurysm formation (Cases 5 and 6), which may occur as late as thirty years after the removal of a cervical rib [6].
8. A tender swelling of the main artery of the limb, commonly the lower brachial, with fading of the pulsations at this point, is strongly suggestive of an embolus at this point.

A Note on Cerebral Ischaemia from Cervical Rib [4, 8A, 21, 22]

Embolism into the right carotid artery (Fig. 12.5) is

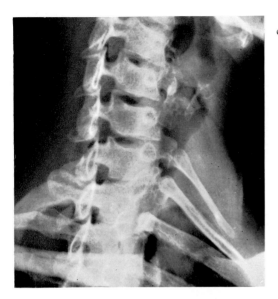

(*a*) Oblique plain radiography shows a long left cervical rib.

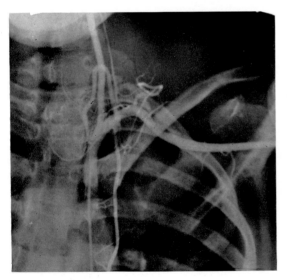

(*b*) Selective trans-femoral left subclavian arteriogram shows slight compression of the artery at rest, and early post-stenotic dilatation.

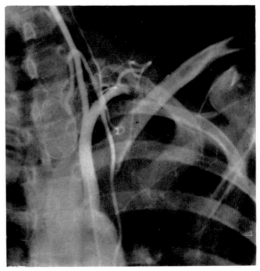

(*c*) Complete obstruction of the artery on bracing the shoulders back.

Case 2. A woman aged twenty-eight had noticed pain in the left shoulder arm and hand for ten years becoming continuous recently and always made worse by raising the limb or by turning the head to the right.

Mr Nigel Harris's case. Fully relieved by exploration confirming the compression and removing the rib.

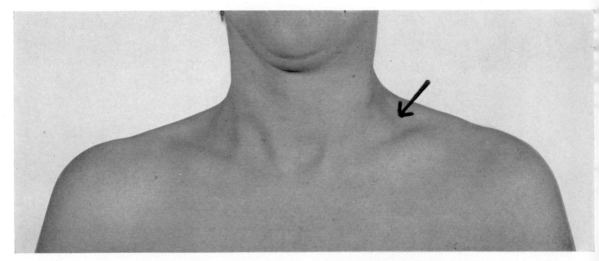

(*a*) Visible swelling in the left posterior triangle and raised trapezius outline.

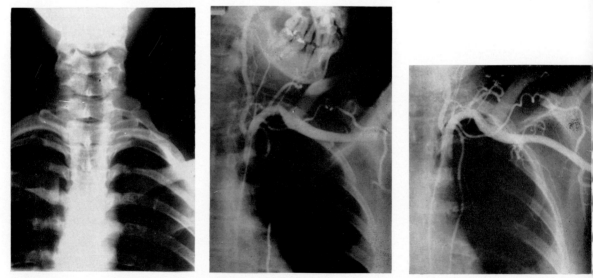

(*b*) Selective subclavian arteriograms showing compression at the cervical rib joint and post-stenotic and fusiform post-stenotic dilatation extending far down into the axillary artery.

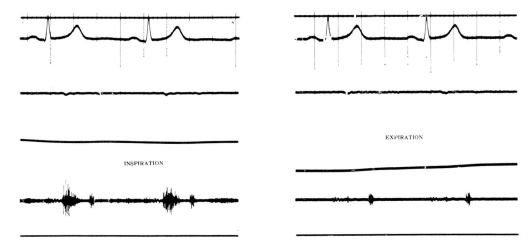

EXPIRATION

INSPIRATION

(*c*) Phonocardiogram reading taken at the point marked by the arrow. A loud systolic murmur was present on inspiration.

Case 3. Left-sided cervical rib of the large, articulated type in a woman aged thirty-six.

The condition in this case was uncomplicated requiring removal of the rib only. The murmur disappeared after operation.

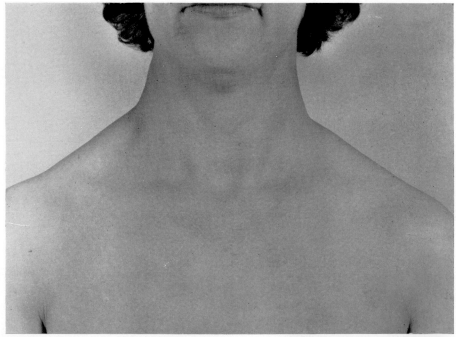

(a)

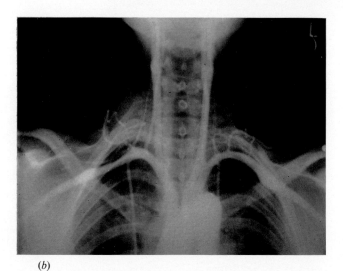

(b)

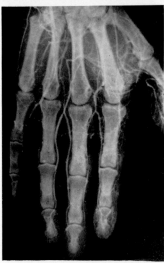

(c)

Case 4. Bilateral cervical rib with early vascular symptoms.

(a) Typical clinical appearance of shoulders.

(b) Trans-femoral catheter aortogram showing bilateral post-stenotic aneurysms larger on the left side.

(c) Painful secondary Raynaud's phenomenon shown by brachial arteriography to be due to multiple digital arterial occlusions (radialis indicis, and ulnar three digitals) most probably from small emboli arising in the aneurysm.

Treated by strip resection of the aneurysm and cervicodorsal sympathectomy. Symptomless right side remains under observation.

226

responsible for the most serious of all complications, which, in six of the nine reported cases left the patient, usually at an age younger than thirty, with a permanent left hemiplegia, and irreversible damage to the arteries of the right arm. Typically, the victim is a young woman in whom pain in the right arm is followed by attacks of pallor and discoloration paronychia and, perhaps, superficial gangrene of the right hand, when after six months to three years there is sudden onset of left hemiplegia with loss of consciousness, from which only partial recovery is made. A palpable cervical rib, prominent subclavian pulsation or aneurysm, or solid thrombosis are present, and the right arm blood pressure is reduced or unrecordable.

There is a resemblance to the young female type of aortic arch syndrome (see Chapter 7, p. 141) though in neither this nor the vertebral steal lesion of the subclavian are the brachial effects so severe.

As with cerebral infarction from extracranial carotid occlusion, surgery can be of little help in the completed lesion; its value is in prevention. It may not be sufficient to remove the rib and free the compressed artery; delayed cerebral embolism has occurred two years after such an operation [23]. Much better is a full correction of the arterial lesion in the neck [6, 21, 24], which need add little more to the severity of the procedure.

INVESTIGATIONS

Skilled arteriography is of the greatest possible help. Indirect methods are preferable to subclavian puncture, which might precipitate local complications and fail to show the lesion. A retrograde femoral catheter is passed up to the arch of the aorta, and one or both subclavians can be well shown. Good selective filling is obtained with the catheter tip at the opening of the innominate or left subclavian. Irregularity, narrowing, and post-stenotic aneurysm are demonstrated together with their relationship to the cervical rib or the first rib. To show the more distal lesions, brachial puncture is required, under general anaesthesia (Case 4c, p. 226).

SURGICAL TREATMENT

Indications

The presence of an uncomplicated symptomless cervical rib is, of course, no indication for its removal, even if an arterial bruit may be demonstrable in some positions of the upper limb. A more difficult decision must be made when a patient has already had arterial decompression or reconstruction on one side, but symptomless, and then shows minimal signs of vascular involvement on the other.

The writer believes that a preventive operation is justified in these circumstances because simple measures will usually be sufficient to halt the disease at this early stage. Again, the arteriographic appearances may help, but a normal picture need not necessarily contra-indicate operation. Pulse or blood pressure deficits are signs of an established lesion and fully indicate the need for surgery on the second side, as indeed they do in the unilateral case.

Technique of Exploration of the Thoracic Outlet, and Sympathectomy

With adequate anaesthesia and a good light, the steps of this dissection are straightforward, and the exposure should be sufficient for the successful completion of any of the corrective measures to be described, as well as for cervico-dorsal sympathectomy. Many of the arterial complications may be dealt with in this limited operation field, but the more extensive thromboses and most aneurysms will require displacement or removal of the clavicle.

The incision (Fig. 12.6a) is made just above the inner four-fifths of the clavicle by drawing the skin down over it and cutting on to the deep fascia, which is divided a little higher up to avoid bleeding and to expose the fatty contents of the posterior triangle of the neck. Sometimes, a large transverse cervical vein or connection with the external jugular will cross the field, also the omohoid muscle. These structures should be divided and taken aside with a self-retaining retractor, together with the fatty pad in which they run.

Muscle bellies to be divided are the clavicular head of the sternomastoid (Fig. 12.7) and, beneath it, the scalenus anterior, the latter to be displayed with caution by stroking the fat and fascia upwards over it to reveal the phrenic nerve (Fig. 12.7a), which should then be freed over its whole length in the field and gently retracted medially and upwards into the more superficial layers of the dissection (Fig. 12.7b). Phrenic paralysis can be a common complication unless considerable care is taken. The scalenus is studied carefully before and after it is divided, for it may be the main compressing structure. The line of division should be near the rib; scissors are used to snip progressively through the muscle fibres until the posterior, aponeurotic layer is seen. This can be well displayed by wiping, up and down, the remaining

227

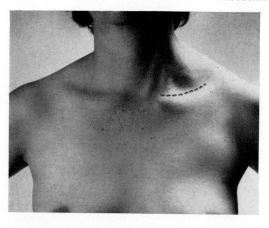
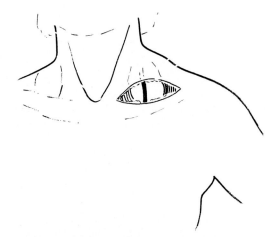

Fig. 12.6. Exploration of the thoracic outlet for neurovascular compression and for cervicodorsal sympathectomy. The incision.

In the patient shown, the prominence of the cervical rib is clearly visible, also raising of the left trapezius profile. This patient had pain in the arm and hand which was relieved by excision of the cervical rib, there being no evidence of structural neurovascular complications.

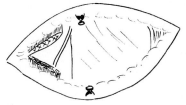
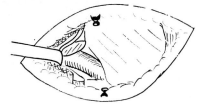

(*a*) Division of superficial structures and identification of phrenic nerve, lying on scalenus anterior.

(*b*) Division of scalenus anterior to reveal subclavian artery.

Fig. 12.7. Exposure of the subclavian artery.

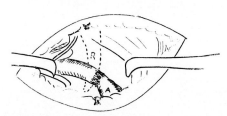
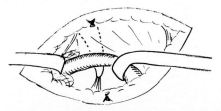

(*a*) Mobilisation of the brachial plexus to expose the site of arterial compression.

(*b*) Mobilisation of the artery to gain access to the cervical rib or to begin the deep dissection phase of cervical sympathectomy.

Fig. 12.8.

muscle, with a dental cotton swab on an artery forceps. It is then picked up with dissecting forceps, and the underlying subclavian artery should then be seen before these strong tissues are cut. There may be adherence at this point.

The subclavian artery can now be freed from its surroundings, and the dissection of the remaining normal and abnormal structures of the region is not difficult. The medial part of the brachial plexus is defined and gently retracted laterally (Fig. 12.8*a*).

Any *abnormal aponeurotic layers* or slips of scalenus anterior or medius are divided. At this point a *cervical rib*, already recognised by previous X-ray examination, will be fully displayed, and can at once be excised as soon as the neurovascular structures have been lifted up from the bone, using a retractor or broad linen tape. Bone nibbling forceps are best for completing the bony decompression. When the bundle is let down again there must be no projection against its under surface. Some further nibbling may be needed to ensure this. If there is doubt about the clearance of the artery, or if there should be an arterial lesion extending out of the field distally, the *clavicle should be freed* and divided or resected, if necessary. An osteoma or a malformation of the first rib, or excessive callus from a fracture should be removed in the same way as described for cervical rib.

Cervico-dorsal sympathectomy may now be performed, the indication being any case of persistent peripheral ischaemia in which there is no evidence of local arterial damage at the outlet, and in which systemic disease has been excluded as a cause (*see* Chapter 11).

With the tip of the index finger, the front of the proximal end of the first rib is felt, and the suprapleural membrane (Sibson's fascia), which runs down from here across the apex of the pleura, is clearly seen; it is divided high, away from the pleura, which may then be stroked gently downwards to display the upper dorsal vertebral bodies and adjoining ribs.

The subclavian artery must be retracted aside at this stage (Fig. 12.8(*b*)) either upwards or downwards as may be found best in the individual.

The light must now be carefully adjusted to focus on the upper vertebrae. The sympathetic chain can usually be picked up without difficulty, using a blunt nerve hook, just distal to the stellate ganglion, which can be made out as a pale, rounded elevation about 0·5 cm in diameter, under a layer of extra pleural fascia near the neck of the first rib. The chain is thick and strong at this point and can be firmly drawn forward off the parietes; long scissors are used to free it as far down the posterior extrapleural tissues as is possible. Care should be taken of the intercostal vessels, particularly on the left, where a large superior intercostal vein may cause difficulty, particularly if the pleura has been opened in error. Diathermy or McKenzie's clips are useful here. Opinion is divided upon whether to remove the chain or to suture it up into the neck (*see* Chapter 11,

p. 212). Removal is necessary if tissue histology is required. With the aid of a Nelson's malleable light the chain is cut across as distally as possible, and proximally across the lower tip of the stellate ganglion.

Complications of cervico-dorsal sympathectomy include:

1. Post-sympathectomy neuralgia, which is common, and like that which follows lumbar sympathectomy, affects both the trunk and the limb neurotomes corresponding to the denervation. Although temporary, it may be quite troublesome. On the left side the pain may cause some anxiety over the possibility of coronary ischaemia. Sympathectomy, however, tends to relieve myocardial pain [2].

2. Brachial plexus neuritis, with weakness or paraesthesia, should be avoidable with careful technique and gentleness in retracting the nerve trunks.

3. Pneumothorax, from pleural injury that was not followed by catheter suction to remove the air during wound closure.

4. Haemothorax, where pleural injury was further complicated by damage to an extrapleural blood vessel during the dissection of the sympathetic chain. This may lead to continued and troublesome bleeding, which seldom happens if the pleura is intact and the blood is confined to the extrapleural space.

Except for the first, none of these complications should occur with care and experience on the part of the operator, except on rare occasions with some unusual technical difficulty or anatomical abnormality, usually in the extrapleural stripping phase. When the subclavian artery itself is the main concern of the surgeon, there may be no need for sympathectomy, and postoperative bleeding will be much less troublesome if the pleura has not been mobilised.

The posterior [17A] *and axillary* [1, 2, 20A] approaches to the sympathetic chain and thoracic outlet have been little used in Great Britain. Better exposure of the first rib, and of the upper thoracic ganglia can be obtained than from the front. This may lead to their wider use in patients with recurrent neurovascular compression, or a return of Raynaud symptoms after the cervical operation for these conditions has failed.

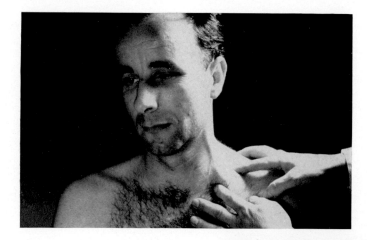

(a) Large tender aneurysm above the left clavicle and weakness of the left hand were the presenting features.

(b) Normal appearance of hands.

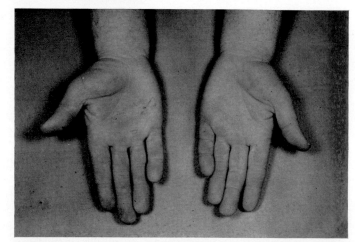

(c) Striking pallor of left hand after exercise elevation test on both sides.

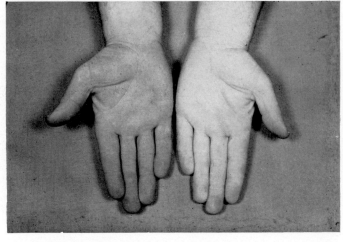

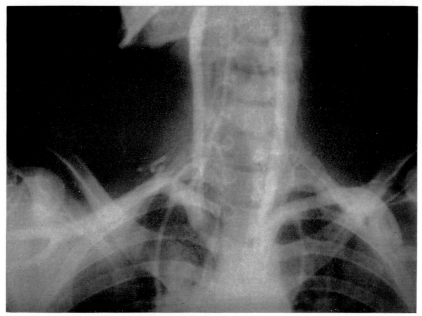

(*d*) Pre-operative arch aortogram showing large left post-stenotic aneurysm containing thrombus and a fusiform dilatation beyond the rib on the right side.

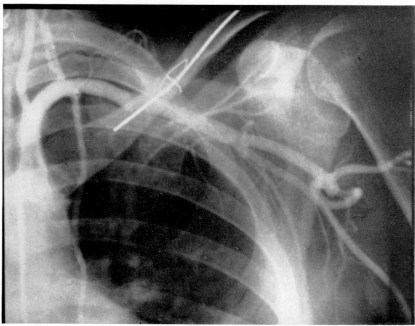

(*e*) Postoperative selective left subclavian arteriogram after excision of the aneurysm which proved to be completely thrombosed by that time. Grafted with saphenous vein. Note occlusion of brachial artery at its origin—a typical appearance, due to previous embolism. Pulsations had been noticed to cease at this point before operation. Reconstruction of the clavicle may constitute a major difficulty, excision often being preferable.

Case 5. Bilateral cervical ribs in a lumberjack aged twenty-six, with severe thrombo-embolic complications on the left side.

231

(a) Trans-femoral aortography shows a point of stenosis in the second part of both subclavians, and unusually large carrot-shaped post-stenotic aneurysm on the right, rising well above the clavicle.

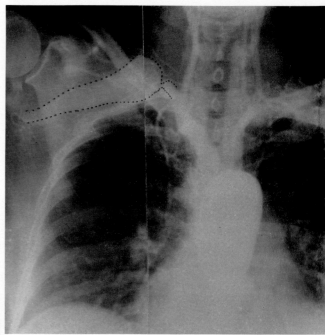

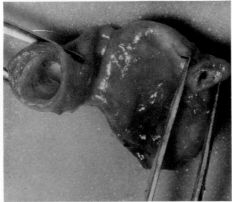

(b) Excised aneurysm in anatomical position showing marked stenosis at the point of compression and thrombus within the distal part of the sac. There were no embolic complications in this case.

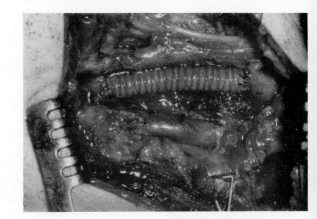

(c) Reconstruction by excision of clavicle and insertion of knitted dacron graft.

Case 6. Bilateral arterial compression by scalenus aponeurosis in a hypertensive woman aged fifty-eight who complained of a large pulsating swelling above the right clavicle, with some local aching.

Subsequent preventive decompression on the left side revealed similar anatomy but no aneurysm.

Direct Arterial Surgery

One of dos Santos's thrombo-endarterectomy patients, in 1947 [5], was a young woman with sub-clavian artery thrombosis from compression by the scalenus anterior. The occlusion extended down to the brachial and was removed through two arteriotomies, one at each end of the blocked segment. The reconstruction remained patent, and was fully effective, though previous distal obstruction prevented a full revascularisation of all the normal main channels. This contribution was forgotten by some of those who, later, undertook arterial reconstruction for this condition, including the writer, who is glad to have this opportunity to acknowledge dos Santos as the first in this field.

The following procedures have proved satisfactory in the writer's experience:

1. Thrombo-endarterectomy (for stenosis or complete occlusion).
2. Strip resection of a dilated subclavian, with linear suture repair.
3. Resection of a saccular subclavian aneurysm with end-to-end anastomosis.
4. In a young patient, resection of the aneurysm and replacement with a saphenous vein graft [24].
5. Resection of a large aneurysm in an older subject with poor veins, and replacement by a prosthetic arterial graft (see Case 6, p. 232).

Technique of Arterial Reconstruction

With good exposure by the anterior route, as described, the arterial lesion is inspected (Fig. 12.8) and freed from all compressing structures. *Thrombo-endarterectomy* is satisfactory provided there is a clear plane of cleavage. A short, dense local block without dilatation can be quickly cleared out with the artery held between the left thumb and index finger while being incised lengthwise, as in pyloromyotomy; the arterial clamps need not be applied until the plane of cleavage is defined as far as the patent part of the artery. If the retrograde flow is brisk and the arteriotomy short and tidy, there is no need to heparinise the patient, for to suture the opening takes only a few minutes. This simple procedure adds little to the thoracic outlet operation, but it may greatly improve the results.

If there is tight stenosis, involving all layers of the wall at the point of compression, some form of resection will be needed. Usually, in such a case there will also be a post-stenotic aneurysm, which must be fully dissected free, taking care not to dislodge any of the contained thrombus onwards into the arm. Often, it will be necessary to divide or resect the clavicle in order to expose and to control the distal artery, where it has become the axillary. Once the dissection is completed, the patient should be heparinised, but if a prosthetic graft is to be used it is better to pre-clot its mesh with fresh arterial blood before heparin is given.

The arterial clamps are then applied, Craaford's being much the best for control of the proximal sub-clavian, though a bulldog clip is preferable for the softer, more dilated distal end. Clips may also have to be placed on large nearby branches such as the internal mammary and the costocervical trunk. The aneurysm can then be removed. The resected specimen should include the stenosis at its commencement (see Case 6).

Graft replacement is by autogenous vein (see Case 5) or knitted dacron cloth prosthesis (Case 6) according to circumstances. An attempt should be made to remove any distal thrombus or embolus, using a Fogarty catheter. This may restore the wrist pulses.

Once the flow from the proximal and distal ends has been proved by a final, brief unclamping, the last few sutures of the distal anastomosis are inserted, the heparin having been reversed by protamine sulphate solution given intravenously by the anaesthetist.

Strip resection of a widened, patent subclavian can be combined with the clearing out of any contained layer of thrombus. In both this, and the similar procedure of patch grafting for a sclerosed and narrowed artery, trimming and suturing take rather longer than after simple endarterectomy. The use of heparin is advisable, as it also is in any acute case, or others in which the back flow is poor.

Other Upper-limb Occlusions

Any of the thrombo-embolic conditions that affect the lower limbs may also occur in the upper limbs, though much less often; and perhaps because the main artery is nearer the heart, and shorter, with rich collateral branching systems around the shoulder and elbow joints, ischaemia tends to be less severe. Nevertheless, if the occlusions are repeated or progressive, their effect is cumulative and serious, as in cervical rib. Such a possibility applies to the patient with Buerger's disease, though here the occlusions are thrombotic rather than embolic.

Furthermore, if, ultimately, an amputation

should become necessary, the patient is worse off than if the lower limb had been affected, for the substituted prosthesis is functionally much less efficient than the extremity it replaces for any skilled movements, particularly of the right hand, compared with the simpler needs of mobility and strength of the artificial lower limb.

Causes

1. INJURY

The causes and mechanisms of this are discussed in Chapter 13. Late cases do not usually require repair, for the acute phase is normally concluded with the formation of a good collateral circulation, and a complete block which affords no risk of embolic deterioration later.

Exceptionally, a fractured clavicle may produce a late thrombosis after many years; as in a man of fifty-nine, a patient of Professor Rob's and the author's who, in 1953, presented with severe ischaemia of four month's duration, and thrombosis of the right subclavian artery beneath a childhood fracture.

Stress fracture of the first rib, from severe coughing, may heal with excess callus and damage the artery, with similar late effects [20].

2. CHRONIC MECHANICAL DAMAGE

(a) Crutch thrombosis [19] occurs in life-long cripples; nearly all reported cases are in people who have used a crutch for fifty years, and the typical age is in the middle fifties. The pattern of the disease is strikingly like that of the cervical rib with arterial involvement, and premonitory embolisation [3A] and secondary Raynaud phenomenon are usual.

(b) Traumatic thrombosis of the superficial palmar arch occurs in heavy manual workers whose job requires them to strike repeatedly with the palm of the hand against some heavy or fixed object, thus the artery sustains occlusion or aneurysm or both (Fig. 11.6b, p. 206).

A similar condition was recognised by Osmond Clarke and the author in the forearm arteries of an international-class tennis player who developed typical Raynaud attacks while training outdoors in cold March weather. All the major arteries were clinically normal, and the wrist pulses only doubtfully reduced at rest. The exercise-elevation test (see p. 230) produced striking pallor of the right hand, and arteriography (Fig. 11.6a, p. 206) confirmed the presence of obstructive lesions of the middle course of the radial, ulnar, and interosseous arteries, evidently from physical damage due to muscle action over several years of unprecedently hard striking.

3. NEOPLASM

Neoplasm of the lung apex, plus radiotherapy, caused severe ischaemia and painful gangrene in one patient [10] who was fully relieved by a carotid-axillary venous by-pass graft.

4. GENERALISED ARTERIAL DISEASE

(a) arteriosclerosis obliterans (Fig. 4.10, p. 104);
(b) Buerger's disease (Fig. 4.13, p. 106);
(c) pulseless disease of young women (Fig. 12.9);
(d) embolism (Fig. 14.5, p. 264).

These common causes of upper limb ischaemia are each discussed in other chapters. Their diagnosis is not difficult if the age, sex, and general condition of the patient are taken into account. Other peripheral occlusions with identifying features are often found on general examination. Arteriography is usually diagnostic in case of doubt.

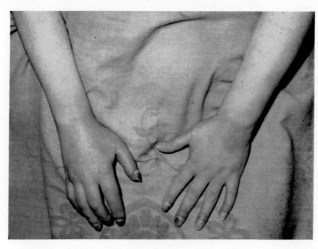

Fig. 12.9. Aortic arch syndrome (female arteritis). Acutely ischaemic right hand and pulseless right upper limb in a 32-year-old woman of gypsy descent. She had previously had both lower limbs amputated through the upper thigh for similar central arterial occlusion. Arm recovery followed loop thrombectomy beneath clavicle.

Treatment: General Measures

General measures to rest the part and prevent further stagnant thrombosis are generally more successful than in the lower limb. Cervicodorsal sympathectomy is the most useful single operative measure, for it takes advantage of the inherent tendency towards improvement and, in the meantime, recovery is favoured by the abolition of vasoconstrictor phases.

Reconstructive arterial operation is seldom applicable, the exception being after embolism, where a limited occlusion affects a major bifurcation of a small but otherwise normal artery. Otherwise, at present, only the aortic arch syndrome or its arteriosclerotic counterpart in older men are suited to arterioplasty. There are, however, a few reports of using saphenous vein grafts successfully in the more distal parts of the upper limb [9].

REFERENCES

1. Atkins, H. J. B. (1954) Sympathectomy by the axillary approach. *Lancet*, **i**, 538.
2. Birkett, D. A., Apthorp, G. H., Chamberlain, D. A., Hayward, G. W. and Tuckwell, E. G. (1965) Bilateral upper thoracic sympathectomy in angina pectoris: results in 52 cases. *Brit. med. J.*, **ii**, 187.
3. Brannon, E. W. (1963) Cervical rib syndrome: an analysis of nineteen cases and twenty-four operations. *J. Bone Jt Surg.*, **45A**, 977.
3A. Danese, C. A., Veleti, D. C., Baron, M. G., Waye, J. D. and Jacobson, J. H. (1969) Recurrent embolism from an occult crutch aneurysm of the axillary artery. *Surgery*, **66**, 680.
4. De Villiers, J. C. (1966) A brachiocephalic vascular syndrome associated with cervical rib. *Brit. med. J.*, **ii**, 140.
5. dos Santos, J. C. (1949) Note sur la désobstruction des anciennes thromboses artérielles. *Presse Médicale*, **57**, 544.
6. Eastcott, H. H. G. (1962) Reconstruction of the subclavian artery for complications of cervical-rib and thoracic-outlet syndrome. *Lancet*, **ii**, 1243.
7. Eden, K. C. (1939) The vascular complications of cervical ribs and first thoracic rib abnormalities. *Brit. J. Surg.*, **27**, 111.
8. Edwards, E. A. and Levine, H. D. (1952) Auscultation in the diagnosis of compression of the subclavian artery. *New Eng. J. Med.*, **247**, 79.
8A. Eriksonn, I. and Hiertonn, T. (1968) The brachiocephalic vascular syndromes. *Acta chir. Scand.*, **134**, 93.
9. Garrett, H. E., Morris, G. C., Howell, J. F. and DeBakey, M. E. (1965) Revascularisation of upper extremity with autogenous vein bypass graft. *Arch. Surg.*, **91**, 751.
10. Gibson, P., Lucas, R. J. and Wilson, G. S. (1965) Subclavian artery occlusion with gangrene. *Grace Hosp. Bull.*, **43**, 103.
11. Gilroy, J. and Meyer, J. S. (1963) Compression of the subclavian artery as a cause of ischaemic brachial neuropathy. *Brain*, **86**, 733.
12. Gunning, A. J., Pickering, G. W., Robb-Smith, A. H. T. and Russell, R. R. (1964) Mural thrombosis of the subclavian artery and subsequent embolism in cervical rib. *Quart. J. Med.*, **33**, 133.
13. Halsted, W. S. (1916) An experimental study of circumscribed dilatation of an artery immediately distal to a partially occluding band, and its bearing on the dilatation of the subclavian artery observed in certain cases of cervical rib. *J. exp. Med.*, **24**, 271.
14. Holst, S. (1963) Cervical rib and associated vascular complications. *J. Oslo City Hospitals*, **13**, 173.
15. Hoobler, S. W. (1942) The syndrome of cervical rib with subclavian arterial thrombosis and hemiplegia due to cerebral embolism. *New Eng. J. Med.*, **226**, 942.
16. Kerley, P., Twining, E. W., Dow, J. and Holesh, S. (1962) 'The cardiovascular and respiratory systems.' *In A Textbook of X-ray Diagnosis by British authors* (Ed. Shanks, S. C. and Kerley, P.). Vol. 2. London: Lewis, p. 376.
17. Lewis, T. and Pickering, G. W. (1934) Observations upon maladies in which the blood supply to digits ceases intermittently or permanently, and upon bilateral gangrene of digits; observations relevant to so-called 'Raynaud's disease'. *Clin. Sci.*, **1**, 327.
17A. Longo, M. F., Clagett, O. T. and Fairbairn, J. F. (1970) Surgical treatment of thoracic outlet compression syndrome. *Ann. Surg.*, **171**, 538.
18. Pickering, G. (1963) Arterial occlusion especially of the coronary arteries and of the subclavian and carotid arteries. *Bull. Johns Hopkins Hosp.*, **113**, 105.
19. Platt, H. (1930) Occlusion of the axillary artery due to pressure by a crutch. Report of two cases. *Arch. Surg.*, **20**, 314.
20. Rob, C. G. and Standeven, A. (1958) Arterial occlusion complicating thoracic outlet compression syndrome. *Brit. med. J.*, **ii**, 709.
20A. Roos, D. B. (1971) Experience with first rib resection for thoracic outlet syndrome. *Ann. Surg.*, **173**, 429.
21. Shucksmith, H. S. (1963) Cerebral and peripheral emboli caused by cervical ribs. *Brit. med. J.*, **ii**, 835.
22. Symonds, C. P. (1927) Cervical rib: thrombosis of subclavian artery. Contralateral hemiplegia of sudden onset, probably embolic. *Proc. Roy. Soc. Med.*, **20**, 1244.
23. Traphagen, D. W. and Marshall, F. (1961) Subclavian artery thrombosis six years after rib resection. *Arch. Surg.*, **83**, 700.
24. Wickham, J. E. A. and Martin, P. (1962) Aneurysm of the subclavian artery in association with cervical abnormality. *Brit. J. Surg.*, **50**, 205.

13 Arterial Injuries

The incidence of arterial injury in traumatic practice is low, and the event unexpected when it happens, but the damage caused soon becomes serious beyond all normal experience of limb injury, often ending in crippling disability, amputation, or a fatal train of complications. Once such a patient begins to go wrong, there is often little that can be done. Transfer to a special unit then offers no solution at all. On the other hand, correct early treatment at the receiving hospital should normally be followed by a straightforward recovery, even though the surgeon dealing with the case may have little experience of arterial work.

Historical Notes
Throughout the ages, penetrating wounds in war have divided arteries. Ambroise Paré, in the sixteenth century, established the ligature for the lifesaving control of arterial haemorrhage. Described hundreds of years earlier by Galen, it was then forgotten, and until Paré, the wounded were forced to submit to the brutalities of the simpler, though less effective, heated cautery. Hallowell, in Yorkshire, in 1759 [33], repaired a brachial artery by transfixing it tangentially with a pin, and winding silk about it as a figure of eight. John B. Murphy of Chicago, in 1897 [64], seems to have been the first to reconstruct a completely transected human artery, though, in the early years of the twentieth century, Carrel and Guthrie achieved consistently good results with experimental vascular repairs and grafts in animals [31]. Application of their work to acute arterial injury in man was slow to follow, but between 1912 and 1914 there were some reports, mainly in the German literature [14, 54, 55, 81, 82], of primary repairs and vein grafts for peripheral aneurysm and arteriovenous fistula, and in Glasgow, in 1912, Hogarth Pringle [75] used a saphenous vein graft to replace a recent traumatic aneurysm in two patients, both of which succeeded. Very little more

seems to have been recorded except for an almost forgotten series of fifty-one vein grafts from Weglowski, in 1925 [89], on German First World War casualties, until a notable paper by Gordon Murray of Toronto in 1939 [65], mainly concerning the use of heparin, but giving details of some patients with reconstruction of the lower-limb arteries by vein grafting.

The incidence of arterial injury in the First and Second World Wars was about 1 per cent of all wounds [20], and the practice of ligation remained general with a 50 per cent incidence of amputation following this method, the only one that could be used in the operational conditions of the bitter campaigns during which these wounds were sustained.

The Korean war opened with similar experience in vascular injuries, which were more common than during the World Wars [40]. Just at that time, the academic surgical world was rediscovering the work of Carrel, and experience in experimental laboratories and in some clinical units was showing that reconstruction was simple and practical for dealing with arterial defects. It was decided to try these methods out in casualties, and in the spring of 1952 repair was undertaken wherever possible, the conditions of the campaign being well suited to it, with quick evacuation and a more steady incidence of wound cases so that the surgeons had time in which to carry out the precision work required for success in vascular repair. The results were striking. The amputation rate fell from 50 to 13 per cent [39] and late results in veterans examined several years later were well maintained [45]. Early repair was also found to be valuable in the treatment of traumatic false aneurysm and arteriovenous fistula (*see* Chapters 15 and 16). Civilian experience since that time [1, 21A, 63, 73], and during the Viet Nam war [7B, 14A, 75B] has confirmed the superiority of reconstruction at the time of injury. All dealing with accident casualties should now be trained in this technique.

Types of Injury

To the Vessels (Fig. 13.1)

Arterial spasm ⎫
Thrombosis in continuity ⎬ Distal ischaemia
Complete severance ⎭
Lateral defect in artery — False aneurysm
Lateral defect in artery and
vein — Arteriovenous fistula

To the Surrounding Parts

Open or closed

Limbs or body cavity

Localised or with severe soft tissue or bony injury
(penetrating or blunt)

Differences between Civil and War Injuries

Civil arterial injury [21A]	*Arterial injury of war* [14A]
1. Closed bony injury with traumatic arterial spasm.	
2. Clean, small, open laceration from glass or knife, into artery but with minimal shock and blood loss, unless into a body cavity; often iatrogenic [1,1A].	Severe, open contaminated injury involving skin, soft tissues and bone; much shock and blood loss, internal external.
3. Extensive limb or body-crushing injury from road traffic accident, partly open but with mainly intact skin cover; severe shock from soft tissue damage, fractures and internal bleeding.	

Effects of Injury

Local and general effects are closely interdependent, for blood and fluid loss into the injury tend to reduce peripheral blood flow and the local obstructive effect of the arterial injury or the surrounding haematoma produces a progressive reduction in the circulation in the injured extremity, so that the local tissue damage is worsened.

Loss of blood and fluid → Local injury → Anoxia, from fall in blood flow → Hypovolaemia → Loss of blood and fluid

Renal failure may follow in the worst cases if resuscitation is delayed or inadequate. Hypotension and toxaemia cause acute tubular necrosis after crush injury or massive limb ischaemia, or anerobic or blood sepsis.

Acute ischaemia from trauma in no way differs from major arterial occlusion due to other causes, except that its effects are usually aggravated by shock and haemorrhage. This is why, in subjects of any age, limb-loss is more likely to follow arterial injury or major arterial surgery than after a non-traumatic thrombosis. Occlusion may be due to any one of the three degrees of injury (Fig. 13.1); or to compression by a false aneurysm over a lateral arterial defect, although this condition is compatible

with a good limb circulation until the late stage is reached, when the pressure in the enlarging false sac obliterates surrounding collateral channels; the distal pulses in the affected limb now become weaker,

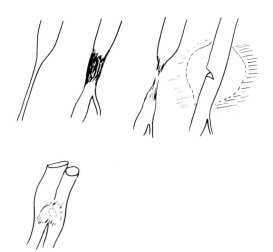

Fig. 13.1. Degrees and types of arterial injury; spasm, contusion, avulsion rupture, lateral injury with false aneurysm, and acute arteriovenous fistula.

while those in the other extremities are well maintained.

Muscle contracture is a common, serious complication signifying irreversible ischaemic damage (*see* Fig. 13.13) (*see* Chapter 2, pp. 19, 20, Figs. 2.1, 2.2).

Assessment of Injury

Experience in trauma is essential for the correct appraisal of the state of the patient and the effects of this upon the injured part. Timing in management is crucial; associated injuries must be taken into account, for while a damaged artery should have high priority, any suspicion of continuing bleeding within the chest, skull or abdomen constitutes a greater threat to life. Two surgical teams may be needed, a possibility that should be envisaged early in the resuscitation period so that extra staff can be notified in time.

Clinical signs in arterial injury may be few, and are often obscured by the other features of the injury, such as pain, swelling, sensory loss or shock. Diagnosis is helped by a high index of suspicion in penetrating wounds sited anywhere near the line of major vessels, in the presence of certain fractures whose displacement approaches the main artery or, when dealing with complex fractures or crush injuries, to the distal part of the limb. *Absent distal pulses* are diagnostic if swelling is not yet present, though the converse is not always true: easily palpable pulses are retained in about 25 per cent of patients [73], and are often normal in volume when compared with the other extremities. An *increasing or pulsating haematoma* is good evidence in such patients (Fig. 13.12). Sometimes a bruit may be heard, due to the blood surging through an incomplete occlusion, or through an acute, recently established arteriovenous fistula.

An arterial injury is highly likely if, during resuscitation, the circulation in the injured limb lags behind the others in its recovery as the patient improves.

Arteriography [7, 16, 25A, 56, 79]

Although in principle this investigation should be decisive and of definitive value in management there are serious drawbacks, which mean that clinical suspicion must remain the chief basis of the diagnosis of arterial injury in the acute phase. Sometimes, however, it is possible to carry out arteriography at the time of the bone X-ray examination.

Objections to arteriography are its inconvenience, and the delay that is inevitable even if the emergency should arise during normal hours. Extra handling of the patient and his injured limb may increase shock and local damage. Dressings and splints may impede access to the injection site. Leakage of the contrast medium may not occur at the point of injury [56]. The medium itself, or the injection, may do harm. The films obtained tend to be of poor quality. Vasoconstriction may limit the filling in a cool injured limb with the patient in mild hypovolaemia, and a false interpretation may be made for the same reasons as in the preceding clinical examination. Yet where there has been real doubt after the clinical examination, or where opinion has settled against exploration for accessory reasons such as the presence of extensive associated injuries or, regrettably, a lack of vascular experience by the surgeon in charge, or when a difficult fracture has been well reduced and there is sufficient swelling to account for non-palpable distal pulses, arteriography can be decisive. An arteriogram showing major arterial injury should reverse all these considerations and point to the need for early exploration of the artery. Other patients with good peripheral circulation in the injured limb may be shown to require arterial surgery, as for example a concealed false aneurysm or an unsuspected acute arteriovenous fistula. Conversely, in any of these conditions or the suspicion of them, a good clear normal filling may avert the serious mistake of an unnecessary arterial exploration as a further complication to an already serious injury.

Management of a Known Arterial Injury

Delay is wrong once the diagnosis has been made. These patients travel poorly, and complications tend to occur during the journey. Resuscitation is best carried out in the operating theatre. If ischaemia is a feature, operation should be aimed at the earliest possible moment, for irreversible tissue damage will usually mar the results of even successful arterial surgery not completed until after eight hours from the time of injury.

Steps in the Surgical Care

1. In the severely shocked case, diagnosed and admitted early, a short period of resuscitation and assessment is allowed, during which time antibiotic cover and tetanus prophylaxis is arranged, and blood is cross matched.

2. X-ray films of the injured part and of other suspected associated injuries should normally be seen before the arterial lesion is exposed, though not at the cost of delay. The limb examination can be combined with an operative arteriogram.

THE ASSOCIATED FRACTURE

This should normally be dealt with first, whether manipulation is sufficient or an open reduction is necessary. Occasionally, simple reduction brings back the pulses, but the reverse may happen, as when manipulation breaks down the wall of a false aneurysm, or when in a late case with stable circulation the fracture or its callus obstructs the artery for the first time.

ARTERIAL SPASM AND ITS CORRECTION

This is a special risk with injuries to the muscular arteries, such as the brachial (Fig. 13.2) and popliteal. Large central arteries, being mainly composed of elastic tissue, seldom show spasm with injury. In the limbs, a mild and localised contraction is common and should soon correct itself spontaneously, e.g. when an arteriography needle is withdrawn, or a fracture is reduced, but even so the condition of the extremity must be closely observed afterwards, for if any signs should persist suggestive of continued or more serious spasm the artery should be exposed without delay.

Exposure of the artery may be sufficient, the effect of decompression perhaps [5]. The full length of the affected part of the artery must be seen up to the pulsating lower end of the normal portion. Since the milder degrees of this condition tend to pass off on their own accord, it is not surprising that claims have been made for various methods of treating it. Controlled animal experiments seem to give first place to the superficial application of $2\frac{1}{2}$ per cent papaverine solution [50], which is more effective than intra-arterial or systemic administration.

Distension by saline injection (Mustard's manoeuvre) [66] can be recommended. This is based upon the same principle as instrumental dilatation of a small artery or vein in repair by anastomosis. The contracted portion of the artery is distended by injection through a fine needle, segment by segment between light bulldog clamps (Fig. 13.3) progressing distally, and admitting the pulsation down into each portion of the artery as it is opened up, until the lower limit of the spasm is reached, thus confirming the effectiveness of the measure. Experimentally, this method compared favourably with local papaverine, and clinical experience was satisfactory in children with fractures of the lower limb, as well as after intra-arterial thiopentone injection.

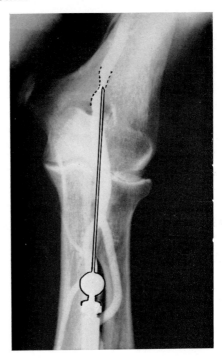

Fig. 13.2. Moderate spasm of brachial artery at the point of entry of an arteriogram needle.

Arterial laceration must be excluded; no doubt in the past some cases labelled 'irreversible spasm' were, in fact, suffering from a lesion in continuity containing curled up intima and thrombus [79A]. There is sub-adventitial bruising and induration of the segment, both most marked just beyond the lower limit of normal pulsation. Arteriotomy is essential to the recognition and correction of this lesion.

Fasciotomy helps to relieve compression at the elbow or popliteal fossa, also distally in the muscle compartments, where incipient ischaemic contracture may be prevented [5]. Arterial surgery on its own may not be enough to do this [34, 79A].

Repair of the Arterial Injury

The worst complications of an injured artery are ischaemia from thrombosis, and secondary haemorrhage from infection. These are also complications of a failed arterial repair, and so there will be times when the surgeon dealing with a massive injury should decide to take the simpler course of ligating the artery at the lowest accessible point, usually at the injury. Complicated, extensive soft-tissue wounds with multiple fractures, in the distal part of the limb may require proximal ligation through normal tissues, or, sometimes, to avoid a prolonged and dangerous illness in such a patient, a primary amputation.

Minor arteries can be ligated; no harm should

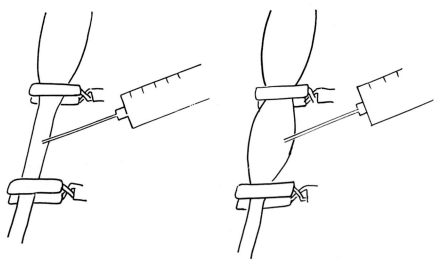

Fig. 13.3. Mustard and Bull's method for relieving traumatic arterial spasm.

result from this, for at this distance from the main artery there are many alternative paths for the blood flow, and in any case the uncertainty of patency following the repair of an artery smaller than 5 mm in diameter means that there will be slight extra risks in reconstruction without compensating benefit. The exception to this is when the main artery itself is small, as in the upper limb, especially in children, or when the other arteries to the extremity are hopelessly damaged so that vitality seems likely to depend upon any that may appear to be reparable, though small.

General Principles of Technique

1. Damage is usually worse than the external appearance of the artery suggests. Therefore, when in doubt open the artery.
2. Lateral suture is unsatisfactory except for a large artery or a small clean and uncontused injury.
3. Primary repair, using arterial tissue only, is preferable to any other method.
4. Adequate back flow from the distal end must be ensured before repair is attempted; a Fogarty catheter is passed distally to remove stasis clot. (It is wise to pass it proximally also.) Heparin may be required, locally or systemically.
5. Fasciotomy is advisable in limb cases; it reduces resistance to distal run-off.
6. The peripheral circulation must at all costs be maintained. Further blood loss during the necessary manipulations of the repair must be fully replaced. For the same reason it is nearly always wrong to operate with tourniquet control or with any form of hypotensive anaesthesia. Success is most likely in cases repaired within ten

hours of the injury, or sooner still if there is acute ischaemia. Some patients with false aneurysm or a good collateral circulation will do well much later than this.

Repair in Continuity (Fig. 13.4 i)

This is often possible when dealing with a small, clean incised lateral wound, or in closing an arteriotomy made in order to remove obstructing material from the lumen. Lateral suture is permissible only if it produces no narrowing. In order to avoid this, insertion of a patch of autogenous vein is often necessary. The presence of more than one lateral wound, or any contusion of the wall, particularly the inner layers, are contra-indications to this conservative type of repair. The whole segment of damaged artery must be resected, and a full reconstruction is carried out by one of the following methods.

End-to-end Anastomosis (Fig. 13.4 i–v)

At the flexures, or when the artery is wide and tortuous, as in some older people, 2–3 cm or even more of the damaged artery can be resected, yet the ends will meet sufficiently well for anastomosis, for artery, unlike most other structures, heals well in moderate tension. Also, though strong apposition may have been needed during the suturing, when the clamps are removed the elastic tissue of the artery is stretched and elongated by the pressure of the blood within, and the repaired artery will resume its normal position and tension. The limb need not be kept in flexion, although this may have helped considerably during the repair.

240

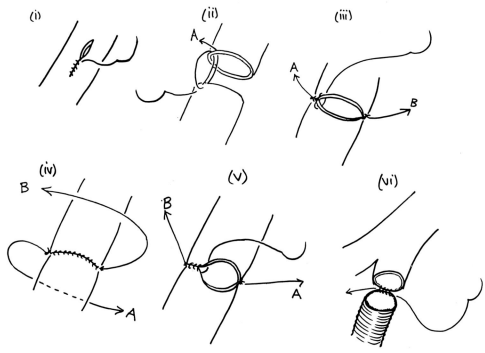

Fig. 13.4. Methods of arterial suture.

(i)   Lateral repair in continuity.
(ii) First slinging stitch, which need not evert.
(iii) Anterior continuous layer through all coats with maintained traction of slinging stitches
      A and B.
(iv) Rotation of the anastomosis.
(v)   Closure of posterior layer.
(vi) Single suture method where rotation of the anastomosis is impossible.

Except in very small arteries, in which eversion of the cut ends may be important, any convenient form of suturing may be used as long as there is good haemostasis, without narrowing, on removal of the clamps. A simple continuous stitch through all coats is quickest and easiest and best adapted to the correction of irregularities and setbacks such as the cutting out of a stitch. The steps in the operation are shown in Fig. 13.4. Where access is limited, it is usually better not to attempt to rotate the artery, but to place the posterior layer from within the lumen, beginning from a slinging suture on the far side of the anastomosis (Fig. 13.4 vi), and progressing with a continuous stitch towards the operator until the point opposite the first stitch is reached. The suture is tied here, and is used for traction, and the anterior layer of the anastomosis is then easy to complete, although care must be taken to include the whole of the region of the far traction stitch, which tends to be out of sight at the closing stage.

Replacement by a graft gives poorer late results, but much better at any time than ligation. In the Korean experience [39, 45] autogenous vein was the best, both early and on late follow-up examination. In Viet Nam it was the commonest operation performed on 1,000 cases in the Vascular Registry: 45·9 per cent compared with 37·7 per cent treated by end-to-end anastomosis [75B]. The superficial femoral was the most usual site. Here the soft tissue damage is often severe and a long graft is required (Fig. 13.5). Nevertheless, a suitable vein can usually be found, and dacron prosthetic replacement has less value in the limbs than in the large arteries of the body cavities.

Injury and the Diseased Artery
A sclerotic artery may thrombose after an accident or operation. The injury need not directly involve the artery. With conditions, already perhaps becoming marginal for patency, and flow already diminishing before injury, the additional stasis which this

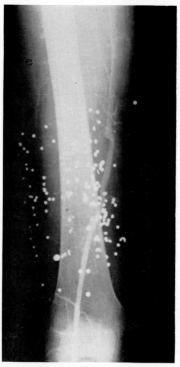

Fig. 13.5. Shot-gun injury to the femoral artery in a security guard who tackled some bank raiders. Extensive soft tissue damage, deep vein destroyed, calf already tense and foot blue. Good recovery after vein grafting and fasciotomy.

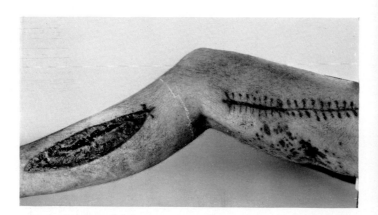

imposes upon peripheral circulation, and the subsequent changes in the blood itself, both favour acute thrombosis.

CASE REPORT 1

A painter, aged sixty-six fell from a ladder and was taken to hospital with a back injury, from which he recovered well, though he had been collapsed and hypotensive at first and was recumbent for two weeks more before being allowed up in the ward. He then experienced intermittent claudication for the first time, and the feet were noticed to be cold. Both superficial femoral arteries had thrombosed. In the subsequent law suit in which the author appeared for the plaintiff, judgement was made in his favour, it being accepted that though the legs were not injured, the accident had caused a premature deterioration.

If the artery, already affected by occlusive disease is directly involved in the injury, the consequences tend to be worse still, as the following show:

CASE REPORT 2

A rugby footballer aged thirty-five sustained a direct injury to the lower, inner left thigh and was unable to continue the game. There was severe pain, and 'deadness' of the limb, and the foot remained cold.

Exploration showed a recent thrombosis of the upper popliteal at the site of an arterial plaque, but extending distally over several centimetres. Thrombo-endarterectomy restored the ankle pulses.

CASE REPORT 3

A soccer footballer aged thirty-two noticed coldness, numbness and pallor of his right leg after a practice. He remembered only mild damage to the part. The limb was acutely ischaemic, and operation revealed an extensive thrombosis centred on a plaque beneath the adductor magnus tendon. A poor back flow was obtained and thrombo-endarterectomy resulted in a failure to restore the circulation despite two further explorations during the next twenty-four hours. A mid-thigh amputation was subsequently required, during the recovery from which he developed a severe myocardial infarct.

In these two cases the severity of the ischaemia appears to have been aggravated by the previous muscular exertion, which perhaps may have increased the metabolic debt (*see also* Fig. 13.13); stasis from vasodilatation in the distal muscles from both causes may explain the large amount of spreading thrombus present.

Special Arterial Injuries and Their Treatment

1. The Thoracic Aorta

Two forms of injury occur from which survival is possible:

(a) Penetrating wounds from missiles such as a small-bore bullet or pellet from a shot-gun, or a narrow-bladed knife or glass splinter.

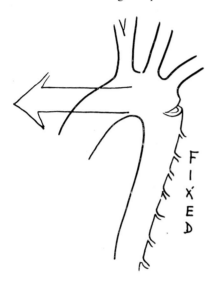

Fig. 13.6(a). Mechanism of production of common posterior tear of aorta just beyond left subclavian origin. The mobile arch and great vessels are dragged forward by the weight of the heart against the resistance of the firmly tethered descending aorta.

(b) Deceleration rupture (Fig. 13.6), the 'steering wheel injury' at or near the origin of the left subclavian artery, and caused by violent onward movement of the heart and great vessels so that the arch is wrenched and partly or completely torn at its junction, with the tethered and less mobile descending aorta.

The second type is becoming more common, and though mainly of forensic interest as the principal injury in motor and air crash victims [88], it is now known that about 20 per cent survive long enough to reach hospital [87]. In these, the haemorrhage is confined by the mediastinal tissues, especially the parietal pleura, and by the adventitia, which may be intact or nearly so. Few cases show dissecting aneurysm, however, perhaps because the aorta is healthy [80]. Clinically, there may be remarkably little to show for such a serious injury, and patients have been allowed home after negative physical examination and chest X-ray films which were only realised to be abnormal in retrospect [80], perhaps

because at this early stage the extravasation was still concealed by the normal shadows of the heart and great vessels. Within a few hours, however, the haematoma or false aneurysm may enlarge and rupture to cause sudden death. Before this, there should be clear radiological signs of the injury. The

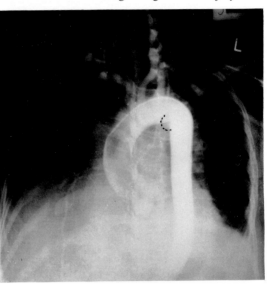

Fig. 13.6(b). A typical aortic deceleration injury in a woman aged thirty-six, whose husband was killed beside her from the same injury. Operation delayed by right rib fractures and respiratory insufficiency. Good recovery after trans-aortic suture of a 2 cm medial tear. (Case treated with Mr L. L. Bromley.)

mediastinum is widened and there is a left upper chest opacity with a rounded, irregular and, in places, hazy left border, and sometimes a basal effusion. A systolic murmur may be heard. Blood pressure is sometimes found to be rising in the arms and falling in the legs, perhaps from thrombotic obstruction to the outflow from the false aneurysm. Paraplegia, no doubt for similar reasons, is a grave sign. Several cases are reported in which arteriography was used to confirm the diagnosis [8] but, as with other arterial injuries, other evidence should be sufficient to decide upon emergency operation without further delay.

Provision for aortic cross-slamping is essential, and must be ready before work is begun on the false aneurysm, for the protection of the spinal cord and the kidneys. Hypothermia [72], a sutured by-pass shunt from the left subclavian to the aorta [87], a pumped atrio-femoral left heart by-pass circuit [10], or a simple ventriculo-aortic tube, not requiring a pump or heparin [46A, 74B].

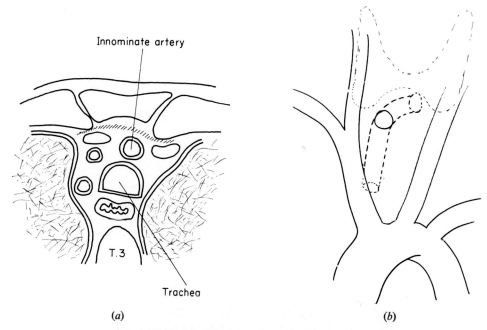

Innominate artery

T.3

Trachea

(a)   (b)

Fig. 13.7. Injury of the innominate artery by tracheostomy.

(a) Close relationship of artery to trachea at the level of the thoracic inlet.

(b) An infra-thyroid tracheostomy may bring the end or the cuff of the tracheostomy tube into relationship with the postero-medial surface of the innominate artery.

The common injury, the posterior tear, if recognised within hours of the accident, may be repaired by direct suture or by transection and end-to-end anastomosis [10]. After the first day the aorta becomes friable and takes the sutures badly, or may undergo dissection, and a replacement graft must be used in place of the excised portion. A low porosity plastic cloth reduces the risk of oozing following heparinisation and massive transfusion. Consistently good results are now reported [46].

Penetrating injury has been successfully repaired over 40 times in the past fifty years [7B, 70, 87A]. Presentation is much the same as in closed laceration; emergency operation is the only hope for survival. By-pass is not always essential, but if available it should be ready as the operation gets under way. Meanwhile, the condition should be managed in the same way as a stab wound of the heart, with rapid exposure, forced blood transfusion, a finger upon the hole, and suture repair once the situation has become manageable.

A narrow stab injury to the ascending aorta may become temporarily sealed off by compression of the mediastinal haematoma beneath the sternum, so that the patient lives to reach hospital, and may be saved by immediate operation. A sternum splitting thoracotomy as for pulmonary embolectomy (*see* Chapter 14) provides rapid exposure. There may be cardiac tamponade, causing troublesome venous bleeding, which ceases as soon as the pericardium is emptied of blood and clot. Such low aortic wounds are difficult to repair, but it may be possible to secure the rent with a lateral aortic clamp, and then to place a second clamp behind it, lifting the aorta up with it, to suture the hole. Care must be taken not to injure the coronary artery, the thin right ventricular wall, or the aortic valve cusp beneath the clamp.

A few patients with acute aortic injury have shown a coarctation-like picture, with rising blood pressure in the arms and hypotension in the lower limbs, perhaps from thrombotic occlusion of the outflow from the false sac [87]. A systolic murmur may be present at this stage [68]. Months later, a true post-traumatic coarctation has been explored and reconstructed [68]. Patients with repaired aortic injury require intensive postoperative care; usually with a tracheotomy, pump respirator, and free bilateral pleural drainage to prevent respiratory acidosis during the first 24 to 48 hours.

2. Innominate and Other Great Vessels Arising from the Aortic Arch

Partial avulsion due to deceleration injury may lead to a similar condition. The confining effect of the thoracic outlet, especially the manubrium, favours the formation of a false aneurysm here. Operative cure of this type of lesion should be easier than in the aorta [13, 42, 46], although the possibility of multiple clamping of the cranial blood supply makes it advisable to use hypothermia as well as making preparation for by-pass for the exploration. The author's earliest case affected the right common carotid of a man of fifty-six who was thrown through a car window and developed a large false aneurysm

arising from behind the right sternoclavicular joint (Fig. 9.14, p. 189). Excision with homograft replacement succeeded and the patient remained well ten years later.

Nearly 100 cases are on record of fatal damage to the innominate artery after tracheostomy [78]. In most of them the site of the opening was below the thyroid isthmus, i.e. the third tracheal ring or as low as the sixth, where the artery is closely related to the trachea (Fig. 13.7). The tube may be seen to pulsate before perforation takes place. Yet even this serious accident can be overcome: prompt over-inflation of the tube cuff may control the arterial haemorrhage for long enough to prepare for emergency operation to control and repair the damage [7A, 22].

Fig. 13.8. The injured subclavian.

(a) Old occlusion of right subclavian artery following fracture of the right clavicle many years before in a middle-aged woman undergoing arch aortography for transient ischaemia cerebral attacks. Thrombus from the upper face of the occlusion might have entered the right vertebral or carotid.

(b) False aneurysm of the right subclavian artery in a twenty-six-year-old man who sustained severe closed injury in a car smash a month before. After treatment of a haemothorax he developed increasing pain and weakness of the right arm and hand, with signs of brachial plexus involvement, but normal wrist pulses. Grafting the affected proximal part of the artery with a dacron replacement prosthesis gave immediate relief, and power quickly returned. This was probably an avulsion of the internal mammary origin with compression of the lower brachial trunks by the expanding false aneurysm. Condition satisfactory, with normal wrist pulses, four years later.

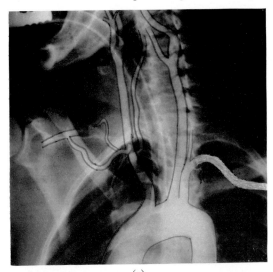

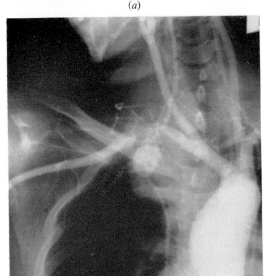

(a)

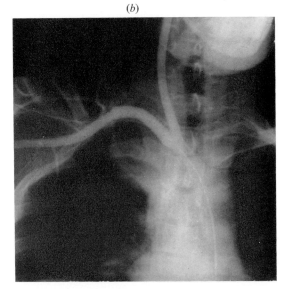

(b)

3. The Subclavian Artery

The distal part of the subclavian artery may be damaged by a fractured clavicle, though narrowing or late thrombosis are often discovered only later (Fig. 13.8a); early expanding aneurysm (Fig. 13.8b) will usually require urgent treatment. Resection of the clavicle is advisable to obtain access to the artery and to prevent further injury after the reconstruction. The first part of the subclavian may become occluded after blunt injury, with fracture of the first rib and clavicle. Vertebral ischaemia from embolism or subclavian steal may be demonstrable [77].

4. Closed Injuries to the Normal or Diseased Cervical Carotid

These have already been considered (p. 155). *Gunshot wounds* of one [73] or even both [32] carotids have been successfully repaired in apparently hopeless circumstances. End-to-end anastomosis is easy in the common carotid, but the internal carotid may require replacement by the proximal part of the external carotid. Venous bleeding and injury to the air passages are serious dangers. In Viet Nam, patients without neurological defect before operation did well [14B].

5. The Abdominal Aorta

This, with its branches, when injured, bleeds freely into the peritoneal cavity, and few such patients reach the surgeon. Some cases have been reported, however, of longer survival, and repair of penetrating aortic wounds below the level of the left renal vein [3] has been completed, even after cardiac arrest [30]. In two other patients the aortic wound sealed off sufficiently to allow them to reach hospital, but in both, the bullet migrated as an embolus to the left common femoral artery, where it caused acute leg ischaemia. In one patient gangrene resulted [44]; in the other, a child, the missile was successfully removed [83]. In fact, though not uncommonly gunshot and other foreign bodies reach the veins and the heart itself, patients in which there has been arterial migration of such objects are more rare [2,18,83]. Body position may determine the path [21].

As with the small penetrating aortic wound in the

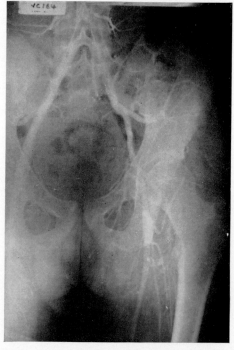

(a) Early phase showing internal iliac and gluteal filling only.

(b) Late phase showing filling of common femoral and its branches via the hip-joint anastomosis. This patient's symptoms were fully relieved following the insertion of an ilio-femoral dacron bypass graft, though a thrombo-endarterectomy at the time of the injury had previously become occluded. He is now able to play first-class Rugby football again.

Fig. 13.9. Closed rupture of the left external iliac artery in a naval rating injured by the handlebar of his motor scooter.

chest, the simplest possible operative method should be adopted. Lateral suture of the aorta is not difficult to carry out after a rapid exposure and finger-tip control of the arterial opening; manual compression of the vessel above and below the opening saves time and blood loss. In Viet Nam, two-thirds of such casualties survived [7B].

Closed aortic injury in the abdomen may cause a typical arterial lesion in continuity with flap dissection and associated acute thrombosis, as in the limb arteries [69].

The renal artery may be thrombosed [28A] or avulsed, presenting usually with haematuria and a non-functioning kidney on an emergency pyelogram [85]. If a renal aneurysm was previously present, rupture may follow minor injury, massive intra- or extra-peritoneal haemorrhage whose cause is revealed at laparotomy for the acute injury.

The hepatic artery, previously thought indispensable, and demanding reconstruction if damaged [53, 62], may be less important than this, provided the portal blood supply is still intact, judging from experience with hepatic ligation and perfusion in the treatment of primary and secondary tumours [55A, 74A]. Bacterial invasion from the gut must, however, be offset by giving broad-spectrum antibiotics.

The superior mesenteric artery may be lacerated by closed [48] or penetrating [62] injury. Spontaneous rupture has also been described [60]. Survival is reported following ligation [60] and after reconstruction for injury [62].

The normal splenic artery may rupture spontaneously in late pregnancy [26] (*see* Chapter 15). More of these patients are surviving early operation now that the need for upper abdominal exploration is better recognised.

The external iliac artery is easily damaged. Contusion of an otherwise normal artery with concealed dissection within the lumen was present in two patients referred to the author following the use of a self-retaining abdominal retractor, and it has also been seen when a tape sling beneath the artery was drawn up too tightly, or after arterial clamping, usually in the course of exploration for occlusive arterial disease.

Closed injuries of the external iliac and common femoral arteries are due to *severe blunt violence to the groin*, as when falling against or crushed by a large object (Fig. 13.9). The lower end of the common iliac, and even its internal branch, can be damaged in the same way [86]. Haemorrhage is usually limited by the injury itself or, if the lumen is open, by the surrounding fascial layers. Ischaemia is often incomplete when the lesion is above the inguinal ligament, because of the good collaterals around the hip and the profunda femoris. Delayed repair may still save such a limb, or if already safe, restore its full function.

Femoral Arteries

The common femoral artery, because it is accessible to puncture and close to so many routine operative procedures, is liable to damage and figures in litigation against the hospitals in which such misadventures occur.

1. THE SELDINGER CATHETER INJURY [4, 6, 25] occurs in one to two per cent of examinations [31A, 52A]

(*a*) *Traumatic Thrombosis with Ischaemia*
An arteriosclerotic patient requiring a contrast examination of the arteries of the lower half of the body is catheterised via the right common femoral artery, usually after some difficulty over the thickness of the arterial wall and, perhaps, some reduction in the pulsation even before puncture. Later, he is found to have a pale, pulseless right lower limb. In the younger patient sustaining this accident similar difficulty may have been experienced during the puncture and catheterisation, e.g. in a small woman under investigation for suspected renal artery disease or some abnormality of the thoracic aorta or its branches. In such people the ischaemic picture is often quite mild and may pass off spontaneously. However, if improvement is slow or incomplete or there is any sign of relapse and the diagnosis of 'arterial spasm' is abandoned, the thrombosis at the puncture site should be suspected, and exploration must be undertaken without further delay. Arteriotomy soon shows the type of damage present, and when the thrombus (usually friable platelet material) has been removed and any distal clot sucked out, a patch graft from one of the nearby saphenous vein tributaries is applied, conserving the main vessel for possible later use as a by-pass if the local repair should fail.

(*b*) *False Aneurysm at the Groin*
Bruising is usual after this investigation, especially in hypertensive subjects in whom it is so commonly required. Haematoma is common. If the discoloured swelling persists, and certainly if it should increase, a false aneurysm must be suspected (Fig. 13.10). This may be caused by avulsion of one of the large branches of the lower end of the external iliac, where they are tightly placed across the small gap beneath the parent artery and the inguinal ligament, a fact that leads to operative hazard in formal dissection of this segment of artery. The tense, expanding haematoma may pull the deep epigastric off, and augment the aneurysm, as it did in the patient shown.

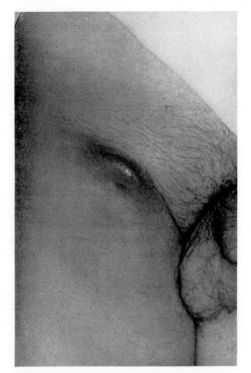

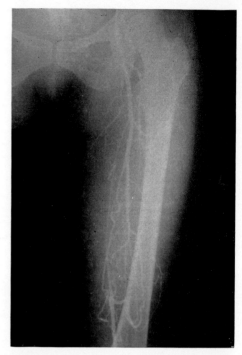

Fig. 13.10. Large false aneurysm of right common femoral artery four weeks after Seldinger catheterisation for hypertension. The aneurysm was of the diameter and height of half a grapefruit.

Fig. 13.11. Femoral arterial occlusion in a woman of twenty-eight following arterial cannulation at the left groin during cardio-pulmonary by-pass. Patency was restored after insertion of a femoro-popliteal saphenous vein by-pass graft.

2. OPERATIVE INJURY

This may not be recognised by the inexperienced surgeon whose misfortune it is to cause it. The artery may be ligated in error during a varicose vein procedure. Usually, there are unusual circumstances, either the patient's build, or difficulty over bleeding, or an unusual anaesthetic may have been used, such as the epidural block, which may suppress the normal difference in appearance between the artery and vein; likewise, with inadequate local analgesia the patient may be syncopal from pain, and the pulsation of the artery may not be felt.

Cannulation in the course of cardiac by-pass may damage the artery [47] more than is evident at the time of repair of the arteriotomy afterwards, acute ischaemia may not be noticed, especially if the superficial femoral has been used for the perfusion, though, as in the Seldinger injury, progressive thrombus formation may follow, both at the site of the injury and, later, along the course of the artery in the adductor canal, and may even reach the upper popliteal region (Fig. 13.11). Anterior tibial compartment ischaemia may occur [34]. A proximal dissecting injury also occurs (*see* Chapter 15).

The butcher's injury, already referred to in the external iliac, also typically affects the right common femoral: the inexperienced victim, using great force with a short, very sharp knife, and omitting perhaps to wear his protective apron, misjudges the cut and plunges the blade into his own groin. The copious external bleeding that follows will prove fatal unless digital compression can be applied. Even when such a patient has been taken to hospital there may be real difficulty over the securing of haemostasis, due to the welling up of blood through the concealed profunda femoris, so that the patient may present to the vascular unit, as did an early case of the author's, with ligatures in place both above and below the profunda and, therefore, requiring two arterial reconstructions.

A similar, though closed injury to the common femoral, caused by a kick from a horse, later presented with thigh claudication in the 26-year-old girl victim upon whom the author operated, using a replacement saphenous vein graft, with return of pulses and relief of symptoms.

SUPERFICIAL FEMORAL AND UPPER
POPLITEAL ARTERIAL INJURY WITH
FRACTURED SHAFT OF FEMUR, OR THE
BONES OF THE KNEE

The recognition of this important complication
bristles with difficulties. The fracture and surrounding soft tissue swelling may have compressed the
artery, or be providing a stimulus to reflex vasoconstriction throughout the limb. Either should
improve with reduction of the fracture, resuscitation, and relief of pain. These things, however, take
time, and if actual structural injury of the artery is
present, the delay may mean the loss of the limb.
Local arterial spasm, a very different state from the
regional vasoconstrictor response to injury, may not
be reversible or, if it is, the release may come too late
to prevent ischaemic muscle contracture in the calf,
(see Chapter 2, p. 19) (Fig. 13.13). It is best regarded
and treated as a probable arterial injury.

Absent distal pulses in lower limb injury should
always suggest an arterial obstruction requiring
operation. Exceptions to this are unimportant; they
have already been discussed, and should never be
made the excuse for procrastination. Only the most
pressing considerations such as burns, chest, or head
injury should ever be allowed to contra-indicate
early operation. With these, and also in elderly, ill
subjects, the decision is most difficult. Arteriography may be of the greatest value [56, 79, 79B].

Of nine patients seen late with damage to the main
lower limb artery from bony injury, all ended with
severe disability or gangrene requiring amputation
[57]. Figure 13.13 is a typical example.

Of nine patients seen early with the same type of
injury [9, 16, 51] all did well after immediate primary
arterial repair.

Operation is planned in stages: an exploratory
assessment of the state of the femoro-popliteal
artery, first by manipulation, which may improve the
circulation (though skeletal traction may worsen it
[35]); then open reduction of the fracture, which
may be seen to relieve the obstruction to the artery,
followed, if possible, by internal fixation by whichever method involves the minimum manipulation of
the injury. The artery is then re-examined and, if
there is no return of pulsations, an internal contusion
is probably the reason, and arteriotomy is essential.
This may need to be several centimetres in length [9].
Thrombectomy by Fogarty catheter is now routine
[79B]. The type of reconstruction best suited to the
lesion is then completed.

Fracture of the lesser trochanter may damage the
profunda femoris artery [36]. In an elderly patient
with occlusive disease already present in the superficial femoral, loss of the profunda will seriously
reduce the limb circulation, which mainly depends

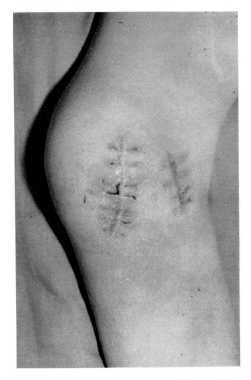

Fig. 13.12. Pulsating false aneurysm and haemarthrosis
of right knee in a girl of sixteen, twelve days after
medial meniscectomy. There had been difficulty over
the removal of the posterior end of the cartilage.

upon it. The same may explain the severe ischaemia
that sometimes complicates hip operations involving
sub-trochanteric osteotomy, as well as with screw
fixation of the lesser trochanter [19].

At the level of the knee joint, the artery may be
penetrated during the removal of the posterior end of
the medial meniscus [74], an injury that tends to
remain hidden until the time of the first dressing,
when a large posterior haematoma is discovered
(Fig. 13.12), and either then or later is noticed to
possess an expansile pulsation. The injury is a short
and simple one to repair; the operator, first secures,
by tape control, the proximal popliteal, the haematoma is entered. The opening in the artery is located
by the spurting haemorrhage, which is easily controlled with finger tip pressure. The distal artery is
then secured with a bulldog clip, and the slit in the
artery can then be closed by lateral suture, with fine
close stitches to avoid narrowing the lumen.

Fracture of an exostosis at the knee level has, on
several occasions, set up an exactly similar condition
[12]. The false aneurysm may continue for months
before being recognised. Earlier effects will be

produced in those patients in which the injury is occlusive rather than aneurysmal.

The inferior lateral geniculate artery may be injured during lateral meniscectomy: it runs within the joint capsule close to the attachment of the meniscus [24]. Because the operation is carried out under tourniquet control the injury is not recognised and, like the main popliteal injury in medial meniscectomy, it presents with unexplained swelling and haemarthrosis at about the twelfth day. Later, a small pulsatile lump appears at the point of injury, sometimes with a murmur or thrill which explains the recurrent, persistent bleeding into the joint [36]. Surgical cure is simple once the condition has been recognised.

Damage to the distal popliteal artery occurs with posterior dislocation of the knee (Fig. 13.13) and in high, oblique fractures of the upper end of the tibia (Fig. 13.14) in as many as five out of seven cases [90]. *This is a very serious lesion, which often leads to amputation.* Since the nerves and large veins are also likely to be involved, and the patient cold and shocked, numbness and blueness of the foot will tend to confuse the diagnosis, and perhaps delay the decision to operate. The repair will usually be

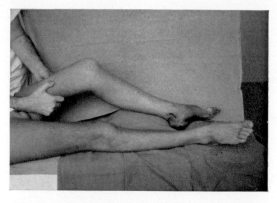

Fig. 13.13. Dry gangrene of left foot and ischaemic contracture of calf five weeks after traumatic posterior dislocation of left knee still seen to be subluxated. Patient was playing rugby football at the time of his injury; the ischaemia may have been worsened thereby. Exploration had not been possible until two days after accident.

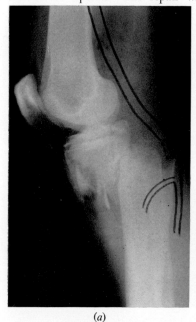
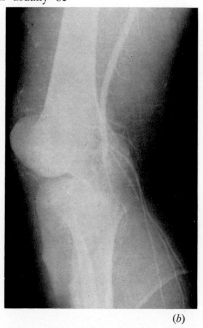
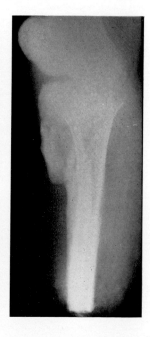

(a)   (b)

Fig. 13.14.

(a) Transection of the popliteal bifurcation in a man aged fifty with a compound fracture dislocation of the knee. Primary repair of the artery was carried out at the time of initial wound and fracture treatment. Successful outcome.

(b) Traumatic occlusion of popliteal artery seen late, after an upper tibial fracture at ice hockey. Repair on second day: distal arteries extensively thrombosed—below-knee amputation required. (Mr Andrew Desmond's case.)

difficult. It must always be accompanied by catheter thrombectomy. Yet even after good management in an experienced vascular unit, civilian [9A] or military [75A], the amputation rate was about one-third. In limbs that survive, recovery of the popliteal nerves is often slow and incomplete, though if the foot has a good circulation the neurological effects are less troublesome.

Another bad end-result commonly seen with this injury is ischaemic contracture, or even complete loss of the muscle bellies [57], with the intact skin and some fibrous tissue as the only investment of the bones of the leg, now healed, the foot being well supplied with blood, though perhaps numb and dropped into equinus. Damage of this kind may follow tibial osteotomy in children [83A], as well as in an arteriosclerotic adult [90A].

Contusion of the tibial arteries and their branches tends to be extensive and multiple in patients with severe comminuted fracture of the tibia and fibula, and ischaemia develops in the plaster during the first night, with muscle contracture or frank ischaemia of the foot, requiring amputation below the knee. The plaster may be wrongly blamed for what has happened [71].

A misdirected sclerosant injection of 3 per cent sodium tetradecyl sulphate into a varicose vein near the ankle may enter a tibial artery, producing severe ischaemia of the toes [22A, 56A].

Arterial Injury in the Upper Limb

In disease, the upper limb tolerates ischaemia fairly well, so that a false sense of security may lead to complacency in the management of some of the more serious forms of ischaemia (*see* Chapter 12). The arterial lesions of trauma are particularly liable to be mistreated for the same reason [76].

The main danger is ischaemic muscle contracture, for though the limb survives, it is useless. It can follow arterial compression at any level from the axilla to the forearm.

The subclavian may be damaged by gunshot or other penetrating injury [17], or by a fractured clavicle (Fig. 13.8). In a young subject an acute, complete thrombosis should be well tolerated, for the collateral circulation at this level is very good. Chronic, progressive damage with incomplete obstruction is more serious; occurring later in life, it may give rise to repeated emboli, with worsening ischaemia as in cervical rib (*see* Chapter 12). Pulmonary embolism may also result from associated vein injury [17]. With closed injury, haemorrhage is fortunately a less common complication than occlusion, but may be highly dangerous when it does occur because of the large potential capacity of the open, injured pleura where bleeding may be missed, an

accident that is better known when this fracture perforates the subclavian vein. Control may be possible from the neck, otherwise the clavicle must be opened up or resected. With a more proximal injury, a flap of chest wall should be turned up; there need be no hesitation in making a median sternotomy with extension through the third intercostal space [84].

The axillary artery is close to the neck of the humerus in its lower course. Here, a dislocation or a fracture with much displacement may impale the artery. Exposure is direct and simple, and an early repair gives good results (Fig. 13.15). More proximally, the artery lies deep; the pectoral muscles must be divided to expose it. The cords of the brachial plexus may share in the injury.

Brachial artery injuries in the arm are the result of fractures of the humeral shaft, or of blunt violence to the inside of the arm. Left heart catheterisation can damage the artery in 10 to 12 per cent of cases (1A, 10B).

Lower down, near the bifurcation, the classic lesion is seen, in which a supracondylar fracture of the lower end of a child's humerus displaces backwards and pulls the artery against the sharp lower end of the proximal fragment (*see* Fig. 11.5, p. 204) producing severe local spasm or contusion, either of which will require operative treatment to ward off the onset of Volkmann's ischaemic contracture. (*See* Chapter 2, p. 19.)

Good results should follow the simpler measures for brachial spasm (*see* p. 239). If they fail, then arteriotomy is essential, and a reconstruction must be undertaken if internal damage is confirmed.

Extending thrombus in the forearm can be cleared out, either with a fine Fogarty catheter, or by flushing back through the radial artery at the wrist, which then can be repaired using 7/0 sutures. An embolectomy catheter may be used.

Intra-arterial Injection of Thiopentone

The files of the Medical Defence Union [29] contain nine cases of extravenous injection during the years 1961 to 1963. In six there was residual weakness, numbness or wasting, usually in the hand. The effects of an arterial injection can, however, be disastrous (Fig. 13.16). Factors that make an intra-arterial injection possible include:

(*a*) A superficial course of the ulnar artery at the elbow, [27] usual in cases of high bifurcation of the brachial.

(*b*) The use of thiopentone in strengths greater than $2\frac{1}{2}$ per cent [49].

(*c*) Uncertainty or haste on the part of the anaesthetist.

The pharmacology of this injury has been studied in rabbits [49]. The drug itself exerts serious irritant

251

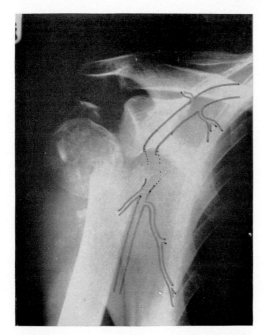
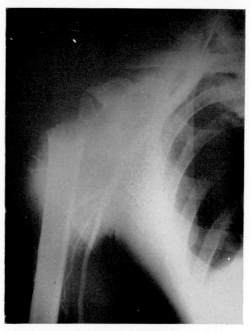

Fig. 13.15. Spike transection of the right axillary artery in a man aged sixty-five from lower fragment of a fractured dislocation of the shoulder. Immediate operation with excision of loose humeral head and repair of artery by end-to-end anastomosis was successful, and full arterial patency was retained eleven years after the accident (Mr Grahame Henson's case). The author has had a similar case due to simple dislocation, also repaired by simple anastomosis.

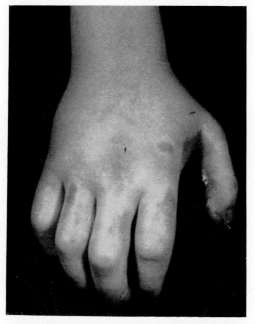
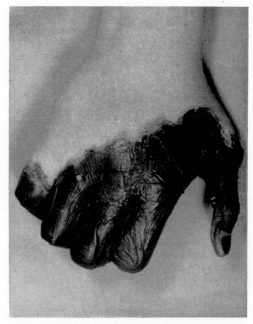

Fig. 13.16. Result of thiopentone injection into the right brachial artery in a young man undergoing sub-mucous resection of the nasal septum. Early acute ischaemia with muscle contracture; later, mummification and good recovery of circulation to line of demarcation. (Case as referred to Professor Rob.)

effects, and not through its alkalinity. It does, however, lead to the production of large amounts of catecholamines in the arterial and arteriolar walls, and it is these that close down the arterial tree, causing an acute intractable ischaemia. Previous administration of reserpine abolishes the mural concentration of adrenalin bodies and prevents the shut down. Intravascular deposition of microcrystals of thiopentone are now believed to play a part in the peripheral circulatory arrest [10A].

Clinical features [15] include severe burning pain in the hand within seconds of the injection. This is followed by intense vasoconstriction, which persists until stagnant, patchy cyanosis develops within three hours or so, or in the mild type of case, until a slow recovery of normal skin circulation is re-established. Hyperaemia is seen in the recovery phase, usually in the junctional areas between affected and normal skin. The radial pulse may at first persist; later it fades away and, finally, the artery can be felt as a thrombosed cord. Ischaemic muscle contracture occurs early as a grave sign. Swelling of the proximal part of the forearm is probably due to occlusion of the venous side. Finally, a black mummification of the extremity shows itself; its extent and the actual line of demarcation depends upon the degree and duration of the ischaemia and the site of the injection, according to which one of the antecubital arteries was punctured, most probably depending upon its anatomical plane in the subject concerned [15, 27]. There may be outlying patches of gangrene with swollen, unhealthy areas of skin between. The usual amputation in this condition is through the forearm, and often must be quite high. In a mild case with low dosage or after effective emergency treatment, recovery may be complete, though years later Raynaud's phenomenon may persist.

IMMEDIATE TREATMENT

As soon as the accident is suspected or recognised the following measures should be adopted:
1. Leave the needle in place.
2. Give 15,000 units (150 mg) heparin through it.
3. Abandon any but a life-saving operation.
4. Maintain the general circulation by treating shock or exposure.
5. Give reserpine 0·5 mg.

Other measures to be considered include brachial plexus block, which provides vasoconstrictor release and opens up arteriovenous shunts as well as relieving pain. Stellate ganglion block is less sure, and in the heparinised patient may cause hidden bleeding into the pleura, and hypotension, which may seriously affect the prognosis of the limb. Full sedation and a restful sleep assist recovery by allowing vasodilatation. Excessive reflex heating should be avoided. It is exhausting to the patient and there is little evidence that it helps.

Exploration of the artery is of debatable value. If done, it should be early. The object is to define, and if possible, relieve local arterial damage or thrombosis at the injection site: this could be of medico-legal importance if the patient was restless during the injection. If clinical examination localises the block at this point, operation is justified, the heparin need not be stopped, but subsequent oozing from the wound may require this, perhaps with adverse effects on the course of the condition.

At the stage of established thrombosis the problem differs little in its features or in its management from any other severe acute ischaemia. Heparin should be given by a continuous method (*see* Chapter 2).

The full extent of the damage may not be certain for a week or more; it is often less than seemed likely at the beginning.

The Severed Upper Limb [23A, 56B]

When an upper limb is cleanly transected or avulsed, and the patient is seen early, with the amputated part retrieved, wrapped up cleanly and still viable, the situation calls for opportunist action: reattachment or 'replantation' should be the treatment of choice.

Carrel and Guthrie showed this to be possible in experiments on the hind leg of small dogs [31]. They encountered the problem of massive early oedema, which was shown in modern experiments of the same kind [23] to be due to large plasma losses into the operated limb, producing fatal shock, the loss of plasma volume equalling the weight increase in the limb. The effect was most marked when the separation time exceeded six hours. This was also the time limit for muscle contractility, but nerves withstood

longer periods of ischaemia (*see also* Chapter 2). Cooling by perfusion may greatly extend the possible interval before replantation [91].

Before embarking upon this surgical *tour de force* in man, it must be considered whether the long and complex course of treatment will be justified by a real benefit to the patient, or whether a primary reamputation would better serve the purpose. The same decision may have to be taken after replantation, when an objective view of the problem may be difficult for the surgeon who may have achieved some limited success towards his objective.

At least forty cases are now on record, mostly from China and the USA]11, 37, 41, 52, 59, 61], and already several important technical points have emerged:

1. Provided the limb is kept cool and clean, there is no reason why a delay of up to six hours should not be compatible with successful replantation.

2. The severed arm should be taken to the operating theatre first, where it is cleaned and prepared for surgery. The line of section should be thoroughly excised, the limb being shortened, if necessary [11, 41], and the vessels milked free of thrombus, after which a brief perfusion with cold heparin saline is made.

3. Bone fixation has first priority as in simpler forms of arterial injury, for unless full stability of the limb is ensured, vascular repair will not succeed.

4. Re-union of the blood vessels is by whichever means is most familiar to the operator. Most often, this means suture anastomosis, preferably using the new, fine grades of silk or plastic, 6/0 or 7/0. Stapling has been used experimentally in Russia, but not, as yet, in any reported human replantation case. Simple intubation, using eversion-invagination over a polythene tube, succeeded in one of the Chinese cases. There is the need for haste if the ischaemic period should be nearing the six-hour limit. A simple technique is then valuable, and should even precede bone fixation. Coupling over a rigid ring is recommended for the venous union. It is quick, and prevents compression by the soft tissues by postoperative swelling. Success was also obtained after suture anastomosis of the veins. A local vascular defect can often be overcome by tension, cross-over anastomosis between radial and ulnar, or with the aid of

bone and soft tissue shortening. In avulsion cases, longer neurovascular defects are likely, and these may require grafting. Autogenous vein and nerve are recommended.

5. Primary suture of nerves is advisable when the division is clean. The best recoveries have followed this method. Severely contused soft tissue injury involving a length of nerve is better dealt with later, having marked the nerve ends with black silk.

6. Postoperative care and observation should be intensive. Elevation reduces the tendency to swelling. Heparin is a debatable adjunct, for it increases the swelling from continued oozing. Arterial patency may be adversely affected, but venous thrombosis is prevented (this may be the deciding factor). Experimentally, low molecular weight dextran infusion after operation reduced the incidence of venous as well as of arterial closure [23], and may be preferred to heparin in future. In this large series of dog-limb replantation operations in which it was employed there was a negligible incidence of vascular occlusion.

In this new field of traumatic surgery most things depend upon the nature of the injury; for the rest, patience and resolution on the part of surgeon and patient should, as in the more established field of renal transplantation, and also with the revascularised colon transplant to the cervical oesophagus (*see* Chapter 17, p. 385), bring rewarding success sufficiently often to make the undertaking worth while.

REFERENCES

1. Annetts, D. L., Harris, J. D., Jepson, R. P., Ludbrook, J., Miller, J. H. and Tracy, G. D. (1970) Arterial injuries in civil practice. *Aust. N.Z. J. Surg.*, **39**, 340.

1A. Armstrong, P. W. and Parker, J. O. (1971) The complications of brachial arteriotomy. *J. thorac. cardiovasc. Surg.*, **61**, 424.

2. Barrett, N. R. (1950) Foreign bodies in the cardiovascular system. *Brit. J. Surg.*, **37**, 416.

3. Beall, A. C. (1960) Penetrating wounds of the aorta. *Amer. J. Surg.*, **99**, 770.

4. Bell, J. W. (1962) Treatment of post-catheterization arterial injuries. *Ann. Surg.*, **155**, 591.

4A. Bengmark, S. and Rosengren, K. (1970) Angiographic study of the collateral circulation to the liver after ligation of the hepatic artery in man. *Amer. J. Surg.*, **119**, 620.

5. Benjamin, A. (1957) The relief of traumatic arterial spasm in threatened Volkmann's ischaemic contracture. *J. Bone Jt Surg.*, **39B**, 711.

6. Bergentz, S.-E., Hansson, L. O. and Norbäck, B. (1966) Surgical management of complications to arterial puncture. *Ann. Surg.*, **164**, 1021.

7. Berk, M. E. (1963) Arteriography in peripheral trauma. *Clin. Radiol.*, **14**, 235.

7A. Biller, H. F. and Ebert, P. A. (1970) Innominate artery haemorrhage complicating tracheotomy. *Ann. Otol.*, **69**, 301.

7B. Billy, L. J., Amato, J. J. and Rich, N. M. (1971) Aortic injuries in Viet Nam. *Surgery*, **70**, 355.

8. Blazek, J. V. (1965) Acute traumatic rupture of the thoracic aorta demonstrated by retrograde aortography. *Radiology*, **85**, 253.

9. Bonney, G. (1963) Thrombosis of the femoral artery complicating fracture of the femur. *J. Bone Jt Surg.*, **45B**, 344.

9A. Brewer, P. L., Schramel, R. J., Menendez, C. V. and Creech, O. (1969) Injuries of the popliteal artery; a report of sixteen cases. *Amer. J. Surg.*, **118**, 36.

10. Bromley, L. L., Hobbs, J. T. and Robinson, R. E. (1965) Early repair of traumatic rupture of the thoracic aorta. *Brit. med. J.*, **ii**, 17.

10A. Brown, S. S., Lyons, S. M. and Dundee, J. (1968) Intra-arterial barbiturates. A study of some factors leading to intravascular thrombosis. *Brit. J. Anaesth.*, **40**, 13.

10B.Campion, B. C., Frye, R. L., Pluth, J. R., Fairburn, J. F. and Davis, G. D. (1971) Arterial complications of retrograde brachial arterial catheterisation. *Mayo Clin. Proc.*, **46**, 589.

11. Ch'en, C., Ch'ien, Y., Pao, Y., Lin, Y. and Lin, C. (1965) Further experiences in the restoration of amputated limbs. *Chinese med. J.*, **84**, 225.

12. Clark, P. M. and Keokarn, T. (1965) Popliteal aneurysm complicating benign osteocartilaginous exostosis: review of the literature and report of one case. *J. Bone Jt Surg.*, **47A**, 1386.

13. Clarke, D. B. (1964) Traumatic aneurysm of the innominate artery at its origin from the aortic arch. *Brit. J. Surg.*, **51**, 668.

14. Coenen, H. (1913) *Verh. dtsch. Ges. Chir.*, **42**, 54, 116.

14A.Cohen, A., Baldwin, J. N. and Grant, R. N. (1969) Problems in the management of battlefield vascular injuries. *Amer. J. Surg.*, **118**, 526.

14B.Cohen, A., Brief, D. and Mathewson, C. (1970) Carotid artery injuries; an analysis of 85 cases. *Amer. J. Surg.*, **120**, 210.

15. Cohen, S. M. (1948) Accidental intra-arterial injection of drugs. *Lancet*, **ii**, 361, 409.

16. Collins, H. A. and Jacobs, J. K. (1961) Acute arterial injuries due to blunt trauma. *J. Bone Jt Surg.*, **43A**, 193.

17. Cook, F. W. and Haller, J. A. (1962) Penetrating injuries of the subclavian vessels with associated venous complications. *Ann. Surg.*, **155**, 370.

18. Cooper, F. W., Harris, M. H. and Kahn, J. W. (1948) Ligation and division of the abdominal aorta for metallic embolus from the heart. *Ann. Surg.*, **127**, 1.

19. Dameron, T. B. (1964) False aneurysm of femoral profundus artery resulting from internal fixation device (screw). *J. Bone Jt Surg.*, **46A**, 577.

19A.David, D. and Blumenberg, R. M. (1970) Subintimal aortic dissection with occlusion after blunt abdominal trauma. *Arch. Surg.*, **100**, 302.

20. DeBakey, M. E. and Simeone, F. A. (1946) Battle injuries of the arteries in World War II. *Ann. Surg.*, **123**, 534.

21. Dillard, B. M. and Staple, T. W. (1968) Bullet embolism from the aortic arch to the popliteal artery. *Arch Surg.*, **98**, 326.

21A.Drapanas, T., Hewitt, R. L., Weichert, R. F. and Smith, A. D. (1970) Civilian vascular injuries, a critical appraisal of three decades of management. *Ann. Surg.*, **172**, 351.

22. Dundee, J. W. (1967) Emergency treatment of tracheotomy haemorrhage. Personal communication. To be published.

22A.Eastcott, H. H. G. and Martin, P. G. C. (1971) Sclerosant injection for varicose veins. *Brit. med. J.*, **4**, 555.

23. Eiken, O., Nabseth, D. C., Mayer, R. F. and Deterling, R. A. (1964) Limb replantation: I. The technique and immediate results; II. The pathophysiological effects; III. Long-term evaluation. *Arch. Surg.*, **88**, 48, 54, 66.

23A.Engber, W. D. and Hardin, C. A. (1971) Replantation of extremities. *Surg. Gynec. Obstet.*, **132**, 901.

24. Fairbank, T. J. and Jamieson, E. S. (1951) A complication of lateral meniscectomy. *J. Bone Jt Surg.*, **33B**, 567.

25. Fogarty, T. J. and Krippaehne, W. W. (1965) Vascular occlusion following arterial catheterization. *Surg. Gynec. Obstet.*, **121**, 1295.

25A.Freeark, R. J. (1969) Role of angiography in the management of multiple injuries. *Surg. Gynec. Obstet.*, **128**, 761.

26. Furler, I. K., Robertson, D. N. S., Harris, H. J. and Pryer, R. R. L. (1962) Spontaneous rupture of the splenic artery in pregnancy. *Lancet*, **ii**, 588.

27. Gagnon, R. (1966) Superficial arteries of the cubital fossa with reference to accidental intra-arterial injections. *Canad. J. Surg.*, **9**, 57.

28. Gerbode, F., Braimbridge, M., Osborn, J. J., Hood, M. and French, S. (1957) Traumatic thoracic aneurysms: treatment by resection and grafting with the use of an extracorporeal bypass. *Surgery*, **42**, 975.

28A.Grablowsky, O. M., Weichert, R. F., Goff, J. B. and Schlegel, J. H. (1970) Renal artery thrombosis following blunt trauma: report of four cases. *Surgery*, **67**, 895.

29. Gray, C. J. and Robb, D. (1967) Extravenous injection of thiopentone. Personal communication.

30. Gryska, P. F. (1962) Major vascular injuries. Principles of management in selected cases of arterial and venous injury. *New Eng. J. Med.*, **266**, 381.

31. Guthrie, C. C. (1912) *Blood Vessel Surgery and Its Applications*. A reprint (1959) (Ed. Harbison, S. P. and Fisher, B.) University of Pittsburg Press. Pittsburgh, Pennsylvania.

31A.Hall, R. (1971) Vascular injuries resulting from arterial puncture or catheterisation. *Brit. J. Surg.*, **58**, 513.

32. Haller, J. A. (1962) Bullet transection of both common carotid arteries with immediate repair and survival. *Amer. J. Surg.*, **103**, 532.

33. Hallowell, (1761) Cited by Lambert, in *Observations on Aneuryism.* (Ed. Erichsen, J. E.) London: Sydenham Society, 1844, p. 265.

34. Hanlon, C. R., Paletta, F. X., Cooper, T. and Willman, V. L. (1965) Acute arterial occlusion in the lower limb. Clinical and experimental studies of muscular ischemia. *J. Cardiovasc. Surg.*, **6**, 11.

35. Hardy, E. G. and Tibbs, D. J. (1960) Acute ischaemia in limb injuries. *Brit. med. J.*, **i**, 1001.

36. Harty, M. and Kostowiecki, M. (1965) Vascular injuries in limb surgery. *Surg. Gynec. Obstet.*, **121**, 339.

36A.Hewitt, R. L. and Grablowsky, O. M. (1970) Acute dissecting aneurysm of abdominal aorta. *Ann. Surg.*, **171**, 160.

37. Horn, J. S. (1964) Successful reattachment of a completely severed forearm. *Lancet*, **i**, 1152.

38. Howard, F. M. and Shafer, S. J. (1965) Injuries to the clavicle with neurovascular complications: a study of fourteen cases. *J. Bone Jt Surg.*, **47A**, 1335.

39. Hughes, C. W. (1958) Arterial repair during the Korean War. *Ann. Surg.*, **147**, 555.

40. Hughes, C. W. and Bowers, W. F. (1961) *Traumatic*

Lesions of Peripheral Vessels. Springfield, Illinois: Charles C. Thomas.

41. Huang, C., Li, P. and Kong, G. (1965) Successful restoration of a traumatic amputated leg. *Chinese med. J.*, **84**, 641.

41A. Hunt, T. K., Blaisdell, E. W. and Okimoto, J. (1969) Vascular injuries at base of neck. *Arch. Surg.*, **98**, 586.

42. Imamoglu, K., Read, R. C. and Huebl, H. C. (1967) Cervicomediastinal vascular injury. *Surgery*, **61**, 274.

43. Inahara, T. (1962) Arterial injuries of the upper extremity. *Surgery*, **51**, 605.

44. Iskeceli, O. K. (1962) Bullet embolus of the left femoral artery. *Arch. Surg.*, **85**, 184.

45. Jahnke, E. J. (1958) Late structural and functional results of arterial injuries primarily repaired. *Surgery*, **43**, 175.

46. Jahnke, E. J., Fisher, G. W. and Jones, R. C. (1964) Acute traumatic rupture of the thoracic aorta. Report of six consecutive cases of successful early repair. *J. Thorac. Cardiovasc. Surg.*, **48**, 63.

46A. Jamieson, C. W., Goodwin, D. P., Storrs, J. A. and Bromley, L. L. (1970) Emergency by-pass of the thoracic aorta. Experimental evaluation of a simple method. *Brit. J. Surg.*, **57**, 661.

47. Jones, T. W., Vetto, R. R., Winterscheid, L. C., Dillard, D. H. and Merendino, K. A. (1960) Arterial complications incident to cannulation in open-heart surgery, with special reference to the femoral artery. *Ann. Surg.*, **152**, 969.

48. Killen, D. A. (1964) Injury of the superior mesenteric vessels secondary to nonpenetrating abdominal trauma. *Amer. Surg.*, **30**, 306.

49. Kinmonth, J. B. and Shepherd, R. C. (1959) Accidental injection of thiopentone into arteries. Studies of pathology and treatment. *Brit. med. J.*, **ii**, 914.

50. Kinmonth, J. B., Hadfield, G. J., Connolly, J. E., Lee, R. H. and Amoroso, E. C. (1956) Traumatic arterial spasm. Its relief in man and in monkeys. *Brit. J. Surg.*, **44**, 164.

51. Kirkup, J. R. (1963) Major arterial injury complicating fracture of the femoral shaft. *J. Bone Jt Surg.*, **45B**, 337.

52. Kleinert, H. E., Kasdan, M. L. and Romero, J. L. (1963) Small blood-vessel anastomosis for salvage of severely injured upper extremity. *J. Bone Jt Surg.*, **45A**, 788.

52A. Kloster, F. E., Bristow, J. D. and Griswold, H. E. (1970) Femoral artery occlusion following percutaneous catheterisation. *Amer. Heart J.*, **79**, 175.

52B. Larrey, D. J. (Baron) (1798) cited by Dible, J. H., in *Napoleon's Surgeon*. London: Heinemann (1970), p. 142.

53. Lenzenweger, F. (1965) Hepatic-artery reconstruction. *Lancet*, **i**, 21.

54. Lexer, E. (1912) 1, Zur Gesichtsplastik. 2, Gefässplastik. *Verh. dtsch. Ges. Chir.*, **41**, 132.

55. Lexer, E. (1913) Ideale Aneurysmaoperation und Gefässtransplantation. *Verh. dtsch. Ges. Chir.*, **42**, 113.

55A. Lucas, R. J., Tumacder, O. and Wilson, G. S. (1971) Hepatic artery occlusion following hepatic artery catheterisation. *Ann. Surg.*, **173**, 238.

56. Lumpkin, M. B., Logan, W. D., Couves, C. M. and Howard, J. M. (1958) Arteriography as an aid in the diagnosis and localization of acute arterial injuries, *Ann. Surg.*, **147**, 353.

56A. MacGowan, W. A. L., Holland, P. D. J., Browne, H. I. and Byrnes, D. P. (1972) The local effects of intra-arterial injections of sodium tetradecyl sulphate (S.T.D.) 3 per cent. *Brit. J. Surg.*, **59**, 101.

56B. McNeill, I. F. and Wilson, J. S. P. (1970) The problem of limb replacement. *Brit. J. Surg.*, **57**, 365.

57. Makin, G. S., Howard, J. M. and Green, R. L. (1966) Arterial injuries complicating fractures or dislocations: the necessity for a more aggressive approach. *Surgery*, **59**, 203.

58. Makins, G. H. (1919) *On Gunshot Injuries to the Blood-vessels*. Bristol: John Wright & Sons.

59. Malt, R. A. and McKhann, C. F. (1964) Replantation of severed arms. *J. Amer. med. Assoc.*, **189**, 716.

60. Martorell, R. (1963) Spontaneous rupture of the superior mesenteric artery. *Ann. Surg.*, **157**, 292.

61. Mathiesen, F. R. and Gammelgaard, A. (1963) Traumatic arterial injuries. *J. Cardiovasc. Surg.*, **4**, 308.

62. May, A. G., Lipchik, E. O. and DeWeese, J. A. (1965) Repair of hepatic and superior mesenteric artery injury. *Ann. Surg.*, **162**, 869.

63. Morris, G. C., Creech, O. and DeBakey, M. E. (1957) Acute arterial injuries in civilian practice. *Amer. J. Surg.*, **93**, 565.

64. Murphy, J. B. (1897) Resection of arteries and veins injured in continuity. End-to-end suture. Experimental and clinical research. *Med. Rec.*, **51**, 73.

65. Murray, G. (1940) Heparin in surgical treatment of blood vessels. *Arch. Surg.*, **40**, 307.

66. Mustard, W. T. and Bull, C. (1962) A reliable method for relief of traumatic vascular spasm. *Ann. Surg.*, **155**, 339.

67. Nelson, D. A. and Ashley, P. F. (1965) Rupture of the aorta during closed-chest cardiac massage. *J. Amer. med. Assoc.*, **193**, 681.

68. Newby, J. P., Gesink, M. H. and Newman, M. M. (1966) Post-traumatic acquired coarctation of the descending thoracic aorta. *J. Thorac. Cardiovasc. Surg.*, **51**, 883.

69. Ngu, V. A. and Konstam, P. G. (1965) Traumatic dissecting aneurysm of the abdominal aorta. *Brit. J. Surg.*, **52**, 981.

70. Ochsner, J. L. and Zuber, W. (1963) Immediate repair of penetrating wounds of the thoracic aorta. *J. Amer. med. Assoc.*, **186**, 1170.

71. Owen, R. and Tsimboukis, B. (1965) Incidence of ischaemic contracture following closed injuries to the calf. *J. Bone Jt. Surg.*, **47B**, 184.

72. Parmley, L. F., Mattingly, T. W., Manion, W. C. and Jahnke, E. J. (1958) Nonpenetrating traumatic injury of the aorta. *Circulation*, **17**, 1086.

73. Patman, R. D., Poulos, E. and Shires, G. T. (1964) The management of civilian arterial injuries. *Surg. Gynec. Obstet.*, **118**, 725.

73A. Patman, R. D. and Thompson, J. E. (1970) Fasciotomy in peripheral arterial injury. *Arch. Surg.*, **101**, 663.

74. Patrick, J. (1963) Aneurysm of the popliteal vessels after meniscectomy. *J. Bone Jt Surg.*, **45B**, 570.

74A. Plengvanit, V., Chearanai, K., Damroksak, D., Tuchinda, S. and Viranuvatti, V. (1972) Collateral blood supply to the liver after hepatic artery ligation; angiographic study of 20 patients. *Ann. Surg.*, **175**, 105.

74B. Powley, P. H. (1971) Ventriculo-aortic shunt for traumatic rupture of the aorta. *Proc. Roy. Soc. Med.*, **64**, 1085.

75. Pringle, J. H. (1913) Two cases of vein grafting for the maintenance of a direct arterial circulation. *Lancet*, **i**, 1795.

75A. Rich, N. M., Baugh, J. H. and Hughes, C. W. (1969) Popliteal artery injuries in Viet Nam. *Amer. J. Surg.*, **118**, 531.

75B. Rich, N. M., Baugh, J. H. and Hughes, C. W. (1970) Acute arterial injuries in Viet Nam: 1,000 cases. *J. Trauma*, **10**, 359.

75C. Rienhoff, W. F. (1951) Ligation of hepatic and splenic arteries in treatment of portal hypertension with report of 6 cases; preliminary report. *Bull. Johns Hopkins Hosp.*, **88**, 368.

75D. Risley, T. S. and McClerkin, W. W. (1971) Bullet transection of both carotid arteries. Delayed repair with recovery. *Amer. J. Surg.*, **121**, 385.

76. Rob, C. G. and Standeven, A. (1956) Closed traumatic lesions of the axillary and brachial arteries. *Lancet*, **i**, 597.

77. Rojas, R. H., Levitsky, S. and Stansel, H. C. (1966) Acute traumatic subclavian steal syndrome. *J. Thorac. Cardiovasc. Surg.*, **51**, 113.

78. Silen, W. and Spieker, D. (1965) Fatal hemorrhage from the innominate artery after tracheostomy. *Ann. Surg.*, **162**, 1005.

79. Sinkler, W. H. and Spencer, A. D. (1960) The value of peripheral arteriography in assessing acute vascular injuries. *Arch. Surg.*, **80**, 300.

79A. Slaney, G. and Ashton, F. (1971) Arterial injuries and their management. *Postgrad. med. J.*, **47**, 257.

79B. Smith, R. F., Szilyagi, D. E. and Elliott, J. P. (1969) Fracture of the long bones with arterial injury due to blunt trauma. *Arch. Surg.*, **99**, 315.

80. Spencer, F. C., Guerin, P. F., Blake, H. A. and Bahnson, H. T. (1961) A report of 15 patients with traumatic rupture of the thoracic aorta. *J. Thorac. Cardiovasc. Surg.*, **41**, 1.

81. Soubbotitch, V. (1913) Military experiences of traumatic aneurysms. *Lancet*, **ii**, 720.

82. Subbotitch, V. (1914) Kriegschirurgische Erfahrungen über traumatische Aneurysmen. *Dtsch. Z. Chir.*, **127**, 446.

83. Stanford, W., Crosby, V. G., Pike, J. D. and Lawrence, M. S. (1967) Gunshot wounds of the thoracic aorta with peripheral embolization of the missile. *Ann. Surg.*, **165**, 139.

83A. Steel, H. H., Sandrow, R. E. and Sullivan, P. D. (1971) Complications of tibial osteotomy in children for genu varum or valgum. Evidence that neurological complications are due to ischaemia. *J. Bone Jt. Surg.*, **53A**, 1629.

84. Steenburg, R. W. and Ravitch, M. M. (1963) Cervico-thoracic approach for subclavian vessel injury from compound fracture of the clavicle: considerations of subclavian-axillary exposures. *Ann. Surg.*, **157**, 839.

85. Steiness, I. and Thaysen, J. H. (1965) Bilateral traumatic renal-artery thrombosis. *Lancet*, **i**, 527.

86. Stiles, P. J. (1965) Closed injuries of the iliac arteries. *J. Bone Jt. Surg.*, **47B**, 507.

87. Stoney, R. J., Roe, B. B. and Redington, J. V. (1964) Rupture of thoracic aorta due to closed-chest trauma. *Arch. Surg.*, **89**, 840.

87A. Symbas, P. N. and Sehdera, J. S. (1970) Penetrating wounds of the thoracic aorta. *Ann. Surg.*, **171**, 441.

87B. Symposium on Traumatic Injuries of the Great Vessels of the Chest (1971). *J. Cardiovasc. Surg.*, **12**, 83.

88. Teare, D. (1951) Post-mortem examinations on air-crash victims. *Brit. med. J.*, **ii**, 707.

89. Weglowski, R. (1925) Über die Gefässtransplantation. *Zentbl. Chir.*, **52**, ii, 2241.

90. Watson-Jones, R. (1955) *Fractures and Joint Injuries*, Vol. 1. 4th Edn., pp. 118–9. Edinburgh: E. & S. Livingstone.

90A. Waugh, W. (1972) Popliteal artery thrombosis following tibial osteotomy. Personal communication.

90B. Whittaker, D. and Williams, E. (1971) Femoral and tibial fractures combined with injuries to the femoral or popliteal artery. A review of the literature and analysis of 14 cases. *J. Bone Jt. Surg.*, **53A**, 56.

91. Worman, L. W., Darin, J. C. and Kritter, A. E. (1965) The anatomy of a limb replantation failure. *Arch. Surg.*, **91**, 211.

14 Embolism

Since the late seventeenth century it has been known that material formed in the heart may break away and lodge in the neck or limb arteries [21a] and for at least 150 years the association between heart disease and peripheral gangrene has been explained in this way [21a]. Virchow introduced the term 'embolus' (i.e. 'something thrown in'), and showed that not only thrombus but other preformed bodies could be propelled to the distant vessels and impact at a point where the width of the lumen would hold it loosely in place, there to become the starting point for a new thrombus, formed locally [21a].

Emphasis has always been upon those patients in whom the ischaemia came on suddenly and progressed to massive gangrene. Attempts to avert this catastrophe by removal of the obstruction were sporadic and mainly unsuccessful, for it was not until the early years of the twentieth century (*see* p. 266) that modern methods of arterial repair could be applied, and even then with only limited success, to what had come to be considered a matter for surgical virtuosity and good luck. Until quite recently this view was still fairly generally held and taught. As late as 1960, a Hunterian Lecturer stated (in an otherwise valuable contribution) that it was a never-failing source of wonder to him that with so few worthwhile results in the published literature the operation was so widely practised [36]; while in 1958, in the United States, the view was expressed that even the diagnosis of embolism was irrelevant because embolectomy was of no practical value [57].

Today, the picture has changed: embolectomy is accepted and is routine for the major arteries with 'success to be expected, and failure explained' [4]. General surgeons everywhere have become familiar with the technique of arterial suture, and extended clearing methods for secondary clot have brought good results on an increasing scale.

Another new development is an understanding of the reasons for the common occurrence of silent embolus, and the features of late ischaemia in a viable limb that make for success or serious general complications after late surgical intervention.

Cardiac and Other Causes of Embolism

Most patients with arterial embolism have serious heart disease; in fact, many are already in hospital under medical treatment for cardiac failure [11]. Some patients who are well compensated and able to get about in their homes develop emboli of the same size and in the same situation without symptoms of any kind, remembering nothing wrong with a limb which later, on routine examination, is found to have a major pulse missing. This was so in 27 per cent of Jacobs's series of patients with mitral stenosis and atrial fibrillation [21b]. Such a condition of 'silent embolism' has been known for many years [18, 29] though only recently has it been recognised as common. Even the aortic bifurcation may be chronically occluded in this way [49] in middle-aged or younger patients with good collaterals.

The following are the heart conditions most often complicated by embolism.

1. *Rheumatic mitral stenosis*, usually with atrial fibrillation. The thrombus forms in the atrium, and a loose portion breaks away. Patients with a large atrial appendage may be more likely to develop embolism [48], and saddle embolus of the aortic bifurcation is commoner in rheumatic than in ischaemic heart disease. There is a known association with over-digitalisation [21c]. Too vigorous treatment with diuretics may cause haemoconcentration, increased blood viscosity, and a raised fibrinogen level [13], all of which also favour thrombo-embolic complications. During and after mitral valvotomy the risk is increased (Fig. 14.1).

2. *Ischaemic heart disease*, often with recent myocardial infarction (Fig. 14.2), which may have been silent [36], with the embolism as the first sign that anything is wrong. Later, embolism may complicate persistent atrial fibrillation or a ventricular aneurysm [58]. In some centres, coronary thrombosis is almost as common a cause as rheumatic heart disease [4, 51]; the prognosis is worse in this arteriosclerotic group [4, 36, 46] but, of course, they are older.

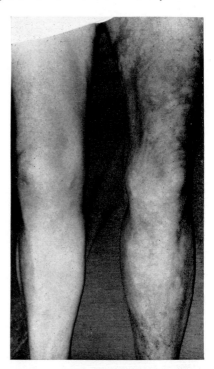

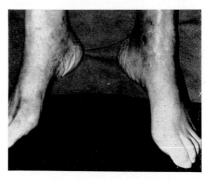

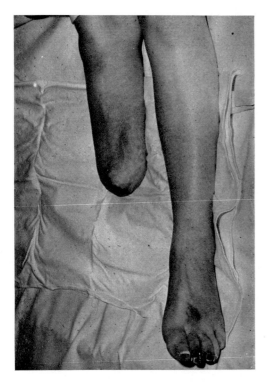

Fig. 14.1. Bilateral embolism following mitral valvotomy. Necrosis of amputation skin flaps and severe ischaemia of remaining limb fourteen days after thorocotomy. Swelling and rubor extend to mid-calf level, with ischaemic contracture of the calf, and the commonly seen anterior skin staining on both sides. (*See also* Fig. 2.3, p. 22 and Fig. 10.8, p. 197.) In these young and middle-aged rheumatic subjects, general recovery is common, but often with limb-loss.

Fig. 14.2. Common iliac embolus on left, following a major cardiac infarct. There is waxy pallor of the left fore-foot and cyanosis of most of the remainder of the limb. Duration uncertain, but limb recovery still possible for there was no ischaemic contracture. Embolectomy restored the circulation at once, but the patient died a few days later of his heart condition. Another typical case contrasting in its prognosis with that of the patient shown in Fig. 14.1.

3. *Other causes of atrial fibrillation* including hypertensive heart disease, with or without cardiac infarction [21*d*] and thyrotoxicosis.

4. *Subacute bacterial endocarditis* produces multiple arterial emboli, most of which are small, although in as many as 33 per cent of patients [42] larger fragments may become detached and may occlude as large an artery as the internal carotid artery at its origin and the common femoral bifurcation, as in the case reported in Chapter 7, page 135. Plastic heart-valve prostheses are frequently complicated by embolism from adherent thrombus.

5. *Less common cardiac causes* include atrial myxoma, and paradoxical embolus from a lower limb [15B]. Thrombus migrating from a patent ductus may cause massive lower limb ischaemia in childhood [16A].

6. *Iatrogenic emboli* into the vertebral artery from irrigation of a clotted forearm Scribner shunt [15A]; cotton fibres reaching brain, kidney or gut after arteriography [23A]; and mercury in the finger tips after brachial manometry [3A].

7. *Peripheral arterial disease.* Mural thromboembolism is a basic mechanism of progressive disease of almost every kind, and as such, therefore, probably the commonest type of arterial embolism.

The Time Factor, Collateral Circulation, and Limb Survival. The outcome in peripheral arterial embolism is determined by the rate at which the collateral circulation extends distally. Once the extremity is perfused again, however sluggishly, there is an increasing chance that it will survive.

Recovery becomes a race between the time of onset of tissue disintegration at the periphery and relief provided by the arrival of a returning proximal collateral circulation. A familiar instance of this in everyday experience is the recovering lower limb, in which at each examination the lowest limit of skin warmth extends farther down the limb, yet meanwhile the toes are showing a steady deterioration from blue to black discoloration, until by the time the extremity is hard and mummified, the skin across the line of demarcation may be quite hot.

In other patients the race never begins. There is little sign of any attempt to open up collateral channels, and massive gangrene occurs early, sometimes with evident deep venous thrombosis as an indication that the circulation in the limb has totally failed [36].

It is usual to blame consecutive thrombosis in the main artery for this, but there is little to show that spreading arterial thrombosis is any more a cause of the gangrene than the venous occlusion in these advanced cases; both are more likely to be the effect rather than the cause.

In some amputated limbs, in early acute ischaemia

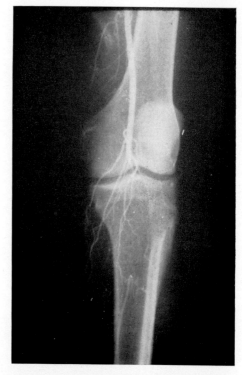

Fig. 14.3. Left popliteal embolism in a girl aged nineteen with mitral stenosis. Surgery was refused for both conditions until below-knee amputation was needed for control of pain. Thereafter, a good recovery, generally, with mitral valvotomy.

in ill patients, there is little consecutive thrombus to be found [21*f*]. Yet bleeding from the line of section is minimal, so that in these fulminating cases central haemodynamic factors must play the major part.

In a fitter, younger patient, recent exertion, though it may not actually cause the embolism [21*e*], could certainly aggravate its peripheral effects; this might explain the unexpected severity of some relatively minor emboli early in life (Fig. 14.3).

Probably, the issue is mainly decided by the state of the general circulation during the hours that follow the embolism. Absence of consecutive thrombosis may mean that asphyxia is too severe for normal clot formation, or that formed clot may have been removed by increased fibrinolysis due to acidosis in the ischaemic area. Patients with good limb recovery have shown extensive and even multiple occlusions [21*f*]. This, of course, does not mean that the limb might not have been even better if such obstructions had been removed.

Table 14.1. Site of Impaction (per cent) of 2,237 Cases of Arterial Embolism

	Key	Haimovici	Warren et al.	Metcalfe	Young et al.	Martin et al.	Cranley et al.	Thompson et al.	Fogarty et al.
	1936	1950	1954	1960	1963	1969	1970	1970	1971
	[24]	[18]	[55]	[36]	[58]	[35A]	[9A]	[50A]	[14A]
Axillary	11·8	4·5	17·5	—	4·0	4·0	5·0	6·4	—
Brachial	—	9·1	—	—	12·0	9·0	5·0	6·4	3·0
Aortic	4·5	9·1	9·0	22·0	19·0	7·0	10·0	9·4	15·2
Iliac	17·3	16·6	9·0	7·0	19·0	14·0	19·0	18·7	19·8
Femoral	54·5	38·5	23·7	45·0	30·0	45·0	56·0	41·9	50·0
Popliteal	11·3	14·2	9·8	19·0	15·0	21·0	5·0	13·8	12·0
Total cases	382	330	200	270	134	88	300	203	330

Site of Embolism

Most emboli lodge at the opening of a large branch or bifurcation. At these places the diameter of the main artery diminishes at once in proportion to the size of the branch. The bifurcations of the aorta, common femoral, and popliteal are the commonest sites for an arterial embolism to come to rest, though the force of the pulse beat may break the embolus into two or more smaller fragments which then are free to pass down the branches; thus, the signs of a saddle embolus may change to those of bilateral obstruction farther down both lower limbs. This, incidentally, is the most acceptable explanation of the condition of 'pseudo-embolism'.

Table 14.1 shows the anatomical distribution of the sites involved in 2,237 cases from the literature. Femoral emboli are the commonest in almost all reported series, with the iliac next, and then the aortic bifurcation. The smaller arteries do not figure prominently in these series, perhaps because at these sites embolism is often silent. They may be the commonest of all [21b].

Clinical Features of Arterial Embolism

Few subjects in the field of vascular disease are more beset with traditional error, confusion, and myth than this. It is still taught that embolism is necessarily attended by sudden acute pain, and is always followed by a sequence of specific appearances; that the diagnosis, in fact, rests upon the study of the affected limb.

We cannot dispel these misconceptions better than in the words of Sir Thomas Lewis:

'So far as is known there is no difference between the symptomatology of embolic and of thrombotic obstruction of an artery. With very few exceptions the symptoms and objective manifestations of both forms of obstruction are the direct or indirect results of ischaemia.'

Recognition of embolism, therefore, depends upon the elicitation of a cause for its occurrence; in most instances this is some serious cardiac condition. Pain will occur with muscular movement, but if the patient is at rest, or as is common, asleep at the moment of embolism, he will not be disturbed. The first effect of which he will be aware will be the numbness which soon comes with impaired nerve conduction in all acute ischaemic states (*see* Chapter 2).

With restlessness or alarm, ischaemic muscle pain may become intense, but mostly it remains as a continuous severe aching. Lewis pointed out that 'pins and needles' seldom occurred in complete ischaemia, but with a slight inflow. This is the state of most limbs in clinical ischaemic states.

Muscular weakness is usually noticed, and is an early symptom. With the numbness that accompanies it, and loss of use of the toes or fingers, it is often described as 'deadness' by the patient. These complaints should be taken as clear warning that severe ischaemia may be present, and such a message should ensure an emergency visit from the responsible doctor and a thorough examination in a good light, for this feeling of deadness, if it persists, may be followed by actual death of tissues in the part affected.

Pallor, which is waxy, or corpse-like (Fig. 14.2), is an early sign on inspection and is accompanied by collapse of the superficial veins, shown only as thin blue lines beneath the pale skin, which may be depressed into a linear groove over the larger channels. Stroking the line of the vein displaces no blood, and none returns into this segment from either end.

Anaesthesia is confirmed by gentle pin-prick testing. It is of the stocking type, without relation to the territory of the cutaneous nerves or nerve roots. Nerve tissue is the most sensitive indicator of local anoxia. There is strong correlation between the presence or absence of skin sensation and the subsequent life or death of the part [4].

Pulses are absent, by definition, with a few unimportant exceptions (*see* p. 263).

This is the stage at which the diagnosis of peripheral embolism must be made, for unless regression of pallor and anaesthesia begins within two hours of their onset, some death of tissue is certain without positive action [21].

The later features are easy to recognise, but are of mainly descriptive interest, though they do provide a guide in deciding the level of the amputation which by now will certainly be needed. These features include:

(*a*) *Ischaemic muscle contracture*, which is usual in all but the most peripheral occlusions. It appears, as a rule, early on the second day, and though it may at first involve only the toes or fingers, and thus be missed because of the preceding stage of weakness or the inhibiting effect of pain, soon the calf or forearm muscles become prominently contracted and very tender under the cold skin. Often, the anterior tibial compartment alone is affected [15, 33] (Fig. 2.3, p. 22); this happens in the recovering case with incomplete return of the collateral circulation, or after successful embolectomy in a fairly advanced case [33], when it is usually followed by a drop foot (Fig. 2.2*a*, p. 20).

(*b*) *Patchy cyanosis* of the previously pallid area means certain skin loss. It often becomes confluent into a true post-mortem lividity. Blisters may form in the agonal stages where some feeble skin circulation persists or has returned too late.

(*c*) *Gangrene* is either dry or moist according to the severity and rapidity of the necrosis, which depends upon the degree of collateral return and, to some extent, upon the patency of the venous side of the circulation. In late cases with delayed recovery of the accessory circulation, the skin may be warm and pink quite close or even right up to the line of demarcation, even though ischaemic muscle may be felt beneath. In this event the overlying skin may actually achieve inflammatory vasodilatation. Such an appearance should suggest to the examiner that embolectomy during the earlier, acute stage might have saved the limb.

Differential Diagnosis

This should not be difficult. Other causes of acute limb ischaemia present special features, which have already been described in Chapter 2 (p. 23). The main conditions that resemble embolism are:

1. *Acute arterial thrombosis*, which occurs mostly in a previously fit subject without evidence of cardiac disability, though arteriosclerotic signs may be present in other parts of the body.

2. *Dissecting aneurysm* sometimes produces an acute pulseless ischaemia of one lower limb soon after the onset of severe pain in the chest and abdomen. This may be confused with femoral embolism following a myocardial infarction, but in this, the history is longer and there is no clinical or X-ray evidence of aortic widening or leakage in the mediastinum, the usual finding in dissecting aneurysm, in which also hypertension, the underlying cause, often persists into the acute illness. The electrocardiogram is usually helpful.

3. *Venous gangrene* (*phlegmasia cerulea dolens*) is often sudden in onset in an ill patient, but the ischaemia is congestive with much early swelling and oedema, blistering, and also increased heat. Waxy pallor never occurs. A white form is commoner in the puerperium (phlegmasia alba dolens) and there may possibly be an element of arterial insufficiency here, from reflex vasospasm in smaller vessels, though this is never severe or progressive. Only the silent, subacute or pseudo-embolic forms would be resembled, and in these swelling does not occur.

4. *Arterial injury* is seldom hidden or unsuspected, except, perhaps, after operation. Postoperative arterial embolism might then be suggested, but this generally occurs after operations upon the heart and aorta, though sometimes operative disturbance of a diseased peripheral artery may cause distal embolism. Here, of course, an arterial injury may also have occurred.*

5. *Pseudo-embolism and recurrent acute ischaemia* are interesting and important conditions, both

---

* Bullet embolus has been described, lodging at the aortic bifurcation having entered the heart a month before, causing slow ischaemia, as in the youthful type of saddle embolus, and requiring removal months later [7]; also at the common femoral, with acute ischaemia and gangrene (*see* Chapter 13, p. 246).

representing a sequel of haemodynamic events in patients with incomplete or compensated arterial obstruction.

(*a*) In pseudo-embolism, an incomplete obstruction, possibly embolic, is overcome by an improvement in cardiac function, or may improve following heparin administration, perhaps with the occluding thrombus slipping onwards down the artery or into branches—this would explain most cases of pseudo-embolism.

(*b*) In recurrent acute ischaemia, a previous major obstruction, well compensated by collaterals adequate under normal conditions, becomes an effective resistance zone once again during any hypotensive or low output state such as may follow injury, or more important, major surgery such as a mitral valvulotomy. Unless the preoperative case assessment contains a good account of the state of all the peripheral pulses, unnecessary and damaging arterial surgery may be embarked upon, when all that was needed was restoration of the blood volume or cardiac output.

The site of the embolism can usually be recognised from the clinical features, chiefly the position of the absent pulses and the extent of the ischaemic, anaesthetic skin. The skin level is always lower because, unless the patient is generally deteriorating, branches arising just above the block should contain a vigorous and increasing circulation that warms the skin well beyond (Fig. 14.3). Yet these signs are wholly conditional on the patient's ability to maintain a good general circulation. Those already in hospital under medical treatment for their heart condition are liable to rapid deterioration, while the fitter subject still able to live at home may have such a good circulation that the diagnosis may be missed, or the condition may not even be reported. This is why observations of the distal limit of skin warmth are more valuable in assessing prognosis than in diagnosing the level of the block.

Absent pulses beyond the embolus lead the examiner to a careful consideration, which proceeds proximally up the line of the main limb artery, to determine if possible the point of embolism. This may show the following features:

(*a*) A tender swelling of the artery corresponding to the embolus itself.

(*b*) A bounding, obstructed pulse immediately above this point, often stronger than in the opposite limb at the same level.

(*c*) A weak axial pulsation transmitted through the embolus.

(*d*) A weak, true pulsation through a narrow channel alongside the embolus (often seen arteriographically).

(*e*) Rarely, in recovering cases, a true pulsation beyond the embolus, due to strongly developing collateral circulation.

In summary, it is the point of transition of pulsation from easy palpability to weakness or absence that marks the position of the embolus: if this can be made out with certainty, as it often can be in thin elderly subjects, the accuracy of clinical localisation equals that of an arteriogram, and with greater safety and no delay.

Arteriographic Appearances in Peripheral Arterial Embolism (Figs 14.3, 14.14, and 12.4, p. 221)

1. The proximal, patent arteries are well filled and normal looking.
2. A sharply defined, usually transverse or convex upper limit to the occlusion.
3. Thin channels of contrast medium passing onwards alongside the embolus.
4. Occlusion is at an unusual site for thrombosis.

Limb-prognosis

Factors affecting limb survival are shown in Fig. 14.4. Many of them can be favourably influenced by correct case management.

Typical Embolic Sites and Their Clinical Presentation: Notes and Surgical Implications

Common femoral. Tender artery. Pulse present near inguinal ligament and proximally. Cold anaesthetic foot, sometimes to mid-calf or higher. Risk of gangrene high. (Common femoral ligation in fit young subjects has 50 per cent amputation sequel.) Anterior tibial syndrome in recovering cases (*see* p. 262).

Saddle embolus at aortic bifurcation. Elderly, ill subject, massive ischaemia, even buttocks discoloured, with general deterioration, and death. Operation scarcely practical. In less severe cases, a sensation of defaecation [23]. In younger patients, with slower onset, prognosis may be good, fair circulation in legs, perhaps weak femoral pulses; operation to improve prognosis and avoid future disability, particularly if mitral condition can be corrected. In most patients with moderate to severe ischaemia the cardiac condition permits an attempt to remove the embolus from below, using a balloon catheter, for the outlook is poor and secondary regression is common [21*h*].

Popliteal. Probably the commonest, if silent cases

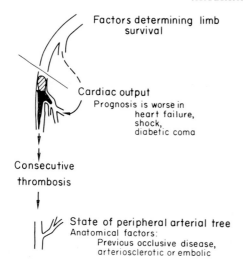

Factors determining limb survival

Cardiac output
Prognosis is worse in
    heart failure,
    shock,
    diabetic coma

Consecutive thrombosis

State of peripheral arterial tree
Anatomical factors:
    Previous occlusive disease,
    arteriosclerotic or embolic

Local demands of peripheral bed increased
Poorer outcome:
e.g. exercise, local heat,
      recent acute ischaemia

Fig. 14.4. Factors determining limb survival.

are included. Unless the patient is ill or postoperative, recovery is to be expected. Transient pallor, sensory impairment and weakness of foot and toes with early improvement. If this does not occur, operation is essential. If noted at conclusion of aortic grafting operation for aneurysm, immediate operation if waxy pallor does not turn to cyanosis of low flow within half an hour. One of the few examples in which the true duration of the condition is known—it occurs at the moment of unclamping.

Axillary brachial. (*a*) from the heart: an isolated incident in a short limb with good collateral potential; transient coldness, pallor and weakness with numbness which soon passes. Outlook good. Often silent. In the elderly, or where cardiac reserve is poor, or if there has been a previous episode, risk of massive gangrene is real (Fig. 14.5).

(*b*) from the aortic arch; in middle-aged females tendency to be repetitive to same limb. Increasing

severity of ischaemia with each occlusion. Limb prognosis poor.

(*c*) from thoracic outlet syndrome, likewise repeated and of serious significance (*see* Chapter 12, p. 221).

Tibial. (*a*) in cardiac patients, mostly symptomless, an incidental finding in a well-nourished limb.

(*b*) from popliteal aneurysm; extensive or multiple occlusion, filling of the plantar arterial system. Risk of gangrene high, though usually confined to toes (*see* Fig. 15.36, p. 312).

Cerebral and visceral embolism are described in Chapters 8 (p. 148) and 17 (p. 372).

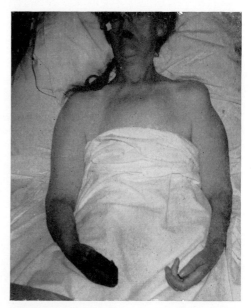

Fig. 14.5. Massive gangrene resulting from a right brachial embolism in a woman aged eighty with advanced congestive heart failure. Limb prognosis at this site is normally favourable if the cardiac status can be maintained.

Subsequently, this old lady rallied sufficiently for amputation of the right arm to be required. An earlier arterial intervention here might have been worth undertaking.

Treatment

The principles are as follows:

1. To maintain the cardiac output and blood pressure.
2. To limit or remove the local obstruction.
3. To reduce the metabolic requirements of the ischaemic extremity.

Every aspect of treatment should be directed at these objectives; equally important is the aim of preventing deterioration in patients in which these conditions have been satisfied, for neglect may lead to an unforeseen late relapse, and success may then turn to failure.

1. Support to the Heart and General Circulation

This is probably the most important of the three. Limb survival may depend on this, the main variable factor in patients with arterial embolism, which seems to determine why in two patients with apparently identical anatomical occlusions one will go on to peripheral gangrene and the other will make a good recovery. Furthermore, the high mortality of arterial embolism is chiefly due to circulatory failure. The terminal stages may be accompanied by the development of multiple areas of ischaemia, peripheral and central.

It may not be possible at the present time to provide much effective support to the failing *ischaemic myocardium*, although accessory cardiac pumping by various methods is now being developed. Reduction of the cardiac work load still depends on good nursing and medical care. The co-operation of a cardiologist is essential. In decompensation from other causes such as *hypertensive disease* and *mitral stenosis* he will be able to provide early assistance to the failing heart and may perhaps turn the scales for the limb as well as for the patient. In an emergency, the surgeon or anaesthetist will himself prescribe digitalis and diuretics. *Thyrotoxic* heart failure is amenable to treatment of the same kind, with anti-thyroid agents in addition.

Preventive measures are important. In a patient with recoverable ischaemia in good circulatory status any excessively severe operative intervention will undoubtedly impair his chances by lowering the cardiac function. This applies most particularly to transperitoneal aortic embolectomy.

Pain should be controlled. The room should be kept warm and free from draughts. In this way generalised vasoconstriction can be prevented. Vasopressors are absolutely contra-indicated, though adreno-cortical replacement may sometimes be decisive. Transfusion requires considerable judgement and caution even in patients with recent blood or extracellular fluid loss. Haemoconcentration, on the other hand, greatly increases the resistance effect of vascular occlusion and so must be overcome.

2. Treatment against the Thrombus

(*a*) anticoagulants and low molecular weight dextran.

(*b*) fibrinolysins.

(*c*) embolectomy.

Anticoagulant treatment occupies a crucial place in the treatment of arterial embolism, but its role and the methods for its application change as the disease runs its course. It is given in the hope of checking the spread of the thrombus within the stagnant blood columns of the main artery and vein. This may give time for the processes of spontaneous recovery to establish themselves.

Heparin is indispensable. It should be given at once, in full effective dosage* as soon as the diagnosis is made. Clinical experience has repeatedly shown the value of this emergency treatment. It can be started by the practitioner before the patient's transfer to hospital. The effect of heparin is to prolong the 'period of grace' during which any essential preliminary medical measures can be taken and the patient moved to a place where surgery is possible. Sometimes, from the moment of heparinisation the limb seems to begin to recover. A vasodilator action, which indeed, judging from the response to its administration in limbs with chronic ischaemia or venous occlusion, heparin does seem to possess, could hardly be expected to work in this way in acute ischaemia. It might, however, be due to the potentiation of natural fibrinolysis when the concurrent, normally equal rate of fibrin formation is inhibited. This is believed to be one of heparin's most useful secondary properties, and it may account for much of its value in the early stages of arterial embolism, certainly as far as freshly formed local thrombus is concerned (*see also* pseudo-embolism, p. 262).

Heparin should prevent the spread of consecutive thrombus in the main artery and keep open the mouths of important collaterals, not only those that are already functioning, which the returning blood flow should hold patent, but also those within the zone of stasis awaiting the return of an improved limb perfusion as the new circulatory bed opens up, which will then find them patent and ready.

Low molecular weight dextran (*LMDX*), next to heparin, is one of the most valuable adjuncts in the treatment of embolic ischaemia. Stasis affecting main channels and collaterals must also apply to smaller branches, and to the capillary bed. Sedimentation and aggregation of the red cells in the static blood in these vessels will cause a sharp rise in peripheral resistance and a further impediment to

---

* *Heparin dosage:* 10,000 units (100 mg) intravenously six-hourly; or 20,000 units (200 mg) by continuous infusion in isotonic saline or LMDX; or for patients in transit or with poor veins, 15,000 units (150 mg) by deep intramuscular injection into the unaffected lateral thigh eight-hourly. Clotting times are unnecessary.

recovery. LMDX is known to stabilise red cell suspension *in vivo*. Its intravenous administration almost always initiates a striking improvement in ischaemic states. Caution must be observed in cardiac patients with peripheral embolism in whom the dosage volume (500 ml every twelve hours, using the 10 per cent solution) must not be exceeded. The writer's practice is to add heparin 200 mg to each 500 ml bottle, which gives an even rate of administration of these two invaluable drugs.

Fibrinolysin treatment is still in the experimental stage. Its principle, the removal of recently deposited fibrin by depolymerisation should be effective in any advancing ischaemia, though it cannot deal with organised thrombus. Although a good many emboli are composed of such material, the consecutive thrombus is always fresh. Remarkable success has been obtained in a few clinical cases [8, 53], often in conjunction with embolectomy, but there are still many drawbacks [1], chiefly from the toxic properties of bacterial products in streptokinase; also overdosage may cause haemorrhage at infusion or operation sites. Human activator (urokinase) may prove to be more suitable, though, perhaps, in a supporting role to proved therapeutic measures. It is extremely expensive.

Late Anticoagulant Treatment. Whether or not operation has been undertaken, there is the need to reduce the risk of late intravascular thrombosis, particularly of veins, even after the ischaemia may have been overcome. Although heparin may be given for almost indefinite periods, and some recommend this as primary treatment [57], there are practical objections, mainly the pain, bruising or actual haemorrhage at the injection sites. As a continuing postoperative measure heparin is usually contra-indicated [43].

Phenindione and the other prothombin depressor drugs are better suited to postoperative use; venous thrombo-embolic complications are reduced, and the circulation is conserved. A good plan (except after operation) is to continue to give heparin with LMDX for at least three days, and then to make the transition to the oral anticoagulant. The aim should be to double the control prothrombin time. Patients with mitral stenosis and atrial fibrillation should be kept on anticoagulants until after mitral valvotomy and amputation of the appendage have removed the risk of further emboli.

Local measures are important; the limb should be cared for and the patient nursed as described in Chapter 2 (pp. 25–7).

Embolectomy

Recent refinements and extension of the scope of embolectomy, in particular the use of the Fogarty balloon catheter, have greatly increased its local effectiveness without adding to the severity of the procedure. Even before these advances were made, the operation offered the simplest and most direct means of removing a serious obstruction, and it is curious that there should ever have been any hesitation over the need to remove an embolus from a severely ischaemic limb. Unfamiliarity with arterial repair and the high hospital mortality, whether or not the embolus was removed, may have deterred surgeons in the past, but should no longer do so.

Early attempts by Moynihan [37], and Sampson Handley [19] were made during the opening years of this century at a time when the technical principles of vascular repair had just been placed on a firm scientific basis by Carrel and Guthrie [17]. Labey, in Paris [24], in 1913, was the first to succeed in removing a femoral embolus from a patient with mitral valve disease, while Key, in Stockholm [24], in 1923, made the first report of a successful series of cases. This achievement stood alone for many years. The first successful British case, a brachial embolectomy, was Sir Geoffrey Jefferson's [22].

Improvement in results everywhere followed the introduction of heparin by Murray and Best in Toronto [38]. Even so, disappointments continued to offset the advantages of surgery. Mostly these were due to the morbidity of the underlying heart condition, and its secondary effect on the limb circulation, and from the multiple and scattered secondary emboli and thrombi often present in these serious cases [36]. We shall later discuss recent technical advances that appear to be at least a partial solution of this last difficulty.

Cardiovascular deaths, however, continue to take a heavy toll of patients with embolism, amounting to some 35 per cent [36] or more [26], whether treated medically or surgically, so that operation is still contra-indicated if the patient's general condition is very poor or is obviously deteriorating; although it should not be forgotten that the reason for decline may be the ischaemia itself, bringing pain and distress as well as the general metabolic effects of massive tissue infarction. In such a patient operation, if quickly and simply completed, may actually improve his chance of survival. Careful judgement is needed before any patient is given up as hopeless (Fig. 14.5).

The Time for Operation

Much has been written about a time limit (8 to 10 hours) after which embolectomy seldom succeeds. This is correct, but it applies only to patients with acute massive ischaemia. It is not a therapeutic axiom for all circumstances, and the following reservations should be made:

(*a*) The actual moment of embolism is seldom known, as Sir Thomas Lewis pointed out; only the time of onset of symptoms.

(*b*) When the embolism can be timed, as happens with the release of the clamps after resection of an abdominal aortic aneurysm, the return of a sufficient alternative circulation, if it happens at all, seldom takes longer than an hour or two. Most aortic unclamping cases are best regarded as massively ischaemic and requiring operation at once. For these, the six to eight hour rule sets far too long a time. Changes of early ischaemia are already present even before the unclamping. (The same applies to acute ischaemia in younger subjects when it follows exertion which (*see* p. 260) likewise produces a 'blood debt'.)

(*c*) Sometimes ischaemia, although severe, is just compatible with survival of the extremity; the skin, and resting muscle (if not compressed by the weight of the limb or a fascial compartment) remain in a state of minimum metabolic activity requiring the least possible amount of blood to maintain life. Any local insult, such as applying even moderate warmth to the surface, may cause tissue death in that area (Fig. 2.8, p. 26) and the same is true of the muscle damage in the anterior tibial syndrome (Fig. 10.8, p. 197) [15, 33]. Both these conditions are capable of full recovery with the return of a better blood supply. Their presence can be taken as an indication that marginal severe ischaemia is present, with a potential for recovery with effective treatment, or even sometimes spontaneously. The important point is that the 'armistice' may be quite prolonged, which means that extensive closure of the vascular circuit has not yet taken place; the occlusion may still be limited to the major branch or bifurcation where it first lodged, and a trickling collateral flow is keeping the lesser arterial branches patent and limiting the spread of consecutive thrombus. In such a patient embolectomy may succeed long after the usual time when it is considered to be worth trying. The following two cases are instructive:

CASE REPORT 1

A frail lady of eighty with atrial fibrillation developed ischaemia of the right lower limb with severe pain, tenderness, and skin discoloration over the anterior tibial region. With expectant treatment for three weeks there was very little improvement. A Stokes-Gritti amputation was performed. When the popliteal artery came to be divided, its upper end was found to be pulsating vigorously, and its lower part was obstructed by thrombus, which on subsequent examination of the specimen was confirmed as a popliteal embolus. It still lay loose and free in the artery, with almost no consecutive thrombus beyond the bifurcation. Clearly a late embolectomy could have been attempted here, even in the third week.

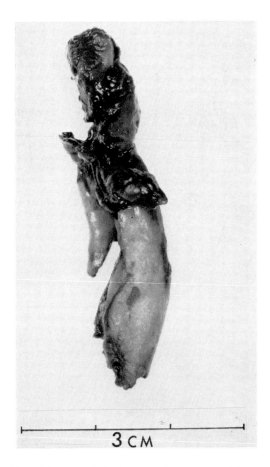

Fig. 14.6. Late embolectomy specimen, removed from the right common iliac artery of a man aged seventy-five who had developed subacute ischaemia of the right lower limb three months before, following soon after a mild cardiac infarction.

Trans-femoral instrumental approach was employed using loop strippers and balloon catheters. Full patency and pulsation restored to all lower limb pulses.

Note the small amount of consecutive thrombus.

CASE REPORT 2

A fit, thin man of seventy-six developed coldness and aching of the left lower limb soon after the resection of his abdominal aortic aneurysm. The limb was viable, and its condition remained unchanged during the next ten days. Ankle pulses had been present before operation but, afterwards, were absent beyond the lowest palpable course of the superficial femoral. The popliteal artery was explored, and a limited embolus was removed without difficulty with subsequent complete restoration of the distal pulses and a normal circulation and function in the limb.

Late Embolectomy

There are many published cases in which operation was fully successful on the second day or later [6, 12, 26, 40, 58] and some in whom the acute ischaemia had become chronic much later (Fig. 14.6). In these, arteriography sometimes helped by showing the diagnostic features of embolic occlusion (see p. 263) where clinical suspicion might have been turning towards arteriosclerotic thrombosis, in which the prospects of clearing the obstruction by simple surgical means are far less good.

Late Revascularisation Syndrome

The fact that the skin is still viable does not guarantee the state of the deep tissues, as is shown when ischaemic muscle contracture occurs without gangrene. If the limb circulation is restored at a time when muscle damage is already established, a severe toxic confusional and oliguric state may follow, closely resembling the crush or tourniquet syndrome, with renal failure as its most serious feature. Metabolic acidosis, hyperkalaemia from damaged cells, and, later, the full picture of acute tubular necrosis with anuria and uraemia have been reported after late embolectomy [27, 51] and it is possible that some of the high mortality of embolectomy in the earlier stages may be contributed to by a degree of this complication.

The best prevention of this 'reopening phenomenon' is, of course, the avoidance of embolectomy in advanced states of tissue damage, and muscle contracture should be reckoned as one of these. In other cases, operated upon late, but with hopes of full recovery, it may be possible to prevent or ameliorate the dangers of acidosis and hyperkalaemia by giving 100 mEq sodium bicarbonate intravenously. In the severest cases, with cardiac arrest shortly after removal of the arterial clamps, a larger than usual dose should be given (up to 500 mEq) [50]. There will be doubtful cases, but if true acute ischaemia with very severe signs has persisted longer than forty-eight hours, or if muscle contracture or other obvious tissue necrosis has already begun, amputation is safer than revascularisation. It is in the slower case with mild ischaemia that late embolectomy is indicated. As always with arterial embolism, the patient's general condition is a valuable guide to limb prognosis at every stage before and after operation.

TECHNIQUE OF EMBOLECTOMY

The basic operation is simple and should now be familiar to surgeons of all degrees of experience, and to their theatre staff. The main points are as follows:

(a) *Anaesthesia*. Local anaesthesia is ideal for a cardiac patient in whom only the common femoral artery need be exposed. Extended manipulations from the groin to distant parts of the arterial tree are now possible, using the Fogarty catheter (see p. 271).

General anaesthesia must be accepted in restless patients, or those with complex, or multiple emboli if the catheter method has failed or cannot be adopted for other reasons. It has the great disadvantage in embolectomy patients that a fall in blood pressure occurs almost immediately after induction and may reach dangerously low levels well before the stage of blood loss is reached. It is particularly important, therefore, to avoid drugs with a known hypotensive action, such as tubocurarine or halothane. Spinal anaesthesia is unsuitable for the same reason.

(b) Exposure should be generous and be capable of extension. Limb cases must be draped in such a way that secondary access can easily be obtained to other points along the main artery (Fig. 14.7). Longitudinal incisions are preferable to those in the skin crease. Self-retaining retractors are valuable. A good light is essential.

(c) The incision should be centred over the lowest point at which pulsation can be felt, for here the artery can be quickly and easily exposed by sharp dissection 'on to the pulse'. It is then under-run and picked up gently over a tape loop. It is important not to apply any compression in these early stages, otherwise the embolus may be broken or its tail of consecutive clot separated.

(d) When the main artery and branches have been

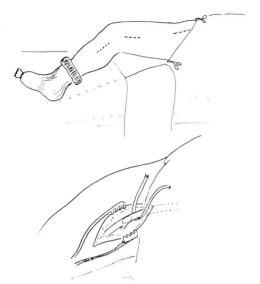

Fig. 14.7. Embolectomy in the lower limb. Draping and exposure of possible arteriotomy sites. For clarity, a longer than usual incision is shown.

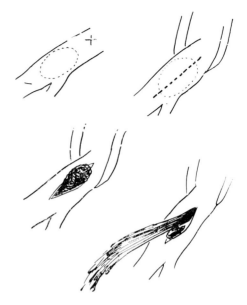

Fig. 14.8. Common femoral embolectomy. The essential procedure is carried out without clamps until a spurting flow has been obtained from the proximal artery.

fully exposed and mobilised, the previous dose of heparin should be supplemented, if necessary by a further injection of 50 mg given intra-arterially into the pulsating segment.

(*e*) *No clamps should yet be applied.*

(*f*) The main artery should be incised using a No. 15 scalpel blade, over the embolus, near the bifurcation, but not beyond it. The dark blue lump of obstructing material can easily be seen through the normal artery, and as soon as the lumen is entered the contents begin to be pumped gently up into the opening (Fig. 14.8). With a little assistance, if necessary, by gentle digital compression at the lower limit of the pulsating upper part of the main artery, or gently freeing the impaction with a Watson Cheyne dissector, the embolus then delivers itself by shooting out, followed by the full force of the arterial blood at normal pressure, checked instantly by the finger tip, which is less damaging than traction upon the upper tape. Only now is the proximal clamp applied.

(*g*) The distal artery may begin to bleed back if there is little consecutive thrombus. In such a case the distal clot can be freed and distal patency confirmed by means of firm bimanual squeezing of the limb along the line of the lower course of the main artery (Fig. 14.9), a simple manoeuvre which is preferable in the first instance to suction or other intra-arterial manipulations. *A back flow must be obtained or the embolectomy will fail.* In effect, this means that arterial blood, albeit under reduced pressure,

must be able to flow into the newly patent main artery from large branches connecting with a fully patent distal circuit for this same flow to be reversible after removal of the clamps (Fig. 14.4). Limited back-flow is due either to fragmented or consecutive

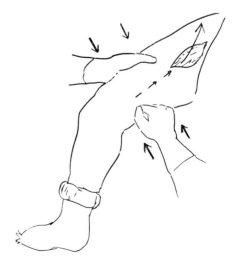

Fig. 14.9. Manual compression of the lower femoral artery for the removal of consecutive clot.

269

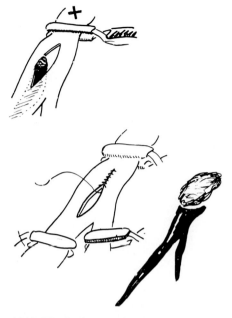

Fig. 14.10. The final stage of embolectomy, the rule being—clamp only a patent artery.

clot, which will require removal by one of the accessory methods described below, or to previous occlusive disease. Usually the appearance of the artery, and its feel during manipulations of its lower course, will tell the surgeon which.

(*h*) Bulldog clips may now be applied to the branch and the distal main vessel, provided all clot has been removed from each (Fig. 14.10).

(*i*) In embolectomy a simple continuous arterial closure is nearly always sufficient. These patients' arteries are usually in good condition, so that narrowing after suture is not a problem. This is, usually, also true in arteriosclerotic subjects, perhaps because there has been no prolonged closure and contraction and no definite siting of the disease at the point of embolism. Even the popliteal can be closed in this way, using 5/0 arterial silk or 6/0 in a small subject. With this material a brachial embolectomy incision can sometimes be safely repaired without having recourse to patch grafting.

(*j*) The distal clamps are removed, and any significant leaks attended to (in a simple repair of a normal artery there should be none) and the proximal clamp is taken off without further delay. The heparin is now reversed by a systemic intravenous injection of protamine sulphate (2 mg per 1 mg of heparin).

(*k*) At this stage the anaesthetist keeps a close watch on the patient's general condition. Loss of circulating blood volume into the dilated peripheral bed may cause a fall in pressure, particularly after aortic saddle embolectomy. Although contra-indicated before operation, aramine (metaraminol, 1 mg intravenously) can now be given with safety and is preferable to rapid transfusion in this type of patient. Bicarbonate infusion should be considered.

(*l*) An assistant should now inspect the extremity. An improvement, though quite slight, means that the wound may be closed. If there is no obvious change, the main artery should be watched for diminishing pulsation (taking into consideration the hypotensive effects of removal of the clamps and comparing with other pulses in unaffected areas).

(*m*) If in doubt, close the wound and remove all drapes so that the limb and the rest of the patient may be fully and repeatedly assessed. The signs of returning blood flow (*see* p. 21) should soon be evident.

(*n*) An intravenous infusion of low molecular weight dextran is started, provided the patient is not in heart failure.

Removal of Secondary Thrombus

The embolus itself should be easy to remove, being limited in size and non-adherent to the artery wall. Consecutive thrombus, however, is often in the form of a tapering, whip-like strip, that extends down a considerable length of the artery, and is more adherent to it. Separated pieces of the embolus, in fact, tend to be impacted and glued into the remote sites where they lodge by this sticky stasis clot. To overcome this serious complicating condition, which would otherwise doom the embolectomy to failure and bring death to the limb, the following improvements have been adopted:

(1) Retrograde arterial flushing.
(2) Extraction of the thrombus with the Fogarty balloon catheter and other instruments.
(3) A combination of both these methods.

Retrograde arterial flushing was a major contribution that greatly contributed to the success of embolectomy when it was introduced [44, 45], and still remains of value when modern methods of direct extraction may fail, or if the equipment is not available; it will therefore be described. Exposing the main artery at a distal point along its course (and possibly at more than one), the operator opens it just sufficiently to admit the nozzle of a 20 ml Luer gauge syringe. A strong gush of saline is flushed proximally up the artery towards the open upper arteriotomy, through which the long consecutive thrombus then delivers itself (Fig. 14.11), followed by a free, clear

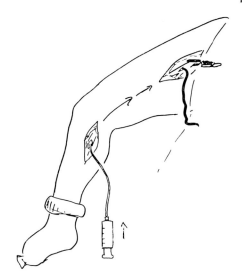

Fig. 14.11. Retrograde flushing for the removal of adherent consecutive thrombus. This method is particularly useful in late embolectomy.

jet of saline. The irrigation should be repeated once or twice, and any further pieces removed. The patient should already be fully heparinised as part of the routine of embolectomy. Retrograde bleeding often begins as the circulation restores itself; the margins of the lower wound become pink with capillary oozing, contrasting with their white or cyanotic colour when the skin was first incised. If necessary, the small arteries at the ankle or wrist can also be opened and flushed.

Instrumental methods in embolectomy may be used when retrograde flushing has failed to clear the channel. Recommended instruments include: vein strippers [2]; endarterectomy loops [3, 16B]; ureteric catheter baskets [20]; and miniature corkscrews [45]. Each of these has been used successfully, though they may harm the artery or further impact the remote clot, from over-energetic and increasingly desperate attempts to clear the obstruction.

The Fogarty Balloon Catheter [14, 14A] (Fig. 14.12)

It is to such conditions that this ingenious instrument is ideally adapted. Through a single arteriotomy (Fig. 14.13), distal and also proximal manipulations can be safely and effectively carried out, the principle being to pass the slim stiff catheter along the artery through the thrombus to its full extent, and then, inflating the balloon to the correct size of the lumen, to exert gentle traction which brings the balloon up towards the arteriotomy and the intact, complete thrombus before it. A flushing type is also available with which to complete the clearance of small fragments.

With this technique it is possible to reach and clear the aortic bifurcation proximally and distally to the popliteal or its branches (Fig. 14.14), all from the common femoral arteriotomy. The early results were good. Fogarty and his colleagues had 50 patients, average age 69·5 years, with 56 emboli, who required amputation in only two instances. The overall mortality of the series was low at 20 per cent. Since then, worldwide experience of the balloon catheter has fully confirmed its value in limb salvage for all sites of embolism and it has been responsible for a reduction in mortality, in the aorto-iliac group in particular [9A]. A few false aneurysms of tibial arteries have been reported [14B, 35B].

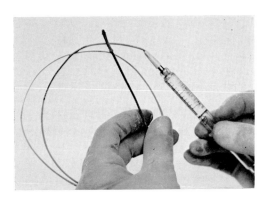
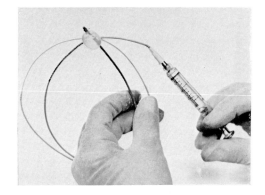

Fig. 14.12. The balloon embolectomy catheter.

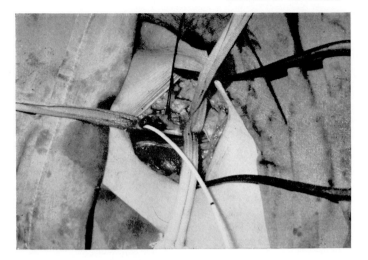

Fig. 14.13. Left common femoral arteriotomy seen from the patient's left side. A Craaford clamp is in place above the arteriotomy and a loose tape beyond it. The balloon catheter is being withdrawn and thrombus from the popliteal can be seen appearing in the arteriotomy.

Results of Arterial Embolectomy

Between 20 per cent [14] and 40 per cent [26] of patients die in hospital, nearly all from associated cardiovascular disease, often during or soon after operation in which difficulties over general or spinal anaesthesia may precipitate collapse [51] or this may result from ill-advised blood transfusion [51] or from the 'reopening phenomenon' (see p. 268), [50] which is a potent cause of cardiac arrest.

After an apparently satisfactory embolectomy with good improvement in the limb circulation there may be only limited or partial return of the peripheral pulses. This may be due either to fragmentation or multiplicity of the emboli, or to previous arteriosclerotic obliteration. The condition of the main artery at the point of exploration, and also the resistance felt to instruments passed down its course, will often give prior warning of the latter possibility.

As in the medically treated group, further emboli are common, and widespread, often affecting vital and clinically difficult areas such as the brain or the intestine [16, 58].

In mitral cases, with adequate treatment, the mortality is lower [46].

Limb salvage among operative survivors is high; over 95 per cent in recent series [14, 16, 51] though, again, the arteriosclerotic patients fared much worse in this respect [14].

Late follow-up has shown a steady loss, mainly from cardiovascular complications, with only 40 per cent alive five years after leaving hospital. The mitral group, however, if fully treated have a better prospect [28].

Yet, repeated limb embolism, and operations for it, figure in most published series sometimes in spite of supposedly adequate treatment of the mitral valve [47], and subsequent emboli have been removed from the aortic bifurcation, for example, on several occasions [47, 56]. For visceral embolectomy, see Chapter 17.

Some Notes on Pulmonary Embolectomy

Opinion is once again changing in favour of surgery for some patients with pulmonary embolism, and it may now come within the scope of the general and peripheral vascular surgeon as a planned emergency procedure which, like injury or embolism to the limb arteries and some patients with leaking or dissecting aneurysm, are often much better dealt with in the receiving hospital than by being transferred to a special surgical unit.

Trendelenburg's brave concept, in 1908, of a desperate attempt to remove the total pulmonary block to the circulation [52] first succeeded in 1924 when Kirschner [25] of Heidelberg saved his patient, a woman of thirty-eight, in this way. Craaford of Stockholm, four years later, reported two recoveries [9], while in Great Britain, Ivor Lewis, in 1938, was successful in a patient who lived another twenty years [30]. By 1964 there were twenty-eight reports

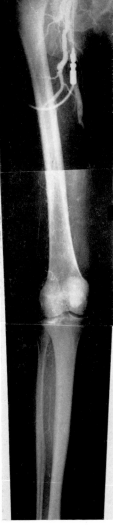
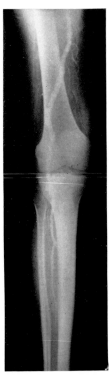

Fig. 14.14. Femoral embolism in an ill man aged seventy-three with congestive heart failure and atrial fibrillation. Separate fragments of secondary clot can be seen in the proximal femorals. Poor filling of the geniculate and anterior tibial arteries. The foot was blue and anaesthetic.

Following catheter embolectomy under local anaesthesia the main arteries were restored as far as the mid-calf, and the foot became hot. Condition maintained since.

[35] of long-term survivals, and results are steadily improving [54], especially when the facilities of a special unit are at hand [41].

Indications

1. The patient should be free from severe intercurrent disease such as advanced malignancy or previous heart failure.
2. The diagnosis must be beyond reasonable doubt.
3. Collapse,* cor pulmonale, and hypotension resistant to vasopressors lasting more than two hours (i.e. a fatal outcome is likely without intervention).

Special concern will arise when the victim is a young woman in early pregnancy, a time in which vascular catastrophes of several kinds are particularly significant and deadly (*see* Chapters 7 and 15) and pulmonary embolism is one of these [5].

The Tactics of Surgical Intervention

1. Urgent, immediate operation is undertaken when there is imminent risk of death, without delaying investigations, or cardiopulmonary by-pass, unless already set up.
2. Serious deteriorating general condition with diagnosis certain; here there should be time to organise by-pass, particularly if the new disposable apparatus is available, requiring no blood-priming [1A].
3. In an otherwise suitable case, where the diagnosis is in some doubt, operation should not be undertaken until clear evidence of pulmonary artery obstruction can be obtained from either right heart catheterisation and pressure measurements, or pulmonary angiography, or both [1A, 39].

Operative Technique

In cases of the second and third types described above, the cardiopulmonary by-pass circuit is prepared, priming with glucose saline.

Vertical, full-length median sternotomy is preferable for all cases other than those of the most urgent and deteriorating kind in which the Trendelenburg incision, which may also divide the sternum, though transversely, is quicker and gives direct access over the pulmonary artery.

Cannulation of the venae cavae and the femoral artery—or in emergency blood may be taken from the right ventricle itself [34]—enables by-pass to be started, after which the operation may assume a more deliberate tempo. Partial perfusion may,

---

* In all Paneth's cases the peripheral veins were collapsed but the central venous pressure was high [41].

alternatively, be begun via the femoral vein, using a long atrial cannula, and the adjacent artery [1A, 3B].

If by-pass is not available, the superior and inferior venae cavae are clamped to reduce the strain on the right ventricle [54].

The dilated pulmonary artery and the aorta are under-run with the right index finger and a broad tape is passed beneath to give control of the artery for suturing after the embolectomy.

The embolus may not be palpable. The artery should not be squeezed in a search for it.

A 2 cm longitudinal incision in the trunk well beyond the valve ring bleeds little, for the embolus prolapses into the arteriotomy. Desjardin's bile duct forceps are used to lift it out, and a wide sucker is then passed into both main pulmonary arteries, taking care not to injure their thin walls. Direct pulmonary massage may help to return distal fragments to within sucker range [1].

The tape sling is released to flush the ventricle outlet. The arteriotomy is repaired with a continuous suture of 4/0 silk. By-pass may now be discontinued

or, if not used, the caval clamps are removed, first the upper, and then the lower, the latter gradually until the right ventricle recovers from strain.

If opened, the pleurae should now be drained, and the chest securely closed. Sodium bicarbonate should be given intravenously (10 to 15 G).

Anticoagulants must be given for several months after recovery. Rarely, recurrent embolism requires that the vena cava should be exposed through a lateral abdominal incision and ligated just above its bifurcation [54]. A constricting clip may be preferred.

Results of Pulmonary Embolectomy

These are encouraging to further attempts as experience is gained and facilities improve for a more regular intervention.

Without by-pass, using median sternotomy, four out of seven patients made a full recovery [54].

Disposable pump-oxygenator cardiopulmonary by-pass has proved highly successful on many occasions [1A, 35, 41, 41A].

REFERENCES

1. Amery, A., Deloof, W., Vermylen, J. and Verstraete, M. (1970) Outcome of recent thromboembolic occlusions of limb arteries treated with streptokinase. *Brit. med. J.*, **4**, 639.

1A. Beall, A. C., Cooley, D. A. and DeBakey, M. E. (1965) Surgical management of pulmonary embolism. *Dis. Chest.*, **47**, 382.

2. Bellman, S. and Jonson, M. (1961) On the effect of mechanical cleansing in embolic arterial occlusion with extensive distal clot formation. *Acta. chir. Scand.*, **121**, 391.

3. Bergan, J. J. and Trippel, O. H. (1965) Simplified removal of propagated intra-arterial thrombus. *Surgery*, **58**, 653.

3A. Berger, R. L., Madoff, I. M. and Ryan, T. J. (1967) Mercury embolisation during arterial pressure monitoring. *J. Thorac. Cardiovasc. Surg.*, **53**, 285.

3B. Berger, R. L. (1971) Pulmonary embolectomy for massive embolisation. *Amer. J. Surg.*, **121**, 437.

4. Blum, L. and Rosenthal, I. (1960) Embolectomy in arteries to extremities. *J. Amer. med. Assoc.*, **172**, 794.

5. Breckenbridge, R. T. and Ratnoff, O. D. (1964) Pulmonary embolism and unexpected death in supposedly normal persons. *New Eng. J. Med.*, **270**, 298.

6. Brock, R. (1962) Late arterial embolectomy. *J. Cardiovasc. Surg.*, **3**, 39.

7. Cooper, F. W. Harris, M. H. and Kahn, J. W. (1948) Ligation and division of the abdominal aorta for metallic embolus from the heart. *Ann. Surg.*, **127**, 1.

8. Cotton, L. T., Flute, P. T. and Tsapogas, M. J. C. (1962) Popliteal artery thrombosis treated with strep-tokinase. *Lancet*, ii, 1081.

9. Craaford, C. (1928) Two cases of obstructive pulmonary embolism successfully operated upon. *Acta chir. Scand.*, **64**, 172.

9A. Cranley, J. J., Krause, R. J., Strasser, E. S. and Hafner, C. D. (1970) Catheter technique for arterial embolectomy: a seven-year experience. *J. Cardiovasc. Surg.*, **11**, 44.

10. Crawford, E. S. and DeBakey, M. E. (1956) The retrograde flush procedure in embolectomy and thrombectomy. *Surgery*, **40**, 737.

11. Daley, R., Mattingly, T. W., Holt, C. L., Bland, E. F. and White, P. D. (1951) Systemic arterial embolism in rheumatic heart disease. *Amer. Heart J.*, **42**, 566.

12. De Girardier, J. and Aupècle, P. (1959) Les possibilités de l'embolectomie dans les embolies artérielles des membres vues tardivement. *Lyon chir.*, **55**, 655.

13. Eisenberg, S. (1964) Changes in blood viscosity, hematocrit value, and fibrinogen concentration in subjects with congestive heart failure. *Circulation*, **30**, 686.

14. Fogarty, T. J. and Cranley, J. J. (1965) Catheter technic for arterial embolectomy. *Ann. Surg.*, **161**, 325.

14A. Fogarty, T. J., Daily, P. O., Shumway, N. E. and Krippaehne, W. (1971) Experience with balloon catheter technique for arterial embolectomy. *Amer. J. Surg.*, **122**, 231.

14B. Foster, J. H., Carter, J. W., Graham, C. P. and Edwards, W. H. (1970) Arterial injuries secondary to the use of the Fogarty catheter. *Ann. Surg.*, **171**, 971.

15. Freedman, B. J. and Knowles, C. H. R. (1959) Anterior tibial syndrome due to arterial embolism and thrombosis. *Brit. med. J.*, ii, 270.

15A.Gaan, D., Mallick, N. P., Brewis, R. A. L., Seedat, Y. K. and Mahoney, M. P. (1969) Cerebral damage from declotting Scribner shunts. *Lancet*, **ii**, 77.

15B.Gazzaniga, A. B. and Dalen, J. E. (1970) Paradoxical embolism: its pathophysiology and clinical recognition. *Ann. Surg.*, **171**, 137.

16. Goldowsky, S. J. and Bowen, J. R. (1960) Arterial embolectomy. *J. Amer. med. Assoc.*, **172**, 799.

16A.Gross, R. E. (1945) Arterial embolism and thrombosis in infancy. *Amer. J. Dis. Child.*, **70**, 61.

16B.Gruss, J-D., Laubach, K. and Vollmar, J. (1969) Le traitement chirurgical de l'embolie artérielle. Un rapport sur 361 cas. *J. Chir.*, **98**, 231.

17. Guthrie, C. C. (1912) *Blood Vessel Surgery and its Applications*. A reprint (1959). (Ed. Harbison, S. P. and Fisher, B.) University of Pittsburgh Press.

18. Haimovici, H. (1950) Peripheral arterial embolism. A study of 330 unselected cases of embolism of the extremities. *Angiology*, **1**, 20.

19. Handley, W. S. (1907) An operation for embolus. *Brit. med. J.*, **ii**, 712.

20. Henson, S. W. and Wise, J. K. (1965) Exploration of the arteries during embolectomy. *Surg. Gynec. Obstet.*, **121**, 589.

21. Jacobs, A. L. (1959) *Arterial Embolism in the Limbs*. Edinburgh and London: E. & S. Livingstone Ltd., p. 28. Other page references: *a:* p. 1, *b:* p. 14, *c:* p. 26, *d:* p. 23, *e:* p. 25, *f:* p. 43, *g:* pp. 53–55, *h:* p. 93.

22. Jefferson, G. (1934) Arterial embolectomy. *Brit. med. J.*, **ii**, 1090.

23. Jepson, R. P. (1955) Peripheral arterial embolism. *Brit. med. J.*, **ii**, 405.

23A.Kay, J. M. and Wilkins, R. A. (1969) Cotton fibre embolism during angiography. *Clin. Radiol.*, **20**, 410.

24. Key, E. (1936) Embolectomy on the vessels of the extremities. *Brit. J. Surg.*, **24**, 350.

25. Kirschner, M. (1924) Ein durch die Trendelenburgsche Operation geheilter Fall von Embolie der Art. pulmonalis. *Arch. klin. Chir.*, **133**, 312.

26. Krause, R. J., Cranley, J. J., Baylon, L. M. and Strasser, E. S. (1959) Recent advancements in the treatment of peripheral arterial embolism. *Arch. Surg.*, **79**, 285.

27. Larcan, A., Rauber, G., Mathieu, P., Masse, P. and Calamai, M. (1965) Le syndrome métabolique gravissime secondaire aux revascularisations trop tardives après ischemies prolongées. *Presse méd.*, **73**, 1819.

28. Leading article (1964) Embolism in mitral valve disease. *Brit. med. J.*, **ii**, 1149.

29. Learmonth, J. R. (1948) Arterial embolism. *Edinburgh med. J.*, **55**, 449.

30. Lewis, I. (1939) Trendelenburg's operation for pulmonary embolism: a successful case. *Lancet*, **i**, 1037; and personal communication (1966).

31. Lewis, I. (1960) 'Problems in diagnosis and management of pulmonary embolism.' In *Modern Trends in Cardiac Surgery*. (Ed. Harley, H. R. S.). London: Butterworth's, p. 56.

32. Lynch, G. (1963) Retrograde embolectomy. *Lancet*, **i**, 751.

33. Lytton, B. and Blandy, J. P. (1960) Anterior tibial syndrome after embolectomy. *Brit. J. Surg.*, **48**, 346.

34. McGuire, L. B. and Smith, G. W. (1965) Pulmonary embolectomy. Report of a case, with a note on indications and technic. *New England J. Med.*, **272**, 1170.

35. Makey, A. R. and Bliss, B. P. (1966) Pulmonary embolectomy: a review of five cases with three survivals. *Lancet*, **ii**, 1155.

35A.Martin, P., King, R. B. and and Stephenson, C. B. S. (1969) On arterial embolism of the limbs. *Brit. J. Surg.*, **56**, 882.

35B.Mavor, G. E., Walker, M. G., Dahl, D. P. and Pegg, C. A. S. (1972) Damage from the Fogarty balloon catheter. *Brit. J. Surg.*, **59**, 389.

36. Metcalfe, W. J. (1960) Arterial embolism in the lower limbs. *Ann. Roy. Coll. Surg. Eng.*, **27**, 407.

37. Moynihan, B. G. A. (1907) An operation for embolus. *Brit. med. J.*, **ii**, 826.

38. Murray, D. G. W., Jaques, L. B., Perrett, T. S. and Best, C. H. (1936) Heparin and vascular occlusion. *Canad. med. Assoc. J.*, **35**, 621.

39. Oakley, C. M. (1970) Diagnosis of pulmonary embolism. *Brit. med. J.*, **2**, 773.

40. Olwin, J. H., Dye, W. S. and Julian, O. C. (1953) Late peripheral arterial embolectomy. *Arch. Surg.*, **66**, 480.

41. Paneth, M. (1967) Pulmonary embolectomy. An analysis of 12 cases. *J. Thorac. Cardiovasc. Surg.*, **53**, 77. Also: (1967) Pulmonary embolectomy. *Ann. Roy. Coll. Surg. Eng.*, **41**, 370.

41A.Paneth, M. (1970) Surgical management of massive pulmonary embolism. *Brit. med. J.*, **2**, 778.

42. Rabinovich, S., Evans, J., Smith, I. M. and January, L. E. (1965) A long-term view of bacterial endocarditis: 337 cases, 1924–1963. *Ann. Int. Med.*, **63**, 185.

43. Salzman, E. W. (1965) The limitations of heparin therapy after arterial reconstruction. *Surgery*, **57**, 131.

44. Shaw, R. S. (1956) A more aggressive approach toward the restoration of blood flow in acute arterial insufficiency. *Surg. Gynec. Obstet.*, **103**, 279.

45. Shaw, R. S. (1960) A method for the removal of the adherent distal thrombus. *Surg. Gynec. Obstet.*, **110**, 255.

46. Shumacker, H. B. and Jacobson, H. S. (1957) Arterial embolism. *Ann. Surg.*, **145**, 145.

47. Slade, P. R. (1963) Repeated aortic saddle embolectomy. *Brit. J. Surg.*, **50**, 979.

48. Somerville, W. and Chambers, R. J. (1964) Systemic embolism in mitral stenosis: relation to the size of the left atrial appendix. *Brit. med. J.*, **ii**, 1167.

49. Starer, F. and Sutton, D. (1960) Aortic occlusion (Leriche's syndrome) in mitral stenosis. Report of six cases. *Brit. med. J.*, **ii**, 644.

50. Stewart, J. S. S., Mostert, J. W., Hilton, D. D. and McGrath, D. (1965) Bicarbonate therapy during embolectomy. Prevention of acidosis shock and acidosis arrest. *Lancet*, **ii**, 1320.

50A. Thompson, J. E., Sigler, L., Raut, P. S., Austin, D. J. and Patman, R. D. (1970) Arterial embolectomy: a 20-year experience with 163 cases. *Surgery*, **67**, 212.

51. Tibbs, D. J. (1965) Technique of arterial embolectomy. *Proc. Roy. Soc. Med.*, **58**, 1032.

52. Trendelenburg, F. (1908) Operative interference in embolism of the pulmonary artery. *Ann. Surg.*, **48**, 772.

53. Verstraete, M., Amery, A. and Vermylen, J. (1963) Feasibility of adequate thrombolytic therapy with streptokinase in peripheral arterial occlusions. *Brit. med. J.*, **i**, 1499.

54. Vossschulte, K., Stiller, H. and Eisenreich, F. (1965) Emergency embolectomy by the transsternal approach in acute pulmonary embolism. *Surgery*, **58**, 317.

55. Warren, R., Linton, R. R. and Scannell, J. G. (1954) Arterial embolism. Recent progress. *Ann. Surg.*, **140**, 311.

56. Weismann, R. E. and Ellsworth, W. J. (1958) 'Saddle' emboli requiring multiple embolectomies. *Ann. Surg.*, **147**, 75.

57. Wessler, S., Sheps, S. G., Gilbert, M. and Sheps, M. C. (1958) Studies in peripheral arterial occlusive disease: **iii.** Acute arterial occlusion. *Circulation*, **17**, 512.

58. Young, J. R., Humphries, A. W., DeWolfe, V. G. and LeFevre, F. A. (1963) Peripheral arterial embolism. *J. Amer. med. Assoc.*, **185**, 621.

15 Aortic and Peripheral Aneurysms

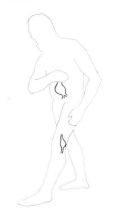

Historical Introduction (eurys Gr. = wide)

Galen [50], in the second century AD, described an aneurysm as a localised swelling with pulsation, from which, if it was wounded, bright blood spurted with much violence. Four hundred years later, Aëtius admitted this overwhelming objection to surgical treatment when the aneurysm lay in the head or the neck, but recognised a less dangerous type at the bend of the arm, from blood letting, and giving the surface marking of the brachial artery showed how to expose and ligate the artery in its upper course before opening the antecubital aneurysm. He then turned out the clot and delivered up the opening of entry with a hook, in order to apply a second ligature there [4].

Ambroise Paré, in 1582, realised that aneurysms could be caused in many ways besides phlebotomy, and described their formation by anastomosis, diapedesis, rupture, and erosion. He also observed progressive hardening of the sac, even to the point of bone formation, thrombosis with loss of pulsation and, later, gangrene of the extremity [114].

William Hunter, in 1757, [71] distinguished between a true aneurysm due to dilatation and a false aneurysm due to rupture, citing Paulus as the originator of this idea. He also recognised bone erosion of the spine, thoracic cage, and skull from aneurysmal pressure. John Hunter [67] understood the importance of local arterial disease in the causation and treatment of aneurysm of the lower limb, and this led him to apply the high ligation method to the cure of popliteal aneurysm. Anel (1714) [6] had previously succeeded in curing what was probably a traumatic brachial aneurysm in a friar, just as it was on the point of bursting through the skin, by applying his ligature as near the sac as possible.

In 1761, Lambert, who with Hallowell had earlier given the first account of a repair of an arterial wound (*see* Chapter 13), considered means of eliminating the circulatory impairment from ligation operations for aneurysm and hoped that by some form of stitch it might be possible to close the opening in the artery and thus retain its patency.

First to ligate the human aorta was Astley Cooper [17] who, in 1817, placed a silk ligature just above the bifurcation in a man aged thirty-eight with a rapidly expanding left iliac aneurysm. He had already, in 1805 and 1808, ligated the common carotid for a similar condition in the neck.

Reconstructive surgery for aneurysm, however, had to await the control of sepsis over a century later, and the work of Carrel and Guthrie [62] on suture and grafting of vessels. Matas, in 1903, performed endoaneurysmorrhaphy [105] with the maintenance in some cases of a lumen for the arterial blood flow. In 1912, Subottitch [141] repaired traumatic arteriovenous fistulae and aneurysms from the Serbian Wars. Graft replacement with saphenous vein was successfully carried out by Lexer of Jena in 1913, and by Hogarth Pringle, in Glasgow, later in the same year [88, 89, 119].

The first excision and graft replacement for abdominal aortic aneurysm was by Dubost of Paris, in 1952 [38]. Ten years later many hundreds of successful cases had been reported from all over the world.

And so, for nearly 2,000 years aneurysm has threatened its victims with a painful and terrible death, and surgeons must deal with such extremes of behaviour as violent haemorrhage and ischaemic gangrene. The incidence of degenerative arterial disease continues to rise; certified deaths from arteriosclerotic aneurysm have increased sevenfold in Great Britain during the past twenty years. In Sweden, the incidence of non-dissecting aneurysm in a group of over 5,000 post-mortems was 1·8 per cent [24]. The surgical aspects of this eminently treatable disease will therefore be considered in detail.

Pathology

Aneurysms have long been classified into true and false;* a useful and still-valid distinction. Both kinds are regularly seen; true aneurysms as a dilatation of the arterial coats which, though thinned out, are still intact; false aneurysms form where there is a breach in the arterial wall and are, therefore, formed of soft tissues and clot. Most true aneurysms are caused by disease; most false aneurysms by injury or operation.

will tend to enlarge where the adverse condition is most marked, and aneurysmal dilatation, saccular or fusiform, may eventually result.

Congenital Medial Defects [99]

(a) *Marfan's syndrome* consists of what has been called the El Greco body build, slender and with long extremities, especially the digits (arachnodactyly) (Fig. 15.1). Also shown are a high arched

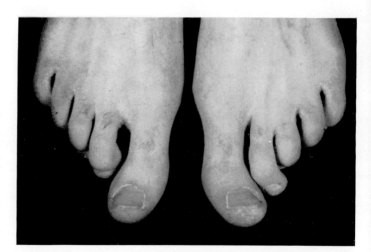

Fig. 15.1. Arachnodactyly and Marfan's syndrome.

This twenty-five-year-old man ruptured an abdominal aneurysm, which was successfully grafted [74] although it later required regrafting. At operation, all his central arteries were grossly enlarged, thin-walled, and elongated. Seven years later he died of a further aortic leakage. (Mr Sinclair Irwin's and the author's case.)

Damage or degeneration affecting the medial coat is thus the common factor. The toughness and resilience of arteries in health is due to the strong layers of elastic tissue. If this material is congenitally malformed, or broken up by inflammatory foci, or worn out by age or local insult, the arterial diameter

palate, dislocated lenses, and a generalised fault in the elastic tissues which in the arteries is associated with cystic medio-necrosis and, because of this, a tendency to partial aortic rupture and extensive dissecting aneurysm between the split layers of the already dilated weakened aorta. Saccular, non-dissecting aneurysm also occurs [63] and may rupture, yet recover with surgery [74]. Some of these features are also present in homocystinuria.

(b) *Ehlers-Danlos syndrome* has a different clinical appearance, with hypermobile joints; inelastic 'bloodhound' skin, notably of the ears; gaping scars of recent injury, especially on the knees in the childhood case; severe bleeding and healing disorders after minor surgery, from a defective formation of collagen or its arrangement, which also predisposes to dissecting aneurysm; spontaneous

---

* Sir William Osler [110] wrote as follows about Antyllus: 'not a fact of his life is known, yet through the mists of eighteen centuries he looms large as one of the most daring and accomplished surgeons of all time.' Osler cites him thus: 'There are two kinds of aneurysms, the one where there is a local dilatation of the artery, and the other from a rupture of the artery and the discharge of blood into the flesh beneath it. Aneurysms due to dilatation are longer than the others. Those due to rupture are rounder.' Then follows a lucid account of how to operate on the two varieties.

rupture of large arteries [10A, 98]; and the development of spontaneous arteriovenous fistula [95]. Multiple neurofibromatosis may also be present [147].

In both conditions the serious arterial complications may not occur until maturity so that marriage tends to perpetuate this often lethal defect, which is inherited as a Mendelian dominant. Patients have been described in which the features of both diseases were present [56], and other members of the same family were affected with one or both diseases. Identical twins may be affected and develop aneurysmal complications [36].

(c) *Localised medial weakness in the cranial arteries* is the cause of 'congenital' or berry aneurysms. The arteries are normal, except at the bifurcation where medial support is deficient and there is herniation of the inner layers. The aneurysm that may result is the commonest cause of spontaneous subarachnoid haemorrhage. Yet the unsupported internal elastic lamina of a healthy artery is sufficient to stand normal arterial pressure, as John Hunter showed [70]. If the lamina is defective [25] these aneurysms form and steadily increase in size. Arteriosclerosis could explain this well [29]. Comparison in 177 cases with a series of 100 patients without aneurysm showed that 35 per cent (or twice as many) had irregularity or stenosis of other parts of the carotid tree [39].

Injury and Other Mechanical Factors, including Post-stenotic Dilatation

Most traumatic aneurysms are false from the outset, growing as the haematoma or the scar tissue stretches. Various injuries causing these and also traumatic arteriovenous fistulae are considered in Chapter 13 and 16. In most cases the lesion develops within a few days or weeks (Fig. 13.10 and 13.12) but in some the course is so slow that the original injury or operation may be almost forgotten (Figs 15.2 and 15.3). Today, one of the commonest false aneurysms is that due to a slow failure of a major arterial reconstruction [140] (*see* Fig. 3.69, p. 76).

The superficial palmar arch may become locally aneurysmal in manual workers; an exostosis of a long bone may interfere with the vascular bundle as it passes over it; these, and post-stenotic aneurysms beyond a severe compression of the main artery are true aneurysms with remnants of the normal muscle and elastic layers, as well as abundant scar tissue. The same is true of distal aneurysm in coarctation of the aorta and of arteriosclerotic stenosis or beyond a complete block where the narrow openings of high-pressure collaterals enter the main vessel.

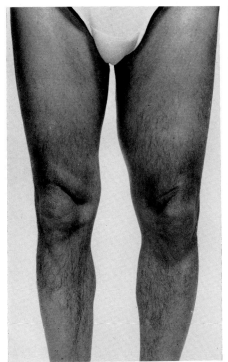

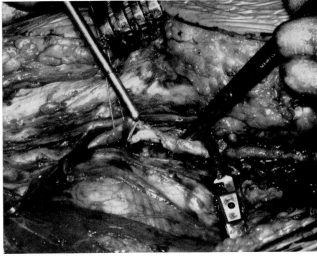

Fig. 15.2. Large false aneurysm of left femoral artery of recent appearance, although it was caused by a gun-shot wound four years before.

The small size of this arterial defect is typical; reconstruction is simple, and the large excluded sac, which here can be seen bulging beneath the thigh muscles between the two bulldog clamps, can be drained externally without fear of bleeding.

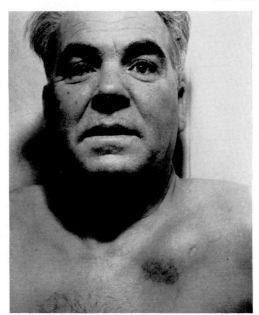

Two of the commonest sites for post-stenotic dilatation are shown in Fig. 15.4.

Mechanical factors must play a part in the topography of the common arteriosclerotic aneurysms. Whether or not the intriguing theory of arterial resonance is correct [103] (Fig. 15.5), it is a fact that nearly all these aneurysms occur in a segment of artery that is unfixed by major branches. Moreover, a nodal pattern is frequently seen in the main artery in which an aneurysm has formed (Fig. 15.9, also Case 3, p. 326). Regular, larger bulges are often present in elderly patients with multiple peripheral aneurysms (Figs. 15.5(b) and 15.7). Certainly, vibrations that coincide with the natural resonant frequencies of the artery can be demonstrated beyond an arterial stenosis [47A].

Fig. 15.3. Traumatic subclavian aneurysm on left side due to a gun-shot wound sustained in the Spanish Civil War twenty years earlier, although the history of aneurysm was much shorter. Excision of the left clavicle and adherent aneurysmal sac with homograft replacement in 1956.

In this and in the patient shown in Fig. 15.2, the deep situation of the initial lesion probably account for the slow clinical course. Some traumatic thoracic aneurysms remain symptomless indefinitely.

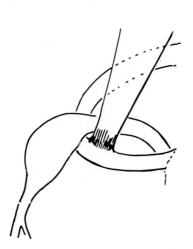

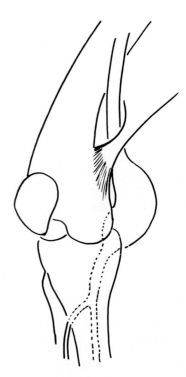

Fig. 15.4. Two common sites for post-stenotic aneurysm. The sac is nearly always elongated and fusiform, tapering distally until it resumes its normal size. This feature allows the surgeon to choose his point of distal division so as to match the diameter of the proximal end in size for grafting or direct anastomosis.

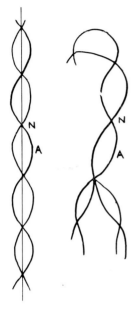

Fig. 15.5(a). The theory of arterial resonance and its possible relationship to the typical sites of aneurysm formation, and of arterial stenosis—the latter being at a fixed point where major branches arise. N = node; A = anti-node.

Medial Degeneration from Age, Infection, and Other Inflammation

By far the most important cause of aneurysm today is degenerative arterial disease; the incidence of this form is rising (*see* Chapter 1, Table 1.1). The abdominal aorta and the popliteal artery are the commonest sites; both lesions are potentially dangerous, and they often occur together. Little is known about the causes of arteriosclerotic medial disease, which are thought to be mainly constitutional, from ageing and degeneration with long-continued mechanical work forces, especially hypertension.

Widening and lengthening of all the arteries, clinically most conspicuous in the limbs, may nevertheless in one and the same patient be associated with local narrowing by arteriosclerotic plaques near and remote from the widening. We have considered the effects of stenosis in causing distal arterial dilatation; in some cases stenosis beyond an arteriosclerotic aneurysm may be even more important mechanically. Any effective occlusive lesion in the 'run-off' area may, from its tendency to thrombose during or shortly after aneurysm surgery, cause early failure from reduced flow and thrombosis or, later, a leakage or rupture from a secondary aneurysm of the graft or one of the suture lines.

Mycotic aneurysm develops insidiously from infective damage to the artery wall (*see* Chapter 7, p. 136), often long after the endocarditis or other septicaemic condition which gave rise to it.

Syphilitic aneurysms are relatively less common today. The classical peripheral type has virtually disappeared; it may, in fact, never have existed as a common condition; for example the clinical pattern of popliteal aneurysm has hardly changed since Hunter's time, although pathologically all cases are now arteriosclerotic.

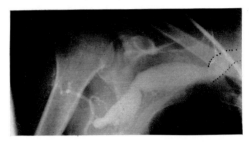

Fig. 15.5(b). Nodal pattern in subclavian and axillary aneurysms in a man aged seventy-five, who also had a similar change on the left side.

Only in the thoracic aorta is syphilis an important persistent cause of aneurysm nowadays (Fig. 15.6). Annual deaths in Great Britain remain at about 500; relatively much less common than arteriosclerotic cases, which now number over 3,000.

From the surgical point of view [9] they may be:

(a) Localised to one part of the aorta; the arch, descending portion, or at the level of the diaphragm.

(b) The whole aorta may be affected, diffusely or with multiple aneurysms.

(c) A saccular aneurysm arises from a narrow opening at a weak point on the convexity of the aorta whose main structure is much less affected.

The sac expands to compress and erode the vertebral bodies (Fig. 15.6); the trachea or oesophagus may be obstructed; involvement of the left recurrent laryngeal nerve, and the left innominate vein produces hoarseness and swelling of the face. Later, there is erosion of the thoracic cage and the aneurysm presents beneath the skin, though usually before this time the aneurysm will have ruptured into the pericardium, bronchial tree or oesophagus. There may be warning haemorrhages before the terminal event.

Active syphilitic aortitis is present throughout the thoracic aorta with generalised medial fibrosis. Serological tests are nearly always positive. The ESR may be grossly raised. For many months this may be the only manifestation of the disease. The course is between six months to three years, with an average of one.

Non-infective arteritis (*see* Chapter 7, p. 138) is associated with aneurysm formation more commonly than is often supposed. The great vessels of the arch are chiefly affected in women in middle life, and in young native Africans [2, 115]. This type of aneurysm is only slowly progressive, often with a long history, and radiologically shows calcification of the wall of the sac.

Post-irradiation arteritis may so damage the elastica as to lead to aneurysm many years later [121B].

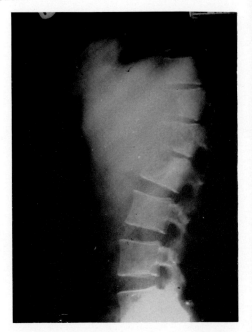

Fig. 15.6. Advanced vertebral erosion from a syphilitic thoraco-abdominal aneurysm. An early patient of Professor Rob's and the author's who survived for three months after resection and homografting. Death from massive secondary haemorrhage due to osteo-myelitis causing local breakdown of the lower anastomosis (*see also* [11]).

Bone erosion is uncommon in arteriosclerotic aneurysm, and is never as extensive as this.

Pregnancy and Arterial Rupture

Arteriosclerosis is rare during the childbearing period, yet arterial rupture is a known risk in pregnancy with or without aneurysm [49]. Hormonal factors have been blamed, such as those that may contribute to the development of varicose veins and haemorrhoids, and also a degeneration of the medial coat [129]. Pregnant women are liable to dissecting aneurysm (*see* p. 316) [124], and the patient with co-arctation of the aorta, either before [57] or after operation [76], may rupture or dissect her arterial coats during pregnancy. The parallel with young female arteritis is striking, but no relationship has been established.

Natural Course and Complications

1. Benign Forms

Arteriosclerotic aneurysm may present as an incidental finding without symptoms. Such aneurysms may be multiple, elongated (Fig. 15.7), and with dilatation of the adjoining artery above and below, which makes it difficult to determine the limits of the lesion; indeed, all the main elastic arteries may be much wider than normal. This is a benign disease of old age; slow and well compensated, with a low incidence of local mechanical complications, and unless these occur, the prognosis is more related to the general cardiovascular status than to the aneurysmal condition. In such a patient, arterial surgery carries unexpected risks (Fig. 15.8).

Spontaneous cure was recognised in 1772 by Guattani of Rome [60] in three cases of popliteal aneurysm: one twenty years after the patient had refused an amputation; another following compression after it had mistakenly been incised; and the third after an acute bout of pain in the aneurysm (*see also* Fig. 15.34.)

This is a common end to the life history of a popliteal and also to a subclavian aneurysm (*see* Chapter 12, p. 222), and is encouraged by obstruction to the outflow, due to previous emboli from the sac. In the central arteries it is unusual, though the author has several patients in which occlusion of the iliac end of an abdominal aortic aneurysm appeared to have provided the opportunity for the thrombus in the sac to obliterate it (*see* p. 292).

2. Disruption

Often, the behaviour of arterial aneurysm is less benign. With obvious progressive enlargement or the onset of symptoms of local pain or compression, the patient is threatened with dangerous and agonising complications which will certainly require surgical intervention, and then at the least opportune moment.

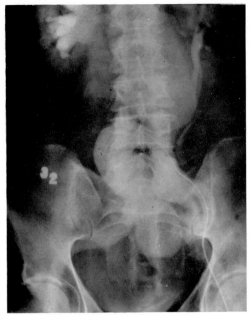

Fig. 15.7. Multiple compound aorto-iliac aneurysm in a man of sixty-five apparently in perfect health. The following sites of aneurysm formation were recognised: abdominal aorta, right and left common iliac, right internal iliac, and left popliteal arteries.

The right iliac complex has compressed the right ureter—the chief complication at this site.

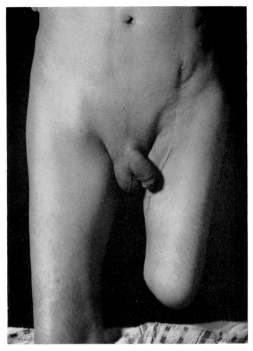

Fig. 15.8. Bilateral common femoral aneurysms. This patient was referred for consideration of his remaining right-sided aneurysm, excision and re-construction having failed on the left. No further operation was indicated in this symptomless case.

Fig. 15.9. Athero-embolism in a patient with a right popliteal aneurysm.

His aneurysm, of moderate size, can be seen with the leg extended, also the scabbing granulomatous lesion over the lower fibular region which had begun as a tender red subcutaneous swelling some weeks before. On an earlier occasion, this patient had been seen with extensive livedo reticularis of the lower calf and foot; both skin conditions were thought to be due to small emboli from the proximal artery, either the aneurysm or one of the beaded stenoses could have been the site of origin. (*See also* Fig. 1.10, p. 11 and Chapter 3 [22].)

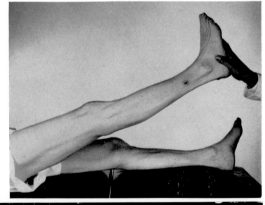

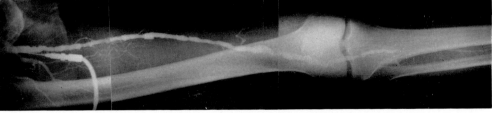

Unfortunately, it is also common for leakage and rupture to occur without warning, particularly in obese or senile patients in whom the earlier physical signs and milder symptoms, if present at all, might easily be missed. Infection may be responsible (*see* Chapter 7, p. 138 and this chapter, p. 291).

3. Embolism from the Contents of the Sac

First recognised as a cause of ischaemia of the hand in patients with subclavian-axillary aneurysm due to local compression (*see* Chapter 12), detachment or discharge of the contents of other aneurysms has since been observed on many occasions. Large portions of thrombus may block the major distal branches, or even the whole outflow tract of the sac, leading sometimes to rupture or to spontaneous thrombosis. Smaller pieces lodge in the digital

vessels, causing one form of secondary Raynaud phenomenon (*see* Chapter 11), while still finer material, semi-fluid cholesterol-containing substance may be discharged from time to time, producing the special appearance in the skin of livedo reticularis [30] which, though similar in some ways to that of acute patchy ischaemia, is more transient, widespread and even; e.g. for a while the whole foot is involved, or even the lower calf, in a case due to popliteal aneurysm; and both lower limbs as high as the buttocks when the complication arises from the abdominal aorta [78]. Biopsy studies have shown a scattered pattern of small arterial occlusion and foreign body giant cells with clear cholesterol clefts in the lumen (Fig. 1.11 p. 11). Skin necrosis may over-lie these lesions in the toes, or on the leg (Fig. 15.9).

Management of Aneurysms in General

1. The Assessment

Many arteriosclerotic, fusiform aneurysms are multiple, symptomless, and require no treatment, but the patient should be seen once or twice a year, and should come earlier if local symptoms should develop. Some abdominal aortic aneurysms and a larger number of those in the femoro-popliteal artery can safely be managed in this way. A proportion will undergo spontaneous cure without developing limb ischaemia.

Conservatism is also preferable in some other symptomless patients who, although their aneurysm may be solitary and conspicuous, have such poor cardio-respiratory reserve, or a history of serious myocardial insufficiency, or other dominating incapacity, that they cannot be offered the safe conduct through surgery expected today in any non-emergency case. Nevertheless, if in such a patient the aneurysm begins to cause severe symptoms, operation must be advised; it may be possible to obtain a good result other than by arterial reconstruction, e.g. by ligation for peripheral aneurysm, or wiring if within the abdomen or pelvis. It is important to exclude other common causes for symptoms in the region; a carcinoma of the body of the pancreas, producing abdominal pain and transmitted aortic pulsations; and an osteo-arthritic hip, or secondary deposits from a prostatic carcinoma being mistaken for pain from a dilated lower-limb artery.

The clinical examination in patients with suspected aneurysm should review all systems in which these other common causes for aneurysm-like symptoms and signs may arise. Useful screening investigations include X-ray films of the chest and of the region of

the lesion, also the haemoglobin level, and a stool test for occult blood.

Arteriography may eliminate the diagnosis of abdominal aneurysm, but in the limbs the narrower central channel through the aneurysmal thrombus may give a falsely normal appearance (Fig. 15.9), or a lateral sac may fail to fill.

2. Choice of Operation

Figure 15.10 shows the classical and the newer procedures and their indications. Preference should be for the simplest effective plan, though today most patients will require an arterial reconstruction. In a fit patient this should not only give the best functional result but fewer complications and a shorter time in hospital.

LIGATION

For centuries, ligation was the standard operation for limb aneurysm, and in the early nineteenth century extended by Astley Cooper and his American pupil, Valentine Mott, to the larger, proximal arteries [17]. It has now given place to arterial reconstruction except for small, peripheral aneurysms (e.g. in the forearm, hand or scalp), and those within the cranium. It remains, however, the treatment of choice for large complicated popliteal aneurysms in elderly, poor-risk subjects (Cases 2 and 3). The merits of the Hunterian principle of ligation above the first large collateral branch are as acceptable today as 150 years ago, and lives can still be saved by it. The closer approach used by Anel has lost none of its difficulties for any large aneurysm, while distal tying, as suggested by Brasdor in Hunter's time [16], was occasionally successful in the past in patients in

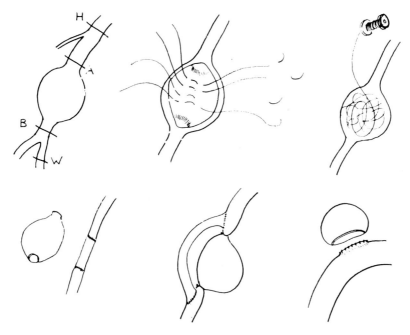

Fig. 15.10. Operations for aneurysm.

The classical ligations: H = Hunter (above first collateral); A = Anel: immediately above aneurysm; B = Brasdor: immediately below aneurysm; W = Wardrop: one of the main branches is tied.

Also shown are endoaneurysmorrhaphy; intrasaccular wiring; excision and graft replacement; by-pass grafting and ligation above and below; excision and lateral suture.

which the proximal site was inaccessible, as in the innominate. No doubt it acted in the same way that a distal embolic obstruction produces a spontaneous cure, though likewise, not without a period of increased risk of rupture.

ENDOANEURYSMORRHAPHY (obliterative and reconstructive)

Matas of New Orleans, in 1903, introduced his method of obliterating the aneurysmal lumen by many sutures [105]. It could be used with safety in patients in whom the sac was closely adherent to important nerves or veins, and in whom there might already be occlusive complications beyond, threatening gangrene with a Hunterian ligation. In this 10 per cent of cases in which Hunter's operation may be expected to fail, Matas's method should be safe. It may, because of existing impairment in the outflow, be preferable to attempting reconstruction by grafting. If one of the main draining branches of the sac should still be patent, this can be preserved by appropriate placing of the obliterating sutures; a good channel through the operated segment can

thus be maintained. Such a patient may after a few months even cease to be troubled by intermittent claudication.

INTRASACCULAR WIRING

Another method of encouraging slow obliteration of the sac is by filling it with wire. Colt [118] originally achieved this by inserting his umbrella-like 'wisps' via a trocar and cannula, often without exposing the sac.

A more extensive procedure is now preferred, using a great length of fine stainless-steel monofilament [19]. Exposure need be only limited. A few inoperable or bad-risk cases of aortic or iliac aneurysm may be treated with success in this way (Fig. 15.11). Three hundred feet or more of a reel of 36 gauge stainless-steel is inserted, beginning with a hypodermic needle puncture in the front of the sac.

This technique is mainly useful for the bad-risk abdominal aortic aneurysm (Table 15.1). Combined with the retro- and para-aortic injection of 10 per cent phenol in water (*see* Chapter 10, p. 199), it often gives good lasting relief of pain.

Table 15.1. Wiring of Abdominal Aortic Aneurysms (14 cases)

Long-term survival	3
Died of other causes	2
From aneurysm	9

REPLACEMENT GRAFTING OR BY-PASSING

These are now standard practice. Choice of method and material depend upon local conditions, including the mobility of the part, size and adherence of the aneurysm, and the size and flow within the artery in which it has formed. Operative details are described with each aneurysm in the sections below.

END-TO-END ANASTOMOSIS

Occasionally this procedure is possible, and a number of traumatic and some degenerative aneurysms can be dealt with in this way. The aorto-iliac channel can be restored by direct suture, making use of the elongation and tortuosity of the iliacs to free a sufficient length to make the ends meet with the correct degree of tension. The course of the subclavian artery in the posterior triangle can be shortened for the same purpose, and the popliteal can be anastomosed with the knee flexed; extension is at once regained on removal of the clamps as the repaired segment fills and lengthens.

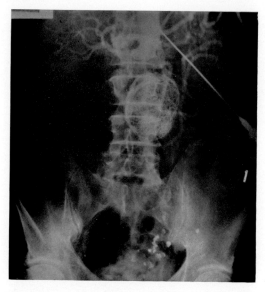

Fig. 15.11. Cure of an obstructed abdominal aneurysm by the insertion of 300 feet of 36 gauge stainless-steel wire in a man of fifty-two with a long history of Leriche syndrome, who had lately developed a painful expanding abdominal aneurysm above his occluded bifurcation.

COMMON ANEURYSMS

I Abdominal Aortic Aneurysm

Excluding all cases of prominent pulsation, tortuous aortic bends and soft tissue mass transmitting the aortic impulse (to do this may require aortography), abdominal aortic aneurysm has become a common condition in hospital practice, though often only as an incidental finding. There are three clinical groups:

(a) Symptomless: unnoticed by the patient, but usually associated with hypertension and heart disease, and often detected during routine examination for these or other conditions. Fever, or a hot bath, may draw attention to the pulsation, 'like another heart'. (Case 1, p. 324.)

(b) Pain in the abdomen or back, often with urological or gastro-intestinal symptoms, and sometimes discovered at exploratory laparatomy.

(c) Leaking or ruptured: presenting as an acute abdominal emergency or with general collapse.

A patient may pass through each of the stages, or any two of them in turn. Some, perhaps one fifth, [54] remain symptomless for the remainder of their life, and eventually die of other causes [123] (*see also* p. 292).

Table 15.2. Clinical Features of Abdominal Aortic Aneurysm (100 patients)

Pain		72
Abdomen	21	
Back	31	
Legs	11	
Discovered by doctor		21
Noticed by patient		11
Genitourinary		6
Gastrointestinal		4

Clinical Presentation (Table 15.2)

Osler, in 1905 [109], had seen 16 cases in his wards at the Johns Hopkins Hospital during the same number of years, and cited the experience of Guy,s

Hospital with 54 cases between 1854 and 1900. Although today we see many more such patients there is little to add to Osler's description of the clinical presentation of this predominantly male disease, with pain as the commonest early symptom and throbbing the most obvious sign. He also realised that it is often wrongly diagnosed, and what is more important today, that it can easily be overlooked because of the obscure nature of the symptoms it may produce.

The author's experience includes several examples of each of Osler's types: e.g. resembling renal disease with colic, haematuria, or a large swelling in the loin; also, appendicitis, with or without peritonitis (sepsis is often imitated by early extravasation insufficient to produce shock). Other patients had testicular pain or swelling, spinal-type pain from vertebral erosion, with root reference to the lumbar or sciatic areas, also with motor effects such as quadriceps weakness or drop foot.

Abdominal pain is seldom severe before rupture. It was present in only 24 per cent of one large series specially examined for this evidence [138], and its true cause may be difficult to detect; in this way a number of aneurysms remain unrecognised until an exploratory laparotomy is undertaken, with or without the support of a diagnosis from clinical investigation. 6 per cent of the author's 200 cases had undergone an operation shortly before referral.

Backache. Lumbo-sacral pain varies from slight to excruciating, in moderate degree, and when combined with the abdominal throbbing and tenderness of the aneurysm it forms the typical presentation in the diagnosis of which aortography is unnecessary. In the worst cases the patient takes large amounts of codein, or even pethidine may be needed throughout the night and day. He may become suicidal [54]. When an operation is suggested he accepts it at once without any question of the risk.

True root compression by the sac may produce a well-defined neurological picture of sciatic pain with areas of sensory loss, quadriceps paralysis, or foot-drop. Myelography may have been done (Fig. 15.12).

Swelling of the left lower limb can be caused by obstruction to the left common iliac vein by the enlarging sac.

Ureteric obstruction by compression or fibrosis is commoner on the left, often producing a non-functioning kidney (Fig. 15.13). Fixed left renal pain is caused, sometimes with haematuria, and less often, renal colic [31]. Both sides may be affected, producing chronic renal failure.

Renal ischaemic hypertension. Either pressure from the aneurysm or occlusive disease in the renal artery may cause obstruction to the renal blood flow, usually on the left side. This can lead to a percept-

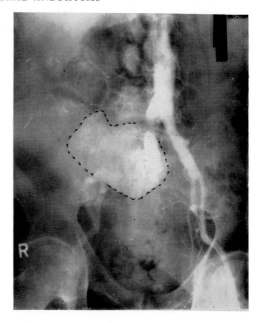

Fig. 15.12. Neurological presentation of abdominal aneurysm.

A man of sixty-four was under investigation for right sciatica and foot drop. Myelography (the central opacity) showed no root lesion. It was then observed that the patient had a pulsatile swelling in the right iliac fossa. Left transfemoral aortography confirmed the presence of a slowly leaking aneurysm of the right common iliac artery, found at operation to be compressing the lumbo-sacral trunk against the ala of the sacrum. Excision and homograft replacement. He survived fourteen years, until a coronary thrombosis at the age of 78. (Patient of Professor Rob, Mr Sol. Cohen, and the author.)

ible increase in the size of the aneurysm, with increased risk of rupture [3]. The left renal vein may also be compressed.

The testicular vessels may be compressed on the left side, causing pain or swelling in the testis or cord, varicocoele, or hydrocoele.

Sexual disturbances [31] may be distressing, with impaired or painful orgasm or spontaneous crises of a similar kind, as in one patient of the author's who, at operation, showed a gross periaortitis with dense adherence of all surrounding structures, including, no doubt, the lumbar sympathetic trunks and presacral nerve plexus.

Bladder symptoms may also be neurologically caused, or there may be compression by a large iliac aneurysm filling much of the pelvis, thereby causing increased frequency of micturition, and occasionally pulsation of the stream.

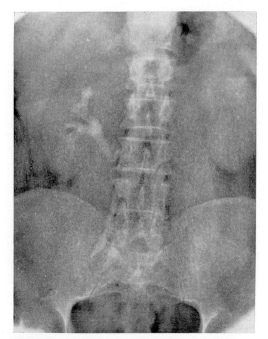

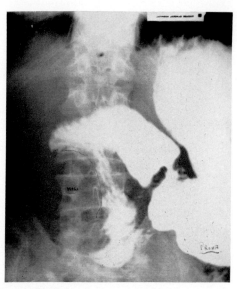

Fig. 15.13. Left ureteric compression by abdominal aneurysm. A gardener, aged sixty, complained of pain in the left loin with slight haematuria. Pyelography showed a non-functioning left kidney, and the lightly calcified left border of a left abdominal aneurysm, which proved at operation to be the cause of the obstruction to the left kidney. Resection of the aneurysm with left nephrectomy in 1961. Patient remains well.

Fig. 15.14. Duodenal obstruction by abdominal aortic aneurysm. From the right side: incomplete obstruction associated with dense adherence of the displaced and stretched out second and third parts of the duodenum. Relieved by aortic resection. (Patient referred by Mr Ivor Lewis.)

Duodenal obstruction was described by Osler [109], but it is unusual [138], though there may be considerable angulation and displacement of the duodenum across the upper part of the aneurysm (Fig. 15.14). It is one of the few clear physical signs of increasing expansion and imminent rupture. It may follow aortic surgery, especially palliative procedures such as wiring.

Inferior mesenteric arterial insufficiency may be caused by tight compression and adherence of the origin of this artery to the left side of the sac, or by thrombus obstructing its opening.

Constipation, irritable bowel, left-sided pain and tenderness are noticed, and are often aggravated by large doses of codeine or pethidine for pain. Colonic symptoms may be due to inferior mesenteric ischaemia (*see* Chapter 17, p. 382).

Loss of weight occurs in about 20 per cent of patients [138] and is somewhat difficult to explain, for frank insufficiency of the superior mesenteric artery is rare. Some other disturbances of the small

bowel or its vessels may be implicated, or pain and anxiety. In one patient, wasting was due to obstruction of the duodenum.

RADIOLOGICAL INVESTIGATION OF A
SUSPECTED ABDOMINAL ANEURYSM

1. A plain film of the abdomen, often shows the curved, partly calcified outline (Fig. 15.15) of the left border of the aneurysm, while sometimes the left psoas shadow is lost. The lateral view is generally clearer and gives a more accurate estimate of the size of the sac. (Fig. 15.16.)

2. Barium meal series show displacement of the duodenum or small bowel by the sac [Figs 15.14, 15.17].

3. Intravenous pyelography may show displacement or compression of the left ureter or both, with or without hydronephrosis, and non-function of the left kidney is common (Fig. 15.13). One of the author's patients had unsuspected polycystic disease, and three others, silent renal calculi. This is of

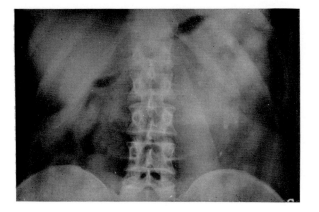

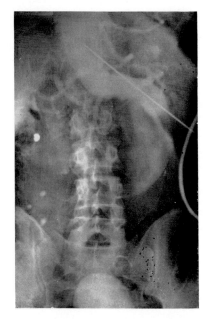

Fig. 15.15. Curved and slightly calcified left border of a large abdominal aneurysm. Size and position confirmed by lumbar aortography during preoperative assessment.

practical importance, for pyelolithotomy can be undertaken at the same time as the grafting operation [31]. Horse-shoe kidney, no longer considered a rare condition*, may simulate, or accompany abdominal aneurysm (Fig. 15.18) [31, 47B]. Most cases show up at pyelography [80].

4. Ultrasonic scanning [55A] provides both the diagnosis and an approximate measurement of the sac in tense or obese patients.

AORTOGRAPHY IN ABDOMINAL ANEURYSM
This need not be routine. The patient should, if possible, be spared the discomforts and slight risk that may lessen his fitness for the major procedure; also, the haematoma may form around the upper part of the aneurysm, which will obscure the dissection at operation, or increase oozing, or adherence if there is to be a delay before the resection.

Aortography, however, can provide information to important questions that may determine the whole course of management:

1. The diagnosis of abdominal aneurysm may be uncertain (*see* p. 287).
2. The position of the renal arteries and their state may be in question if the sac is very large or unusually high in the abdomen.
3. Occlusive disease in the iliac or femoro-popliteal

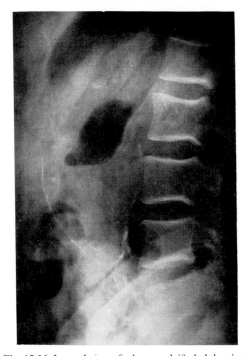

Fig. 15.16. Lateral view of a large, calcified abdominal aortic aneurysm in a man of sixty-eight. Note close relationship of back of sac to body of 3rd lumbar vertebra. Patient declined operation. He remained well until his death, from coronary thrombosis, six years later. (Mr Sinclair Irwin's case.)

* Incidence is now given as 1 in 200 to 400 individuals [80].

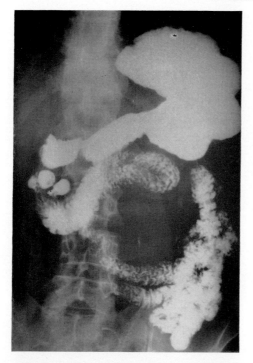

Fig. 15.17. Duodeno-jejunal displacement by abdominal aneurysm. Lesion thus recognised during barium examination for abdominal symptoms.

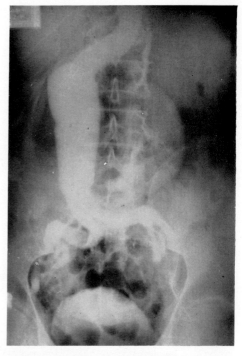

Fig. 15.18. Abdominal aneurysm with horse-shoe kidney. (Mr Andrew Desmond's case. Successfully grafted and remains well eight years later.)

arteries, or a coincident popliteal aneurysm may require study.

4. Any question of aortic dilatation above the renal arteries, or of the common or internal iliacs within the pelvis, any of which may, in an obese patient, be obscured during clinical or plain X-ray examination: such factors weigh against operation, and without aortography might be missed.

The choice between translumbar aortic puncture and percutaneous retrograde catheterisation from the common femoral will depend upon the experience and inclinations of the radiologist; at St Mary's Hospital, Dr David Sutton [142] prefers to use the lumbar route in most cases of arteriosclerosis, because plaques, stenosis, or kinking so often impede the passage of a femoral catheter. However, if there should be the need for selective renal or mesenteric study as well as a general view of the aneurysm the retrograde method will be adopted. Lateral films can be taken, which show the anterior outline of the sac as well as the superior mesenteric artery.

THE RISK OF RUPTURE?

This is the most important problem in any patient with abdominal aortic aneurysm, yet one that cannot often be solved with confidence, least of all in the symptomless case.

Rupture comes as a catastrophe, without previous warning in perhaps a quarter of the patients seen in hospital. At operation, or at post-mortem examination the sac is almost always large; 6–7 cm was found to be the critical diameter in four studies [54, 81, 123, 143], with the incidence of rupture rising steeply above this size. The morbid anatomy of an unruptured abdominal aneurysm shows thinning of the wall at the wide part of the sac (Fig. 15.19).

A history of pain is more usual (*see* p. 286). It can safely be stated that from the time when pain develops in a case of abdominal aortic aneurysm, rupture takes place in a matter of months, not years, and often within a few weeks.

Hypertension probably increases the risk [54], but this factor is obscured in the fulminating cases by their shocked state on admission. Patients with renal artery stenosis appear to be specially liable [3].

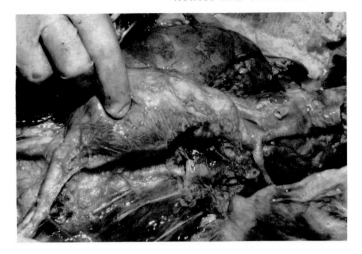

(a) Post-mortem examination showed the neck of the sac curving forwards to open up the retro-aortic plane of dissection and clamping.

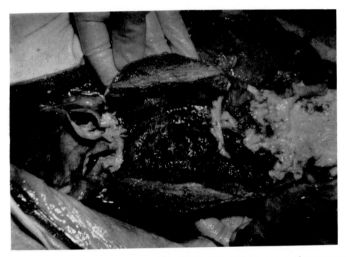

(b) The opened sac shows the relatively healthy arterial wall at the neck and the bifurcation. At its equator, however, the wall is thinned and ulcerated with adherent thick thrombus deposition. This would have been a good case for the unbranched, inlay type of graft (Figs 15.25 and 15.26).

Fig. 15.19. Morbid anatomy of an unoperated case.
A man of sixty was admitted with a view to resection of his abdominal aneurysm, but died two days later from an overwhelming influenzal pneumonia.

Infection in or near the sac has been shown to be a factor in some patients [137], either blood-borne or from an adjoining lesion such as an osteomyelitis of the lumbar spine (which may have begun as pressure erosion). The aneurysm itself may be mycotic. Staphylococcal, salmonella and tuberculous infections have been demonstrated (*see* Chapter 7, p. 135). Clinically, rupture often follows a febrile illness.

Obstruction of the iliac outflow of the aneurysm has not been given the prominence that it deserves as a cause of rupture or leakage. Two opposing pathological processes are at work (Fig. 15.20):

1. Progressive dilatation from increased strain upon the wall of the partly obstructed aneurysm.
2. Stagnant thrombosis in the wide channel whose slowed stream is further reduced by the diminished outflow.

According to which of these is more active, the aneurysm will either give way or undergo a spontaneous cure, though until the final closure up to the lower level of the renals (Fig. 15.11) the risk of disruption is still present.

Thrombosis of the inferior vena cava may, in the

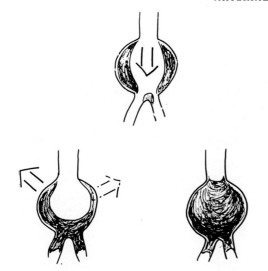

Fig. 15.20. The mechanism of rupture of an obstructed aneurysm and of spontaneous cure.

while in the other group 50 per cent survived, although most of the deaths were from the aneurysm [123].

At Barnes Hospital, St Louis, 30 patients were followed up for five years or until death. Twenty-seven per cent were alive at the end of the study; 15 of the 21 deaths had been from ischaemic heart disease or stroke. Only 2 died of ruptured aneurysm, neither of whom had other evidence of cardiovascular disease [81].

Perhaps the most striking evidence on prognosis in the type of case seen by surgeons was in a group of 68 untreated patients seen during the post-war years in King's County Hospital, New York; of those with symptoms 33 per cent were dead within a month, 74 per cent within six months, and 80 per cent at one year [54].

same way, increase tension within the aneurysm; the extensive circulatory obstruction caused by phlegmasia cerulea dolens has been suggested as a cause of rupture [22].

Prognosis in Abdominal Aortic Aneurysm

In 707 cases, studied by Colt [27], of aortic aneurysms at all levels the average duration of life from first onset of principal symptom was 18 to 24 months.

The mortality of rupture, untreated, is virtually 100 per cent. Leakage, also, is usually fatal, although if it is slow and of minor extent the patient may survive for several weeks; not always with continuing symptoms; advice may not be sought, when a second, fatal leak is then probable.

We have seen that rupture is related to the size of the sac and the severity of symptoms, but if all cases are taken into account, small and large, silent or symptomatic, the prognosis may mainly depend upon whether there is associated cardiovascular disease, for not only may this decide the outcome of any surgery but, in the untreated case also the mode of death tends to be determined in this way. At the Mayo Clinic, in a series of 141 patients seen during the 1950s, including many in which the aneurysm was silent or coincidental, the survival rate at five years was 20 per cent in those with cardiovascular disease, most of the deaths being from this cause,

Indications for Resection of Abdominal Aortic Aneurysm

Absolute:	Leakage or rupture
	Uncontrollable pain
Early necessity:	Very large sac
	Suspected enlargment of sac
	Moderate, persistent pain, or tenderness
	Pressure effects on other viscera
Debatable:	Symptomless
	Small
	Elderly, frail or unfit subject
	Other aneurysms present
Contra-indications:	Proved carcinoma by investigation or laparotomy (but *see* p. 293)
	Advanced cardio-respiratory insufficiency or other manifest major cardiovascular disease (unless absolute indications also present).

This still leaves cases in which the policy is in doubt, e.g. a medium-sized symptomless aneurysm in a fit patient. Age, and the patient's inclinations should help the decision.

Special Features of Leaking or Ruptured Abdominal Aneurysm

Much depends upon the size and situation of the opening in the wall of the sac (Fig. 15.21).

A free, extensive anterior rupture into the general peritoneal cavity is quickly fatal, the initial pain and collapse being so sudden that as a rule the doctor will arrive only in time to pronounce death. There will have been little in the way of warning symptoms for, except for the duodenum, there are no adherent structures to be compressed by the expanding thin-walled convexity of the front of the sac; vomiting, which may be blood-stained is sometimes an early effect in such a case.

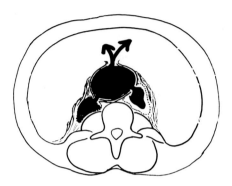

Fig. 15.21. Ruptured and leaking abdominal aneurysm. Bursting of the anterior wall of the sac causes immediate exsanguinating intra-peritoneal or gastro-duodenal haemorrhage. Posteriorly, the leakage is usually more gradual. Any or all of the retroperitoneal structures may be affected, including ureter, sympathetic chain [42A], vena cava [124A], or the lumbar plexus [82A, 120A].

Extraperitoneal rupture is more common in surgical experience, fortunately, for such a patient may be able to travel a considerable distance to reach hospital, still in fair condition. The anterior part of the sac is often found to be thick-walled, although the back is weakened by friction upon the lumbar vertebral bodies, and eventually may disappear altogether, its part in the aneurysm being taken by the bone, which by that time is obviously eroded, a feature that is present in from 3 per cent (author's experience) to 6 per cent [54] of all cases. The discs are less quickly worn down, one foot may be warm and dry from damage to the sympathetic trunk (Fig. 15.22). Posterior rupture occurs either where the sac is attached to the bone area, or earlier, during compression against it. Haemorrhage is extraperitoneal and, therefore, often relatively confined (Fig. 15.23), which explains the latent period during which patients remain fit for transfer for surgery. A few hours or days later sudden collapse may take place, if the retroperitoneal false aneurysm should burst into the major peritoneal cavity. This may happen during the early stages of operation (not always with the diagnosis made) or during the anaesthetic induction from relaxation or straining.

Earlier, during the preoperative, quiescent phase, gentle abdominal palpation often shows up this type of lesion; the true central aneurysm may not be palpable, being obscured for example by increased abdominal muscle tone. Yet, far out in the flank, as

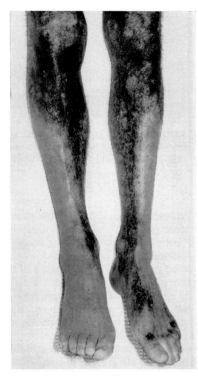

Fig. 15.22. Sympathetic neuropathy due to abdominal aneurysm in a consultant physician aged sixty-four. False aneurysmal extension posteriorly caused compression of the lumbar chains on both sides, though more on the right, as the area of anhidrosis would suggest. The right foot was much warmer before operation. Postoperatively, the condition was symmetrical. Left sympathectomy signs are very common after resection of the sac, and the relative coldness of the right foot may cause concern.

far as the mid-axillary line, right or left, will be felt a large tender swelling (often mistaken for an inflammatory mass [144], unless the hand is kept still for a few moments, when the arterial pulsation will be perceived. Thus, the tragic classical error of incision, the greatest perhaps in all surgery, may, as Pirogoff showed, be avoided (for his words, *see* p. 307).

Sepsis (appendicitis, cholecystitis, perinephric abscess, or other inflammation, especially pancreatitis) is also suggested by the association, in an elderly and often obese patient, of fever and abdominal rigidity, both due to extravasated blood, with no

blade inferiorly. This gives an excellent exposure of the entire field.

If the evisceration method is not considered necessary, the duodenum is dissected off the front of the aneurysm. A dry pack is tucked into the upper end of the field to hold this and the reflected duodenum behind a Deaver's retractor. Now the area of exposure is isolated, using three or four large dry packs, and the Goligher's retractor is inserted with its deep third blade in the pelvis. The left renal vein is then identified and can usually be lifted away without difficulty from the front of the neck of the aneurysm. The inferior mesenteric vein is divided high, to complete the anterior exposure of the upper end of the aorta, behind which gentle dissection with the right index finger (if the tissues are free) or cholecystectomy forceps (if there is adherence or lack of room) soon provides space for a broad, moist, linen tape in readiness for the application of the upper aortic clamp. A pair of lumbar arteries may be in the way and must be kept to one side of the dissection space above or below, whichever is easier. Later, they may need to be divided. An abnormal, postaortic left renal vein [145A], or left vena cava [7], or both together, may be the site of unexpected and quite profuse bleeding, which must be completely secured before proceeding further.

A less serious anatomical difficulty concerns the aberrant lower pole renal arteries which, if present, must be divided. The author and others [31] have not yet seen hypertension to follow from this cause.

The common iliac arteries are now exposed near their origin from the aneurysm. The peritoneum over each, or between them, is divided and moved away to both sides, and the anterior surface of each iliac is cleared for a few centimetres to find the easiest place at which to pass the encircling tape. It is important not to injure the iliac vein. Often, it is easier to take the artery just beyond the adherent part of the vein.

Either ureter, though more often the left, may be compressed by the aneurysm, usually at the region of its maximum diameter, about the level of the origin of the inferior mesenteric artery. Although it is often possible to dissect it free from the sac, it may be buried fairly deeply, and in some cases it is so flattened and atrophic that it is better to leave it alone and to preserve this part of the sac. This degree of ureteric involvement is compatible with perfect function.

SHOULD HEPARIN BE GIVEN?

When all three clamps are ready to apply, it must be decided whether or not the patient is to be heparinised. 100 mg would now be given into the aorta. Factors for and against are shown below:

Heparin advisable	Heparin may be omitted
Many elective cases.	All leaking or ruptured cases.
Prolonged clamping anticipated.	Short period likely.
Occlusive or aneurysmal lesions present in lower limbs.	Lower limb arteries in good condition.
Early experience of operator.	Experience extensive in this procedure.

We have found the measured blood loss and replacement requirement to be more than doubled when heparin was used. A large adherent aneurysm, requiring extensive operative dissection with clamps applied for much of the time, would suggest the need for heparin, but it is this type of case that bleeds most during the removal phase of the operation; thus, the two requirements of haemostasis and avoidance of stagnant thrombosis beyond the clamps are to some extent incompatible. Every effort should be made to shorten the procedure; the simplest way being to limit the extent of the resection.

The Operation

1. It is often possible (in 50 per cent of my patients) to preserve the bifurcation so that a simple tubular graft can be used (Figs 15.25 and 15.26), one large inferior anastomosis being much quicker than two smaller ones. Exceptionally, it is possible to secure a satisfactory end-to-end aortic anastomosis after removal of the aneurysm in a case in which the iliacs are tortuous, and when dissected this permits the aortic bifurcation to be drawn up to meet the aortic stump. The same is sometimes possible with an iliac aneurysm, the aorta also being mobilised and brought across to the side of the resection.

2. No attempt is made to dissect the sac from the inferior vena cava; in fact it is usually better to leave most of the aneurysm undissected, and once the three main clamps are in place to open the front of the sac longitudinally. When the thrombus has been turned out, and any bleeding lumbar branch orifice dealt with by suture-ligation, the graft may either be inserted within the cavity of the aneurysm (Fig. 15.25b), which is then closed over the front of it, or if the lumbar vertebral bodies are exposed and irregular or appear possibly to be infected, a culture is taken from the denuded bone and the sac is folded across the front of the vertebral column and secured there to form a firm, fibrous bed for the graft.

3. An extensive, complicated aorto-iliac aneurysm (Fig. 15.7) may be densely adherent at the pelvic brim, and so involve the internal iliac arteries so that a complete resection is out of the question. Since ligation of both the internal iliacs, in addition to the

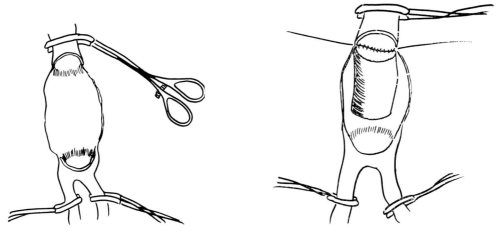

Fig. 15.25. Tubular inlay-graft.

(a) The sac is opened longitudinally, and the sites for the two anastomoses are inspected.

(b) The upper anastomosis is made beginning with the posterior layer; similarly for the lower anastomosis with tension on the graft maintained with a fourth clamp.

inferior mesenteric, means almost certain left colon necrosis, some provision must be made to maintain the pelvic blood supply:

(a) A very large compound or calcified aorto-iliac sac should be left *in situ*; the aorta is transected at the neck of the aneurysm and the distal end closed with a strong suture. Of the several possible ways of arranging the outflow, the simplest is to graft as for extensive occlusion, with the two limbs of the bifurcation prosthesis brought through the femoral canal on either side and anastomosed to the common femoral (Fig. 15.30). Usually one of the iliac arteries can be ligated proximal to the internal iliac origin, so that the distal colon receives a supply from this side, backwards up the external iliac. The more aneurysmal iliac on the other side can then be taken out of circulation by ligating the external iliac beneath the inguinal ligament.

(b) Internal iliac aneurysm on its own is uncommon and rather difficult to deal with except by ligation or exclusion and suture, for the sac is closely adherent to most of the pelvic structures. Wiring is a good solution to this difficulty.

The operation from this point is straightforward. Only if the sac is freely mobile should it be removed; it is easier, standing on the patient's left, to dissect it distally (caudally), taking each pair of lumbar branches as they present. This gives a good view of the adherent zone of the bifurcation. Now

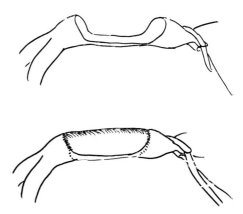

Fig. 15.26. Inlay-graft, lateral views. Redundant sides of aneurysm have, for clarity, been excised: sufficient is usually kept to cover the graft later.

it must be decided whether the reconstruction requires a bifurcation prothesis. In most instances the iliacs will already have been controlled separately so that the operator can make a trial section of the lower end of the aorta near the bifurcation to assess the suitability of the aortic wall at this point for a single anastomosis to the lower end of an unbranched graft. The decision must be made now, so that the graft can be chosen and cut to size.

The upper anastomosis is constructed as shown in Fig. 15.27; if the neck of the sac has been transected it is usually best to place the front row first.* The posterior part of the aortic stump is usually thinner and more difficult to handle, thus it helps to have the anterior half already securely sutured in place. A second line of sutures may be inserted if any gaps or small rents are thought to be present, particularly at the back. If the graft is to be sutured into the opened-out aneurysm (Fig. 15.25), the posterior row of the upper anastomosis is inserted first, beginning at the centre and continuing round both sides, choosing the line that best matches the graft to the aorta for size.

The neck may be flush with the right renal artery, or may tear away at the line of the clamp. Figure 15.28 shows one way in which this difficulty may be overcome.

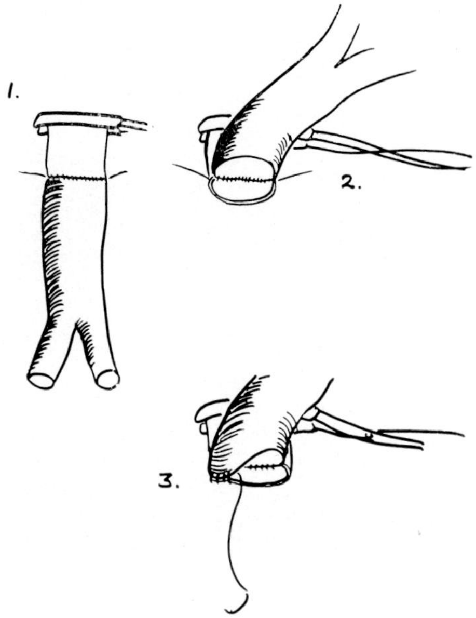

---

* Choice of suture material is important. The author still prefers silk; 4/0 for a transected stump, and 2/0 with deep posterior bites for an inlay anastomosis.

Fig. 15.27. Bifurcation aortic replacement. The upper anastomosis

(1) The anterior layer is completed: (2) The graft is turned upwards to expose the posterior aortic margin: (3) The posterior layer of the anastomosis is completed suturing towards the operator.

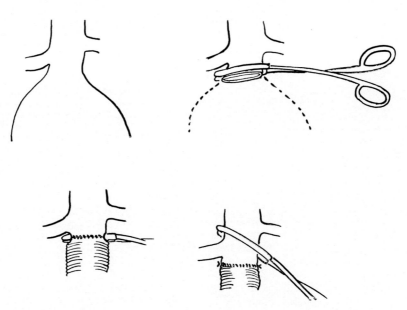

Fig. 15.28. Anastomosis over the proximal clamp, where the neck of the aneurysm is close to the right renal artery. Alternatively, a 30 ml Foley catheter can be inflated in the stump [121A].

The upper anastomosis must be tested for leaks, releasing the aortic clamp with the graft clamped below.

The lower anastomoses (Fig. 15.29) may be difficult because of calcification, which may interfere with suturing. Spicules can be removed where necessary, and large bites of the artery wall beyond the calcified

heparin) slowly, beginning a few minutes before completion of the last anastomosis. Unless the graft has been preclotted, and sometimes with a knitted dacron graft even if it has, bleeding may be free through the mesh of the material on removal of the first lower clamp. Several more minutes may have to be allowed for the mesh to become sealed by clot, though this

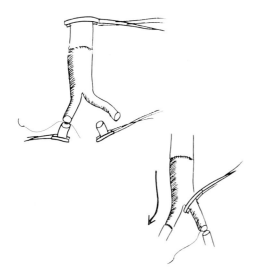

Fig. 15.29. The lower anastomoses. The right iliac is joined first, using one stitch, preferably beginning at the back. If heparin has not been given, it is an advantage to unclamp the aorta and the right iliac artery while completing the left iliac anastomosis.

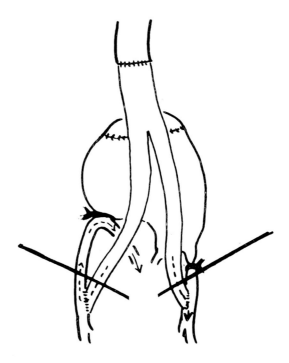

Fig. 15.30. Aorto-femoral by-pass graft for extensive aorto-iliac compound aneurysmal sac, adherent to main pelvic veins, showing method of iliac ligation to exclude sac and preserve blood supply to hind-gut.

margin will usually bring the two sides together with satisfactory haemostasis later, or removal of the clamps.

Whether a single or double distal anastomosis is required, it is usually best to suture from within, placing the back row first (Fig. 13.4 (vi), p. 241).

As in all arterial grafting, moderate longitudinal tension is necessary. A clamp on the graft enables the first assistant to approximate the ends during the suturing.

It is worth passing a Fogarty catheter down each lower limb at this stage, to remove debris or stasis clot before the final unclamping.

REMOVAL OF THE CLAMPS

If heparin has been used, the anaesthetist must now give intravenous protamine (2 mg for each mg

happens much more quickly in the unheparinised patient, and with a woven graft. So, too much time should not elapse with the graft filled with blood, but with no flow through it; all clamps must be removed at the earliest possible moment once free-clotting blood has been admitted to the lumen of the graft. A good plan is to allow an occasional beat through to keep the channel clear and to offset the rapid shift of much of the blood volume into the widely dilated vessels of the ischaemic lower limbs. At this point there is usually a fairly sharp fall in blood pressure, which must be measured and charted, and checked against the recent blood loss figures.

The causes of hypotension on removing the clamps may be any of the following:

1. The reactive hyperaemia flow [120] into the previously clamped area. This should not last more than five to ten minutes.
2. Unreplaced blood loss at this time or earlier in the operation.
3. The effect of protamine.
4. 'Washout acidosis' [19] in patients already anoxic from shock, or acidosis from the infusion of stored blood [21].
5. Citrate intoxication [93].

With correct management, each of these factors should be offset before the hypotension can reach any dangerous level or duration. Before the clamps are removed, blood replacement of previous measured losses must be complete, plus 250 to 500 ml above the amount lost.

Further rapid replacement must be possible, using pressure; for this a Martin's pump is effective and simple.

Protamine must be given slowly. Heparin titrations are seldom necessary. The state of the blood-clotting mechanism can be fairly accurately judged from the appearance of the operative field, and the blood in the packs. Small soft clots should appear within five minutes of giving the protamine.

If the blood pressure tended to be low during the earlier part of the operation, though the blood loss may have been small, the additional fall on unclamping can usually be safely controlled by further rapid transfusion. The surgeon can effectively conserve the patient's condition by staged release of the upper end of the reconstruction. First, the clamp is quickly but carefully withdrawn from the wound, and the aorta above the anastomosis is at once held between the thumb and first finger; this control, gentler and safer than with the clamp, is only intermittently released, first for one beat in ten, then one in seven, and so on, until within five to ten minutes all the beats can be allowed through. A useful indication of the patient's condition is the force of the pulse within the surgeon's grip. When he begins to tire, the patient is doing well. During the released beats the field is watched for any continuing bleeding from one place, which is best dealt with by local pressure, until the unclamping is completed. If this is not possible, a strip of haemostatic absorbable material is wrapped around the anastomosis or other bleeding point. Extra sutures are not often needed and should never be used in any inaccessible position, for worse bleeding usually results. Only the most serious leakage should bring the operator to reapply the clamps. One iliac may be reclamped, if absolutely necessary, but rarely the aorta itself, for fear of thrombo-embolic complication in the graft and beyond.

Once the graft is fully functioning it should be covered snugly with dry abdominal pack for a few minutes until local haemostasis is complete.

The iliacs and common femorals are checked for pulsation. If these are fully present the closure can begin. If not, the cause must be found and dealt with. A kink may require correction. The iliac branch of the graft or the iliac artery beyond it may have to be opened and sucked and flushed free from clot or atheroma, and quickly resutured with large but non-constricting bites of a thicker suture material. A fine technique here is out of place; breakage or other delays prolong the secondary clamping time, and re-occlusion is likely to take place.

THE CLOSURE

The field is closely checked for bleeding from the dissection zone. It is best not to retract or disturb the graft in any way.

The posterior peritoneum or the remaining part of the sac should be closed over the graft, using continuous atraumatic 2/0 catgut. If little of either of these structures remains, it is a good plan to interpose the omentum between the graft and the back of the duodenum as a barrier to infection and late haemorrhage from the anastomosis.

A secure abdominal suture method is essential. Strong tension sutures of wire or thick nylon are routine; 34 gauge stainless-steel wire is suitable for the rectus sheath, continuous or interrupted as preferred, avoiding kinks.

After skin closure, the tension sutures are tied over a substantial anchor-dressing of gauze roll. This provides comfort and security, protects against haematoma and is an effective barrier against infection from the outside.

If not already in place, a naso-gastric tube should be passed.

Modified Technique for Leaking Aneurysm

Such patients often travel badly; so the operation should be at the receiving hospital, if facilities permit [5A]. The same general operative plan is followed but with all possible emphasis on speed and control of blood loss. At least ten pints of blood will be required. *Heparin should not be given.*

The prime, life-saving objective is to clamp the proximal aorta, which should be achieved within a few minutes of opening the abdomen. Relaxation under anaesthesia may open up the soft tissues confining the haematoma; fresh arterial bleeding may then begin. At this point cardiac arrest may occur; yet, in one of the writer's patients it was possible to re-start the heart and quickly to proceed to a successful grafting operation.

Usually, there is little difficulty in isolating the neck of the aneurysm by passing the right index finger behind the aorta, through the ready plane of cleavage made by the extravasated blood or oedematous tissues near the haematoma. The left index finger is then introduced between the vena cava and the aorta to meet the right, so as to open up a space for the immediate application of a Craaford aortic clamp. If the main mass of the extravasation appears to centre on the neck of the aneurysm, or when active bleeding is seen to be coming from this area, it is dangerous to attempt this dissection, for the full aortic pressure may burst out into the field.

This is the situation in which aortic clamping above the renals is advisable [135]. The stomach is drawn downwards, and the lesser omentum is divided. With a deep retractor above, the aorta is felt high in the lesser sac. It is easier to isolate the aorta if the nearby crus of the diaphragm is quickly divided with long scissors. Digital dissection is often possible, or a gall-bladder forceps may be passed gently behind the aorta. The clamp is applied, often vertically, which requires less opening-up of the tissues behind the aorta (Fig. 15.31).

The front of the aneurysm should now be opened, and the first two fingers of the left hand are passed up into the neck of the sac, which can then be easily defined and clamped in the correct position. The high aortic clamp is removed, the time during which it has been in place being noted.

High aortic clamping should only exceptionally be necessary. It is more difficult, and increases the danger of renal ischaemia, which is one of the chief complications in patients who survive operation. Once the proximal clamp is in position the patient's condition should immediately improve; otherwise the outlook is grave.

Important measures to be taken at this time are:

1. *Rapid transfusion*, preferably of fresh donor blood, warmed if possible. Central venous pressure measurement is a useful guide when accurate figures for blood-loss or blood-volume change cannot be obtained [19, 84, 85].

2. *Calcium gluconate*, 100 mg should be given intravenously for each litre of blood transfused. This should prevent citrate intoxication [93], which may otherwise show as hypotension resistant to further transfusion or to pressor amines, or as myocardial depression with prolonged QT interval eventually leading to asystole. Hypothermia and occlusion of the hepatic artery both accentuate the citrate effect by interfering with metabolic clearance of the radicle,

80 per cent of which, in man, is disposed of in this way. The remaining 20 per cent is cleared by the renal tubules, which are themselves depressed at this time.

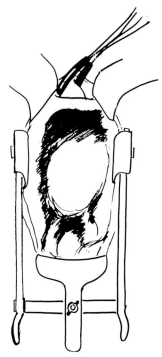

Fig. 15.31. Leaking aortic aneurysm. The aorta is quickly defined above the left renal vein and a vertical clamp is applied without fully immobilising the vessel. As an alternative the thumb and index finger of the right hand can be used.

3. *Mannitol*, 200 ml of the 20 per cent solution should now be given. There is much to suggest that the risk of renal tubular damage may be minimised by this substance [92, 104, 125]. It acts not only as an osmotic diuretic, but also as a means of directly stimulating renal blood and urine flow [90], probably by reducing blood viscosity along with the haematocrit. This may be from a fluid shift from the red cells, which have been seen to be crenated in the renal vein. For this reason, mannitol should not be mixed with blood in a transfusion set. Agglutination and irreversible crenation have been demonstrated *in vitro*, using the 10 per cent solution [121].

4. *Blood pH measurement.* Metabolic acidosis is a major accompaniment of aortic resection for leaking aneurysm; from shock, peripheral vascular

stasis, acute ischaemia of the lower half of the body due to the aortic clamping,* and the infusion of large quantities of stored blood. Tracheal 'tug' and hypotension are both present. An estimation should be taken from just above the clamp as soon as it is in position, to compare with a later value after it is removed, as a guide to bicarbonate dosage (an average requirement is 150 mEq).

5. *Anti-fibrinolysin* (EACA = epsilon-amino caproic acid, 5 G), when given intravenously, will check many cases of defective haemostasis when there is no possibility of laboratory testing for excessive fibrinolysis. Further dosage is 1 G/hour [101].

6. *Fibrinogen* may also be given (8 G, intravenously) if there is clotting defect.

7. Hydrocortisone (100 mg, intravenously) may offset hyperplasminaemia [101] and give physiological support to an elderly over-stressed subject. Problems of massive blood replacement are many and complex, but mostly correctable [139].

Low molecular weight dextran must *never* be given at this stage. Renal tubular stasis may cause an irreversible obstructive anuria; the viscous polymer may glue up the lumen (*see* Chapter 2, p. 27).

DE-CLAMPING AND CLOSURE

Intermittent release of the aortic clamp (*see* p. 300) is even more important in the emergency case. With the blood pressure constantly under observation the time taken to reach full release may be fifteen minutes or more. No free bleeding can be tolerated.

Provision must be made for gastric decompression. A nasogastric tube should have been passed before operation; its patency must now be checked. Temporary gastrostomy is sometimes recommended, but is has the disadvantage that if the tube becomes blocked early in the postoperative period a fatal aspiration into the bronchi may still occur; for this reason a nasal tube should be used as a reserve during the resuscitation period.

If by now the patient is in better condition, and is of a suitable build and still well relaxed, a formal layer closure is begun.

For many other cases a better method is to use through-and-through sutures of strong material such as thick, braided nylon or No. 22 stainless-steel wire, as for a burst abdomen.

Intensive postoperative care is necessary, sometimes with tracheotomy and mechanical ventilation. Many deaths from ruptured or leaking abdominal aneurysm occur during the operation, either from

bleeding before the application of the clamps or from hypotension shortly after their removal. Some later deaths are from renal tubular necrosis, or massive ischaemia of the lower limbs, or both; yet most of those who leave the table in acceptable condition make a good recovery.

The late survival rate of such patients is much the same as after elective operation for unruptured aneurysm.

Postoperative Care and Complications of Resection

Most complications can be avoided by careful technique. The following are those most often seen (Table 15.3):

Table 15.3. Abdominal Aortic Aneurysm Operations: Morbidity (190 cases)

Lower limb ischaemia		10
Embolectomy, recovery	6	
Thrombectomy, recovery	1	
Amputations	3	
Ischaemic colitis		2
Intestinal obstruction		2
Burst abdomen		3
Anuria or uraemia		3
Infected graft		1

ILEUS

Although to some extent inevitable, this should not usually be more troublesome than after any other major abdominal operation. Exteriorisation of the mid-gut loop does not increase its severity; rather the reverse, for strong continued retraction of the gut within the abdomen is probably more damaging.

Intravenous infusion and gastric aspiration will be required for at least two to four days, with strict limitation of oral fluids at first. Gastrostomy drainage is not advised: as in the elective procedure the risk of leakage is too great, and the consequences of failure of the tube to empty the stomach disastrous.

WOUND DEHISCENCE

The incidence of this setback falls with the experience of the surgeon in this work, and as operation time and trauma are reduced. It will, however, remain likely to occur within hours of the removal of sutures unless a durable type of abdominal closure is routine, and unless tension sutures are allowed to remain in place until the twelfth to fourteenth day, by

---

* During aortic clamping there is a sharp fall in leg muscle pH. It returns to normal when the blood flow is restored [28A].

which time convalescence will, in all other respects, have begun.

LOWER-LIMB ISCHAEMIA

(a) Thrombosis

Warning of this risk should be taken when a patient already has missing pulses before aortic clamping, or if a popliteal aneurysm is present. Occlusion of these diseased segments of the main artery is highly likely to occur unless the patient was fully heparinised during the time of clamping. Prevention is much easier than cure.

(b) Embolism

Careful clamping and flushing technique appears to have reduced this risk. Care should be taken to remove all loose clot or debris from upper and lower ends of the artery before completely closing the anastomosis.

If at the end of the operation, with the abdomen closed and strong femoral pulses present, one foot appears waxy pale, a popliteal embolism has probably taken place. Immediate removal is almost invariably successful.

RENAL COMPLICATIONS [147B]

A close check is kept on the urinary output in the first 24 to 48 hours. Most patients should be catheterised. A daily output of less than 1,000 ml with a urine urea of less than 1,100 mg per 100 ml usually means acute tubular necrosis; likewise a failure to respond to mannitol infusion [94], or a urea ratio between the urine and blood of less than 14 [115A], or simply a rise in the blood urea level of 45 mg above the preoperative figure by the first postoperative day [11A]. If anuria is confirmed the fluid intake must be limited to the measured daily loss plus an estimated 400 ml for insensible loss. Potassium accumulation can be limited by reducing protein breakdown with glucose administration and treated by ion-exchange resin enemata. Some patients recover spontaneously with a diuresis beginning on about the fifth day (see p. 324). Dialysis is not often successful, for there are dangers of bleeding with heparin during haemodialysis, and of infection of the graft if the peritoneal method is used. Earlier treatment, however, may improve the outlook [83]. Some cases are irreversible, from renal embolisation. Renal scanning may detect these.

COLON NECROSIS

This deadly complication of inferior mesenteric ligation occurs in approximately one per cent of aorto-iliac operations [14, 40]. For the first few days a quiet necrosis of the left colon and rectum may be masked by the normal discomforts of major surgery. Early sigmoidoscopy is advisable if there should be a premature or blood-stained motion, or if abdominal pain or tenderness seem confined to the left side. Reoperation with resection, although theoretically correct, is almost never successful. Proximal colostomy and drainage of the left side may be better (see also Chapter 17, p. 384).

URETERIC DIFFICULTIES

Involvement in the aneurysm, and injury in its separation may lead to late leakage and abscess formation which, unless recognised, will inevitably infect the graft. Late ureteric obstruction has been reported where the iliac limb of the graft was placed in front of the ureter [96].

GENERAL SURGICAL COMPLICATIONS

1. Retention of urine is best managed by catheterisation, with no question of early prostatectomy, which may lead to blood-stream infection by gram negative organisms likely to infect the graft and anastomoses.

2. Haematemesis is not usually due to failure of the upper anastomosis, as it is in later months, but to bleeding from an associated peptic ulcer. Conservative treatment is usually successful.

3. Intestinal obstruction may occur during the distension phase in a patient who has already had abdominal surgery. Radiology, including gastrografin meal, is valuable. When in doubt, with the patient already on aspiration and replacement, the surgeon should decide to re-operate.

GRAFT INFECTION

This, though fortunately rare, may follow an apparently smooth early convalescence. Fever, pain and collapse develop in much the same way as in a patient with leaking aneurysm. The only effective management for this crisis is to remove the graft, suture the aortic and iliac stumps, and after wound closure; then, through a clean field, and with fresh instruments, two axillo-femoral grafts are inserted. This method succeeded in the case mentioned in Table 15.3, after a rescue helicopter flight that enabled operation to be commenced soon after the crisis developed.

The Results of Excision of Abdominal Aortic Aneurysm

Hospital mortality was 15.3 per cent in 3,000 cases collected from the world literature [14A]. Szilagyi and his colleagues [143] have examined the subsequent course of 480 resected patients and concluded that removal of the aneurysm had doubled their life expectancy. Operative mortality fell from the overall figure of 14·7 to 6·3 per cent in the last two years of the study. Of the late deaths, 9·4 per cent were due to ischaemic heart disease. In comparison, 223 untreated patients had a 34·6 per cent death rate

Table 15.4(a). Abdominal Aortic Aneurysm
(150 elective operations)

Hospital deaths	16 (10·6%)
Haemorrhage	4
Coronary	3
Anuria	2
Colon ischaemia	2
Infection	1
Other	4

Table 15.4(b). Leaking Abdominal Aortic Aneurysms
(40 cases)

20 Operative deaths	
Died on table	7
Coronary	4
Anuria	4
Visceral complications	3
Homograft rupture	1
Infection	1

from rupture and 17 per cent from heart disease. Even among the aneurysms judged smaller than 6 cm, 19 per cent ruptured and their survival rate was only a half of the resected smaller aneurysm.

In a collected series of 682 patients, from ten centres, with *ruptured aneurysms* [83A], the average mortality was 54 per cent. Late survival of 100 patients, successfully operated upon, was four years, most deaths being from arteriosclerosis away from the graft site.

Table 15.5. Abdominal Aortic Aneurysm

Survival of 45 cases
followed > 5 years was 5·4 years
(average age 66 years)

Late aorto-intestinal fistula [128A]. This, the most dreaded complication of abdominal aortic grafting, occurred in 3·0 per cent of the author's aneurysm patients. Two developed within four months, one at just under two years and the other three at six and a half [41A], ten and fourteen years. Two, apparently successfully re-operated, recurred and died. Recurrence of the aneurysm, without fistula, occurred in two patients, at eight and ten years.

II Aneurysms of the Visceral Arteries [35A]

Although much less common than the aorta as the site of an abdominal aneurysm, these arteries do pose special individual problems when affected by this disease, and by the time symptoms have developed the outlook is serious. The two main types are set out in the next column.

Splenic Aneurysm

This is the second commonest abdominal aneurysm. Three per cent of one large series of abdominal aneurysms were splenic [54]. A reported incidence of 1 in 2,607 post-mortems [112] may be a low estimate, for some proximal aneurysms may have been overlooked. Calcified ring opacities of the splenic artery are fairly often seen radiologically. In one British hospital, ten cases were clinically recognised in five years [148].

Most splenic aneurysms cause no symptoms. They may be multiple, when they affect the terminal branches of the hilar region, and somewhat elongated when the main course is involved, a fairly common

Non-aortic Abdominal Aneurysms

Arteriosclerotic	*Due to polyarteritis nodosa*
Common	Rare
Seldom more than three	Always multiple
Moderate sized (true sac)	Small (false sac)
Splenic, renal, hepatic and mesenteric in this order of frequency	Renal and mesenteric clinically the commonest
Rupture may mark clinical onset (patient previously well). Often an incidental finding	Rupture terminates the disease (patient ill, for some months, febrile, anaemic with raised ESR)
If unruptured, spontaneous cure by thrombosis and calcification	A progressive disease, steroids may fail to control

finding when, during partial gastrectomy, the lesser sac is explored. Some patients complain of recurring upper and left-sided abdominal pain passing through to the back. This may be due to direct pancreatic involvement by the sac, or from ischaemia of the body and tail (Fig. 17.22, p. 381).

RUPTURE

The most important feature of splenic aneurysm is its tendency to rupture, particularly in pregnancy [49], when the splenic artery may also rupture without evidence of aneurysm. As in aortic rupture, the haemorrhage is often massive and free into the peritoneal cavity, a rapidly fatal ending [129], or, less often, into the extraperitoneal tissues, where it may be confined for some hours, days, or even weeks, until the haematoma ruptures secondarily into the peritoneum. Early in pregnancy the picture suggests a ruptured ectopic gestation; in later months, when the accident is more common, some obstetric complication such as ruptured uterus or concealed accidental haemorrhage is suspected. An emergency operation is essential; many recoveries are now on record. Foetal death is said to be inevitable, but there should be hope of saving the mother. The recommended plan is to obtain access to the abdominal cavity by means of a long incision and a quickly completed caesarian section, and then, delivering the spleen and tail of the pancreas, to excise the spleen and its bleeding pedicle without attempting to identify the aneurysm.

Renal Aneurysm

Similar in its behaviour to splenic aneurysm, and sometimes accompanying it [117], is the renal aneurysm, but it is less common. It, too, may show as a calcified ring shadow on X-ray films, but such a lesion is usually partly or completely thrombosed by the time it is recognised. Here, however, there are other possible explanations for the opacity, e.g. renal calculus, cyst, tuberculoma, lymph node, or arterial calcification, any of which may require aortography to distinguish them from aneurysm. The pyelogram phase should be studied for function and deformity. Even a pea-sized aneurysm may rupture and produce severe intra-abdominal haemorrhage, particularly during pregnancy. In fact, 24 out of 100 non-calcified cases presented in this way [64] with a mortality of 75 per cent. In others, upper abdominal pain, especially with a ring shadow on the right, may be taken to be due to gallstones.

Haematuria is another puzzling type of onset. A few cases develop renal hypertension, especially those in which the aneurysm is post-stenotic, in an artery affected by fibro-muscular hyperplasia. The renal outline may be small; in fact renal atrophy may lead to the diagnosis [23]. This may account for the association of an active, symptomatic aneurysm on one side with an atrophic kidney on the other [133].

A recognised symptomless, uncomplicated renal aneurysm could be treated conservatively because of its tendency to spontaneous obliteration by thrombosis and calcification, but when the condition is discovered unexpectedly at operation a delicate decision must be taken, for, unlike the spleen, the kidney is not dispensable, and nephrectomy, the simplest means of surgical cure, cannot be lightly undertaken. A saccular aneurysm may sometimes be dissected free from the renal artery, and after excision the lateral defect can be closed by simple arterial suture. This was successfully accomplished long before arterial reconstruction had entered into routine surgical practice [23, 108]. In latter years, more cases mostly involving the main branches of the artery, have been cured in this way [48], though, until 1951, nephrectomy proved the safest course [1] in a review of 115 cases treated up to that time. Aneurysm involving the whole circumference of the main renal artery should, today, be excised with end-to-end anastomosis or, if the bifurcation is involved, one branch may be joined end-to-side to the reconstructed main artery and other branch [48], or there may be sufficient spare tissue for a lateral arterioplasty [133].

The crisis of sudden rupture will continue to be managed best by emergency nephrectomy, provided that exploration confirms the presence of the opposite kidney.

Coeliac and Hepatic Aneurysms

Being deeply placed and seldom large, these tend to remain hidden and unrecognised. Exceptionally, they may be noticed, on aortography, for another condition such as hypertension [82]. Most of the reported cases were diagnosed at an operation, either in an emergency for intra-abdominal haemorrhage, or for right upper quadrant pain, usually with the diagnosis of gallstones. Leakage into the bile ducts may cause jaundice and haemobilia. Even so, the lesion may be missed: a story of multiple operations is common [61].

Of the 150 or so cases of *hepatic aneurysm* reported, less than a third were successfully treated and 80 per cent were first seen after rupture [97]. A few were found at an operation for another disease such as gallstones or duodenal ulcer [61]. This is a difficult aneurysm to resect, and reconstruction is seldom possible [91A]. A case seen by the author was of mycotic origin, and closely adherent to the portal vein, which it was compressing and obstructing, with the production of oesophageal varices which had bled severely. A portacaval anastomosis was required during removal of the sac. Simpler measures than these are usually preferable. Ligation may be safer than any other method [73, 136] (*see* Chapter 13, p. 247). Matas's operation has also been used [61, 97].

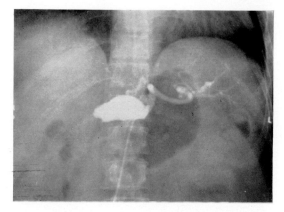

(*a*) Selective coeliac arteriogram shows failure of hepatic filling.

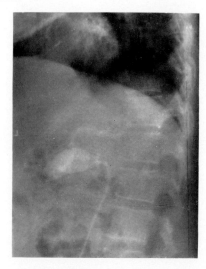

(*b*) Lateral view suggests that the aneurysm has a neck of normal coeliac artery.

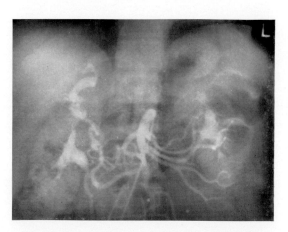

Fig. 15.32. Coeliac aneurysm in a man aged forty-six, recognised at an operation for gallstones.

(*c*) Selective superior mesenteric arteriogram shows good hepatic filling through the pancreato-duodenal arch and other collaterals in the region of the pylorus. Good recovery and remains well five years after ligation of coeliac at its origin. (Patient referred by Mr K. A. Moore.)

Coeliac aneurysm is in many ways more amenable to operative cure: excision with anastomosis of the coeliac itself [146] or of the hepatic to the coeliac [131], perhaps via a graft, into which the splenic can be joined [82].

The coeliac artery has been successfully ligated for acute haemorrhage from an aneurysm at the origin of the splenic or the coeliac itself [106]. In the patient shown in Fig. 15.32*a, b,* the aortic origin was tied for a 6 cm aneurysm of the trifurcation. A left thoraco-abdominal approach was used, and the procedure was well tolerated. In this case there had evidently been previous embolism from the sac to the common hepatic artery, followed by the development of a sufficient collateral supply to the liver from the superior mesenteric via the pancreatico-duodenal arch (Fig. 15.32*c*). The finding of a splenic infarct at operation also supports this view.

III Peripheral Aneurysms

Clinically, it may be difficult to decide whether a patient has an aneurysm, or simply a tortuous, widened artery, part of a generalised deterioration with age, hypertension, or both.

Arteriography may decide, but not if:

(a) The sac contains much thrombus through which the main channel is little wider than that of the adjoining artery (Fig. 15.33).

(b) The main artery is everywhere much widened and the onward flow of the contrast medium slow, and concentration, because of dilution, is poor (p. 326, Instructive Case 3).

In middle-aged or younger subjects, aneurysm is the most likely cause of prominent arterial widening behind the knee or above the clavicle, where a local mechanical fault has damaged the main artery, producing an accelerated though confined form of degenerative disease, or one of the special lesions well known in these situations, for example: cystic adventitial disease, which may go on to premature popliteal aneurysm formation; and post-stenotic dilatation of a thinned-out axillary trunk.

Peripheral aneurysms differ from those of the aorta and other central arteries in their higher incidence of thrombo-embolic complications and lower risk of leakage or rupture. No doubt these differences are due to the lower tension and flow rate in the smaller peripheral arteries.

The diagnosis of complications in a peripheral aneurysm should be more straightforward than recognising the lesion in its quiescent stage. Pitfalls of all degrees of severity do exist, however; for example:

(a) Embolism may be mistaken for arteriosclerotic ischaemia or Raynaud's disease.

(b) The leaking case may be confused with other, hot, expanding peripheral limb conditions such as sarcoma, aneurysmal bone cyst, or, classically,

an acute abscess, leading to the dreadful error of a surgical incision, so difficult to understand or to explain in retrospect, though, in the words of Pirogoff [116]:

'An overweening self-confidence, a preconceived opinion, vanity, and weariness are the causes of these astounding mistakes.'

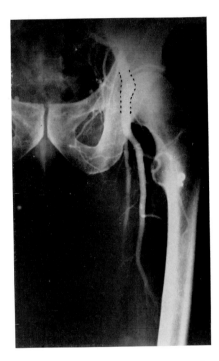

Fig. 15.33. This patient had a common femoral aneurysm 4 cm in diameter, yet his arteriogram shows only slight widening at this point. (*See also* Fig. 3.69, p. 76.)

IV Popliteal Aneurysm

Important features of this historic lesion that are not so well known are that it is:

(a) Very common, but often missed.

(b) Almost invariably arteriosclerotic, but not necessarily signifying the generalised form of this disease.

(c) Frequently bilateral.

(d) Mostly symptomless.

(e) Often self-limiting by spontaneous thrombosis.

(f) Occasionally liable to serious thrombo-embolic complications and to rupture.

After the aorta, the popliteal artery is the second commonest site for arteriosclerotic aneurysm and resembles it in that many cases are unrecognised or have a perfectly benign course in an otherwise healthy, elderly subject.

JOHN HUNTER AND POPLITEAL ANEURYSM
In Hunter's time, as today, it was the large, expanding painful aneurysm that showed itself clinically and gave the lesion so bad a reputation. Previous attempts at surgical cure had mostly been by the logical though highly dangerous direct approach

through the popliteal fossa, with the object of ligation of the entering artery (Anel's method [6]). This difficult procedure often led to uncontrollable operative or secondary haemorrhage, or to a mid-thigh amputation which, in pre-Listerian surgery, carried a very high risk of fatal sepsis.

Hunter's approach to the problem of ligation of the main artery was to avoid the hazards of the direct dissection by applying his ligature to the superficial femoral in the mid thigh, where the short incision in a clean field should be reasonably sure to heal, and where, from his earlier experimental observations on collateral circulation in the deer's carotid [111], there might be a good chance for the limb to survive.

The first successful case was in December 1785 in a coachman, whose large, active aneurysm completely resolved, following femoral ligation, and who was able to return to his work, until his death fifteen months later from a feverish illness. The limb was examined and showed that Hunter's object of selective thrombosis almost confined to the aneurysmal sac had been achieved. Clearly the ligature had so reduced the flow through the sac that the thrombus within it was able to close it off completely; meanwhile the collaterals between it and the high ligature had kept this important part of the main artery open and ensured the survival of the limb. We have no account from Hunter himself of this, his best-known contribution to vascular surgery. His brother-in-law, Everard Home [67], recorded it, and several other cases, with the good results obtained. Hunterian ligation, 150 years later, still has a valuable place in the most dangerous case; an elderly unfit subject, with a complicated aneurysm (see Case 2, p. 325).

Surgical Pathology

The traditional syphilitic popliteal aneurysm of the equestrians of the past may never have been more than a myth. Today, in the thoracic aorta the incidence remains steady, but syphilis as a cause of peripheral aneurysm seems almost to have disappeared. Fewer than 0·5 per cent of a large series from the Mayo Clinic [152] were considered syphilitic. A patient of Professor Rob's and the author's had bilateral popliteal aneurysms, a positive Wasserman reaction, and general paralysis of the insane; yet the histological examination of his material showed only arteriosclerotic changes, with no sign of syphilis.

The configuration of the whole femoro-popliteal artery in a case of arteriosclerotic aneurysm is typically wide and beaded, with more marked distortion as the aneurysm is approached. Although proof is lacking, a standing wave or other oscillatory cause is suggested by this appearance. The fixed point may be provided by the adductor opening, or this may produce the conditions for post-stenotic aneurysm formation (Figs. 15.4 and 15.5). Other cases, with the sac formed lower in the course of the popliteal artery may be due to a similar restrictive effect produced by the oblique posterior ligament of the knee [52].

It is known that degenerative or obstructive arterial conditions other than arteriosclerosis may lead to popliteal aneurysm; for example cystic adventitial disease or popliteal entrapment (see Chapter 3, p. 45). Both conditions can occur in young or middle-aged, previously athletic, subjects. A well-remembered injury is sometimes considered responsible, the accident having brought on an acute thrombosis.

Anatomical Types

There appear to be two distinct kinds of popliteal aneurysm, according to the level of the artery occupied by the sac:

1. High, large, conspicuous and, often, multilobular (Fig. 15.37), as part of the beaded appearance mentioned above. These are commoner in the elderly.
2. Small, lower, clinically hidden, and often bilateral, often in younger men (Fig. 15.34).

These have a separate clinical significance, for the larger type more commonly develops serious complications, while the smaller very often, if not always, undergoes cure by thrombosis [15].

Natural Course

From what has been said, it will be understood that no hard and fast prognosis can be given, much less a universally severe one, although statements to the contrary are common in the surgical literature [10, 53, 86], based, most probably, upon selected cases presenting at surgical centres. Without doubt many of the patients in such series would have had aneurysms of the larger, symptomatic type. It is the author's view [41] and that of others [15, 151] that many patients go on to spontaneous cure undiagnosed. Certainly no harm has yet come in his knowledge to the many patients (approximately 100) in whom the probable clinical diagnosis of early popliteal aneurysm was made on routine peripheral arterial examination.

The truth seems to be that danger lies mainly in the larger, symptomatic case, while the commoner, silent type is usually benign in all its stages.

The Patient with Popliteal Aneurysm

Much of the available information concerns surgical patients requiring operation. In the Mayo Clinic experience [152] of 152 patients with 233 aneurysms, seen between 1961 and 1968, 90 per cent were aged between fifty and seventy-nine. There were only four women. 67 per cent were hypertensive; 59 per cent had bilateral aneurysms; 45 per cent had yet another aneurysm or more, and 44 per cent had ischaemic heart disease. 155 of the aneurysms were conservatively managed, and though among 87 of these followed for an average of 3·7 years, 69 per cent remained symptomless or quiescent, 31 per cent developed complications, 7 of which required operation (including 3 amputations). Of the 78 aneurysms requiring surgery at the outset, 13 had to be amputated for serious thrombo-embolic complications.

The Clinical Picture

Most popliteal aneurysms are symptomless [15, 59]. They may thus escape notice by the patient, and are equally easily missed on routine medical examination. Quite a large sac may cause no trouble and remain hidden and unrecognised behind the knee, particularly if the patient is elderly, obese, stiff-jointed,* or orthopnoeic.

Symptoms (pain, tenderness, increased swelling of knee or leg, also ischaemia of the foot) mean complications or their imminent development; as in abdominal aortic aneurysm, an early straightforward case soon becomes a difficult, advancing, and dangerous one. It is important, therefore, to recognise the larger, significant type of popliteal aneurysm during the early silent phase. It should not be missed if the following method is routinely employed.

PALPATION FOR POPLITEAL ANEURYSM
The normal popliteal pulse is no more than a finger's breadth across when palpated with the four fingers placed along its course. If it feels wider, so that the diameter can be measured with the parallel finger tips of both hands, it is probably aneurysmal.

As with abdominal aortic aneurysm, this method of clinical examination gives positive evidence of a widened arterial impulse, which may be more convincing than the arteriographic appearances that show only the lumen through what may be a large amount of intrasaccular thrombus (Fig. 15.35).

---

* Sometimes a patient with chronic arthritis of the knee develops posterior synovial rupture into the popliteal fossa, with pain and swelling that may suggest an aneurysm or deep vein thrombosis.

Complications include:
(a) Expansion of the sac with slow compression of the neurovascular bundle.
(b) Leakage, or rupture, with rapid compression of these structures and, also, of the collateral anastomosis around the knee.
(c) Embolism to the tibial or plantar arteries.
(d) Thrombosis of the sac.

Each of these presents a typical clinical picture and all but the last require early surgical treatment.

Compression of the popliteal vein produces acute congestion in its tributaries, with aching pain in the calf, worse on standing, and swelling of the ankle. There will not be sufficient time for chronic gravitational lesions to develop over the perforating malleolar veins; arterial complications take place first. In the early phase of vein compression the aneurysm may still be fairly small and unsuspected as the underlying cause of what is assumed to be a primarily venous condition. Phlebography should clearly show the true cause [13].

Damage to the popliteal nerves is a later complication, though some of the earlier pain in the calf or foot may be caused in this way. Also due to a minor degree of motor neuropathy, may be the claw-foot deformity sometimes seen. Much more serious are nerve complications from leakage or rupture of the aneurysm. These include drop foot, or even a complete paralysis of the leg and foot, or, more often, a painful type of sensory loss that may take months to clear up, even after surgical cure of the aneurysm.

Leakage or rupture brings the onset of severe local pain for the first time; up to then there will have been only slight local pain, though tenderness is noticed sooner. Pain increases hourly, and with it comes progressive soft tissue swelling from infiltrating haemorrhage, most marked behind the knee but soon spreading all round the joint, which is held stiff by muscle spasm and usually shows a moderate amount of effusion. The distal pulses are still present, though becoming obscured by the massive oedema, and eventually obstructed by the tension of the haematoma compressing the main artery and the collaterals around the knee. The foot soon becomes cold, and ischaemic recovery is now unlikely. Leaking popliteal aneurysm is a surgical emergency of the first urgency. It may have been brought on by anticoagulant treatment given for the earlier phase of venous obstruction. Sometimes a minor injury may be an immediate cause.

Acute Thrombosis of the Sac

This complication may take the following forms:
1. Commonly, in the smaller type of aneurysm, it is silent, or may later be revealed as the cause of intermittent claudication in the calf.

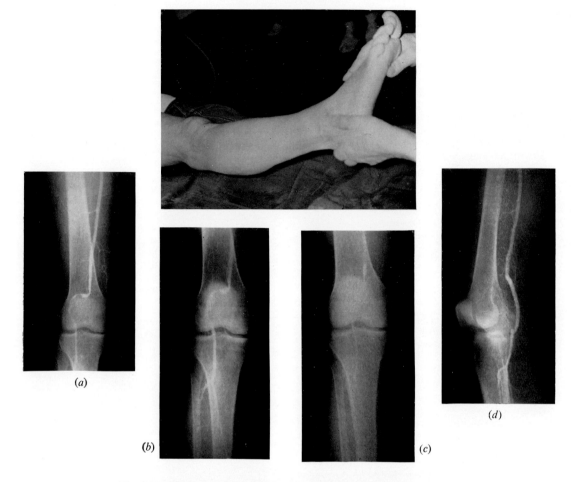

(a)

(b)

(c)

(d)

Fig. 15.34. Painful acute thrombosis of right popliteal aneurysm presenting as a tender lump behind the right knee in a man aged fifty-three.

(*a*) Most of the femoro-popliteal artery is normal for a man of this age.
(*b*) Irregular, almost complete thrombosis of the lumen of the aneurysm.
(*c*) Thrombosis complete. Local pain disappeared at once, but claudication developed at 75 yards.
(*d*) Saphenous vein by-pass inserted with relief of symptoms.

This man's identical twin brother subsequently required grafting for a leaking false aneurysm of the aorta at the level of the main visceral branches.

2. In some elderly patients, an acute thrombosis extends far beyond the sac, then involving most of the wide, now stagnant femoro-popliteal artery (Fig. 15.35), from high in the thigh, perhaps down to its bifurcation. This chiefly happens as a result of intercurrent illness, or local leakage, acute embolism, or during aortic clamping for the removal of an abdominal aneurysm. Gangrene and a major amputation are common sequelae, though in fitter subjects, claudication only.

3. Occasionally, in either type, although more often the larger type, the sac slowly thromboses, with only mild discomfort at first, until a phase is reached of acute obstructive ischaemia, no doubt from thrombotic or embolic obstruction to the outflow of the sac. The aneurysm then becomes agonisingly painful and acutely tender (Fig. 15.34), for the still patent entering artery still continues to beat against the block and to distend it.

There is a risk of misdiagnosis. Abscess, deep

vein thrombosis or synovitis of the knee may be suspected, with inappropriate treatment. One patient referred to the author with a large aneurysm was on anticoagulants and another had just had the sac incised.

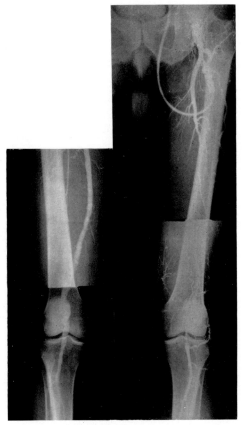

Fig. 15.35. Extensive thrombosis in widened left femoro-popliteal artery in a doctor aged forty-seven with a recent acute history of severe left calf claudication and coldness of the left foot. Good response to left lumbar sympathectomy. Left side almost symptomless four years later when he presented with a large aneurysm in the right popliteal. There had been one earlier incident of pain in the right foot, possibly embolic, for the ankle pulses were diminished. Good recovery following excision and saphenous vein graft.

Embolism to the Tibial Arteries

This is a common and important complication of medium to large-sized popliteal aneurysms (Fig. 15.36). Severe, progressive ischaemia develops in the same way as it does in the upper limb in subclavian aneurysm from thoracic outlet syndrome, first with transient digital changes of secondary Raynaud's phenomenon, often with recovery of the pulses within a few hours [30], and later, as the embolism is repeated, and more of the distal arterial tree becomes occluded, gangrene of the forefoot.

Treatment along general lines for peripheral ischaemia (e.g. lumbar sympathectomy) may not succeed unless the source of the embolic material is rendered ineffective either through completing its own occlusion, by thrombosis (though this, as with ligation in this late stage may seal the fate of the limb), or better, by reconstruction of the popliteal after the aneurysm has been excised. Sympathectomy then fulfils a useful secondary role [151].

Treatment of Popliteal Aneurysm

From what has been said about the frequency of symptomless cases, and their benign course with spontaneous cure by occlusion, it follows that a current trend towards arterial reconstruction of all cases [86] must obviously be questioned [15, 41, 151].

Conservatism now seems the best course when:

1. The aneurysm is small, silent, bilateral, or only one of many others. For such cases nothing need usually be done.
2. A larger aneurysm gives rise to symptoms and/or complications in an unfit subject. For this combination a Hunterian ligation is preferable to arterial surgery involving prolonged anaesthesia and possible blood-loss.

Technique of Operation

1. HUNTERIAN LIGATION

This is still the operation of choice for rapidly expanding, painful and, therefore, probably leaking popliteal aneurysm in the usual type of patient with this condition (*see* Case 2, p. 325) who is already too ill for complicated arterial surgery; for him, the advent of severe local complications does nothing to mitigate this contra-indication.

All that is required is simple ligation, under local anaesthesia if necessary, of the superficial femoral artery at its most accessible point just beneath the sartorius muscle in the mid-thigh, using strong chromic catgut, and taking care to avoid injury to the closely related femoral vein on the deep surface. If this should happen, the ligature should be tied; when the artery is allowed to fall back into its bed, and after pressure for a few minutes, bleeding will cease. Before closing the wound it is important to ensure that no pulsation continues distal to the ligature, as it may, if the surgeon has been over-cautious when tightening the first tie of the knot. It is good practice to add a second ligature a little beyond the first. The femoral artery itself is often aneurysmal

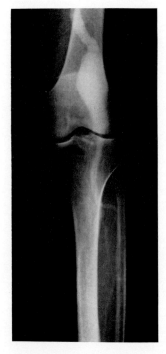

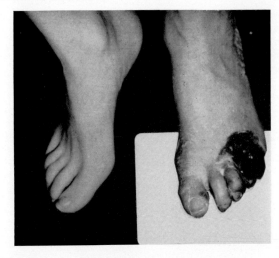

Fig. 15.36. Plantar embolism from popliteal aneurysm.

(*a*) Large but locally symptomless aneurysm.
(*b*) Dry gangrene of outer two left toes and moderate ischaemia of the first three. Ankle pulses still present.

in this type of case, so it is important not to run the risk of cutting through the artery at the ligature point. It is safest to use only such tightness in the two ligatures as will suffice completely to obliterate the pulse beyond them.

Immediately after Hunterian ligation the toes often become pale and cool for a few hours, yet an early return of good skin circulation is the rule. In the 10 per cent or so of patients who go on to develop severe ischaemia the reason is probably a secondary occlusion, involving either the collateral arteries, or of the deep vein.

Anticoagulants are contra-indicated. The use of low molecular weight dextran infusion may be helpful during the first twelve to twenty-four hours. Lumbar sympathectomy has been widely advocated as a support to the collateral circulation after ligation or excision operations but, although it should provide useful freedom from vasomotor tone in the late recovery period, it can scarcely be expected to exert a definitive effect on the outcome of acute post-ligation ischaemia, any more than from other causes (*see* Chapter 2, p. 28).

In most cases recovery is surprisingly rapid and complete, with mild claudication as the only adverse effect of the presence of the ligature. In 1953, Professor Rob and the author treated and studied a sixty-year-old patient whose bilateral popliteal aneurysms were treated on one side by ligation and on the other by replacement arterial grafting. Claudication on the ligated side was only mild, although the post-ischaemic blood flow curves were characteristic of the occluded and open main-artery pattern.

Weeks after ligation of a large or leaking aneurysm there may be alarm over the fact that sepsis has developed in the stagnant contents of the sac. Simple drainage is effective and safe from all risk of secondary haemorrhage. (*See* Case 2.)

ARTERIAL RECONSTRUCTION FOR POPLITEAL ANEURYSM

The following methods are possible:

1. Excision of the aneurysm with end-to-end anastomosis of the artery.
2. Excision of the aneurysm with replacement grafting, using a vein or prosthetic graft.
3. By-pass grafting with vein or prosthetic graft leaving the sac undisturbed (Fig. 15.37).

The choice of technique will depend on the size and adherence of the aneurysm and the state of the adjacent artery.

Excision is best suited to the smaller, more localised aneurysm, e.g. when due to popliteal artery entrapment by the medial head of the gastrocnemius muscle; also for the traumatic false or mycotic aneurysm which is rounded, with a small arterial defect.

be completed, according to the size and adherence of the sac. The chief difficulties with this operation are the prone position which limits access to the rest of the limb and which is poorly tolerated by the elderly; also the risk of damage to the nearby vein and nerves.

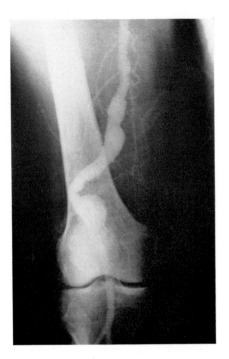 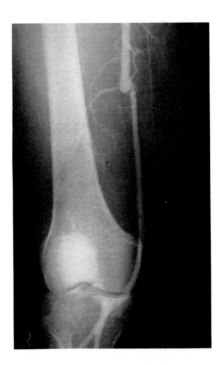

Fig. 15.37. Medial by-pass saphenous vein graft for the relief of a long, lobulated fusiform aneurysm that filled the popliteal fossa.

The posterior approach is by an S-shaped incision with its upper limb medially over the artery as it enters, very deeply, into the popliteal fossa. The middle portion runs across the flexure almost horizontally, to avoid later keloid scarring. The lower limb of the incision is lateral, over the upper fibula, though the deep fascia of the calf must also be divided nearer the mid-line, between the gastrocnemius bellies, where the artery lies much more superficially, though still obscured by crossing veins and calf motor nerves. The aneurysmal sac is often closely adherent to the popliteal vein. Thrombus may have to be extracted from the lower end of the artery, using a balloon catheter. A good length of saphenous vein will already have been taken from the upper thigh before the patient was turned on to his face. By-pass or replacement grafting will then

The medial by-pass (Fig. 15.37) avoids these objections, but does not allow a direct exposure of the aneurysm. This, however, is unnecessary in the long, compound thrombosing type of sac so common in the older patient. The standard, limited approach to the adductor opening is made, as though for an open endarterectomy or a by-pass for thrombosis. The popliteal is then exposed below the knee between the tibia and the medial gastrocnemius. The vein graft can be taken, to the length required, without moving the patient, and the by-pass is inserted, making the lower anastomosis first, passing the graft up through a tunnel along any convenient tissue plane. The aneurysm is then excluded from the circulation, by ligating the main artery with strong thread, on the aneurysm side of each anastomosis.

V Femoral Aneurysm

Although not as common as the popliteal, the femoral artery is an obvious and familiar site for aneurysm formation; frequently the condition is bilateral, and an abdominal aneurysm may also be present (in 28 per cent of one series [113]). Hypertension was also noted in 54 per cent. Complications of earlier arterial surgery have now become a frequent cause. A femoro-popliteal homograft may dilate to produce a true aneurysm of the middle of the thigh. The femoral anastomosis of a plastic cloth prosthesis appears to be specially liable to develop a false aneurysm whether at the proximal end of a femoro-popliteal by-pass (Fig. 3.69 p. 76), or at the distal union of an aorto-femoral graft [140].

Any prominent, well-localised, femoral aneurysm [113] should be excised, and grafted, whether of this new type or occurring spontaneously, even though it may be symptomless, for rupture is probable (Fig. 15.38), and preventive operation is straightforward. The common elongated, bilateral or multiple type is treated conservatively except when causing pressure symptoms; thrombosis alone is no indication for operation unless severe ischaemia is also present. By-passing is better than replacement of the long superficial femoral sac.

A common femoral aneurysm may grow very large, perhaps from its anatomical shortness and its situation in a place of bending strain unsupported by muscle, except deeply; rupture is more likely than with aneurysms lower in the thigh. Reconstruction should include the profunda, if possible, which it usually is in the intact case; after rupture, the graft may of necessity be from the common to the superficial femoral only. Replacement is preferable over this short distance, and with a bulky sac that might otherwise force a by-pass graft up towards the skin incision. Ligation with by-passing are better reserved for the occasion of a rapid operation on a poor-risk patient. It is inadvisable to make any

prolonged search for the profunda opening: haemostatic sutures widely placed will control this possible source of recurrent difficulty.

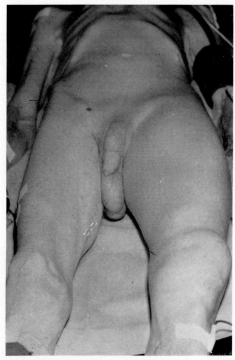

Fig. 15.38. Ruptured aneurysm of left profunda femoris artery in a man aged seventy-two. Massive haemorrhage with pulsating haematoma of groin, swelling of whole thigh and effusion into left knee joint.

Good recovery following operation: external iliac exposed and temporarily clamped while the aneurysm was opened below the groin. Suture of opening of origin and ligation of branches. Femoral patency was thus unaffected.

A Note on Thoracic Aneurysms

Thoracic aortic aneurysm develops where the vessel has been damaged by trauma, syphilis or mycotic infection, or beyond a coarctation. These dangerous lesions may occur in early adult life, and although their surgical treatment is a formidable undertaking that properly belongs to the cardiac surgical team, experience now favours an active policy in most of them, especially the coarctation type, which, with its well-formed collaterals, needs no by-pass; also, the lateral saccular syphilitic aneurysm in which continued aortic flow can be maintained by lateral clamping during the excision [8]. In others in which the ascending portion is unaffected a temporary sutured cloth tube by-pass is attached above and beyond the clamps. This is a good method for distal arch lesions, and has the advantage over the pumped shunt that heparin is not needed. The great vessels can be detached from the aneurysm and moved to the graft in stages, via the shunt, while the main graft is being inserted [33, 68]. The more proximal aortic aneurysm involving the arch ascending portion, and perhaps the valve and coronary openings, poses some of the most difficult operative problems in vascular surgery, but in several centres where special skills have been developed in dealing with many patients, often in native populations, good results are now reported using cardiopulmonary by-pass, with profound hypothermia to protect the vital areas of the cerebral and coronary circulation during cold-induced cardiac arrest [9, 11, 28, 68]. Survival has even followed operations for leaking aneurysm in these sites.

Descending and thoraco-abdominal aortic aneurysms, whether infective or arteriosclerotic, set similar problems to the surgeon. Clamping of the thoracic aorta in its descending portion for more than 45 minutes [29] may cause spinal or renal ischaemia. Hypothermia, a temporary sutured shunt, or preferably left heart by-pass, will avoid these dangers

[32, 34]. Separate perfusion cannulae must be made ready in case the great branches of the middle course of the aorta are arising from the sac, or so close to it that clamping the aorta will occlude them. These will later require reimplantation into the side of the graft or specially constructed branches of it.* If there is vertebral erosion, the sac should be folded over between the bone and the prosthesis.

Woven grafts are preferred for all these operations, as in leaking abdominal aneurysm, for their good haemostasis in the haemorrhagic heparinised patient. Haemostasis is crucially important in these cases, for infection is common and late haemorrhage is fatal. Mortality figures, however, remain high, and operation cannot yet be recommended in all older patients unless symptoms demand it and the prospects seem good.

VII Dissecting Aneurysm

This condition is often confused with leakage from an already formed aortic aneurysm, but the two diseases are by nature and in their behaviour quite different.

Acute dissecting aneurysm is a fresh, spreading, generally uniform widening of a large portion of the aorta, and often of its branches, with extensive recent haemorrhagic splitting within the media, usually the result of degeneration in the arterial wall, the causes of which are not yet fully understood, although hypertension and advancing age are important and probably act through prolonged mechanical fatigue. Other factors not necessarily connected with hypertension, but contributing to the fallibility of the media, are heredity (the congenital connective tissue disorders), pregnancy, which in some way weakens large blood vessels (pp. 141, 282, 305, 316), injury, possibly diet [149], and some drugs [12].

In one respect, however, acute dissecting aneurysm does resemble leaking saccular aortic aneurysm: untreated, most patients die within a day or so.

It is revealed as the cause of death in from 1 to 4 per cent of post-mortem examinations [24].

Pathology

The work of Shennan [128] provided a firm basis for the advances of the subsequent thirty years and bears directly on recent developments in treatment. Shennan studied 300 cases and found that:

1. Most patients died within two days with extensive separation of the aortic coats, and terminal rupture, usually into the pericardium.
2. In approximately three-quarters of the patients the dissection appeared to have originated in the ascending aorta or the arch, most commonly through a short transverse tear approximately 2 cm above the valve; in nearly a half, the damage was still confined to the proximal aorta at the time of death.
3. In 10 per cent, a chronic, stable condition appeared to have been established, several such patients having died from other causes.

Hirst and his colleagues [65] reviewed 505 cases in the English literature over the twenty years following Shennan's account of the disease. The most constant findings were:

1. Cardiac enlargement, present in 86 per cent.
2. Mucoid degeneration of the actual or potential dissecting layer with loss of muscle and elastic tissue in lacunae which healed to become cysts, with consequent loss of strength in the media (cystic medio-necrosis of Erheim) (Fig. 15.39).

These are the effects of sustained hypertension.

The Role of Hypertension and of Medio-necrosis

Hypertension is present in most cases, and may even continue its damaging effects on into the acute dissection phase. It appears to be the principal cause of the medio-necrosis that leads to the dissection. The lesion is also seen proximal to an aortic coarctation, also beyond it in the jet stream, likewise where the outflow from a stenosed aortic valve impinges upon the aortic wall.

---

* With Mr L. L. Bromley and Mr A. E. Thompson of the Cardiac Unit at St Mary's Hospital the author was able to use this method successfully in a 45-year-old nurse whose thoraco-abdominal aneurysm included the coeliac and superior mesenteric arteries.

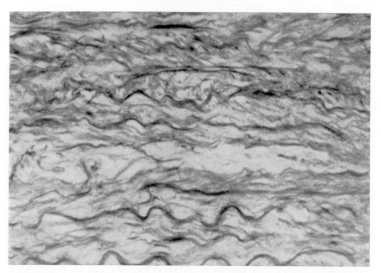

Fig. 15.39. Aorta in cystic medionecrosis (× 220). Cystic mucoid areas with fragmentation of elastic layer in a part of the aorta some distance from the split of the dissection which caused this patient's death. (Photomicrograph by Dr R. Parker.)

Some patients inherit a predisposition to the medial weakening; family series and twin cases testify to this [36]. Certainly the gross hereditary connective tissue abnormalities in Marfan's disease and the Ehlers-Danlos syndrome are associated with a high risk of early development of the lesion.

Thus, it would seem that mechanical fatigue from the pulse cycle is the basis of the medial lesion and of the dissection; either from an increase in the mechanical forces (hypertension) or from a premature failure of the material under stress (inherited tissue defects).

The high reported incidence in negroes [65] may be due to both factors.

Pregnancy [124]

A quarter of all cases below the age of forty years occurred in pregnant women, according to one report [66]; recent confinement also appears to predispose, particularly in women late in the childbearing period [18]; in these patients the coronary arteries were often affected, although no arteriosclerotic plaques were seen.

There may be a connection with other forms of arterial disease more common in females (*see* Chapters 7, p. 137, and 3, p. 40). The fact that, in general, and in the common age group fifty to sixty years, dissecting aneurysm is much commoner in males [65] suggests that when the condition arises in association with pregnancy it may have a separate structural basis.

Arteriosclerosis

At operation or at post-mortem the lining of the inner arterial tube is often remarkably healthy in appearance considering the degree of hypertension that is so common. Some cases suggest that the first penetration of the blood stream between the arterial coats may have been through the breach of an atheromatous ulcer, but the fact that most dissections begin close to the aortic valve, where the aorta is usually fairly free from intimal irregularity, and not distally, where the most severe lesions are found, probably means that arteriosclerosis is not an important factor in the development of dissecting aneurysm.

Other arterial diseases may be associated, e.g. giant-cell arteritis [100, 102], tuberculous arteritis [107] and even hydatid disease [5].

Trauma

Damage to the aortic arch is a fairly common cause of death following deceleration injury (*see* Chapter 13, p. 243), yet in such cases dissection between the coats is rare; apparently the healthy artery is more likely either to withstand the trauma, or to rupture completely or, under the strong adventitia [43], to form a false sac, not a dissecting aneurysm.

There is seldom any history of injury, although recent physical strain is sometimes mentioned [45]. Exceptions to this rule occur mainly in hospital as a result of arterial procedures of various kinds:

1. Translumbar aortography: [51] although intramural injection of the small test dose is fairly com-

mon, only rarely should the main injection gain entrance to the split thus started, although perhaps the initial injury might open up the dissecting plane in a patient with medio-necrosis.

2. Transfemoral catheter aortography [145] may be followed by thoracic aortic dissection, perhaps because of the jet of medium under high mechanical pressure.

3. Cardio-pulmonary by-pass has been the cause of many cases [44, 75, 77, 150]: in patients over forty years of age an incidence of 3 per cent was reported in 378 patients perfused via the femoral artery [77]. The site of the afferent cannula was changed to the ascending aorta, as a result. This is also the correct emergency treatment when the accident is recognised during by-pass, from a rising afferent line pressure and a soft thoracic aorta in the operative field. If the difficulty is encountered at the moment of starting perfusion, a misplaced cannula is suspected, and adjustment or transfer to the other femoral should suffice [150]. Some cases, however, develop late in the operation [44]. Although it is usual for the dissection to begin at the cannula and to run upwards as far as the heart itself, occluding main visceral and other branches on its way [150], the lesion may be localised, e.g. at the aortic bifurcation [44]. It is possible that this type, and that which results from the jet of contrast medium at catheter aortography, may be due to the oscillations of violent standing waves, such as are often seen in peripheral arteriograms (see Fig. 3.36 rt., p. 50), which might serve either to open up an arteriosclerotic lesion into the wall, or to rupture the inner media into the medio-necrotic plane. Such turbulent forces would be less violent with the perfusing cannula into the wide proximal aorta.

The Anatomy of the Dissection

The cleavage plane may be present throughout a large part of the arterial tree; generally, on histological examination the weakness is found to be due to a concentration of the cystic lesions of Erheim's medio-necrosis [46], by no means confined to the region of the actual haemorrhagic dissection (Fig. 15.39); in fact, a dry form of dissection is recognised, which may give rise to mechanical complications at branch openings [20], while medio-necrosis on its own may cause weakening and dilatation of the ascending aorta, and valvular incompetence [87].

Three main types of dissection (Fig. 15.40), mostly originating from the transverse supravalvular tear described by Shennan are:

1. Confined to the ascending aorta or arch, causing severe aortic incompetence.
2. A widespread separation affecting the whole aorta and many of its large branches.

3. A localised, often chronic, almost saccular type beginning at about the level of the left subclavian.

To distinguish between these is of practical importance, for their treatment may be different. Aortography is the most accurate method (see p. 320).

Natural Course and Mortality

Untreated, nearly all patients die of their disease, not at once, as with traumatic aortic haemorrhage or open rupture of the sac of an abdominal aortic aneurysm, but from about the end of the first day, by which time 21 per cent of Hirst's and his colleagues' series had died [65], until at six to twelve weeks only the 10 per cent with 'chronic dissection' remained. Such patients, however, may live for many years [37] (Figs 15.41, 15.43). Those in whom the ascending aorta is unaffected have the best chance of survival.

Death is due to rupture through the outer aortic layer, usually proximally into the chest, often intrapericardially, causing tamponade, or into the pleura, with rapid exsanguination. Later deaths may be due to ischaemia from compression of the lumen of important aortic branches, e.g. coronary, mesenteric or renal. Deaths of both kinds also occur in the surgically treated case, either during clamping, or from recurrent dissection, or from damage already incurred before operation.

Spontaneous decompression of the dissecting channel through the inner aortic layer back into the true lumen, usually distally, is the explanation usually accepted for the 10 per cent of survivors found to have chronic dissecting aneurysm at the site of the former acute dissection.

Double dissections sometimes occur, in which major lesions are separated by a length of normal appearing aorta, in which, however, at post-mortem, the potential cleavage plane can easily be traced.

Exceptionally, a dissecting aneurysm may begin in a situation other than the aorta; the coronaries, especially in recently pregnant women [124], the carotid, as well as the renal and mesenteric arteries [47], have all been described as the starting point, also smaller arteries such as the intracranial and thyroid branches [55]. Most of these cases show cystic medio-necrosis in the splitting layer.

The Clinical Picture

THE BACKGROUND

A history of hypertension and the presence of cardiac enlargement are the most constant general features in the patient who is to develop aortic dissection. A family history of this disease, or the clinical appearance of one of the hereditary connective tissue defects are of more direct significance however.

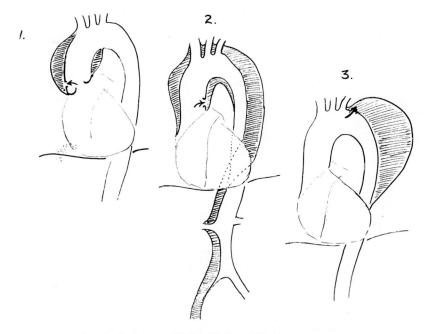

Fig. 15.40. Common types of dissecting aortic aneurysm.

1. Localised to ascending aorta with secondary valvular incompetence. The entry split is close to the valve ring.

2. Extensive, total type with involvement of major branch orifices. The two channels of the 'double-barrelled' aorta often twist in the manner shown.

3. Common localised lesion of descending aorta with entry split just beyond left subclavian. This type is frequently chronic. Not all patients require surgical treatment. The lower limit may extend below the diaphragm.

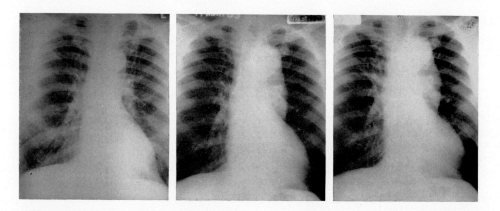

Fig. 15.41. Symptomless chronic dissecting aneurysm of the third type shown in Fig. 15.40, in a hypertensive coronary subject. Note slow progress of lesion during five years under observation. Hypotensive treatment applies particularly here.

318

THE ACUTE ILLNESS

Pain dominates every other feature in the 70 per cent majority of patients in whom it is present. The diagnosis of dissection is strongly suggested by the sudden maximal onset, often described as of a tearing quality, or with the feeling of overwhelming distension or tightness.

In contrast to the pain of myocardial infarction (the principal alternative diagnosis), in dissection the pain usually abates during the first few hours, and often moves downwards towards the subcostal region, abdomen, or lumbar area. However, coronary occlusion may occur as a complication of the dissection. The blood pressure is at first well maintained. There may be no history of pain, even in a fatal case, and in many of those whose condition goes on to become chronic [26, 36].

Acute ischaemia of one lower limb may be the presenting feature; although, more often, it comes on a few hours after the first crisis of chest pain. Clinically, again this may suggest a myocardial infarct that has been complicated by an arterial embolism. The interval is much shorter in acute dissection, and locally the condition of the common femoral artery differs in the two conditions. Although tenderness is present in both types of occlusion, the artery should be softer and more compressible beyond an iliac dissection than over an impacted embolus at the groin.

Hemiplegia is the reason for admission to hospital in some cases. Unequal brachial blood pressures or absent upper limb pulses, or weak or absent carotid or temporal pulses will usually indicate the aortic arch as the site of the lesion, but its nature may not at first be suspected.

THE CHRONIC PHASE

Many patients are symptomless (Fig. 15.41); it is therefore not possible to be sure how large this clinical group may be. From the small number of patients with diagnosed acute dissection who spontaneously recover, though with persistent widening of the mediastinal shadow, and the 10 per cent minority of chronic cases in Shennan's post-mortem series [128], chronic dissecting aneurysm appears to be fairly uncommon, yet once an equilibrium has been established the chronic lesion may be compatible with symptom-free survival for many years.

Late complications, however, include chronic heart or renal failure, and occasionally an unexplained haemothorax.

Diagnosis

The acutely ill, typical patient is easily recognised. Many are diagnosed by the junior medical officer who receives them into hospital from the clinical features described above, although difficulty may arise when the patient is unable to give a history, or in a painless case, or when the dissection shows only isolated features such as abdominal pain, lower limb ischaemia, or hemiplegia.

The susceptible patient must be remembered should one of these more doubtful aspects be presented. The diagnosis of aortic dissection in such circumstances is supported if the patient is acutely ill, with a previous history of treated hypertension often persisting into the acute illness or, has a family history of deaths from vascular catastrophe, or is a woman in late pregnancy. Clinical features of Marfan's or Ehlers-Danlos type (*see* p. 278) are also highly suggestive.

Common clinical findings, mostly of serious significance include:

(*a*) Aortic murmurs, mostly systolic along the arch and distally, though in one-quarter of the cases diastolic and proximal, from valvular incompetence. Murmurs may change or disappear, a favourable sign.

(*b*) A left pleural effusion, blood stained on aspiration.

(*c*) Pulsus paradoxus, suggesting haemopericardium.

(*d*) Tenderness of the abdominal aorta and main arteries at the limb roots.

(*e*) Unequal limb and neck pulses, often changing over a few hours.

(*f*) Red cells in the urine.

CHEST RADIOGRAPHY

This is the most important single diagnostic aid. The routine postero-antero view shows widening of the superior mediastinum with a hazy margin that later becomes clearer and somewhat lobulated [36] (Fig. 15.42). The false channel may be less opaque than the true lumen. Calcification in the inner layer may run parallel with the side band of the false channel along the lateral aortic border. Pleural effusion may be present. Comparable previous films are most helpful. Progress films during the acute illness, however, are of less certain value, for position errors are difficult to avoid in the portable examination in these ill patients [142].

Electrocardiography, though it offers no specific evidence of the condition, may be important in excluding myocardial infarction as the main cause of the illness, for to give anticoagulants in dissecting aneurysm may prove fatal. Ischaemic changes may be present, either recent, from involvement of the coronary ostia, or from dissection along the arteries themselves, or the features may be established along

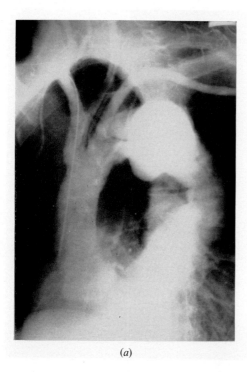
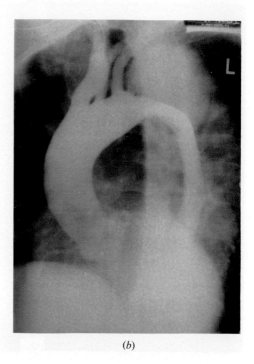

(a)   (b)

Fig. 15.45. 'Forward' aortography in the diagnosis of dissecting aneurysm.

(a) An earlier film in the series taken of the patient shown in Fig. 15.42, more clearly defining the entry split which in both films appears to be just opposite the notch in the inferior border of the aortic arch.

(b) The chronic lesion in the patient whose serial chest X-rays are shown in Fig. 15.41. In this case too, the entry jet appears to be shown, here rather closer to the left subclavian.

Emergency Measures

1. *Pericardial aspiration* may be life-saving in early developing tamponade, or the compression may be relieved by pericardiotomy through the epigastrium under local anaesthesia [134].

2. *Control of blood pressure.* In cardiac tamponade, vasoconstrictors may be required to help sustain the falling blood pressure while decompression is being initiated, but in most cases the need is the very opposite, with hypertension continuing its damaging stresses into the phase of acute dissection; hypotensive treatment is essential whether or not surgery is contemplated. Likewise, though the haematocrit may have fallen considerably, blood transfusion will be contra-indicated.

The Conservative Treatment of Acute Aortic Dissection

Poor results from emergency operation led to a trial by Wheat and his colleagues [149] of a deliberate and drastic hypotensive regime aimed at reducing the tearing stress of the cardiac impulse and of its elastic recoil or 'bounce' upon the intact aortic valve. This it was hoped might not only prevent further stripping, and avoid rupture, but also might allow time for organisation and healing of the limits of the lesion, so as to prepare the case for elective surgery if any progressive lesion could be shown to justify it.

In clinically quiescent patients in poor condition for proximal aortic surgery, the medical control might continue indefinitely as the primary basis of treatment.

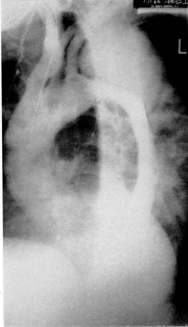

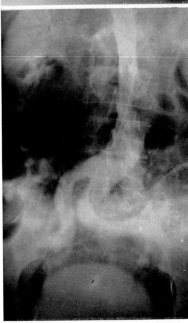

The following routine is advised, preferably in an intensive care unit:

1. Trimethaphan (Arfonad) intravenously. 1–2 mg/ml is given by slow infusion at a rate that should be sufficient to lower the systolic blood pressure to the 100 mm Hg region within 1 to 2 hours*, monitoring of the general condition, blood pressure and ECG tracing are essential. Pain which previously may have persisted in spite of morphine injections may pass off as the blood pressure falls.
2. Reserpine 1 to 2 mg is given intravenously at the same time.† This dose is repeated two to four times daily.
3. Guanethidine (Ismelin) 50 mg twice daily by mouth is given with the object of keeping the pressure down as the patient becomes refractory to trimethaphan.
4. Chest X-ray films are taken every twenty-four hours, for mediastinal size and signs of pleural fluid.
5. Heart sounds are checked for aortic incompetence.
6. Limb pulses are palpated and auscultated for signs of occlusion.
7. Urine output and scrutiny for red cells should give warnings of renal arterial involvement or tubular necrosis.

Further experience of this regime in acute aortic dissection has been good, with 50–80 per cent recovery and late survival in a group of cases that would normally have carried a high mortality untreated or with operation [63A, 97A, 145B, 149A].

Aortography should be carried out in case of doubt over progress after the acute phase, or when major branch occlusion requires investigation [145B]. Late surgical intervention is safer than early [35], so the medical regime may be useful in preparation, e.g. for valvular incompetence.

Fig. 15.46. Combined forward and retrograde aortography to demonstrate the whole and extensive aortic dissection from the left subclavian to the aortic bifurcation occluding the left renal artery. (The same patient as Figs. 15.41 and 15.45*b*.)

---

* Trimethaphan not only lowers blood pressure but reduces cardiac impulse [149]. Hexamethonium, although it lowers blood pressure, increases cardiac impulse, and it has been thought to cause dissecting aneurysm in patients receiving it for their hypertension [12].

† Reserpine has been shown to have a specific action in preventing dissecting aneurysm outbreaks in turkey flocks [149].

Case 1.

An unusually large abdominal aneurysm in a man aged sixty-seven, with recent pain and haematemesis—the latter subsequently shown to be due to a chronic peptic ulcer. A difficult operation was followed by acute tubular necrosis. The blood urea rose to over 300 mg but a spontaneous diuresis developed on 6th day. Uneventful further recovery. Patient remained well six years later.

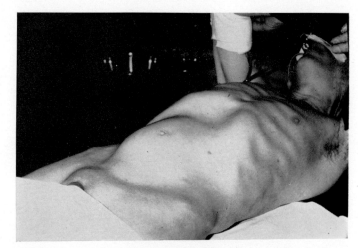

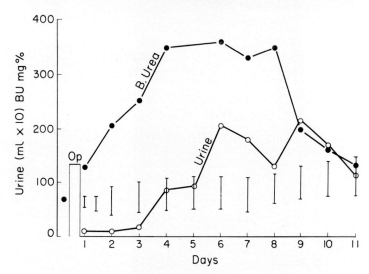

Case 2. Infected popliteal aneurysm.

A man aged seventy, hypertensive and with mild chronic renal failure developed a very large painful throbbing inflamed swelling in his left lower thigh and behind the knee. Forceful pulsation was found on examination, and arteriography showed the lumen of this aneurysm to occupy approximately one-fifth of its total diameter. There was marked slowing in the onward flow of the medium, illustration (*a*), being composed of two serial films.

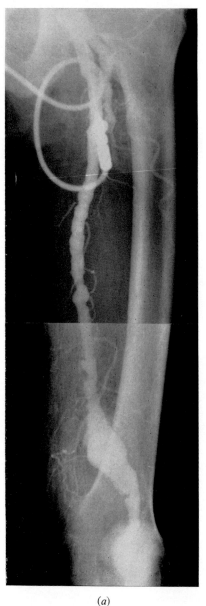

Hunterian ligation was performed in the mid-thigh. Some pulsation remained, however, and a further ligature was applied close to the first. Ten days later, the skin just above the adductor tubercle became inflamed and fluctuant, and a large abscess was drained, which yielded no growth on culture.

(*b*) The sinogram shows the size of the cavity ten days after this. Uneventful healing with good general recovery.

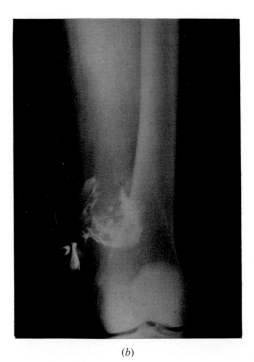

(*a*)   (*b*)

325

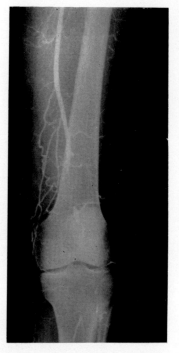

Case 3.

A successful Hunterian ligation. This patient had a painful, expanding, obstructed popliteal aneurysm. It was explored in Sim's position (*see* Fig. 3.70*a*, p. 77) but local adherence, bruising and oedema were extensive. High ligation was therefore carried out and the patient made a good recovery.

Four years later, he is free from ischaemic symptoms, although for most of this time he has been subject to superficial thrombo-phlebitis migrans for which he is on continuous anticoagulant treatment. The lack of arteriosclerotic features in this patient's case suggest that both his vascular conditions may be due to a vasculitis. Recently he had a resection and grafting of a left common femoral aneurysm.

The pattern of the collateral circulation in this arteriogram is almost identical with that of the injected specimen in the Hunterian collection of the Royal College of Surgeons of England.

Operation

The objects of surgery are as follows:

1. to prevent fatal rupture,
2. to relieve ischaemia in major branches,
3. to remedy aortic incompetence.

The methods by which surgery seeks to achieve these include:

(*a*) Opening the aorta, and constructing a re-entry channel between the two lumena (Fig. 15.47*a*).
(*b*) Transecting the aorta below the aneurysmal portion and securing the distal edge of the inner layer (Fig. 15.47*b*).
(*c*) Resecting the aneurysmal segment and replacing it with a graft, the lower anastomosis of which also secures the distal cut end of the dissected layer (Fig. 15.47*c*).
(*d*) This last method can be combined with aortic valvuloplasty or replacement.

CHOICE OF METHOD

This will depend on the site and extent of the dissection, the clinical severity of the condition and its duration, and which of the surgical objectives mentioned above appears to be the most suitable.

A left thoracic exposure of the aorta suits most cases, except those in which the abdominal aorta or the iliacs are involved, or in those severe proximal dissections in which the aortic valve ring has been reached and rendered incompetent.

In the recent, deteriorating thoracic or thoraco abdominal case, the fenestration or 're-entry' operation has given good results [79, 127]. Clinical and plain radiological assessment should indicate where the lower limit of the lesion lies, e.g. abdominal tenderness or ischaemia of a lower limb will require a laparotomy and possible grafting reconstruction [122]. Otherwise, the left chest is more likely to be the right place for a transection. Although the thoracic transection operation carries a higher immediate operative risk than the abdominal fenestration near the bifurcation, extra protection is afforded to the renal and other great visceral branches that may later occlude after the low operation. Before the aortic clamps are applied, the blood pressure should be brought down either by drugs, as described above, or by the more controllable method of exsanguination of up to a litre of blood from an artery in the operative field [79]. Otherwise, the obstructed aorta may rupture into the pericardium. Aortic clamping above the renals cannot be tolerated for more than twenty minutes; damage to the kidneys or the spinal cord is an increasing risk after this time.

Localised, saccular dissecting aneurysm of the thoracic, or the abdominal aorta may be resected and

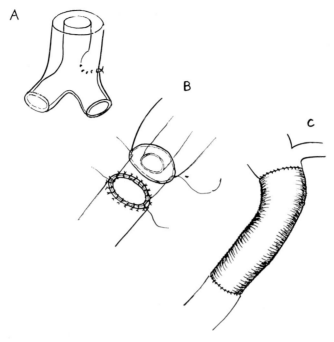

Fig. 15.47. Operations for dissecting aortic aneurysm.

(*a*) Abdominal fenestration. The aortic bifurcation is isolated and clamped and linear aortotomy provides access to the inner tube through which a generous defect is made and its distal end sutured to the outer tube.

(*b*) Transection and circular suture of the two tubes distally, providing decompression of the proximal false channel. End-to-end anastomosis of the outer tube to the repaired lower end.

(*c*) Transthoracic excision and prosthetic replacement is the preferred treatment for localised chronic dissection at this site. DeBakey and his colleagues reported a hospital mortality of only 19 per cent in 142 such cases [35].

grafted [35]. A left heart by-pass will be required for the thoracic cases [35]. Hypothermia on its own is an insufficient protection. The tolerance of the human spinal cord to aortic mobilisation and resection is very variable.

Good results are reported after grafting the chronic localised thoracic type [35], but the replacement of the ascending aorta, valve, and arch is much more formidable, and especially so in the acute phase [69, 72]; in these cases a later intervention after medical control may be more acceptable [149]. Full cardiopulmonary by-pass is required.

IN SUMMARY

1. The extensive, actively spreading dissection with incipient rupture or lower-limb ischaemia calls for emergency decompression operation, usually by simple transection or fenestration, or, occasionally, in the abdomen by grafting replacement, without the need for by-pass techniques.

2. The shorter, wider, and more chronic dissections of the thoracic aorta do well with resection and grafting, using either a tube shunt or a left heart by-pass during clamping.

3. The proximal type, affecting the aortic valve is a problem for the cardiac surgical unit.

4. Intensive medical hypotensive treatment of most acute cases has been proved effective. Control of the blood pressure level is essential in all late survivors.

REFERENCES

1. Abeshouse, B. S. (1951) Aneurysm of the renal artery: report of two cases and review of the literature. *Urol. Cutan. Rev.*, **55**, 451.

2. Abrahams, D. G. and Cockshott, W. P. (1962) Multiple non-luetic aneurysms in young Nigerians. *Brit. Heart J.*, **24**, 83.

3. Abrahams, D. G. and Parry, E. H. O. (1962) Hypertension due to renal artery stenosis caused by abdominal aortic aneurysm. *Circulation*, **26**, 104.

4. Aëtius (sixth century) as translated by Erichsen, J. E. In *Observations on Aneurism*. London: Sydenham Society, 1844, p. 4.

5. Alivisatos, C. N. and Lazarides, D. P. (1965) Dissecting aneurysm of hydatid origin of the bifurcation of the abdominal aorta. *J. Cardiovasc. Surg.*, **6**, 20.

5A. Alpert, J., Brief, D. K. and Parsonnet, V. (1970) Surgery for the ruptured abdominal aortic aneurysm. *J. Amer. Med. Ass.*, **212**, 1355.

6. Anel, D. (1714) as translated by Erichsen, J. E. In *Observations on Aneurism*. London: Sydenham Society, 1844, p. 217.

7. Anson, B. J. and Daseler, E. H. (1961) Common variations in renal anatomy, affecting blood supply, form and topography. *Surg. Gynec. Obstet.*, **112**, 439.

8. Bahnson, H. T. (1953) Definitive treatment of saccular aneurysms of the aorta with excision of sac and aortic suture. *Surg. Gynec. Obstet.*, **96**, 383.

9. Bahnson, H. T. and Spencer, F. C. (1960) Excision of aneurysm of the ascending aorta with prosthetic replacement during cardiopulmonary bypass. *Ann. Surg.*, **151**, 879.

10. Baird, R. J., Sivasankar, R., Hayward, R. and Wilson, D. R. (1966) Popliteal aneurysms: a review and analysis of 61 cases. *Surgery*, **59**, 911.

10A. Barabas, A. P. (1972) Vascular complications of the Ehlers-Danlos syndrome: with special reference to the 'arterial type' or Sack's syndrome. *J. Cardiovasc. Surg.*, **13**, 160.

11. Barnard, C. N. and Schrire, V. (1963) The surgical treatment of acquired aneurysm of the thoracic aorta. *Thorax*, **18**, 101.

11A. Bates, C. P., Pigott, H. W. S. and Stableforth, P. G. (1970) Changes in blood-urea concentration after operation and their relation to the early diagnosis of acute renal failure. *Brit. J. Surg.*, **57**, 360.

12. Beaven, D. W. and Murphy, E. A. (1956) Dissecting aneurysm during methonium therapy. *Brit. med. J.*, **i**, 77.

13. Bergan, J. J. and Trippel, O. H. (1963) Management of giant popliteal aneurysm. *Arch. Surg.*, **86**, 818.

14. Bernatz, P. E. (1960) Necrosis of the colon following resection for abdominal aortic aneurysms. *Arch. Surg.*, **81**, 373.

14A. Blondeau, P. and Santot, J. (1967) Les résultats éloignés de la chirurgie artérielle restauratrice de l'aorte sous-rénale. *J. Chir.* (*Paris*), **94**, 185.

15. Boyd, A. M. (1966) Popliteal aneurysms. *Brit. med. J.*, **i**, 918.

16. Brasdor (1799) cited by Deschamps, translated by Erichsen, J. E. In *Observations on Aneurism*, London: Sydenham Society, 1844, p. 481 *et seq.*

17. Brock, R. C. (1952) *The Life and Work of Astley Cooper*. Edinburgh and London: E. & S. Livingstone. (*a*) pp. 49–55, (*b*) pp. 50 and 57.

18. Brody, G. L., Burton, J. F., Zawadzki, E. S. and French, A. J. (1965) Dissecting aneurysms of the coronary artery. *New Eng. J. Med.*, **273**, 1.

19. Brooks, D. K. (1967) *Resuscitation*. London: Edward Arnold.

20. Burman, S. O. and Geratz, J. H. D. (1958) Non-hemorrhagic cleavage of the aorta. *Ann. Surg.*, **147**, 571.

21. Burton, G. W., Holderness, M. C. and John, H. T. (1964) Circulatory and acid-base changes during operations for abdominal aortic aneurysm. *Lancet*, **ii**, 782.

22. Calem, W. S. and LeVeen, H. H. (1962) Arterial thrombosis complicating inferior vena cava ligation. *Surgery*, **52**, 613.

23. Callahan, W. P. and Schiltz, F. H. (1926) Aneurism of the renal artery. *Surg. Gynec. Obstet.*, **43**, 724.

24. Carlsson, J. and Sternby, N. H. (1964) Aortic aneurysms. *Acta chir. Scand.*, **127**, 466.

25. Carmichael, R. (1950) The pathogenesis of non-inflammatory cerebral aneurysms. *J. Path. Bact.*, **62**, 1.

26. Cohen, S. and Littmann, D. (1964) Painless dissecting aneurysm of the aorta. *New Eng. J. Med.*, **271**, 143.

27. Colt, G. H. (1927) The clinical duration of saccular aortic aneurysm in British-born subjects. *Quart. J. Med.*, **20**, 331.

28. Cooley, D. A., DeBakey, M. E. and Morris, G. C. (1957) Controlled extracorporeal circulation in surgical treatment of aortic aneurysm. *Ann. Surg.*, **146**, 473.

28A. Couch, N. P., Dwochowski, J. R., van de Water, J. M., Harken, D. E. and Moore, F. D. (1971) Muscle surface pH as an indication of peripheral perfusion in man. *Ann. Surg.*, **173**, 173.

29. Crawford, E. S., Fenstermacher, J. M., Richardson, W. and Sandiford, F. (1970) Reappraisal of adjuncts to avoid ischemia in the treatment of thoracic aortic aneurysms. *Surgery*, **67**, 182.

30. Crichlow, R. W. and Roberts, B. (1966) Treatment of popliteal aneurysms by restoration of continuity. *Ann. Surg.*, **163**, 417.

31. Culp, O. S. and Bernatz, P. E. (1961) Urologic aspects of lesions in the abdominal aorta. *J. Urol.*, **86**, 189.

32. DeBakey, M. E., Creech, O. and Morris, G. C. (1956) Aneurysm of thoracoabdominal aorta involving the celiac, superior mesenteric, and renal arteries. Report of four cases treated by resection and homograft replacement. *Ann. Surg.*, **144**, 549.

33. DeBakey, M. E., Cooley, D. A., Crawford, E. S.

and Morris, G. C. (1958) Aneurysms of the thoracic aorta: analysis of 179 patients treated by resection. *J. Thorac. Cardiovasc. Surg.*, **36**, 393.

34. DeBakey, M. E., Crawford, E. S., Garrett, H. E., Beall, A. C. and Howell, J. F. (1965) Surgical considerations in the treatment of aneurysm of the thoraco-abdominal aorta. *Ann. Surg.*, **162**, 650.

35. DeBakey, M. E., Henly, W. S., Cooley, D. A., Morris, G. C., Crawford, E. S. and Beall, A. C. (1965) Surgical management of dissecting aneurysms of the aorta. *J. Thorac. Cardiovasc. Surg.*, **49**, 130.

35A. Deterling, R. A. (1971) Aneurysm of the visceral arteries. *J. Cardiovasc. Surg.*, **12**, 309.

36. Dow, J. and Roebuck, E. J. (1964) Dissecting aneurysms of the aorta. *Guy's Hospital Rep.*, **113**, 17.

37. Drury, R. A. B. (1955) Healed dissecting aneurysm of the aorta. *Brit. med. J.*, **ii**, 1114.

38. Dubost, C., Allary, M. and Oeconomos, N. (1952) Resection of an aneurysm of the abdominal aorta. *Arch. Surg.*, **64**, 405.

39. Du Boulay, G. H. (1965) Some observations on the natural history of intracranial aneurysms. *Brit. J Radiol.*, **38**, 721.

40. Eastcott, H. H. G. (1966) Ischaemic diseases of the colon. *Proc. Roy. Soc. Med.*, **59**, 890.

41. Eastcott, H. H. G. (1966) Popliteal aneurysms. *Brit. med. J.*, **i**, 799.

41A. Eastcott, H. H. G. and Robinson, S. H. G. (1962) Rupture of orlon aortic graft after six years. *Lancet*, **ii**, 75.

42. Eastcott, H. H. G. and Sutton, D. (1958) Chronic dissecting aneurysm of the aorta diagnosed by aortography. *Lancet*, **ii**, 73.

42A. Eastcott, H. H. G. and Gardner, A. L. (1969) Autosympathectomy in abdominal aortic aneurysm. *Ann. Surg.*, **169**, 290.

43. Eiseman, B. and Rainer, W. G. (1958) Clinical management of posttraumatic rupture of the thoracic aorta. *J. Thorac. Cardiovasc. Surg.*, **35**, 347.

44. Elliott, D. P. and Roe, B. B. (1965) Aortic dissection during cardiopulmonary bypass. *J. Thorac. Cardiovasc. Surg.*, **50**, 357.

45. Erb, B. D. and Tullis, I. F. (1960) Dissecting aneurysm of the aorta. The clinical features of thirty autopsied cases. *Circulation*, **22**, 315.

46. Erdheim, J. (1929) Medionecrosis aortae idiopathica. *Virchows Arch. path. Anat.*, **273**, 454.

47. Foord, A. G. and Lewis, R. D. (1959) Primary dissecting aneurysms of peripheral and pulmonary arteries. *Arch. Path.*, **68**, 553.

47A. Foreman, J. E. K. and Hutchinson, K. J. (1970) Arterial wall vibration distal to stenosis in isolated arteries of dog and man. *Circ. Res.*, **36**, 583.

47B. Frawley, J. E., Dickson, G. H., Jamieson, C. W. and Eastcott, H. H. G. (1972) Abdominal aortic aneurysm and horse-shoe kidney. *Brit. J. Surg.*, **59**, 513.

48. Fuller, C. H. and Peters, P. C. (1962) Aneurysm of the renal-artery bifurcation. Resection with restoration of arterial continuity. *New Eng. J. Med.*, **267**, 757.

49. Furler, I. K., Robertson, D. N. S., Harris, H. J. and Pryer, R. R. L. (1962) Spontaneous rupture of the splenic artery in pregnancy. *Lancet*, **ii**, 588.

50. Galen (second century) as translated by Erichsen, J. E. In *Observations on Aneurism*. London: Sydenham Society, 1844, p. 3.

51. Gaylis, H. and Laws, J. W. (1956) Dissection of aorta as a complication of translumbar aortography. *Brit. med. J.*, **ii**, 1141.

52. Gedge, S. W., Spittel, J. A. and Ivins, J. C. (1961) Aneurysm of the distal popliteal artery and its relationship to the arcuate popliteal ligament. *Circulation*, **24**, 270.

53. Gifford, R. W., Hines, E. A. and Janes, J. M. (1953) An analysis and follow-up study of one hundred popliteal aneurysms. *Surgery*, **33**, 284.

54. Gliedman, M. L., Ayers, W. B. and Vestal, B. L. (1957) Aneurysms of the abdominal aorta and its branches. A study of untreated patients. *Ann. Surg.*, **146**, 207.

55. Golby, M. G. S. and Kay, J. M. (1965) Primary dissecting aneurysm of the inferior thyroid artery. *Brit. J. Surgery*, **52**, 389.

55A. Goldberg, D. B. and Lehman, J. S. (1970) Aorto-sonography: ultrasound measurement of the abdominal aorta and thoracic aorta. *Arch. Surg.*, **100**, 652.

56. Goodman, R. M., Wooley, C. F., Frazier, R. L. and Covault, L. (1965) Ehlers-Danlos syndrome occurring together with the Marfan syndrome. *New Eng. J. Med.*, **273**, 514.

57. Goodwin, J. F. (1961) Pregnancy and coarctation of the aorta. *Clin. Obstet. Gynaec.*, **4**, 645.

58. Gordon-Taylor, G. (1950) The surgery of the innominate artery, with special reference to aneurysm. *Brit. J. Surg.*, **37**, 377.

59. Greenstone, S. M., Massell, T. B. and Heringman, E. C. (1961) Arteriosclerotic popliteal aneurysms. *Circulation*, **24**, 23.

60. Guattani, C. (1772) as translated by Erichsen, J. E. In *Observations on Aneurism*. London: Sydenham Society, 1844, p. 279.

61. Guida, P. M. and Moore, S. W. (1966) Aneurysm of the hepatic artery. Report of five cases with a brief review of the previously reported cases. *Surgery*, **60**, 299.

62. Guthrie, C. C. (1912) *Blood Vessel Surgery and Its Applications*. A reprint (1959) (Ed. Harbison, S. P. and Fisher, B.). University of Pittsburgh Press.

63. Hardin, C. A. (1962) Successful resection of carotid and abdominal aneurysm in two related patients with Marfan's syndrome. *New Eng. J. Med.*, **267**, 141.

63A. Harris, P. D., Bowman, F. O. and Mason, J. R. (1969) The management of acute dissections of the thoracic aorta. *Amer. Heart. J.*, **78**, 419.

64. Harrow, B. R. and Sloane, J. A. (1959) Aneurysm of renal artery: report of five cases. *J. Urol.*, **81**, 35.

65. Hirst, A. E., Johns, V. J. and Kime, S. W. (1958) Dissecting aneurysm of the aorta: a review of 505 cases. *Medicine, Baltimore*, **37**, 217.

66. Holesh, S. (1960) Dissecting aneurysm of the aorta. *Brit. J. Radiol.*, **33**, 302.

67. Home, E. (1786) 'An account of Mr. Hunter's method of performing the operation for the popliteal aneurysm. Communicated in a letter to Dr Simmons.' *The London Medical Journal*, **7**, 391. Cited by Erichsen, J. E. In *Observations on Aneurysm*, (1844). London: Sydenham Society.

68. Hou, Y., Shang, T. and Wu, Y. (1964) Surgical treatment of aneurysm of thoracic aorta. *Chinese med. J.*, **83**, 740.

69. Hufnagel, C. A. and Conrad, P. W. (1962) Dissecting aneurysms of the ascending aorta: direct approach to repair. *Surgery*, **51**, 84.

70. Hunter, J., cited by Home, E. (1793) in *Observations on Aneurysm*, (Ed. Ericksen, J. E.) Sydenham Society, 1844, p. 388.

71. Hunter, W. (1757) as edited by Erichsen, J. E. In *Observations on Aneurism*. London: Sydenham Society, 1844.

72. Hume, D. M. and Porter, R. R. (1963) Acute dissecting aortic aneurysms. *Surgery*, **53**, 122.

73. Inui, F. K. and Ferguson, T. A. (1956) Aneurysm of the right hepatic artery, preoperative diagnosis and successful excision. *Ann. Surg.*, **144**, 235.

74. Irwin, J. W. S., Hancock, D. M. and Sharp, J. R. (1964) Ruptured abdominal aortic aneurysm in Marfan's syndrome. *Brit. med. J.*, **i**, 1293.

75. Jones, T. W., Vetto, R. R., Winterscheid, L. C., Dillard, D. H. and Merendino, K. A. (1960) Arterial complications incident to cannulation in open-heart surgery. *Ann. Surg.*, **152**, 969.

76. Jordan, W. M. (1963) Resected coarctation of the aorta and pregnancy. *Brit. med. J.*, **ii**, 224.

77. Kay, J. H., Dykstra, P. C. and Tsuji, H. K. (1966) Retrograde ilioaortic dissection. A complication of common femoral artery perfusion during open heart surgery. *Amer. J. Surg.*, **111**, 464.

78. Kazmier, F. J., Sheps, S. G., Bernatz, P. E. and Sayre, G. P. (1966) Livedo reticularis and digital infarcts: a syndrome due to cholesterol emboli arising from atheromatous abdominal aortic aneurysms. *Vascular Dis.*, **3**, 12.

79. Kenyon, J. R. (1963) Aortic aneurysms. *Ann. Roy. Coll. Surg. Eng.*, **32**, 116.

80. Kilpatrick, F. R. (1967) Horseshoe kidneys. *Proc. Roy. Soc. Med.*, **60**, 433.

81. Klippel, A. P. and Butcher, H. R. (1966) The unoperated abdominal aortic aneurysm. *Amer. J. Surg.*, **111**, 629.

82. Kraft, R. O. and Fry, W. J. (1963) Aneurysms of the celiac artery. *Surg. Gynec. Obstet.*, **117**, 563.

82A. Kubacz, G. J. (1971) Femoral and sciatic compression neuropathy. *Brit. J. Surg.*, **58**, 580.

83. Kulatilake, A. E. (1966) The artificial kidney in acute renal failure following surgery. *Proc. Roy. Soc. Med.*, **59**, 42.

83A. Lagaaij, M. B., Terpstra, J. L. and Vink, M. (1970) Ruptured aneurysm of the abdominal aorta. *J. Cardiovasc. Surg.*, **11**, 440.

84. Leading article (1964) Central venous pressure in oligaemic shock. *Lancet*, **i**, 1143.

85. Leading article (1966) Warm blood for massive transfusion. *Lancet*, **i**, 1193.

86. Leading article (1966) Popliteal aneurysms. *Brit. med. J.*, **i**, 625.

87. Lewis, M. G. (1965) Idiopathic medionecrosis causing aortic incompetence. *Brit. med. J.*, **i**, 1478.

88. Lexer, E. (1907) Die Ideale Operation des Arteriellen und des arteriell-venösen Aneurysma. *Arch. klin. Chir.*, **83**, 459.

89. Lexer, E. (1913) Ideale Aneurysmaoperation und Gefässtransplantation. *Verh. dtsch. Ges. Chir.*, **42**, 113.

90. Lilien, O. M., Jones, S. G. and Mueller, C. B. (1963) The mechanism of mannitol diuresis. *Surg. Gynec. Obstet.*, **117**, 221.

91. Linton, R. R. (1951) Intrasaccular wiring of abdominalarteriosclerotic aneurysms by the 'pack' method. *Angiology*, **2**, 485.

91A. Little, J. M. and Spence, J. W. (1971) Aneurysm of an anomalous hepatic artery. *Brit. J. Surg.*, **58**, 886.

92. Luck, R. J. and Irvine, W. T. (1965) Mannitol in the surgery of aortic aneurysm. *Lancet*, **ii**, 409.

93. Ludbrook, J. and Wynn, V. (1958) Citrate intoxication. A clinical and experimental study. *Brit. med. J.*, **ii**, 523.

94. Luke, R. G., Linton, A. L., Briggs, J. D. and Kennedy, A. C. (1965) Mannitol therapy in acute renal failure. *Lancet*, **i**, 980.

95. Lynch, H. T., Larsen, A. L., Wilson, R. and Magnuson, C. L. (1965) Ehlers-Danlos syndrome and 'congenital' arteriovenous fistulae. A clinico-pathological study of a family. *J. Amer. med. Assoc.*, **194**, 1011.

96. Lytton, B. (1966) Ureteral obstruction following aortofemoral bypass grafts. *Surgery*, **59**, 918.

97. McAlexander, R. A. and Lawrence, G. H. (1966) Operative repair of hepatic artery aneurysm. *Arch. Surg.*, **93**, 409.

97A. McFarland, J., Willerson, J. T., Dinsmore, R. E., Austen, W. G., Buckley, M. J., Sanders, C. A. and DeSanctis, R. W. (1972) Medical treatment of dissecting aortic aneurysms. *New Eng. J. Med.*, **286**, 115.

98. McFarland, W. and Fuller, D. E. (1964) Mortality in Ehlers-Danlos syndrome due to spontaneous rupture of large arteries. *New Eng. J. Med.*, **271**, 1309.

99. McKusick, V. A. (1955) The cardiovascular aspects of Marfan's syndrome: a hereditable disorder of connective tissue. *Circulation*, **11**, 321.

100. McMillan, G. C. (1950) Diffuse granulomatous aortitis with giant cells associated with partial rupture and dissection of the aorta. *Arch. Path.*, **49**, 63.

101. McNicol, G. P. and Douglas, A. S. (1965) Acute fibrinolytic states in surgery. *Proc. Roy. Soc. Med.*, **58**, 259.

102. Magarey, F. R. (1950) Dissecting aneurysm due to giant-cell aortitis. *J. Path. Bact.*, **62**, 445.

103. Malcolm, J. E. (1957) *Blood Pressure Sounds and Their Meanings*. London: Heinemann, p. 84 *et seq.*

104. Mannick, J. A., Brooks, J. W., Bosher, L. H. and Hume, D. M. (1964) Ruptured aneurysms of the abdominal aorta. *New Eng. J. Med.*, **271**, 915.

105. Matas, R. (1903) An operation for the radical cure of aneurism based upon arteriorrhaphy. *Ann. Surg.*, **37**, 161.

106. Mátyus, L., Bodnár, E. and Littmann, I. (1966) Ruptured aneurysm of the splenic artery. *J. Cardiovasc. Surg.*, **7**, 324.

107. Meehan, J. J., Pastor, B. H., and Torre, A. V. (1957) Dissecting aneurysm of the aorta secondary to tuberculous aortitis. *Circulation*, **16**, 615.

108. Orth, O. (1919) Ein Fall von traumatische Anaeurysma der Arteria renalis sinistra und einer traumatischen rupturierten Hydronephrose. *Dtsch. Z. Chir.*, **151**, 272.

109. Osler, W. (1905) Aneurysm of the abdominal aorta. *Lancet*, **ii**, 1089.

110. Osler, W. (1915) Remarks on arterio-venous aneurysm. *Lancet*, **i**, 949.

111. Owen, R. (1879) John Hunter and vivisection. *Brit. med. J.*, **i**, 284.

112. Owens, J. C. and Coffey, R. J. (1953) Aneurysm of the splenic artery, including a report of six additional cases. *Int. Abstr. Surg.*, **97**, 313.

113. Pappas, G., Janes, J. M., Bernatz, P. E. and Schirger, A. (1964) Femoral aneurysms. Review of surgical management. *J. Amer. med. Assoc.*, **190**, 489.

114. Paré, A. (1582) as translated by Erichsen, J. E. In *Observations on Aneurism*. London: Sydenham Society, 1844, p. 185.

115. Penn, I. (1963) Abdominal aortic aneurysm in the African patient. *Brit. J. Surg.*, **50**, 598.

115A. Perlmutter, M., Grossman, S. L., Rothenberg, S. and Dobkin, G. (1959) Urine-serum urea nitrogen ratio; simple test of renal function in acute azotemia and oliguria. *J. Amer. Med. Ass.*, **170**, 1533.

116. Pirogoff, N. I. Cited by Osler, W. (1905) *In* Aneurysm of the abdominal aorta. *Lancet*, **ii**, 1089.

117. Poutasse, E. F. (1957) Renal artery aneurysm: report of 12 cases, two treated by excision of the aneurysm and repair of renal artery. *J. Urol.*, **77**, 697.

118. Power, D. and Colt, G. H. (1903) A case of the abdominal aorta treated by the introduction of silver-steel wire. *Lancet*, **ii**, 808.

119. Pringle, J. H. (1913) Two cases of vein-grafting for the maintenance of a direct arterial circulation. *Lancet*, **i**, 1795.

120. Provan, J. L., Fraenkel, G. J. and Austen, W. G. (1966) Metabolic and hemodynamic changes after temporary aortic occlusion in dogs. *Surg. Gynec. Obstet.*, **123**, 544.

120A. Razzuk, M. A., Linton, R. R. and Darling, R. C. (1967) Femoral neuropathy secondary to ruptured abdominal aortic aneurysms with false aneurysms. *J. Amer. Med. Ass.*, **201**, 817.

121. Roberts, B. E. and Smith, P. H. (1966) Hazards of mannitol infusions. *Lancet*, **ii**, 421.

121A. Robicsek, F., Daugherty, H. K. and Mullen, D.

(1970) The elective use of balloon obstruction in aortic surgery. *Surgery*, **68**, 774.

121B. Ross, H. B. and Sales, J. E. L. (1972) Post-irradiation femoral aneurysm treated by iliopopliteal by-pass via the obturator foramen. *Brit. J. Surg.*, **59**, 400.

122. Savage, C. R. (1959) Retrograde aortography in acute dissecting aneurysm of the aorta. *Lancet*, **i**, 281.

123. Schatz, I. J., Fairbairn, J. F. and Juergens, J. L. (1962) Abdominal aortic aneurysms: a reappraisal. *Circulation*, **26**, 200.

124. Schnitker, M. A. and Bayer, C. A. (1944) Dissecting aneurysm of the aorta in young individuals, particularly in association with pregnancy. With report of a case. *Ann. Int. Med.*, **20**, 486.

124A. Seal, P. V. and Shepherd, R. C. (1970) Rupture of an abdominal aortic aneurysm into the inferior vena cava. *Brit. J. Surg.*, **57**, 904.

125. Seitzman, D. M., Mazze, R. I., Schwartz, F. D. and Barry, K. G. (1963) Mannitol diuresis: a method of renal protection during surgery. *J. Urol.*, **90**, 139.

126. Shackman, R. (1966) Acute renal failure in surgery. *Proc. Roy. Soc. Med.*, **59**, 37.

127. Shaw, R. S. (1955) Acute dissecting aortic aneurysm. Treatment by fenestration of the internal wall of the aneurysm. *New Eng. J. Med.*, **253**, 331.

128. Shennan, T. (1934) *Dissecting Aneurysms*. Med. Res. Council Spec. Rep. Series No. 193. London: H.M.S.O.

128A. Sheil, A. G. R., Reeve, T. S., Little, J. M., Coupland, G. A. E. and Loewenthal, J. (1969) Aorto-intestinal fistulas following operations upon the abdominal aorta and iliac arteries. *Brit. J. Surg.*, **56**, 840.

129. Sherlock, S. P. V. and Learmonth, J. R. (1942) Aneurysm of the splenic artery: with an account of an example complicating Gaucher's disease. *Brit. J. Surg.*, **30**, 151.

130. Short, D. W. (1966) Aneurysms of the internal iliac artery. *Brit. J. Surg.*, **53**, 17.

131. Shumacker, H. B. (1958) Excisional treatment of aneurysm of celiac artery. *Ann. Surg.*, **148**, 885.

132. Simon, A. L., Hipoma, F. A. and Stansel, H. C. (1965) Dissecting aortic aneurysm in Marfan's syndrome. *J. Amer. med. Assoc.*, **193**, 156.

133. Slaney, G., Ashton, F. and Dawson-Edwards, P. (1964) Renal-artery aneurysmectomy with severe contralateral renal hypoplasia. *Lancet*, **ii**, 937.

134. Sleight, P. (1965) Dissection of the aorta with pericardial tamponade: successful relief of tamponade. *Brit. med. J.*, **i**, 1165.

135. Smith, R. F. and Szilagyi, D. E. (1961) Ruptured abdominal aortic aneurysms. *Ann. Surg.*, **154**, Suppl. 175.

136. Smyth, N. P. D. and Teimourian, B. (1964) Resection of hepatic arterial aneurysm following intraperitoneal rupture. *Ann. Surg.*, **160**, 61.

137. Sommerville, R. L., Allen, E. V. and Edwards, J. E. (1959) Bland and infected arteriosclerotic abdominal aortic aneurysms: a clinicopathologic study. *Medicine, Baltimore*, **38**, 207.

138. Sondheimer, F. K. and Steinberg, I. (1964) Gastrointestinal manifestations of abdominal aortic aneurysms. *Amer. J. Roent.*, **92**, 1110.

139. Stewart, J. W. (1962) 'Some problems of massive blood transfusion during surgical procedures.' In *Modern Trends in Surgery*, 1. (Ed. Irvine, W. T.). London: Butterworth's, p. 261.

140. Stoney, R. J., Albo, R. J. and Wylie, E. J. (1965) False aneurysms occurring after arterial grafting operations. *Amer. J. Surg.*, **110**, 153.

141. Subbotitch, V. (1913) Military experiences of traumatic aneurysms. *Lancet*, **ii**, 720.

142. Sutton, D. (1962) *Arteriography*. Edinburgh and London: E. & S. Livingstone, p. 103.

143. Szilagyi, D. E., Smith, R. F., DeRusso, F. J., Elliott, J. P. and Sherrin, F. W. (1966) Contribution of abdominal aortic aneurysmectomy to prolongation of life. *Ann. Surg.*, **164**, 678.

144. Szilagyi, D. E., Elliott, J. P. and Smith, R. F. (1965) Ruptured abdominal aneurysms simulating sepsis. *Arch. Surg.*, **91**, 263.

144A. Szilagyi, D. E., Smith, R. F., Elliott, J. P., Hageman, J. H. and Rodriguez, F. J. (1970) Aorto-iliac atherosclerotic and non-vascular intra-abdominal surgical lesions. *Arch. Surg.*, **100**, 470.

145. Templeton, J. Y., Johnson, R. G. and Griffith, J. R. (1960) Dissecting aneurysm of the thoracic aorta as a complication of catheter aortography: successful surgical treatment. *J. Thorac. Cardiovasc. Surg.*, **40**, 209.

145A. Thomas, T. V. (1970) Surgical implications of the retro-aortic left renal vein. *Arch. Surg.*, **100**, 738.

145B. Thompson, A. E., Spracklen, F. H. N., Besterman, E. M. M. and Bromley, L. L. (1969) Recognition and management of dissecting aneurysms of the aorta. *Brit. med. J.*, **4**, 134.

146. Thompson, J. F., Mazella, S. F. and Thistlethwaite, J. R. (1965) Aneurysm of the celiac artery. Case report of successful management. *Ann. Surg.*, **161**, 83.

147. Turkington, R. W. and Grode, H. E. (1964) Ehlers-Danlos syndrome and multiple neurofibromatosis. *Ann. Int. Med.*, **61**, 549.

147A. Walker, D. I., Bloor, K., Williams, G. and Gillie, J. (1972) Inflammatory aneurysms of the abdominal aorta. *Brit. J. Surg.*, **59**, 609.

147B. Walker, W. F. and Johnston, I. D. A. (1971) *The Metabolic Basis of Surgical Care*. London: William Heinemann Medical Books, p. 172.

148. Ward-McQuaid, J. N. (1961) Splenic aneurysms. *Brit. J. Surg.*, **48**, 646.

149. Wheat, M. W., Palmer, R. F., Bartley, T. D. and Seelman, R. C. (1965) Treatment of dissecting aneurysms of the aorta without surgery. *J. Thorac. Cardiovasc. Surg.*, **50**, 364.

149A. Wheat, M. W., Harris, P. D., Malm, J. R., Kaiser, G., Bowman, F. O. and Palmer, R. F. (1969) Acute dissecting aneurysms of the aorta. Treatment and results in 64 patients. *J. Thorac. Cardiovasc. Surg.*, **58**, 144.

150. Williams, K. R. and Johnson, J. (1964) Aortic dissection after femoral artery cannulation. *Arch. Surg.*, **89**, 663.

151. Woodruff, M. (1966) Popliteal aneurysms. *Brit. med. J.*, **i**, 918.

152. Wychulis, A. R., Spittell, J. A. and Wallace, R. B. (1970) Popliteal aneurysms. *Surgery*, **68**, 942.

16 Arteriovenous Fistulae

Abnormal communication between the arterial and venous sides of the circulation occurs in several disease states, and may involve vessels of all sizes, from the smallest capillaries in some congenital types, to the aorta and vena cava as an acquired condition in adults from penetrating injury. The variety of effects produced by arteriovenous connection is great, yet they differ only in degree; their general picture is constant, and clinical principles based upon these changes should clarify the recognition and management of an individual case, no matter where it occurs.

The Murmur

A typical, continuous 'machinery' murmur can always be heard over an arteriovenous fistula of any significant size, of which it is the most important single diagnostic feature. The murmur, better described as a roaring, is accompanied by a thrill which affords a useful guide at operation. Loudest in systole, and over the actual opening of the fistula, it is conducted freely and extensively around the region, by branching vessels, particularly along the main artery and vein.

EFFECTS UPON THE CIRCULATION [9, 19, 29, 41, 44, 61]

Short-circuiting of part of the peripheral vascular bed produces changes in proportion to the extent of communication. In most congenital cases, though diffuse and multiple, this is small and only of local haemodynamic significance. The larger, solitary opening caused by injury will sooner or later throw strain both upon the local conducting channels and often, also, upon the heart, which is subjected to ceaseless overwork.

Fall in diastolic pressure occurs because the arterial system is unable to support the pulse pressure, except when the heart is in systole. The blood leaks away into the venous side so quickly in diastole that, though the pulse pressure is widened, the mean arterial pressure is reduced and a collapsing water-hammer pulse can be felt, as in aortic regurgitation [29], patent ductus arteriosus, and also the onward fast passage of the peripheral blood from the arterioles and capillaries in thyrotoxicosis, Paget's disease of bone, and in physiological states of vasodilatation, including fever. In the absence of these other causes of collapsing pulse and with a bruit, arteriovenous shunting must exist. Complicated haemodynamic studies are not required.

Increase in pulse rate goes with collapsing pulse; it is in some way related to the increased work of the heart, and is actuated either by the Bainbridge reflex from increase in the venous pressure resulting from the greater return to the heart, or from reduction in the mean arterial pressure (Marey's law) [29]. Arterial receptors could be responsible [16].

Obliteration of the fistula either by digital compression or by operation, or by occluding the afferent artery, causes immediate slowing of the heart (Branham's sign), another important clinical test for functionally significant arteriovenous fistula.

Cardiac dilatation and, eventually, congestive failure are everywhere recognised, but the haemodynamics that lead to this state are less well documented.

The cardiac output is increased in experimental fistulae in animals [19] and in many of the human cases in which it has been measured [8, 9, 14, 44, 52B, 55]. In all cases in which it is raised, closure of the fistula is followed by a prompt return to normal. Dilatation of the heart (Fig. 16.1), increase in stroke

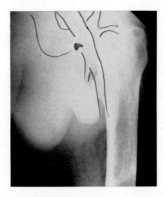 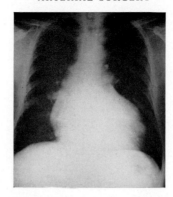 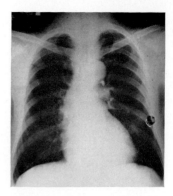

Fig. 16.1. Massive fistula between common femoral vessels, from a gun-shot wound at Dunkirk, for which the left lower limb was amputated through the thigh. Twenty years later, having been breathless on effort for some years, he became totally incapacitated by congestive heart failure.

Quadruple ligation produced immediate relief of all symptoms and signs, a large diuresis and a return to normal heart size.

volume and tachycardia, common features of a large fistula, are also corrected, though at first the heart and aorta may further enlarge [20, 24]. The advent of heart failure, an inevitable complication in patients with a large untreated fistula, is shown by the inability of the cardiac output to increase further in response to exercise [44].

Blood volume is increased if the fistula is large [19, 64]; like the cardiac output it falls soon after closure, which may be followed by a remarkable diuresis [9].

Hyperventilation and respiratory alkalosis occur without heart failure, also an increase in oxygen consumption, which is not fully accounted for by the work of the heart [9]. The arteriovenous oxygen difference is decreased by the shunt without respect to the rate of body consumption. The reverse happens when the shunt is within the lung, for here the passage of much blood direct from the pulmonary artery to vein prevents it from reaching the alveolar capillaries, and cyanosis, polycythaemia and finger clubbing are produced [31].

Subacute Bacterial Endocarditis

This is an important late complication of a large, untreated arteriovenous fistula, which, as in patent ductus arteriosus, may be accompanied by endarteritis at the site of the fistula [21]. No doubt it is due to increased wear and tear and haemodynamic forces due to the accelerated circulation. Experimentally, it can be produced by adding successive fistulae in dogs; infection almost invariably develops at a predicted level of cardiac output [30], preceded by enlargement of the adrenal glands. A case in which septicaemia was also present was cured by excision of the fistula [50].

Local Vascular and Haemodynamic Effects
(Fig. 16.2)

Dilatation occurs in the artery leading to the fistula and in the vein that drains it, clearly due to the increased blood flow but by a mechanism that is not understood.

In late cases there may be severe degenerative and

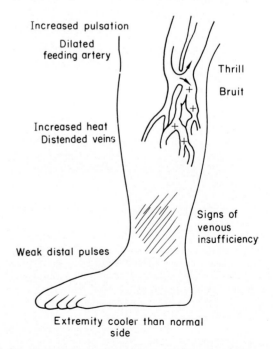

Fig. 16.2. The local effects of an arteriovenous fistula.

aneurysmal changes in the main feeding artery and draining vein, that extend over a great length of these vessels [52B, 55A]. These changes are irreversible even after closure of the fistula, and in fact may need surgical treatment in their own right.

Arterial branches and venous tributaries near the fistula also take part in this dilatation, obscuring the anatomy of the main vessels; at operation they are the main obstacle between the surgeon and the fistula. It is this rich *collateral network* that was the object of surgical attempts to increase limb blood flow for therapeutic purposes [41]. The number and profusion of vessels increases with time, and such fistulae are more difficult to close than to construct. This is the main reason for the early operative closure of recent traumatic fistulae, at a time when the main vessels can still be approached without much difficulty. Nowadays, a reserve of new collaterals is no longer necessary to ensure limb survival, for restoration of the main artery in most patients no longer poses any difficulty.

Overloading of the venous side of the limb circulation will eventually produce the clinical picture of *venous insufficiency*, and this in no way differs from that which follows deep venous occlusion or incompetence, chiefly involving the skin and soft tissue changes at the ankles over the fascial openings of the perforating veins, and with generalised swelling of the limb as well. Aching and ulceration may be the patient's reason in seeking treatment. Spontaneous cure may follow thrombophlebitis [51]. Localised, superficial clumps of aneurysmal varices may, like the familiar, large varicosities of superficial venous incompetence, be quite symptomless. In such a case the fistula is often small and no treatment may

be needed. *Lymphatic involvement* has also been described [45] with lymphoedema, and apparent cure after excision of the fistula.

The distal arterial tree is deprived of blood, a fact that is sometimes forgotten although clearly explained two centuries ago by William Hunter [47], and in recent years confirmed by blood flow studies [61]. Clinical examination shows the affected extremity to be colder and its distal pulses weaker than on the healthy side. Therapeutic fistulae for limb lengthening achieve their object only in the bones proximal to the communication [61].

If a traumatic arteriovenous fistula is sustained by a child, the limb distal to the fistula may actually undergo wasting, presumably from proximal shunting of blood that should have passed through the periphery. Likewise, the circulation of the three normal limbs might be deprived, or at least limited by a fistula in the fourth, since closure of the fistula has been shown to be followed by an increase in blood flow through the unaffected limbs [8, 29] as well as in the distal part of the operated extremity [8].

Creation of a fistula as a treatment for limb ischaemia could scarcely be expected to succeed in its object unless the communication could be made far down the extremity, though in an unfavourable graft operation the rate of flow might be so increased by a short-circuit at the knee that improved patency rates could be hoped for [52]. A more successful application is the surgical anastomosis of an artery and vein at the wrist in patients requiring repeated haemodialysis or frequent blood transfusions: venous enlargement with fast flow makes it easier to obtain access to the circulation with less risk of phlebitis than with an external shunt [6, 40A].

Congenital Arteriovenous Fistulae [36, 57, 59]

Blood vessels are among the earliest specialised tissues to appear in the embryo, whose body they connect with the yolk sac; these delicate red structures can be clearly made out when the embryo is barely visible. The main arteries and veins form later from a primitive capillary network, with an axial artery and two marginal veins [66], which are connected not only by the capillaries but also by some larger anastomotic channels. Both types of vessel may persist as congenital arteriovenous fistulae of various sizes and distribution. Lymphatics are sometimes involved. Most are first noticed in childhood or early adult life. They are commoner than the acquired type, except in wartime.

Clinical Types and Their Treatment

1. *Diffuse* vascular overgrowth (Fig. 16.3) affecting a part or the whole of a limb with swelling, superficial

varicosities and haemangiomata [57], increased heat and over-development of bones and muscles, is the common presentation; though some areas may appear to be worse affected there is no clear division into normal and abnormal. Yet, with the striking appearance of the limb there is little evidence of significant haemodynamic shunting (a bruit was present in only just over a third of one surgical series [57]; cardiac effects are uncommon, and usually the pulse rate is not slowed by compressing the artery at the limb root. Local vascular complications do occur, however, from venous insufficiency, thrombosis, and varicose erosion of overlying skin (Fig. 16.4), and in such patients a certain limited success may follow cautious local surgery, though haemorrhage may be troublesome and healing slow. Diathermy cauterisation is sometimes effective. It is better to regard most of these patients as inoperable

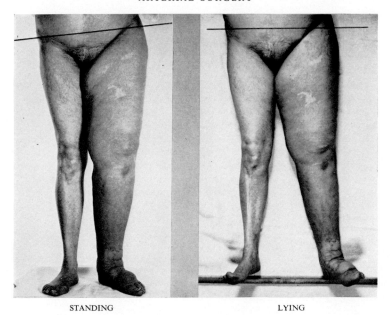

STANDING   LYING

Fig. 16.3. Congenital diffuse arteriovenous malformation of the left hind-quarter showing lengthening, lymphoedema, and haemangioma of most of the skin area. There is usually no bruit in this type of case.

in spite of the pleas of the parents. Simple support is the only effective conservative treatment. Later, in the worst cases, amputation may be an acceptable alternative to pain, disfigurement, sepsis or haemorrhage.

2. *Localised aneurysmal varices* are less common but very characteristic, often affecting the knee region (Fig. 16.5), the foot or the hand (Fig. 16.6) and sometimes the neck. They are often softly pulsatile and are always hot. Tenderness is common. The lesion may be confined to a single muscle, e.g. the deltoid (Fig. 16.7) [59] or the gastrocnemius [67]. The bunch of distended veins can be excised *en masse*, and if there is an arterial feeding channel, possibly suspected clinically because of the presence of a localised bruit or thrill, and then demonstrable angiographically, it too should be dissected out and ligated. This type of operation gives good relief of local disfigurement and discomfort (which may often amount to throbbing pain). In the hand and foot such an operation is more difficult; damage may be done to the function of the extremity; furthermore, recurrence is almost inevitable.

Very occasionally there may be massive shunting within a localised congenital arteriovenous lesion (Fig. 16.8), with severe and increasing cardiac strain. Radical surgery can sometimes be achieved with full correction of the haemodynamic effects.

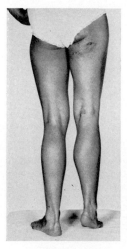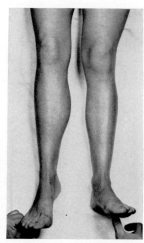

STANDING   LYING

Fig. 16.4. Complications of congenital arteriovenous fistula, in a girl aged nineteen.

On the left, there are the scars of past ulceration of superficial varicosities of the right buttock and popliteal fossa.

Both views show calf swelling and equinus deformity due to a severe recent thrombo-phlebitis in the lower half of the limb.

336

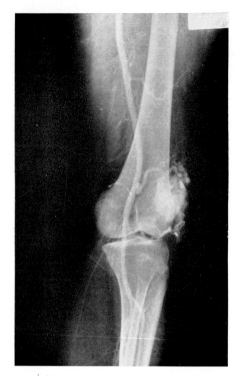
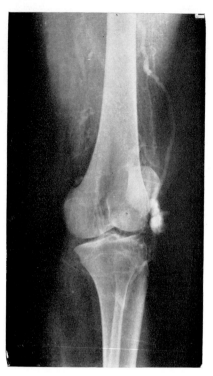

Fig. 16.5. Locally conspicuous aneurysmal varices in a young woman with vascular malformation throughout the left lower limb. Lengthening and moderate hypertrophy of the limb did not trouble her, but pain in the hot, pulsating varicose veins on the antero-lateral aspect of her knee responded well to excision of this clump with ligation of the two large feeding arteries, and of the draining vein on the side of the thigh. Local heat, pulsation and bruit establish the clinical diagnosis in this common type of case (*see also* Fig. 16.15).

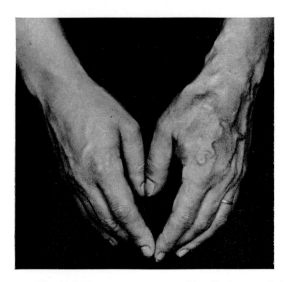
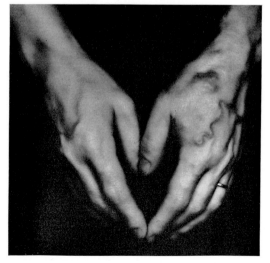

Fig. 16.6. The commonest type of localised congenital arteriovenous fistula. Usually symptomless, except for the large, disfiguring veins. Bruit present over the prominent clump at the base of the first interosseous space (infra-red photograph on right).

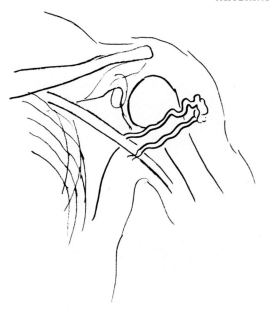

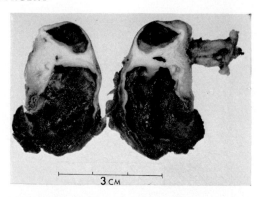

(b) Locally excised specimen with feeding vascular pedicle (there were no other connections). Cause of pain and increased swelling shown on section to be thrombosis in the large blood spaces obstructing the venous outflow and spreading along it.

Fig. 16.7. Monomuscular arteriovenous fistula.

This case closely resembles one of those reported by Tice *et al.* [59]. Venous complications are common in all types of arteriovenous fistula.

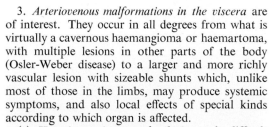

(a) Drawing from the subclavian arteriogram of a school-mistress aged forty-seven who had noticed a tender, walnut-sized pulsating lump in the muscle for some months previously.

3. *Arteriovenous malformations in the viscera* are of interest. They occur in all degrees from what is virtually a cavernous haemangioma or haemartoma, with multiple lesions in other parts of the body (Osler-Weber disease) to a larger and more richly vascular lesion with sizeable shunts which, unlike most of those in the limbs, may produce systemic symptoms, and also local effects of special kinds according to which organ is affected.

(a) *Hepatic arteriovenous dysplasia* may be difficult to distinguish from an acquired lesion of non-traumatic origin when they present with unexplained haematemesis in middle-age due to bleeding gastro-oesophageal varices. Hepatic lobectomy is curative for the lesion that is confined to one lobe [39].

(b) *Pulmonary lesions* produce polycythaemia, finger clubbing, and cyanosis, though these may be late in appearing, or occasionally absent altogether [31]. Many cases have been described [15A, 68] some with complications including infection, haemorrhage, heart failure and stroke, justifying surgical treatment by excision, lobectomy, or even pneumonectomy. The lower lobes are most often affected, and the condition is often bilateral [68].

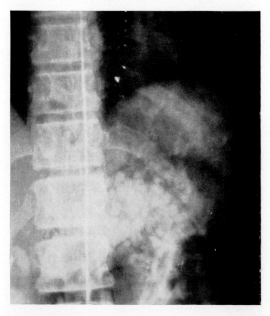

Fig. 16.8. Massive congenital intercostal arteriovenous fistula in a girl aged seventeen whose cardiac condition was still normal ten years after ligation of seven feeding intercostals at their aortic origin, and block resection of the four intercostal spaces and overlying fascia. Before operation the cardiac output was 11 litres/min.

Acquired Arteriovenous Fistula

Here the artery and vein have been opened into one another by some mechanical incident, usually an injury or operation, but sometimes from disease. Although more than two vessels may be involved the fistula is almost always single, and can, therefore, in most cases, be located and closed surgically.

Surgical Anatomy

The terms varicose aneurysm and aneurysmal varix, though archaic and somewhat confusing in their similarity, still serve a useful purpose in distinguishing between the two common anatomical types of acquired arteriovenous fistula (Fig. 16.9) (*see also*

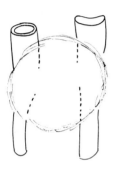
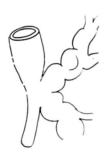

Fig. 16.9. Arteriovenous fistula with sac (varicose aneurysm); and without (aneurysmal varix).

p. 345). This was realised by William Hunter who, in his original description in 1761 [47], not only observed the palpable vascular thrill but also showed that a direct communication produces a pulsating (aneurysmal) varix or varices as its main clinical feature, while a less intimate union, through a passage in the tissues, lacking support of the vessel walls over this distance, will in time expand and dissect among the tissues of the part as though it were a false aneurysm of purely arterial origin. Such a swelling may properly be termed a varicose aneurysm, for it is as a distending pulsatile mass that it presents clinically (Fig. 16.10), and its arteriovenous features may be of only secondary importance, yet the typical, continuous bruit is always present when the swelling is auscultated. This test accurately distinguishes between a false aneurysm with a fistula, and a traumatic aneurysm without one; in the latter, any murmur present will be limited to systole, and localised to the sac.

Arteriography shows clearly whether the lesion

is a false aneurysm, or a varicose aneurysm, or aneurysmal varix.

Systemic cardiovascular effects and complications cannot be depended upon as clinical evidence of arteriovenous fistula in these rapidly expanding cases, for there may not have been time for them to establish themselves. The bradycardia phenomenon may be absent, unless the fistula is large, and in this event there is usually no large false sac, though there are exceptions (Fig. 16.10). In slower cases there

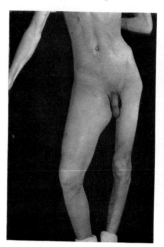
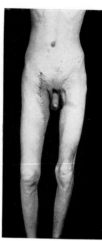

Fig. 16.10. Large arteriovenous aneurysm with false sac containing almost three pints of clot. A good example of the apprentice butcher injury. This youth of nineteen was ill, febrile and grossly anaemic on admission. After excision and repair of the fistula, his condition at once improved, as shown in the early postoperative picture on the right. (Professor Rob's case.)

may be calcification or even bone formation. The fistula may be double [49].

Causes

Anything that destroys the tissue barrier between artery and vein will set up a fistula.

Penetrating injury by knife, bullet, shell fragment, glass splinter, fractured bone end, and surgical instruments, biopsy and arteriography needles; bone screws and nails, as well as certain deep forceful manipulations between bones and ligaments, such as attempts to secure the posterior end of a semilunar cartilage, or to remove a lumbar intervertebral disc: quite a small injury by any of these, if it passes between the artery and the vein, is very likely to open up a fistula. With much soft tissue damage there

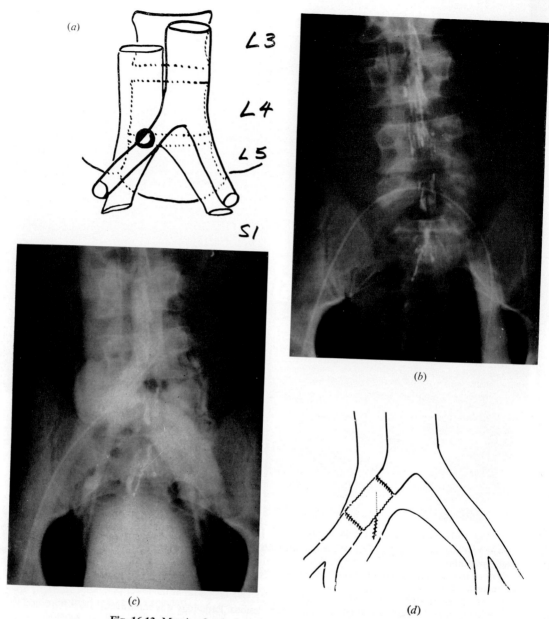

Fig. 16.13. Massive fistula from injury at intervertebral disc operation.

(*a*) The commonest site for this injury is on the right side of the L.4/5 intervertebral space.

(*b*) A right transfemoral catheter has passed through the fistula and down into the left ilio-femoral vein. Note: myodil remnants.

(*c*) Withdrawal of the catheter and advancement to the aortic bifurcation shows the huge distension of the left common iliac vein and vena cava, and the early formation of a moderate sized false sac.

(*d*) Repair of venous defect by simple suture. Dacron graft replacement required for artery, because of tension and loss of part of the posterior wall at the time of injury.

This patient's laminectomy operation was uneventful. It was performed by a most experienced neurosurgeon who recognised the complication when, on the fifth postoperative day, the patient, a man of twenty-six, developed shortness of breath and swelling of the lower limbs. The abdomen was auscultated and the characteristic bruit was heard. The fistula was successfully repaired on the tenth postoperative day by the method shown.

common iliac arteries are locally intimately related to the anterior surface of these great, thin-walled veins, the force needed to cause this injury may not have to be great.

In 15 out of 30 collected cases [38] the fistula involved the right common iliac artery and either of the iliac veins or their junction at the vena cava, most typically the site is the contact area between the right common iliac artery and the left common iliac vein, which, as experience in aorto-iliac reconstruction and of the iliac compression syndrome [7] has shown, is sometimes abnormally 'tight' and fixed.

If the injury is through the third and fourth interspace, the fistula will be aorto-caval.

From the time of injury to re-exploration averaged seventeen months in the reported cases [5]. The earliest was at three days [60c] and the longest interval was eight years [58].

Clinically these patients present in one of the following ways:

1. Early heart failure, with a large fistula or in a frail patient, may be the occasion for full systemic examination during the postoperative period, when the bruit should be detected. This test should, in future, become routine in any patient who is not doing well.

2. Swelling of the lower limbs, especially the left, sometimes with dilated subcutaneous veins; and often wrongly diagnosed as deep venous thrombosis; the veins though insufficient are still patent. Reduced ankle pulsations on the same side as the iliac arterial opening may be obscured by oedema, but detectable by oscillometry. Patients may go on for months or years in this state until—

3. Late congestive heart failure again leads to suspicion of a major cardiovascular cause, and the full re-examination which then takes place reveals the fistula through its murmur and typical accompaniment of high output signs with failure. Even so, mistakes may still occur: the blame may be placed on another cause, such as a non-existent patent ductus arteriosus [5].

Note on the Technique of Repairing this Fistula

A generous supply of ready-matched blood, and a long abdominal incision, and good exposure are essential. The paramedian incision should be made on the affected side. In an early case, the thin-walled lumbar veins and their small tributaries are dangerously tense with full aortic pressure; great care must be taken not to injure them in isolating the aorta and iliac arteries. Later, the risk is still present but is less because of secondary thickening of the veins near the fistula.

To expose the fistulous opening it is usually necessary to divide either the affected common iliac artery (Fig. 16.13*d*) or the internal iliac [5].

Taylor's method [58] of controlling venous haemorrhage from the caval opening is valuable in early or late cases. A Foley's catheter is inserted and the small balloon is inflated: gentle traction then seals the opening. In an early case the vein wall is oedematous and friable and difficult to suture with arterial silk: however, a 2/0 atraumatic catgut suture, taking larger bites and including perivenous soft tissues, is effective, and when the artery is restored its pressure helps to secure the repair.

A defect in the posterior arterial wall, due to loss of a 'bite' with the rongeurs, plus the tension along the divided common iliac will mean that end-to-end anastomosis of the artery will not be possible, the alternatives being replacement grafting with a cloth prosthesis or, failing this, quadruple ligation, which proved successful in the first case of operative cure by Linton and White in 1945 [32], and in subsequent cases [5]. With a well-developed collateral system from the effects of the fistula the effects of loss of the common iliac artery were less severe than they would have been from isolated injury or ligation.

INTRACAVAL RUPTURE OF AN ABDOMINAL AORTIC ANEURYSM

The area between the two great vessels being, as a rule, densely adherent, if rupture should occur within it an aorto-caval fistula is established. Massive shift of aneurysmal thrombus into the cava may cause a fatal pulmonary embolism [23]. A smaller leak will show the same features as the disc operation injury described above, while if there is also extravasation, this may bring the patient to an emergency operation at which the fistula is discovered as a secondary feature [1, 23]. This was so in 4 out of 140 patients seen at Houston, Texas, with leaking abdominal aneurysm [1].

Small-bore gunshot wounding may establish a fistula with or without a false sac [40].

Neoplastic erosion between the aorta and cava can produce a large fistula with an acutely progressive picture of venous insufficiency of the lower limbs and haemodynamic evidence of heart strain. Cure of the vascular complication is reported after resection and bifurcation aortic grafting, and simple linear suture of the vena cava [9].

RENAL ARTERIOVENOUS FISTULA

At least sixty cases are recorded [4, 60a], and apart from expected causes such as nephrectomy by mass ligation [69], and stabbing injury, there are now many cases following needle biopsy [60, 60a]. Renal neoplasms [4] appear to be specially liable to this spontaneous complication which occurs not in the main body of the tumour but in the enlarged and complex vascular pedicle in the renal hilus: tumour invasion of the vein may cause secondary rupture into the adjacent artery [27]. Hypernephroma metastasis may also develop arteriovenous fistula (Fig. 16.12) [67].

Many patients are hypertensive; this may be relieved by removal of the fistula [37]. Loss of pulse pressure, and reduced blood flow beyond the fistula would explain this phenomenon and its surgical cure.

SYSTEMIC-PORTAL FISTULAE [56]
These are uncommon; hepatic and splenic are about equal in incidence, while superior mesenteric is the rarest. They may be erosive, following sepsis in abdominal operations, especially resections such as in gastrectomy, or for Crohn's disease or mesenteric thrombosis; or from stabbing or small-bore gunshot wounding, or from rupture of an arteriosclerotic aneurysm into the accompanying vein; this was the apparent cause of most splenic cases.

Hepatic-portal Fistula
Acquired fistula in this site is less common than congenital from the very nature of the two causes: the complex, slow evolution in utero of the two vascular systems of the liver (as in the lung) must afford free opportunity for connections to persist and compensation for them to take place, whereas upper abdominal injury of the violence required to set up such a deep vascular communication will be likely to prove fatal at the time of injury.

Penetrating or blunt liver injury have both been blamed [55B]. Although these fistulae were large, central haemodynamic changes were not marked, perhaps from interposition of vascular bed of the liver between the fistula and the vena cava [10, 42]. Local changes, however, may be well marked. Large varicose collaterals develop not only in the lower oesophagus and stomach, but also in the duodenum, and in both situations cause severe bright red bleeding.

Ascites, as in cirrhosis, should not occur from portal hypertension alone. Its presence here would suggest either that phlebitis had developed or that liver function or hepatic venous drainage was affected.

In the absence of a known injury the origin of such a fistula may be obscure. A single fistula suggests that it is of the acquired type, though solitary connection between the right hepatic artery and the vena cava [39], and also of the common hepatic to the portal vein [34] have both been described as congenital, and were successfully ligated. Three traumatic cases have been reported [10].

Splenic Arteriovenous Fistulae
These cause splenomegaly and portal hypertension, and like other splenic arterial lesions are commoner in women. They show clearly at aortography and should be cured by splenectomy to include the lesion [28].

Fistula of the Superior Mesenteric Vessels [60B]
If injured near their origin, where some local support may confine the damage and direct the blood loss into the vein, survival is possible and repair may succeed [56]. Auscultation of any injured abdomen should be routine, and so the diagnosis should be possible for the surgeon who is accustomed to listening for arterial as well as for intestinal sounds. As in the case of hepatic-portal fistula, if the patient survives, there will be portal hypertension, with oesophageal, duodenal or even jejunal varices, any of which may bleed. (*See also* Instructive Case, p. 349.)

Peripheral Arteriovenous Fistulae

The long, exposed course of the limb vessels and their closely packed surroundings favour non-lethal injury, which when the early swelling and extravasation have subsided may be found to have set up an arteriovenous fistula. In the distal part of the extremity this may be a small, inconspicuous lesion (aneurysmal varix), perhaps symptomless for many years (Fig. 16.14), but in the limb root where the vessels are larger and the surrounding tissues looser; with room for a more extensive spread of initial damage (*see* Fig. 16.10), a fistula will be more often complicated by early expanding false aneurysm (varicose), and the opening itself is often large.

Diagnosis
Auscultation is the essential step in diagnosis, whether the lesion is small, peripheral, and inconspicuous, perhaps presenting late as a case of deep venous insufficiency or simply as varicose veins; or in the more dramatic, early cases with much soft tissue swelling. Both types then, have misleading features which, on inspection and palpation, are easily misdiagnosed, yet both will be instantly recognisable when the roaring bruit is heard.

This may be of considerable practical importance, for with early repair there are fewer difficulties over separation or repair of nearby structures, particularly

Typical Peripheral Fistulae

1. *Lower Limb*

Vessels	Cause	Type of fistula
Superior gluteal [10]	Intramedullary rod to femur	Direct
Common femoral (Fig. 16.10)	Butcher injury	With false sac
Profunda femoris [67] or both [10]	Osteotomy	With false sac
	Screws	
	Gunshot	
Superficial femoral	Fractured femoral shaft, therapeutic limb lengthening	Small direct communication
Popliteal [51]	Meniscus operation. Therapeutic, for severe ischaemia	Often a false sac; short, direct communication
Tibials	Fractured shaft	Aneurysmal varix
Plantar (Figs 16.14, 16.15)	Crush injury	Aneurysmal varix

2. *Upper limb*

Axillary	Knife stab Glass splinter	False sac. Serious disability common
Brachial [67]	Venepuncture (the classical phlebotomy injury)	Aneurysmal varix
Radial [6]	Therapeutic, for dialysis	Aneurysmal varix

3. *In the neck*

Innominate-caval [10]	Missile fragment or small-bore bullet	Either type
Carotids [67]		
Vertebral [15]	Stabbing or arteriography	Aneurysmal varix
Superior thyroid	Surgical ligature	Aneurysmal varix

4. *In the head*

Carotid-cavernous [17, 48]	Fractured skull Ruptured aneurysm	Aneurysmal varix (with pulsating exophthalmos)
Middle meningeal [65]	Fractured skull	Aneurysmal varix
Scalp (Usually temporal) [43]	Direct blow	Aneurysmal varix (cirsoid means varicose)

5. *In the chest wall*

Internal mammary	Knife stab	Aneurysmal varix
Intercostals [33]	Paracentesis	

nerves, and not the least important, the main vein itself.

Auscultation also localises the site of the fistula, often better than arteriography does.

Arteriography, however, should not be omitted, for it should show the size and position of the fistula and of any false sac or foreign body, and the anatomical relationships of these to the large arterial branches in the region of the opening.

Just as the bruit is the cardinal clinical sign, so arteriographically are conspicuous early venous filling and dilatation of the artery and vein (Fig. 16.15). Distal venous reflux occurs only as far as the next competent valves. There may be evidence of retrograde arterial flow back into the fistula.

Spontaneous Closure

Not all cases require operation. Spontaneous cure [55], for no apparent reason, is sufficiently common (5 per cent in Makins's large case series) [35] to encourage a conservative policy for small, peripheral fistulae without local complications. It has been reported following arteriography [48, 67] and after deep thrombophlebitis after abdominal operation [51] where it seems clear that the fistula becomes occluded from its venous side, the vessel being already damaged by chronic mechanical strain, the haematological changes of the postoperative response then combine to seal the outflow. In the same way, a thrombophlebitis in quite another part of the body (e.g. in varicose veins) may stimulate intravascular thrombosis in the vein draining a fistula [46]. Experimentally, in dogs with prepared popliteal arteriovenous fistulae, these mostly showed late spontaneous closure after obstruction of the draining vein by ligation [52].

Indications for Operations for Arteriovenous Fistula

Apart from the hope of spontaneous cure there is another basis for expectant management: there may never be any complications; in fact, the smaller and more peripheral fistulae, especially aneurysmal varices, are compatible with survival into old age. Positive indications include:

1. Expanding false sac.
2. Severe venous insufficiency.
3. Cardiac failure.
4. Rarely, ischaemic gangrene.
5. The development of endocarditis, endarteritis or septicaemia.
6. Patient distressed by head or neck bruit.
7. Cerebrovascular steal [28A, 52A].

Timing of Operation

Experience in two World Wars led to a policy of delay which had the following merits:

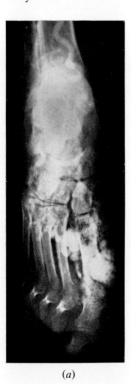 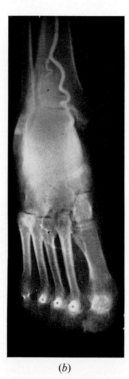

(a)   (b)

Fig. 16.14.

(a) Traumatic fistula in a man aged forty-seven whose right foot had been trodden on by a horse forty years before. Loud localised bruit and dilatation of feeding arteries, and of draining veins.

(b) Postoperative arteriogram shows satisfactory result of local block excision under tourniquet control.

(a) Conditions in the field and along the evacuation line were unfavourable for early operation and transport of these men.

(b) The risk of acute ischaemia, either from the injury itself or as a result of early arterial surgery, became less with the passing of the first few weeks after wounding.

(c) Healing and consolidation of the wound with a well-established collateral circulation offered better material for exacting surgical work than the early, damaged, and doubtfully viable tissues of a war wound.

These are important considerations which should still be given full attention [13, 14, 54], and with a large number of other casualties requiring attention the delayed method would be the only one possible.

Yet, in modern civilian hospital practice or under the special operational conditions of restricted warfare with rapid evacuation, a patient with arteriovenous fistula should be received soon after injury at a vascular unit where it should be possible to undertake the immediate primary repair of the lesion. The merits of this were established during the Korean campaign (*see* Chapter 13, p. 236), for purely arterial wounds, and some fistulae, were also closed early. Among 50 cases received into Houston, Texas, hospitals during the 'transition years' between 1947 and 1962 [2], 8 patients were recognised early, or with bleeding, or with ischaemic complications, and were operated upon at once, with good results that have now established this as the routine method of choice at this centre; 17 were operated on within the first two weeks, when the initial inflammatory reaction had subsided, while most of the remainder were either seen late or had quadruple ligation (*see* p. 349) or both.

In summary:

1. *Early Operation Essential*

   False sac with local pressure effects and general deterioration from anaemia, fever or wasting.

   Aorto-caval or other very large fistula with incipient heart failure.

2. *Early Operation Desirable*

   Any favourable acute case where facilities and experience permit. Most centrally situated fistulae.

   Associated nerve, tendon or other potentially disabling limb damage.

   Retained and possibly dangerous foreign body.

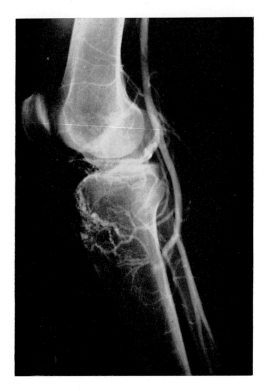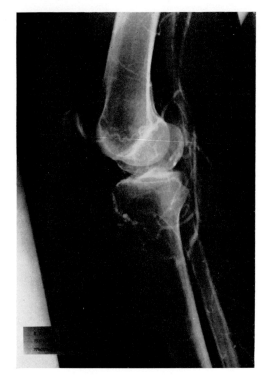

Fig. 16.15. Congenital a/v malformation of the knee showing aneurysmal varices and early venous filling. (Wing Cdr. T. R. Beatson's case.)

3. *Observation*

Small or moderate-sized fistulae with direct communication.

Injuries of more importance affecting other parts.

4. *Late Operation*

Mainly for missed cases, and some from group 3 above.

Severe late complications as listed on page 346.

Technique

General dissection procedure and haemostasis.
Identification of the fistula.
Methods of dealing with the fistula.

The operative cure of these lesions is one of the most exacting in the whole of vascular surgery. Neither the acute nor late cases should be undertaken by those without special training or experience in this work. The tradition of transferring such cases is wise and well established.

RECOMMENDED METHODS

Haemostasis must be carefully preserved, otherwise many large vessels will be opened and control of the dissection will be lost. Dangerous increasing haemorrhage is then likely in situations such as the limb-root.

Two methods of control are practised:

(*a*) *Tourniquet* application where the fistula is sufficiently far down the limb to allow the whole operative field to be kept clear for skin preparation and any necessary proximal extension of the dissection. In general, it is true that modern techniques in vascular surgery should make use of the observation and negotiation of haemodynamic conditions in the blood vessels of the region, and that wherever large, reconstructable vessels are concerned, the completely bloodless field produced by the tourniquet is out of favour. In the hand or foot the method is ideal.

(*b*) *Proximal arterial clamping* through a separate incision, e.g. the subclavian or external iliac. A more distal lesion can be approached direct, with a pneumatic tourniquet in position but not inflated, and the main artery may be isolated and taped, ready for clamping, through the same incision as when extended downwards will expose the fistula region.

Although ample blood should be ready-matched, and loss measured by swab weighing, replacement should be avoided in these subjects whose blood volume is abnormally high, and whose heart is in many cases under strain.

Exposure must be generous, for as A. K. Henry said [18], 'in the dissection of the main arteries a long incision needs no defence'. His intermuscular planes can often be used to gain access both to the main artery proximally and to the part involved in the fistula.

Dissection must be deliberate, with sharp division of the tissues, which is preferable to blunt separation, which may open up large, irregular, and profusely bleeding defects in major branches or the thin-walled main vessel itself. Gentle stroking of the perivascular tissues is permissible once the vessel has been defined, isolated, and lifted up.

All vessels must be finely ligated and divided as they enter or leave the suspected fistula region. The main feeding artery and draining vein are to be fully exposed as close as possible to the block of tissue containing the fistula, after which they, too, will be either ligated with stout catgut, which is preferable to non-absorbable material; or clamped, if the vessels are to be reconstructed. Care should be taken not to include nearby structures such as nerves or tendons. In peripheral cases with a tourniquet in use, this should always be released and haemostasis be completed before closing the wound.

Heparin should not be given unless at the conclusion of the dissection stage, with the arterial clamps applied, it is evident that the distal circulation is poor, or that the reconstruction phase may take some considerable time.

Identification of the Fistula

Careful preoperative assessment by auscultation for the point of maximum bruit, confirmed by the demonstration of the bradycardia effect on compressing this; also study of the arteriograms and of the radiological anatomy of any bone injury or retained foreign body; all these should prepare the surgeon for what he is to find at operation.

Early in the operation, before the main artery has been clamped, the intensity of the fistulous thrill is the best guide to its location. A finger-tip is placed at successive points along the pulsating artery, compressing it fully, and the test repeated until a point is reached where this localised pressure not only

reduces the thrill but stops it completely. This is the site of the fistula.

Later, after clamping the artery and when the thrill has disappeared, the main vein, now soft and more or less collapsed, is compressed so as to empty it. If it refills quickly the fistula is still open.

In case of real difficulty with an inaccessible and uncontrollable fistula, e.g. high in the neck, the method of Reid and McGuire [49] may be effective: the vein is divided and twisted on its axis. The leak is turned off like a tap.

Taylor's method of balloon catheter occlusion of a large opening [58] may be adapted to these smaller peripheral fistulae by using Fogarty's balloon embolectomy catheter in the same way [28A], passed from a distance.

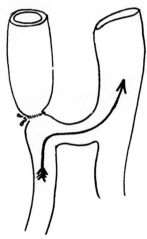

Fig. 16.16. Arterial ligation above the fistula may be followed by severe limb ischaemia, for the entire collateral flow passes back through the low resistance of the fistula and its wide draining vein.

Ligation Operations

These are less used today. The essential preliminaries of dissection and control of the main vessels, and isolating the fistula, which make up the most exacting part of such operations, are essentially the same for the reconstructive procedures which, therefore, have come largely to replace the older methods, except in special situations where working space is insufficient to allow the manipulations of clamping and vascular suture, e.g. in the deeper regions of the neck or pelvis.

Proximal ligation of the feeding artery should never be used. Though simple in prospect to an inexperienced operator, and seeming to control the rush of blood through the fistula, appearing safe in a limb manifestly well supplied with blood, nothing could be more wrong, for as Fig. 16.16 shows, the effect of

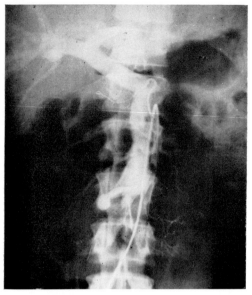 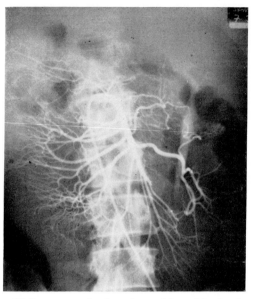

(a) Preoperative selective superior mesenteric arteriogram showing fistula into portal system, and poor filling of small bowel supply.

(b) Repeat examination after excision of the fistula. All branches now fill.

Superior Mesenteric Arteriovenous Fistula

(Mr J. E. Mitchell's and the author's case)

A steel worker aged 30 was caught in a machine which crushed him between itself and the floor. He sustained fractured ribs and pelvis and showed signs of abdominal injury for which he underwent a laparotomy at which a ruptured spleen was removed. Multiple intestinal contusions were noticed and one bowel laceration required suturing. A month later, he presented the picture of acute intestinal obstruction and was again explored: three feet of gangrenous small gut were resected and he made a good recovery, but continued to have bowel trouble in the form of persistent diarrhoea up to nine times a day. However, his general health improved, and he ate normally.

On examination he was found to have a fairly loud continuous full-cycle bruit, typical of arteriovenous fistula, chiefly in the central abdomen, but seemingly conducted up and to the right. With a clinical diagnosis of mesenteric fistula, he was referred for further investigation. Schilling and xylose absorption tests indicated a reduction in small bowel function but fat excretion was normal. Barium swallow showed no oesophageal varices. Selective superior mesenteric arteriography by Dr David Sutton showed a fistula into the portal system (a), a small varicose aneurysm, and poor filling of the mesenteric arterial branches. Transfemoral catheterisation of the hepatic vein showed the wedged pressure to be normal. The oxygen saturation, however, was raised.

Exploration confirmed the presence of a fistula in the middle course of the mesenteric vessels, and a small sac. The feeding artery and draining vein were ligated, and the fistula was excised once it had been confirmed that the distal mesenteric arterial pulses were not affected by the clamping of the base of the lesion. Postoperative arteriography (b) showed a return to normal, except for the stump of the feeding artery (the lower part of the main mesenteric axis).

Comment. This fistula may have been caused either by the initial accident or by the necessary ligation of the mesenteric vessels during the small bowel resection. In the few cases that have been recorded both causes have been described [60B]. In this case, both possibilities were present.

proximal ligation alone is to shunt blood from the remaining patent distal arterial tree back through the fistula.

An exception to this good rule is the intracranial carotid cavernous fistula whose known propensity to spontaneous thrombosis [48] is encouraged in this way, though some cases of hemiplegia may have been due to leak-back rather than to thrombotic ischaemia.

Occlusion by muscle embolus is an ingenious method used by neurosurgeons for the closure of this type of fistula. The cervical carotid is exposed, and a piece of muscle of carefully chosen size is inserted, either free, or on a long fine thread, and is allowed to pass upwards with the blood stream to lodge in the fistulous opening [17, 62].

QUADRUPLE LIGATION

This reliable and well-tried operation gives good results in young subjects in whom it may be followed by an early recovery of distal pulses even in lesions as high as the iliac region [32] and with either mild claudication or none. None of Elkin's 338 cases went on to gangrene [14].

Four ligatures, or more if necessary, are applied as shown in Fig. 16.17 as closely as possible to the

fistula so that no branches remain to sustain it. Complete obliteration is then assured with full relief of venous and cardiac insufficiency and of any local pressure effects from a false sac, which then quickly closes off and heals.

A good modern indication for quadruple ligation is in the control of a large fistula in an amputation stump (Fig. 16.1), also for the cure of most peripheral fistulae situated in the hand or foot, forearm or calf, though with these it may be just as simple to excise the lesion *en bloc* (Fig. 16.14).

Repair of the Fistula with Preservation of the Vessels (Figs 16.18, 16.19)

The fistulous track may be long enough to be doubly ligated and divided, or if shorter may, like some cases of patent ductus, require suture of the two openings.

If the artery and the vein are in direct contact, the opening may be closed by transvenous suture through the large varix which lies over the opening (Fig. 16.18*b*).

Matas's principle (*see* Chapter 15, p. 285) may be used similarly for the intraluminal closure of a fistula with a false sac (*see* Fig. 15.12); this consolidates the separate suture of the openings: if the sac alone is sutured, an arterial aneurysm may later develop.

Reconstruction of the Artery (with suture of the vein) (Fig. 16.19)

This is the modern operation of preference in all cases where the proximal part of the main artery is involved, and when no simple repair is possible.

The arterial defect is almost always short, so that there is seldom any difficulty in restoring arterial continuity. End-to-end anastomosis is more often possible in a limb artery (Fig. 16.19*a*) that has more laxity along its axis, than in the larger, tighter, more central vessel in which, also, the size of the defect contributes to the greater tension. Here a dacron graft is ideal for its durability and good late patency in this situation of high blood flow (*see* Figs 16.13*c*, 16.19*b*). If a graft is needed to replace the defect in a limb artery, a saphenous vein segment is preferable [24].

It is most important to attempt to reconstruct the vein concerned in the fistula. It should be possible to do this with a simple lateral suture in most instances because the vein is already grossly enlarged at this point. As would be expected from the previous phase of venous hypertension, incompetence, and other structural damage, it was found in a late study of cases from the Korean war that swelling and varicosity in the affected limb appeared to be due to venous ligation.

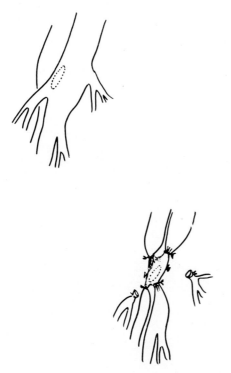

Fig. 16.17. Quadruple ligation.

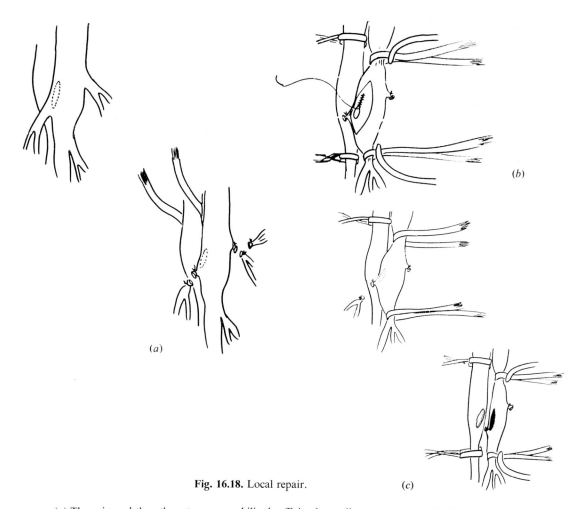

Fig. 16.18. Local repair.

(a) The vein and then the artery are mobilised sufficiently to allow temporary occlusion.

(b) Transvenous suture of the opening. Repair of the vein may not succeed after this operation, but it should be attempted.

(c) A more complete dissection is required if both vessels are to be repaired.

Recurrent or Persistent Fistula after Attempted Operative Cure

Reasons for this may be:

1. incomplete operation, failing to define all branches near the fistula;
2. giving way of a transvenous suture of the opening;
3. stretching of an endo-aneurysmorrhaphy;
4. the presence of a second fistula from the same injury (e.g. the profunda as well as the femoral vessels).

Reoperation, though difficult, should resolve the problem [2].

351

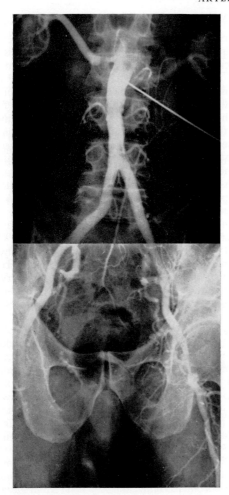

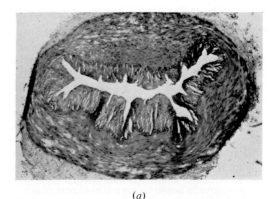

(a)

(b)

Fig. 17.1. Arteriosclerotic stenosis of the right renal artery. Discovered incidentally during translumbar aortography in a man aged sixty for high type claudication of the left lower limb. Stenosis of the left common femoral and of both internal iliacs is also shown.

Fig. 17.2. (a) Fibromuscular hypertrophy. Section (× 40) of the gastroepiploic artery in a thirty-eight-year-old woman with symptoms of mesenteric insufficiency. (b) Extensive beading of both renal arteries also present, but without hypertension.

complications (*see* Chapter 15, p. 287). The same hazards apply to cases of dissecting aneurysm with renal encroachment [49].

Fibromuscular Hyperplasia [45A]

This distal, beaded type of distortion of the renal artery (Fig. 17.2b) would be easily missed at routine autopsy examination. Yet, even when contrast injection and X-ray studies were carried out, admittedly in a mostly normotensive sample, no cases were seen [62]. Though a clinical case had been reported years before [83], the advent of fibro-muscular hyperplasia as a renal arterial lesion coincided with the application of aortography to the investigation of hypertension, and though it was not long before this radiological lesion was surgically explored [118, 170] it now accounts for between 13 and 40 per cent of operations for renal artery stenosis [111, 124, 154A]. Histological examination shows that the arterial lumen is greatly reduced by thickening of the medial coat composed of hypertrophied normal elements (Fig. 17.2a). Post-stenotic dilatation nearly always follows beyond the narrowed portion, and the process is often multiple. The common, medial type is usually non-progressive. Tight stenosis may however develop in the intimal and sub-adventitial forms [154A].

Nearly all patients are women of child-bearing age, though the first reported case [83] and others [105] were in quite young children. The condition may be inherited. Like arteriosclerotic stenosis, it can exist without hypertension (Fig. 17.2).

The ultimate prognosis of fibromuscular hypertrophy and the frequency of extra-renal lesions are not yet established.

Arteritis (Fig. 17.3)

Hypertension is common late in the course of most forms of this broad group of diseases (*see* Chapter 7).

3. *A renal transplant* may develop arterial narrowing, either at the anastomosis, or beyond it, with the production of a bruit and rising blood pressure [148A].

Other Multiple, Diffuse or Obscure Lesions

Experimentally, the injection of microspheres (dia. 30–170 μ) into the renal artery can cause a sustained rise in blood pressure within three days. Though many nephrons are undamaged, the urine may be similar to that secreted by a pyelonephritic kidney [84].

Some cases of pyelonephritic hypertension appear to have just such a vascular basis [70], for microscopy

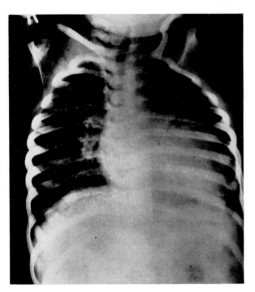 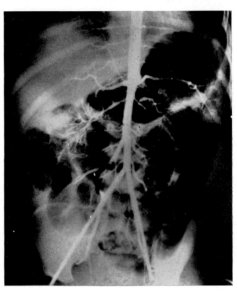

Fig. 17.3. Stenosis of both renal arteries with severe hypertension in a 2½-year-old girl. A probable case of female arteritis. (Dr A. P. Norman's case.)

Renal ischaemia is due either to large or to small arterial lesions:

1. *Aortic arch syndrome* (young female arteritis) with narrowed or occluded branches of the aortic arch may extend into the thoraco-abdominal aorta and one or both renals, causing hypertension [18, 147, 153], which tends to be obscured by the fact that the brachial pressure readings are low.

2. *Diffuse collagen disease* with small intrarenal arterial defects may cause obvious macroscopic patchy infarction, as in polyarteritis nodosa, or with rheumatoid endarteritis (*see* Chapter 7, p. 139), or a more widespread, even damage with failure of excretory function in which hypertension is only a secondary feature of the illness.

shows partial infarcts [121], though clearly, a local infective process can have the same effect as is seen in the 5 per cent or so cases of renal tuberculosis that develop hypertension [74].

Other diffuse damage causing hypertension, probably through ischaemia, includes: diabetic nephropathy, X-irradiation and amyloid disease. A few cases of hydronephrosis develop hypertension.

The important lesson to be drawn from all these examples is that multiple intrarenal ischaemic lesions may be commoner in clinical practice than has been realised, and that the growing concept of parenchymal ischaemia as a result of small arterial lesions should be given full consideration when considering the problem of a hypertensive patient with major arterial disease in the aorto-renal region. Not the least significant possibility may be the occurrence of many secondary arterial occlusions from emboli derived from loose arteriosclerotic debris on the surface of the large proximal artery, as is known to happen in carotid, subclavian, and aortic disease. Pain in the loin and haematuria in such patients may lead to the diagnosis of pyelonephritis.

Clinical Recognition of Renal Artery Disease as the Cause of Hypertension

Mild to moderate stenosis is so common after middle age [62, 135] that there is a tendency to blame it for hypertension of any degree in all patients in whom aortography has shown the lesion to be present. Secondary evidence of structural change and disturbed function in the affected kidney is essential to the diagnosis, and a normal opposite kidney should be a prerequisite to any attempt at surgical treatment.

The Presentation

Patients with hypertension as an isolated or unexpected finding, without a family history, especially the young and early middle-aged; those with known arterial disease in whom hypertension is of rapid onset, especially arteriosclerotic subjects with intermittent claudication [18], and others with upper limb or cerebral ischaemia. Weak limb pulses with widely differing pressure readings are suggestive: hypertension may be masked.

A localised abdominal arterial bruit may be heard above the umbilicus and slightly off the midline.

Renal symptoms such as pain in the loin or haematuria may lead to pyelography, which is often diagnostic (*see* below). There may be a history of renal tuberculosis or of local irradiation.

Polycythaemia may complicate renal artery stenosis [65] and aggravate its hypertensive effects.

Most cases are recognised from an awareness of the possibility when the cause of the hypertension is doubtful, or its presence seems inappropriate to the individual concerned.

Intravenous Pyelography (IVP) [18]

In the search for any type of renal cause for hypertension, this has become routine. The following pyelographic signs of renal ischaemia are fairly reliable:

1. The renal outline may be smaller, either obviously so or on measurement. A reduction of 1·5 cm in the axis-length of the suspected kidney compared with the opposite side is almost always significant, and usually of renal artery stenosis [61].

2. Indentation of the shadow of the upper ureter or lower pelvis may suggest the presence of large arterial collaterals [163], later confirmed as such in the nephrogram phase of aortography.

3. Changes in renal function, due to decreased arterial perfusion pressure resulting in decreased volume and rate of flow of filtrate and increased tubular reabsorption of water, though not of the contrast medium; these often show well on the IVP with either:

(*a*) Delayed excretion on the affected side.

(*b*) Reduction in the apparent volume of the renal pelvis, the so-called 'systolic kidney', in fact due to reduced flow.

(*c*) Increased density of the shadow from tubular reabsorption of water, which may lead to the mistaken conclusion that the more clearly seen kidney is the normal one.

The 'wash-out' or 'water-load' pyelogram [157] accentuates these differences to the point of actually removing the shadow of the normal functioning kidney by dilution during the diuresis, while the slow flow in the ischaemic tubules on the affected side still maintain a dense, clear pyelogram (Fig. 17.4). This phenomenon, if induced inadvertently, can throw suspicion upon the wrong kidney, and unless this important disorder of function is familar to the surgeon it may cost the patient his good kidney, and his life.

If both renal arteries are affected, simple radiological comparison is no longer of much value,

---

Fig. 17.4. Investigation of hypertension in a fifty-five-year-old man with a central abdominal bruit.

Lumbar aortography (*a*) showing tight stenosis of the left renal 1 cm from its origin, and (*b*) a moderate stenosis of the right renal at its aortic opening.

(*c*) The original pyelogram seemed to show a non-functioning right kidney. This was probably due to an unrecognised water-loading eliminating the medium quickly from the right kidney.

(*d*) Subsequent repeat pyelography by infusion and during fluid restriction showed good function on the right side, and a similar dense shadow on the left due to low filtration and relative increase in tubular reabsorption of water.

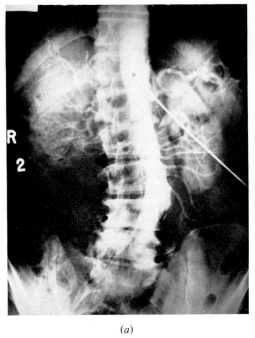

(a)

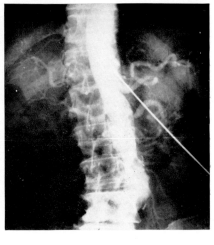

(b)

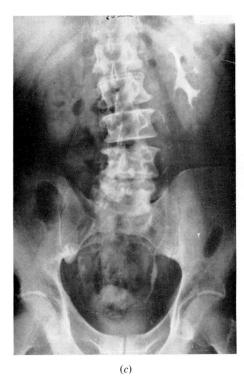

(c)

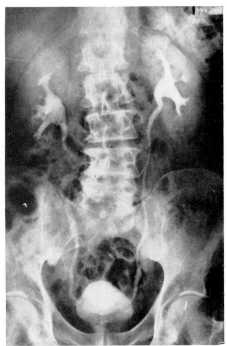

(d)

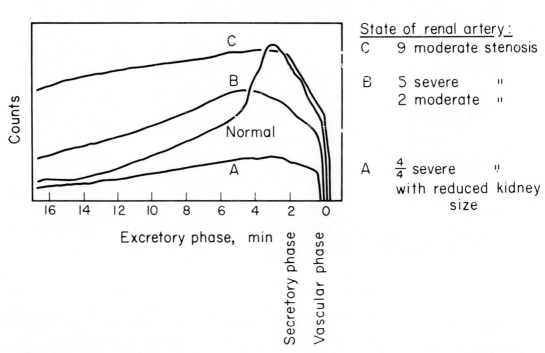

Fig. 17.5. Radioisotope renography showing the various patterns of secretion and excretion in the normal kidney and in twenty subjects with renal artery stenosis. (After Luke *et al.* [82], by courtesy of the publishers of the *Quarterly Journal of Medicine.*)

though all the above-mentioned changes may be present and, later, be confirmed by separate renal function tests.

Radioisotope Renography

A comparative study by external counting over the two kidneys, previously located with accuracy by intravenous pyelography [82], of the arrival pattern of [113]I labelled orthoiodohippurate (radio-hippuran), usually shows a flattening of the counting curve with delay, and a lowering of the peak on the affected side as shown in Fig. 17.5. Vascular, secretory, and excretory phases may each show changes from the normal pattern and from the opposite kidney, though there may be difficulty if this is not normal, as with the excretion pyelogram. For these and other reasons we, at St Mary's Hospital, have preferred the more tangible evidence of the pyelogram, though others have found the renogram to be a simple and fairly reliable screening test [69]; it is, of course, easier and safer than those which involve aortic or ureteric catheterisation. False positive results are sometimes misleading [82]. On the other hand, a normal pattern with a kidney known to have stenosis of its renal

artery is good evidence that the narrowing is not causing renal ischaemia.

Aortography and Selective Renal Arteriography [126, 158] (Fig. 17.6)

Ultimately, any clinical diagnosis, even with positive screening tests, will require confirmation by arterial contrast studies to show the position and the degree of the stenosis and the condition of the intrarenal branches, and to some extent the rate of flow within them. Films taken after a second injection (or, sometimes after th test dose) should show the relationship of the arterial filling to the pyelogram phase of the initial dose (Fig. 17.7). The nephrogram phase shows the size of the kidney better than plain films.

Contra-indications include renal failure (blood urea above 75 mg/100 ml) because of the risk of anuria; also very high blood pressure, which should first be lowered to 180/110 or there may be major bleeding from the arterial puncture site [126] (*see* Fig. 13.10, p. 248).

Translumbar aortography gives useful general information on the state of the abdominal aorta, as well as showing both renal arteries together with

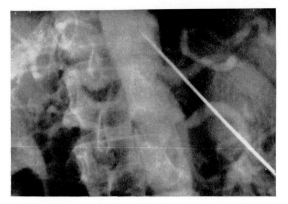

(a) High translumbar injection shows stenosis of both renal arteries and the aorta itself a few centimetres above them. (Same patient as in Fig. 17.4.)

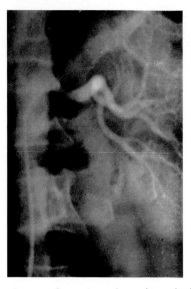

Fig. 17.6. Translumbar and selective renal arteriography.

(b) Selective transfemoral renal arteriography in a different patient provides accurate definition of the stenosis of one renal artery and shows the state of the intrarenal branches.

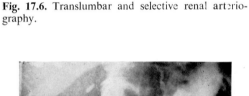

Fig. 17.7. A second translumbar injection showing the relationship of the diseased renal artery to the excretion pyelogram. Note high density of excreted medium in this case, due as in Fig. 17.4, to increased tubular reabsorption of water. (Different patient.)

their pyelogram phase, and it compares the kidney sizes. Some authorities have used it exclusively [124]. If the patient has aortic bifurcation obstruction or narrowing, the volume of contrast medium injected should be reduced because of the risk of mesenteric or renal damage with the normal dose.

Transfemoral catheterisation aortography (Fig. 17.17) provides all this information with the patient supine, the position of choice for renal X-ray photographs and of comfort for the patient. It may, however, be difficult or impossible if there is much arterial disease along the catheter route.

Selective renal arteriography can be carried out in the same way and gives accurate delineation of the state of the artery at and beyond the stenosis; data that may considerably influence the decision to operate, for multiple or extensive occlusive lesions are seldom suitable. The exact position of the stenosis and the post-stenotic dilatation are of crucial importance to the surgeon in planning the operation and choosing the type of reconstruction.

Divided Renal Function Studies [18, 151]

These give direct evidence, comparing the working of the two kidneys, and at St Mary's Hospital we do not normally operate for renal artery stenosis unless this test shows that the narrowing is causing underperfusion of the suspect kidney, and that the opposite kidney is functioning normally.

The principle of the test is simple: reduced arterial perfusion causes a fall in glomerular filtrate. The tubules, though structurally affected by the ischaemia, can still reabsorb water and salt, so that their concentration in the excreted urine is low, but meanwhile the concentration of non-absorbable solutes rises (diodone being an important example as seen in the IVP); creatinine, inulin and PAH* are others that are convenient for chemical estimation [18].

Table 17·4 shows a typical set of findings in a patient with left renal ischaemia; the operative procedure subsequently employed is shown in Fig. 17.10. Positive findings here are: the reduction in volume in each five-minute collection, and increased concentration of PAH and creatinine. Function was good, and the kidney was well worth conserving.

It should be remembered that divided renal studies cannot differentiate between parenchymal renal ischaemia and that which is due to a main artery lesion. When both lesions are present, renal arterial surgery is likely to fail.

* CR = creatinine; PAH = sodium para-amino hippurate.

Table 17.4. Divided Renal Study (by Dr J. J. Brown)

Sample	Urine vol. ml/min	Urine conc. mg%		Clearance ml/min	
		CR	PAH	CR	PAH
L. 1	1·6	30·0	490	52	366
R. 1	2·6	19·3	280	52	326
L. 2	1·6	27·6	420	45	300
R. 2	2·8	18·7	250	55	316
L. 3	1·9	25·2	370	50	320
R. 3	3·4	14·9	190	54	300

	P_0	P_1	P_2	
Plasma CR	0·95	0·95	0·95	mg/100 ml
Plasma PAH		2·20	2·20	

Comments: Both kidneys are functioning well. *Left* kidney is ischaemic.

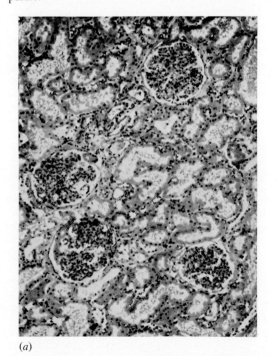

(a)

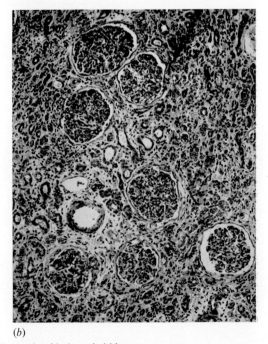

(b)

Fig. 17.8. Renal biopsy in the diagnosis of ischaemic kidney.

(a) A normal renal cortex.

(b) Atrophy and fibrosis of tubular components with consequent crowding of glomeruli. (Microphotographs by Dr R. A. Parker.)

Renal-Vein Renin Estimation

Values in normal and hypertensive subjects do overlap somewhat [68A], but when the two kidneys are compared, and the results of divided renal function studies are also taken into account, there is good correlation between raised renal-vein renin, reduced function and success after the relief of renal artery stenosis [2A, 45A, 68A].

Renal Biopsy

Percutaneous needle biopsy should, in theory, be decisive, though patchy changes are a source of possible error. The atrophy and other damage produced by ischaemia are shown in Fig. 17.8, in which the glomeruli on the affected side, though relatively normal, are more numerous per field because of the damage to the tubular component of the renal cortex. Hypertensive vascular changes are less common than in the 'healthy' opposite kidney, probably because the stenosed renal artery protects its own vessels from the effects of systemic hypertension; in fact, the presence of intrarenal vascular lesions will suggest that correction of renal artery stenosis may fail to relieve the hypertension.

It is desirable that operative biopsy specimens should be obtained with which to compare and amplify the needle specimens. They are a much better guide to postoperative assessment, and to prognosis.

Surgical Treatment of Reno-vascular Hypertension

1. *Nephrectomy* is indicated in poor-risk subjects and for complete renal artery occlusion [18], including that which follows attempted arterial reconstruction [68]. The opposite kidney must have adequate function; even so, it may fail later.

2. *Renal artery reconstruction* aims at cure, and with preservation of what is potentially the better (i.e. protected) kidney [18].

INDICATIONS

A young patient.
Unilateral renal artery stenosis.
Confirmation obtained that renal ischaemia is present.
Failure or intolerance of medical treatment.
Severely symptomatic or accelerated hypertension.
As the only alternative to nephrectomy.
Anuria from arterial occlusion in a solitary kidney [4, 71C].

CONTRA-INDICATIONS

Older patient.
Most bilateral, multiple or focal [6A] lesions.
Renal stenosis without evidence of renal ischaemia [18, 75].
Poor operative risk for a possibly long and exacting procedure (nephrectomy preferable).
Medical treatment effective.
Generalised arteriosclerosis, especially of aorta or splenic artery.
Severely contracted kidney, probably irreversibly damaged.

General Technique of Exposure

A transverse incision is preferable, at the level of the junction of the upper one-third and lower two-thirds of the xipho-umbilical line. A general abdominal exploration should not be omitted. The adrenals are gently palpated for the presence of a secreting tumour.

The kidney is approached through the posterior extraperitoneal plane by dividing the peritoneal reflection lateral to the colon, and retracting the intraperitoneal viscera across to the opposite side. The renal fascia is opened and, after a renal biopsy has been taken, the hilar vessels are exposed, first mobilising the vein, retracting it with a tape loop; the artery is then traced back to its origin. The tissues are adherent here and at the zone of the stenosis, so there is often troublesome small-vessel bleeding. A thrill may be felt over the obstruction.

Electromanometric readings are taken as early as possible in the dissection [117], simultaneously through two needles, one in the aorta and another in the post-stenotic part of the renal artery. The pressure gradient is measured on the oscillograph scan or on the paper tracing (Fig. 17.9). A gradient of 50–100 mm Hg signifies effective stenosis [117, 151]. Readings are repeated after the arterial reconstruction.

When the vessels have been fully exposed and the method of reconstruction to be used seems certain, the patient should be given 50 mg of heparin, into the aorta.

Backflow. Although the renal is an end-artery, and no backflow would be expected from a proximally clamped renal arteriotomy, it is believed that quite low perfusion pressures may keep the kidney alive; such a blood supply might come from the capsular, ureteric, and other anastomotic channels. In fact, if there is no backflow the prognosis is poor [68].

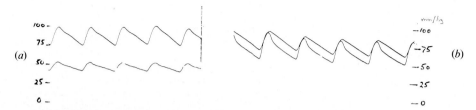

Fig. 17.9. Electromanometric tracings from the aorta (upper) and left renal (lower), (a) before, and (b) after correction of renal artery stenosis; taken from the patient whose operation is shown in Fig. 17.10.

Thrombo-endarterectomy. The first method used [46] is usually difficult because the aorta is so often involved, and unless the renal opening is thoroughly cleared any local restoration of the renal artery must fail. Exposure for this is never easy to obtain, and on the right side the vena cava prevents any safe local access. The left renal vein may impair work on the origin of the left artery. Local tissues are adherent to the segment of artery containing the plaque, and numerous fine anastomotic channels cause troublesome oozing. Nevertheless, with careful technique some good results have been reported [68].

Autogenous arterial shunt, using the splenic artery, is less difficult and should offer a good prospect of revascularising the left renal artery beyond its stenosed part, though it will not reach across to the right. The splenic must be reasonably wide and free from occlusive disease, with a measured pressure equal to, or very near to, that of the aorta. The pancreas is mobilised forwards and the splenic artery detached, with ligation of any local branches to the gland. It should not be tied until the correct length can be assessed. Splenectomy is unnecessary. An end-to-side anastomosis is usually chosen.

By-pass grafting is often used, taking off from the aorta, between the renals and the inferior mesenteric, where exposure is easy and lateral clamping is simple, to either or both of the renal arteries, end-to-side, always choosing the site of maximum post-stenotic dilatation for the distal anastomosis. The recipient artery may be quite thin at this point, so it is preferable to make the distal anastomosis first, using 6/0 sutures. An autogenous vein graft is suitable for this by-pass. A secure and not too wide aortic anastomosis should ensure against overstrain on the graft. Fine, knitted, dacron cloth tube prosthesis have been extensively used [111] with good early results. Late evaluation of this material in this site has yet to be made. The small size of the renal artery and its moderate flow rate may not support long-term patencies here.

Other techniques less often applicable include *resection and anastomosis, reimplantation* of the distal renal artery into the aorta (Fig. 17.10), and

Fig. 17.10. Reimplantation of left renal artery into aorta below left renal vein. This patient had severe hypertension, which persisted after her first confinement. Anaesthesia and operative manipulation explain the low initial readings shown in Fig. 17.9. After two normal confinements her blood pressure and intravenous pyelograms have remained normal during the seven years since the operation. (Divided renal function study—Table 17.4.)

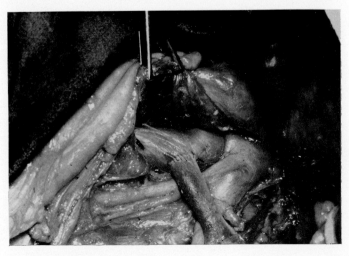

even complete *autotransplantation* of the kidney [140]. Many successful bilateral renal arterial reconstructions have been described with endarterectomy [164] or by-pass [111]; also, several cases in which by-pass methods were effective in revascularising a solitary kidney [86].

Postoperative Care

Special attention is paid to the blood-pressure level, with frequent readings during wound closure and during the first day and night, for a precipitate fall may occur soon after the renal artery has been restored, especially when, previously, the pressure was very high. More often, however, the fall is gradual. The urine output is carefully watched. A diuresis is a good sign that reconstruction may have succeeded. Anuria may mean that damage has been done to the supply to the normal kidney.

Results of Surgical Treatment of Renovascular Hypertension (Table 17.5)

By 1956, when renal revascularisation was still in its infancy, Homer Smith [149] had reviewed nearly 600 cases of nephrectomy for hypertension thought to be due to unilateral renal disease of various kinds, in which definite sustained hypertension was clearly established before operation. A postoperative blood pressure of 140/90 or lower, remaining so for at least a year, was his criterion of success, and nothing short of this should be accepted today. Twenty-five per cent of the early cases were successful by these standards.

Subsequent case series have mostly been for renal arterial disease, now known to be the commonest reversible cause for hypertension, and while renal artery reconstruction has naturally become increasingly common practice, nephrectomy cases still make up a good proportion of today's literature. Against a very proper concern for conserving renal function must be set the reservation that the success rate with ablation is probably higher [68].

Conclusion

With an average success rate of about 50 per cent and a surgical mortality of 5 per cent or more, renal arterial surgery or nephrectomy will, at present, find its main usefulness in the treatment of severe, drug-

Table 17.5. Results of operation for renovascular hypertension

(Kaufman [68] with additional material)

	Patients	'Cured' (%)	% ratio Nephrec-tomy/ arterial operation	Died (%)
Poutasse (1961) [124]	76	62	41/59	10
Stewart et al. (1962) [154]	43	40	51/49	4
DeCamp (1963) [32]	33	45	48/52	6
Baker et al. (1962) [5]	25	39	21/79	9
Kaufman (1965) [68]	70	39	40/60	4·5
Hejnal et al. (1965) [60]	43	68	8/35	2
Morris et al. (1966) [111]	432	41	—	7
Hsuing (1966) [64]	48	56	56/44	8
Owen (1967) [117A]	69	43	31/40	7
Foster et al. (1969) [45A]*	29	87	* Fibro-muscular cases only.	

resistant or accelerated hypertension in young patients. Even in these, the possibility of recurrent stenosis at fresh sites, whether from fibromuscular disease or arteriosclerosis, will to some extent limit the expectation of lasting cure. Moreover, the later death-rate from other cardiovascular causes is higher in hypertensive subjects however treated. There should, however, remain a proportion yet to be finally determined of fully successful results to justify continued selective trial of surgery in well-investigated cases, especially in fibromuscular disease.

MESENTERIC ISCHAEMIA

The Acute Condition

Sudden loss of the superior mesenteric artery (SMA) is normally incompatible with survival. The whole of the mid-gut loop depends upon it for blood supply at a high rate of flow, and no immediately available alternative pathway is sufficient. The inferior mesenteric, however, can usually be ligated without danger, for the left colon is short, has a lower blood requirement, and is nearer to its collateral sources from the middle colic and internal iliac.

Local conditions tend to regulate splanchnic blood flow: measurements of blood pressure in the SMA, a small mesenteric vein, and the main portal vein of the dog, when related to flow show that the total resistance in the mesenteric vascular bed decreased at low flow rates (20–60 ml/min), yet increased with higher flow (90–270 ml/min). Changes in small vessel resistance were chiefly responsible, suggesting that, as in the kidney, a local factor tends to compensate for variations in systemic arterial pressure [161].

EXPERIMENTAL DATA ON MESENTERIC LIGATION IN ANIMALS

Death follows a shock-like state, which develops in two to four hours, and lasts about ten, though survival may be longer under hypothermia, or if heparin or antibiotics have been given. The mechanism of the shock is still in question; the two conflicting views being that:

(a) bacterial endotoxins from the gut enter the general circulation and cause a paralytic vaso-dilatation;

(b) fluid from the general circulation enters the damaged bowel, where it becomes sequestered, causing oligaemic shock.

In some animals, such as the dog, in whom bacterial invasion of the body tissues is present even in health, the dominant role of toxaemia as a cause of the widespread gut necrosis from which the animal dies is strongly supported by the experimental evidence [44]. In monkeys and rabbits, fluid shifts appear to be more important [93]. Removal of the small intestine may protect against shock of this and other kinds [89], either by eliminating the source of vasoactive substances, or by removing the pool into which fluid loss would otherwise occur. The dog is not protected by enterectomy [79], and germ-free rats die as readily as controls after mesenteric ligation [21].

Visible effects of superior mesenteric ischaemia by ligation begin, almost at once, with a transient increase in peristalsis, soon amounting to a general muscle spasm followed by pallor, emptying of the arteries, and, after about three hours, the bowel becomes flaccid and congested. Blood-stained fluid appears in the peritoneal cavity, and oedema thickens the wall of the gut, though there is no necrosis, and rupture does not occur. Gas distension is not marked, though there are bubbles to be seen in the mesenteric veins, the result of gas-forming bacterial activity, so important a feature of the condition in the dog. Muscle contractility may be retained very late, even after death of the animals.

Histological Changes

Serial biopsies during the experiment show that as early as the first hour a membranous slough forms over the tips of the villi, which become necrotic and adherent to a sheet of exudate. This membrane is believed, by some, to be identical with that cast off in the clinical condition known as pseudomembranous entero-colitis [88]. The arteries remain empty but the veins become progressively engorged, probably from the portal venous return from intact portions of the gastro-intestinal tract. Much of the circulating fluid loss may be explained in this way. Early on, there is marked infiltration with polymorph leucocytes, the numbers of which are also greatly increased in the circulating blood. Complete necrosis does not often occur in massive ischaemia, for death of the animal supervenes, in contrast to localised strangulation in which ischaemia survival is prolonged, and death results from rupture and peritonitis.

Changes in the Biochemistry and Body Fluids

These are complex and interrelated, and the several connected vicious circles are shown in Fig. 17.11. Many of the same features are present in human bowel infarction.

(a) *Chemical effects* include the production of catecholamines, serotonin, histamine, and polypeptides [71], all of which are vasoactive. The exact way in which these affect the vessels of the intestine is not yet known. A biphasic action has been demonstrated with intravenous adrenalin [54]; though given into the artery, vasoconstriction is always produced [53]. *Nor*-adrenalin is more potent still. Gangrene of the bowel has been described in phaeochromocytoma [133]. Adrenergic blocking agents can reverse the effects of catecholamines [54], an effect that has also been shown clinically in treatment by using rogitine 5 mg intra-arterially in saline [78]. A polypeptide-like vasodilator is increasingly produced and mobilised in ischaemia of the gut, and on release of the obstruction [71]. Bacterial endotoxins (coliforms) and exotoxins (clostridia) are liberated by the invading gut organisms. Endotoxins are strongly sympatheticomimetic, an effect which, like that of the catecholamines themselves, can be blocked by vasodilators including steroids in massive dosage [80]. Serotonin may be produced by the action of endotoxin on blood platelets [134]. The whole process can be slowed by the previous administration of antibiotics [72].

(b) *Fluid shifts* are well documented. Blood volume is lost via the portal vein at the rate of 5 per cent per hour [91], mostly as plasma, for at the same time the haematocrit rises. Fluid is sequestered in the wall and the lumen of the gut. With this there is increase in blood viscosity, more resistance to flow in obstructed areas, and sludging in marginal zones, which increases the effect of the ischaemia. Meanwhile, there is also a fall in the perfusion of other

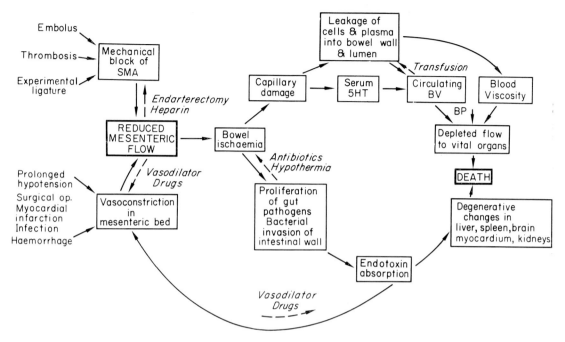

Fig. 17.11. Mechanisms of death in bowel ischaemia. (*From* Marston [88], by courtesy of the Editor of *Lancet*.)

vital organs, which further depresses the circulation in the gut and in the body as a whole.

'IRREVERSIBLE SHOCK' [76]
It is said that this should never be diagnosed in a living patient. It was seldom seen in war casualties [6] in whom adequate blood replacement and control of the effects of the injury, if they were possible, would almost always check the deterioration. In older subjects this is no longer the case (*see* p. 370). In dogs, however, such a state can readily be produced by severe exsanguination, and changes in the bowel are thought to be responsible [44]. If dogs are bled though a cannula and container that later can be used to re-infuse the blood, and the blood pressure is brought down to 35 mm Hg, the animal will survive when the shed blood is returned within the first two hours. After four hours, however, neither the blood in the container nor any extra transfusion can be made to restore the blood pressure, and at this time it is found that the intestines have become congested with haemorrhagic necrosis, an appearance closely resembling acute mesenteric ischaemia.

Endotoxin from Gram-negative bacteria we have already seen to be strongly vasoconstrictive to the

gut, though other substances may be working in the same way (Fig. 17.11). Systemic effects of absorbed endotoxin in overwhelming quantity are thought by Fine [44] to explain why the animal dies though its blood volume has been restored.

Hypovolaemia causes a large increase in circulating catecholamines [55] to which the mesenteric vessels are highly sensitive. Irreversibility could be explained by damage to the gut wall by vasoconstrictive ischaemia leading to damage that allowed the outpouring of plasma and some red cells being able to gain continued access to the affected bowel either from the portal venous radicles (which are seen to be engorged—*see* p. 368) or from the patent arterial inflow from the adjoining live bowel.

Effects of Restoring Circulation to Ischaemic Gut
When the main arterial circulation is restored after prolonged ischaemia most, but not all, of the bowel begins to recover, even in the moribund animal [92]. Massive haemorrhage occurs into the damaged, sloughing, membranous remnant of the mucosa and sub-mucosa. These observations by Marston also included cross perfusion of the ischaemic gut by a healthy dog, which in most experiments died within three hours from whole blood loss, without evidence

of endotoxin damage to its own gut or reticulo-endothelial system. When the donor dog was transfused it usually survived, which is not the response of endotoxin shock.

Other experiments by Fine and his colleagues [114], however, suggest that, in dogs and in rabbits, coeliac blockade and dibenzyline protect the gut from vaso-constriction, and the liver also, with better survival rates due to these measures for control of endotoxin damage [109].

MESENTERIC LIGATION IN MAN

This is usually fatal, though there have been cases in which a normal superior mesenteric artery has been ligated, as for example to control haemorrhage, and in which no lasting ill effects were suffered. In a surviving case of spontaneous rupture of the artery near its origin, the site of the ligature was later confirmed at an autopsy following accidental death, and the inferior pancreato-duodenal artery was found to have been excluded from the collateral bed by the placing of the ligatures [96].

Enterectomy in man, as in animals, appears to mitigate the effects of traumatic shock. This protective effect has been seen in battle casualties [6] and in cases of criminal abortion in which the small bowel was removed [145].

Morbid Anatomy of Mesenteric Occlusive Disease

Some cases show more or less extensive thrombosis of a diseased aorta at the level of the major visceral branches [97, 112], but in most instances a localised arteriosclerosis of the coeliac, superior, and inferior mesenteric arteries is confined to the orifice and first part of the artery. Fibromuscular hyperplasia is less common but more diffuse. As the obstructive effect of these lesions increases, important anatomical connections between these three territories are called into use; they are shown in Fig. 17.16. The critical zones are the pancreas, the splenic flexure, and the rectum. The stomach is less readily affected by acute or chronic ischaemia than the gut. Abnormal anatomical communications between the three zones are common [16] and are of considerable practical importance, for they may lead to unexpected ischaemic complications in biliary surgery and in staged operations upon the colon as well as with resections for abdominal aortic aneurysm (see Chapter 15). The inferior mesenteric artery may be the only surviving member of the triad [127] and may, as described over a century ago by Chiene of Edinburgh, attain the size of the femoral [23].

Quite apart from major arterial obstruction due to stenosis or thrombosis, diffuse mesenteric arterial narrowing increases with advancing age and the flow-capacity of these arteries may become acutely insufficient either as a result of general illness, shock, local operations or injuries or, most important of all, from cardiac failure.

Mesenteric Ischaemia in Heart Failure

Bowel necrosis is now well known as a terminal event in severe heart disease; in one autopsy series [8] in which 100 cases dying after laparotomy had shown gangrene of the bowel, 23 had no major mesenteric occlusion.

Surgical experience, too, has shown that the site and extent of the infarcted gut need bear no constant relationship to the vascular occlusion [87].

Heart failure patients sometimes develop peripheral gangrene in the extremities, with or without evidence of previous local arterial insufficiency (see Chapter 2, p. 24). Dynamic obstruction in many tissues and organs can be reversed or ameliorated by improving cardiac function [166A]; it seems more than likely that the blood supply of the bowel often behaves in a similar way, though with much potential limitation of recovery by arteriosclerotic narrowing of the arcades which, unlike the same lesion in the limb arteries, will, in the gut, produce hidden, silent damage that, moreover, is to a certain extent self-perpetuating from the effects of the vaso-active substances produced by the ischaemia, as well as from haemoconcentration due to fluid loss. Sympathetic tone is increased in heart failure, with raised levels of nor-adrenalin in the blood and urine [13]. Digitalis causes splanchnic vasoconstriction that can be reversed by glucagon [26A].

It has been suggested by Marston [88], that the reason why severe hypotension in elderly men and postmenopausal women may prove fatal is because of acute aggravation of existing potential ischaemia in the mesenteric territory, so that in these patients the bowel, unlike that of the young healthy casualty, may constitute an important factor in the cause of death. In over a half of 33 such cases there was zonal liver necrosis and focal renal tubular necrosis, as seen in hypotension [103].

Most surgeons will have noticed, during major abdominal surgery, that striking alterations in gut colour and arterial pulsation often occur along with changes in the patient's general condition; both tend to deteriorate and improve together. We may regard the exposed gut as a ready manometer and plethysmograph with which to monitor the peripheral circulation in the vital areas of the body.

Clinical Types of Mesenteric Ischaemia

There is much variation in the clinical pattern [36], much depending upon the morbid anatomical basis of the ischaemia as well as on the age and general condition of the patient (Figs 17.12 and 17.13).

The following aspects of time, anatomical site, and pathological basis of the lesion and the underlying condition (Table 17.6) should be considered; they may occur in almost any combination.

Dunphy [40] found that in 7 out of 12 patients dying of acute mesenteric occlusion there was a

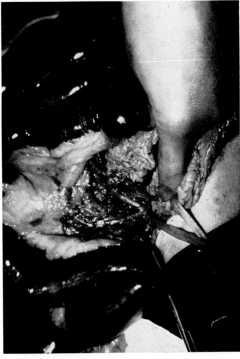

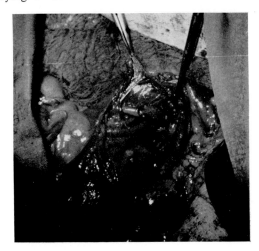

Fig. 17.13. Localised stenosis of the proximal portion of the superior mesenteric artery in a patient with intestinal angina. Intestines appeared normal at operation, though on close inspection it could be seen that the mesenteric branches were not pulsating. Thromboendarterectomy and vein patch graft are shown here. Following this operation the patient has remained free from abdominal symptoms for three years.

Fig. 17.12. Advanced, massive small bowel ischaemia in a man aged eighty with congestive heart failure. Note the good colour of the mesentery. The exposed superior mesenteric and its first branch were shown to be pulsating normally.

previous history of abdominal trouble; this prodromal stage might last weeks, months, or years. Sometimes it is quite short [97]. It should be hoped that more cases might be recognised in this earlier

Mode of onset	Site of ischaemia	Pathological features	
		Causes	*Effects*
Acute		Arteriosclerotic thrombosis	
	Superior mesenteric (mid-gut loop)		Gangrene (rarely perforation)
Chronic		Embolism, large or small	
	Inferior mesenteric (splenic flexure and descending colon)		Stricture
Acute-on-chronic		Arteriosclerotic or dissecting aneurysm	Ischaemic granuloma
			Intestinal insufficiency
		Heart failure (Fig. 17.12)	
		Arteritis (Fig. 17.14)	

Table 17.6

phase when treatment of the arterial lesion could succeed, but the clinical diagnosis of mesenteric ischaemia is difficult in every part of its course, and the number of cases recognised in time for successful surgery is still very small.

Diagnosis of the Acute Condition

No other acute abdominal emergency can match this one, with its dangerous combination of progressive, lethal damage, and so few physical signs. Of the many hundred of reported cases [93, 99] the only regular features were:

1. *Abdominal pain*, usually severe, is nearly always present and should bring the patient under medical observation early, at a time when treatment might still be successful. The pain is sudden in its onset, often colicky but soon becoming constant. It may be referred to the back, as in volvulus, and, similarly, perhaps because of a response to injury within the mesentery.

In a young patient such a complaint, unaccompanied by signs of appropriate severity can lead to a misdiagnosis of hysteria, which may be abandoned only in the face of grave deterioration in the patient's general condition. In fifteen children [34] there was an average delay of 39·5 hours; in which the child might be thought 'not ill enough for appendicitis'.

2. *Tenderness* is sometimes early, but *without rigidity or guarding* it is often disregarded.

3. *Distension* is a late sign indicating extensive intestinal infarction; earlier on, there are seldom any obstructive features either clinically or on plain radiography.

4. *Shock* develops and increases as fluid is lost from the circulation; it is usually a late effect, marking the end of the featureless 'latent period' which is such a dangerous delaying factor in the diagnosis of acute mesenteric. A small rapid pulse probably means that it is too late to save the patient, not so much from 'irreversible shock' as from the extent of the damage to the gut.

5. A loose, bloody stool in a case of this kind should always suggest a vascular cause.

6. *Leucocytosis* is a consistent and early finding. A white cell count of 20,000 or more in a patient with severe abdominal pain and little else should be 'considered to be due to mesenteric infarction until this has been excluded' [93].

7. Plain X-ray films of the abdomen may, where the main artery is occluded, show a striking absence of gas; in the peripheral, cardiac type of infarction with a patent artery there is often ileus [57]. Gas in the portal vein has been described [144], mostly in the finer intrahepatic branches, with a slender

appearance in the translucencies which differs from that of the gas in the bile ducts in gallstone ileus.

8. Serum amylase levels may be reduced [27].

The previous history is often relevant:

(*a*) Rheumatic heart disease with mitral stenosis and *atrial fibrillation* probably mean that the ischaemia is embolic. Major limb pulses may be absent, confirming a history of previous peripheral arterial emboli (*see* Chapter 14, p. 258).

(*b*) Previous abdominal pain after meals, weight loss, and other evidence of chronic mesenteric insufficiency (*see* p. 375) should suggest that a stenosed superior mesenteric artery has finally and acutely occluded, or an important collateral has thrombosed. The patient may have had intermittent claudication [137]. Emergency thromboendarterectomy may succeed [15].

(*c*) *In the aged*, known ischaemic or hypertensive heart disease with worsening attacks of congestive failure may set the stage for the final tragedy of massive mesenteric infarction affecting smaller vessels rather than the main orifices, and precipitated by central failure of perfusion (Fig. 17.12).

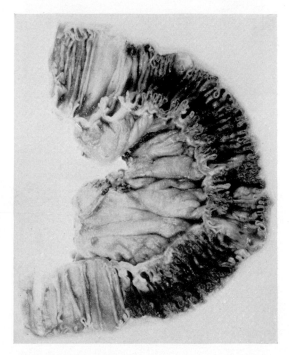

Fig. 17.14. Polyarteritis of the small intestine. Diagnosis made on histological examination of this excised segment which had appeared to be affected with Crohn's disease. (Sir Arthur Porritt's case.)

(*d*) *In children*, though the diagnosis is difficult [34], an embolus from a patent ductus arteriosus is one recognised cause; and, nowadays, embolism or thrombosis may be due to cardiovascular manipulations such as cardiac catheterisation under anaesthesia.

(*e*) In mature adults, a febrile illness may mean that polyarteritis nodosa is the cause (Fig. 17.14). Abdominal symptoms are present in at least 50 per cent, and include steatorrhoea [20]. Multiple, small infarcts are typical. Other arteritis conditions occasionally affecting the mesenteric supply include: systemic scleroderma [83A], amyloidosis [16A] and retroperitoneal fibrosis [24B]. In all these the primary area of vascular symptoms is more often the limbs.

Diagnosis, therefore, rests upon the high probability that severe abdominal pain without impressive clinical or radiological signs, yet with high leucocytosis and, later, shock in an elderly, arteriosclerotic

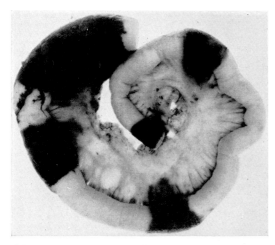

Fig. 17.15. Haemorrhagic/obstructed small bowel due to segmental extravasations following overdosage of phenindione. (Mr Andrew Desmond's case.)

or cardiac subject is due to acute superior mesenteric infarction. Anticoagulant overdose should be remembered as a cause of a similar picture (Fig. 17.15).

The Course of the Illness

The stage of severe pain and milder physical signs may be somewhat prolonged, with more patients developing serious features after twelve hours than before, and. in some, the deceptive early picture lasts seven days or more [99].

Signs of peritonitis are soon followed by cardio-

vascular collapse. This is the stage at which most exploratory operations are performed; such late intervention is no more than an incident that confirms the diagnosis and hastens death, the mortality being over 90 per cent [99].

In other cases the picture is that of a fulminating enterocolitis [103] in which the bowel is found to be oedematous, with patchy congestion, haemorrhages, and superficial ulceration.

Management of Acute Mesenteric Ischaemia

Most patients have severe heart disease with decompensation. The problem is to decide whether this alone is the cause of the condition (*see* p. 370).

In younger patients, and those with atrial fibrillation though not necessarily in heart failure, a major proximal mesenteric occlusion is probable, either embolic or, if there have been prodromal symptoms in a patient who may show other features of peripheral occlusive arterial disease, thrombosis of the narrowed superior mesenteric near its origin. These patients require immediate operation. Superior mesenteric arteriography may become a decisive investigation [1].

Medical Treatment

Based on experimental work mainly in dogs, various agents appear to help towards a natural recovery:

(*a*) Fluid replacement, preferably with plasma [93, 81].

(*b*) Antibiotics, either to work systemically [72, 114, 115] or if non-absorbable, to help sterilise the bowel [114].

(*c*) Heparin, to reduce consecutive thrombosis [115], though it might also aggravate the tendency to haemorrhage.

(*d*) Low molecular weight dextran, to reduce red cell aggregation and perhaps also platelet accumulation [27, 28, 77, 139].

(*e*) Coeliac or splanchnic nerve block [114, 116] (*see* p. 370), which may be repeated or continuous.

(*f*) Hydrocortisone in massive dosage [81].

(*g*) Adrenergic blocking agents [78, 81, 114]; both being aimed at preventing mesenteric vasoconstriction.

(*h*) Glucagon inhibits splanchnic vasoconstriction due to catecholamines, sympathetic stimulation [71B], and by digitalis [26A]. It also has an inotropic cardiac action [71A].

Clinical experience appears to support most of these claims; in particular those of LMW dextran [28, 139], though in one of the reported cases anuria followed the infusion of several litres [28].

Surgical Intervention

The first successful superior mesenteric embolectomy without gut resection was reported by Shaw and Rutledge of the Massachusetts General Hospital, in 1957 [142], in a fifty-four-year-old woman with atrial fibrillation from rheumatic heart disease, a typical case, with a fifteen-hour history of abdominal pain, vomiting, and melaena, who was already under treatment for a stroke, one week before. Though the gut was bluish-grey at operation twenty-five hours after the onset, it improved with embolectomy, and at a 'second look' operation next day was pink, with pulsating arteries. With recovery she showed a late absorptive defect, but eventually did well.

Since then there have been at least twenty-five cases [50, 67A, 173] of recovery after embolectomy, and several others after emergency thrombo-endarterectomy of the superior mesenteric; the first report again being from Shaw, with Maynard, in 1958. This was also a typical case; a man with earlier claudication and peptic ulcer. Later, after recovering from his mesenteric arterial surgery he developed an ischaemic stricture of the descending colon [143].

OPERATIVE FINDINGS IN ACUTE MESENTERIC VASCULAR OCCLUSION

1. Free blood-stained peritoneal fluid is usually, though not always, present.
2. The affected bowel will have lost its normal pink colour, and one or more of the following changes will be noted:

(a) In early cases, a pallor and corrugated spasm.

(b) Later, beginning distension, with a purple suffusion, perhaps patchy and appearing to be becoming confluent. The serous coat still glistens normally (Fig. 17.12). The bowel wall is oedematous and may collapse again, though usually it remains distended.

(c) Finally, the gut becomes greenish black, and dullness at last affects the serosa: this is seen only in cases of locally advanced infarction in whom recovery of other parts of the bowel, with survival of the patient beyond the lethal phase during the second day, after a more massive infarction. It is the appearance to be anticipated at a 'second look' operation. The colon as it dies becomes lighter in colour, patchily at the caecum and, generally, farther on.

(d) Arterial pulsation is absent from the affected segment. This is more easily described in theory than it is to confirm at the operation. Venous thrombosis is easier to see, by transmitted light, and to feel as hard cords, dark in colour in the terminal arcades and straight vessels. Gas

bubbles may be present, drifting sluggishly to and fro within veins or lymphatics. A foetid smell is common. Yet with all these colour changes it is the arterial status of the gut that is crucial. A useful test for this is to lay the affected bowel alongside a healthy segment, for example the ileum, and to compare it with the sigmoid colon, or the transverse colon with the greater curvature of the stomach. The contrast in colour and pulsation between the stagnant and the normal loops is in this way made more striking and obvious.

3. The presence of aorto-iliac arteriosclerosis with plaques suggests that the cause of the ischaemia is a thrombosis. A more normal set of abdominal arteries but with irregular pulses are typical of the patient with mesenteric embolism. Thrombosis is twice as common [93, 99]. Sometimes the two conditions occur together. The outlook is then extremely grave, no doubt because of impairment of the collateral circulation.

CHOICE OF SURGICAL PROCEDURE

1. *If the gut is already gangrenous* resection offers the only hope of survival [165], though the outlook is virtually hopeless in the majority of cases with cardiac insufficiency, and nearly so in any late case whatever the state of the heart. Total removal of the mid-gut loop from a few inches below the duodeno-jejunal flexure to the mid-transverse colon can easily be carried out but is almost incompatible with late survival in the group of elderly patients with which we are concerned.

In a few patients, smaller segments are infarcted, perhaps because of a partial recovery of circulation, either spontaneous or on re-exploration following an arterial reconstruction operation the previous day. Resection of these parts of the gut should be well tolerated.

2. *With the gut still viable* or apparently so, an arterial operation must be attempted provided that a major occlusion can be located with reasonable certainty. This may be difficult, though here again, the best test is the sharply visible contrast between a strongly pulsating aorta or mesenteric root, and the still, even elusive main mesenteric trunk at and beyond the duodenal flexure. An atheromatous plaque may be felt at the origin of the superior mesenteric.

Techniques for Elective Superior Mesenteric Arterial Reconstruction are described on p. 379

In the emergency case, exposure and dissection are the same, though with emphasis on simplicity and expedition, and as short an operation as possible.

A nick in the artery over the embolus allows it to be pushed out by the force of the arterial pulse. There may be very little retrograde bleeding. In a poor-risk case it is justifiable to milk the embolus back into the aorta and to extract it if necessary from one of the lower limb arteries, particularly now that the Fogarty balloon catheter has made most of these emboli accessible from the common femoral (*see* Chapter 14, p. 271). The catheter can also, of course, be used to bring a proximally impacted mesenteric embolus down into the accessible part of the artery [50].

When an embolus lodges in an already narrowed, sclerotic artery the operation becomes more difficult. A local procedure may not be possible; a by-pass is then preferable (*see* p. 379).

LATE REVASCULARISATION PHENOMENA

As with limb emboli (*see* Chapter 14, p. 268), there may be the serious problem of a metabolic acidosis and hyperkalaemia soon after the restoration of mesenteric blood supply [7]. To make matters worse, ablation is no such alternative as it is in the limbs; also, there is real danger of haemorrhage into the damaged gut. A sudden fatal collapse is therefore possible after the clamps are removed, though the gut may appear to be viable [100]. Apart from infusion of sodium bicarbonate solution (250 mEq or more) and adequate blood replacement there is little that can be done to control this serious situation, though perfusion of the mid-gut loop with oxygenated blood has been suggested [101].

RE-EXPLORATION: THE 'SECOND LOOK'

Not all the gut may recover after restoration of its blood supply. The possible need for supplementary surgery in the form of resection of any remaining avascular portions was envisaged by Shaw and his colleagues [142, 143] in the first successful reported cases of arterial surgery for embolism and acute thrombosis, and both patients were re-explored during the first forty-eight hours. Since then, this has become accepted practice. Loosely applied through-and-through sutures are therefore employed at the first closure. Several cases are on record in which gut resection succeeded with the help of the arterial surgery, when it scarcely could have done without it [15, 104, 154]. The opportunity may also arise for a successful revision of an early recurrent arterial occlusion.

LATER MANAGEMENT

1. Survivors of embolectomy who have mitral disease and atrial fibrillation should be considered for mitral valvotomy and removal of the atrial appendage.

2. Malabsorption effects of ischaemia or of massive gut resection may require special care by a gastroenterologist. Prospects for a full recovery should be good. The small bowel remnant achieves an increased absorption [38].

Chronic Mesenteric Insufficiency

As in the limbs, and in the carotid-vertebral circulation, a slow occlusion should almost always be better tolerated than one that is sudden. Thus, the superior mesenteric artery may completely occlude at its origin by a slow increase in thickness of the narrowing plaque, yet with good health and nutrition preserved over many years (Fig. 17.16). The same is

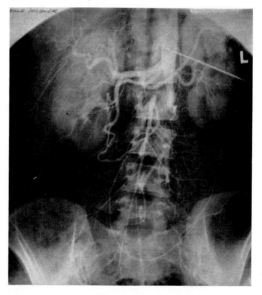

Fig. 17.16. Symptomless complete occlusion of the proximal superior mesenteric artery in a woman aged thirty-six whose main complaint concerned the associated thrombosis of her aortic bifurcation. The latter was relieved by thromboendarterectomy, and the patient continued well for ten years, her only complaint being increasing obesity. Eventual death from coronary thrombosis.

true in dog experiments [93] in which gradual narrowing produced no ill effects, either upon the absorptive function or the general well being of the animals.

If occlusion is gradual, two of the three main arteries to the gastro-intestinal tract must have become occluded before chronic ischaemia is produced.

This may explain why superior mesenteric insufficiency as a clinical entity is rarer than the finding of an anatomical stenosis of the artery. Even with only one of the three main visceral arteries remaining patent there may be no symptoms [129].

Exceptions to this rule are few. Sudden closure by embolism or by major, acute thrombosis of an already narrowed main superior mesenteric are the most important, the clinical evidence, as Dunphy realised, being sudden deterioration after milder prodromal ischaemia. In one of his cases, with both mesenterics already occluded, it was a recent block in the coeliac that determined the fatal outcome [40].

Nearly all cases of chronic mesenteric ischaemia are of arteriosclerotic origin. A few are due to arteritis: these mostly show isolated featues, e.g. steatorrhoea [20], segmental ischaemic stricture [107] haemorrhage (see Chapter 7, [14]), and rarely, perforation [108].

Clinical Features of Chronic Mesenteric Insufficiency

Abdominal
Pain after
  meals ⎫
Small food ⎬ 'intestinal
  capacity ⎭ angina'
Severe weight loss

Intestinal difficulties:
  Diarrhoea, from
    small bowel ⎫
    in SMA ⎬ ischaemia
    colon in ⎪
    early IMA ⎭
  Constipation with
    late IMA ischaemia
  Malabsorption and
    steatorrhoea
  Ischaemic granuloma

  Failure to heal gut
    anastomosis

Epigastric bruit

Constitutional
Premature physiological
  ageing
Commoner in men

History of arteriosclerotic
  troubles
    Coronary insufficiency
    Intermittent
      claudication
    Abdominal aneurysm
    Stroke

Anaemia

Reduced or increased
  glucose tolerance

Sometimes polyarteritis
  nodosa, SLE, or
  scleroderma

Segmental ischaemia of a short length of bowel, either large (Table 17.7, p. 382), or small [59, 122, 169] usually follows within a few weeks of an acutely painful episode, often with distension and general prostration, and though the mucosa has good powers of regeneration it may have been totally destroyed at the central part of the lesion. A stricture will then follow, leading to intestinal obstruction and an operation at which the fibrous, adherent segment is discovered, whose mesenteric branch may be found

to be thrombosed [122]. Arteriosclerotic occlusion is uncommon in vessels of this size; it seems more likely that closure would have taken place either during a period of hypotensive stagnation, or from a small embolus lodging in the branch to the loop.

Intestinal Angina [73, 93, 94A, 106, 107]

This elusive syndrome is easier to describe than to recognise. If it is true that many terminal cases of intestinal gangrene give such a history (though probably the cardiac cases do not [57]), then the condition should be commoner in practice than it seems to be. Unlike most of the other advances in arterial surgery, reports of restorative operations on the mesenteric artery are still relatively few. Stenosis of the origin of the superior mesenteric artery is found at autopsy in approximately one half of all subjects [33, 35, 168]. The incidence and severity of mesenteric arteriosclerosis in 500 consecutive adults dying in Pittsburgh hospitals was found to be closely similar to that found in the renal arteries whether or not the cause of death was a cardiovascular condition [130].

PAIN AFTER MEALS AND SMALL FOOD TOLERANCE

Yet, clinically, the classical picture of intestinal angina, with intense food fear, the small-meal syndrome [125, 128], wasting, and bowel upsets is seldom diagnosed. Other more common causes for these symptoms will rightly be considered first, though sometimes, on aortography, the patient proves to have mesenteric arterial stenosis. Carcinoma of the pancreas and hiatus hernia have both been described in this association [110]. Other abdominal vascular conditions may be suspected in a thin patient with constant, worsening abdominal pain, for example a prominent or deviated aorta may be thought to be aneurysmal. Other patients, with severe symptoms but few signs may be thought to be neurotic, as in some cases of acute infarction (see p. 372).

At the onset there is often an acute phase with severe pain, perhaps accompanied by shock and bloody diarrhoea, suggesting a temporary severe ischaemia with partial recovery. The chronic stage which then follows should be recognisable before it once more relapses into terminal acute ischaemia [166], though it is not certain that all cases of intestinal angina necessarily die of gut necrosis [93], for it may be possible, as in the ischaemic limb, for a sufficient collateral circulation to be established, and with it relief from symptoms. Pain may also be temporarily relieved after taking trinitrin and prednisone [143].

Loss of weight is usually very marked and unmistakable, with scaphoid abdomen and prominent ribs. It is due to reduced intake, and, also, in all probability, to impaired absorption. Over twenty pounds may be lost in four months [97], such rapidity being characteristic of the disease.

Malabsorption, though theoretically to be expected in many cases, is difficult to prove [47]. Carbohydrate handling may be normal as judged by the d-xylose test; or there may be a raised glucose-tolerance from poor absorption, or reduced if there is ischaemic disease of the pancreas. Fat studies are more often positive with ^{131}I-labelled oleic acid or tri-olein as well as faecal fat estimations [167]. Absorption of ^{60}Co-labelled vitamin B12 may be impaired [167]. There may also be radiological evidence suggestive of malabsorption, with puddling of small bowel barium [29]. On the whole, laboratory findings often are of limited importance as far as diagnosis is concerned, with the possible exception of testing for occult blood [73].

Bowel habit is usually changed, either towards constipation or with a loose frothy stool if there is steatorrhoea.

ABDOMINAL BRUIT

A localised epigastric systolic bruit, which is not conducted along the aorta or its other branches, is a highly significant finding in a case of suspected abdominal angina. It may be the first clue to the diagnosis, and certainly justifies aortography. The patient whose operation is shown in Fig. 17.20*a* was recognised in this way. Other causes of localised epigastric murmur must be considered, notably in patients with carcinoma of the body of the pancreas, nearly half of whom show the sign [138] (due to splenic arterial compression), and whose symptoms of persistent chronic pain and wasting over many months closely resemble the abdominal angina syndrome. Occasionally, the two conditions co-exist [110] (Fig. 17.17).

With extreme narrowing of the coeliac or mesenteric artery, or on final completion of the block, the bruit will be lost, as happens in the internal carotid.

Constitutional features of mesenteric insufficiency, apart from the wasting, include secondary anaemia, a raised ESR, reduced glucose tolerance in coeliac ischaemia [47], and pre-senile general deterioration; a previous history of claudication [137] or coronary thrombosis; mental depression, and the signs and smell of excessive cigarette smoking. A poor history is given, which, with the scarcity of the physical signs and inconclusive results of most tests other than the lateral aortogram, constitutes yet another reason for the difficulty of making this particular

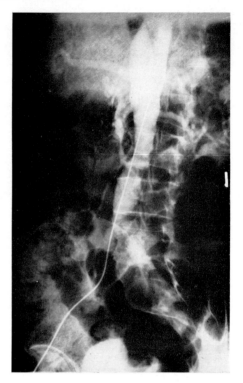

Fig. 17.17. Trans-femoral aortogram in a man aged sixty-five with intractable abdominal pain and a loud central arterial bruit. Poor filling of superior mesenteric and non-filling of splenic arteries found at operation to be due to their compression by a carcinoma of the body of the pancreas.

diagnosis and, also, perhaps for its apparent clinical rarity in the chronic, prodromal phase.

FAILURE TO HEAL INTESTINAL ANASTOMOSES

Adherent, chronically ischaemic small bowel may resemble regional ileitis in appearance [169]. This is one type of ischaemic granuloma, a form of local ischaemia commoner in the colon (*see* p. 383). Resection and anastomosis may be followed by slow leakage and the formation of a cutaneous fistula. A patient of the author's suffered this complication on three occasions and was found at post-mortem to have an occlusion of the superior mesenteric artery. In retrospect, the bowel colour and consistency was poor, and no note had been made of the state of the mesenteric pulsations. Mavor [101] has called this lower ileal region 'the great toe of the mid-gut loop'. In ischaemia it will be no better able to heal a suture line than the bloodless extremity of the lower limb.

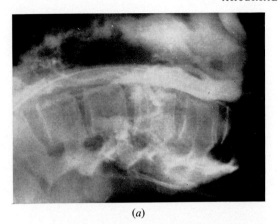 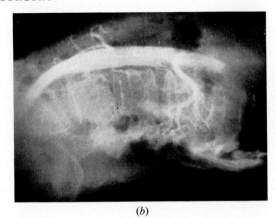

(a)   (b)

Fig. 17.18. Normal lateral trans-femoral aortography.

(a) Early phase showing coeliac and superior mesenteric origins.
(b) Later phase showing left renal and inferior mesenteric trunk and branches. A normal examination.

LATERAL AORTOGRAPHY IN CHRONIC
MESENTERIC ISCHAEMIA [110]

This is the definitive investigation, yet there are risks and difficulties in carrying it out. Postaortographic infarction of the mid-gut loop, worsening of the intestinal angina [29, 143] and, more commonly, either an acute or chronic ischaemia of the inferior mesenteric distribution [58] may be due to an intramural aortic injection with dissection of the branch orifice, or to the passage of an undue concentration of medium into the mesenteric circulation: the risk is greatest in a patient whose abdominal aorta is occluded or narrowed. Either complication tends to show itself up in the early films. Test dosage films

and the use of minimum concentration of medium should eliminate these dangers.

Access to the upper abdominal aorta may be difficult because of limb occlusions or aorto-iliac narrowing and irregularity obstructing the passage of the retrograde catheter. A good delineation can, however, be obtained by translumbar aortography, but with some inconvenience with the patient on his right side.

These disadvantages are minimised with skill and experience, and the coeliac, superior, and inferior mesenteric arteries should be well seen from their origins to main branches in the lateral view (Fig. 17.18). Collateral pathways are better shown in the postero-anterior projection (*see* Fig. 17.16).

Technique of Superior Mesenteric Arterial Reconstruction

Good exposure is essential. A long, left paramedian incision allows the full abdominal exploration which must always be carried out in these uncertain cases. Other and more dangerous conditions may be present, such as carcinoma of the pancreas or colon.

The appearance of the chronically ischaemic small bowel at operation may be normal, or with only such apparent reduction in capillary oxygenation and branch pulsation as may often be seen during a general fall in peripheral pressure and flow in the course of major surgery in a subject with cardiovascular disease (*see* p. 370). In other cases, gut pallor may be more evident, or it may develop at the site of a peristaltic contraction. A grossly abnormal, though rare, finding is the segmental thickening and adherence resembling Crohn's disease, to which we have already referred.

Elevation of the transverse mesocolon shows up the duodenojejunal flexure. The peritoneum between this and the inferior mesenteric vein is divided, and the flexure is mobilised to the right, which brings the superior mesenteric vessels into view as they run beneath the neck of the pancreas. They should be carefully localised, first by palpation, so as to limit the amount of dissection in exposing them; for these tissues are richly vascular with collaterals, and troublesome bleeding may interfere with the process of mobilising the mesenteric artery and its branches. Elevation of the body of the pancreas reveals the aortic origin of the artery, where the firm plaque or roll of atheroma will be felt within the first 2 cm or so.

The inferior pancreatico-duodenal and middle colic arteries are located and their origins on the SMA are dissected out. This is a useful way of identifying the main artery when, because it lies pulseless and ad-herent in the main bulk of the root of the mesentery, its exact position may be uncertain. The middle colic should be easy to find and to trace back in this way.

The free length of SMA between these two branches and the leash of jejunal arteries is then fully mobi-lised, for this is the site of choice for most types of reconstruction.

Choice of Method of Reconstruction

1. THROMBOENDARTERECTOMY AND PATCH GRAFT

Because they offer the simplest solution to the technical problem, these methods are preferable in a suitable case. But if the stem of the SMA is heavily

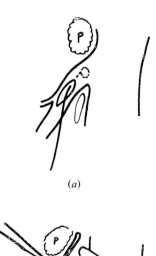

(a)

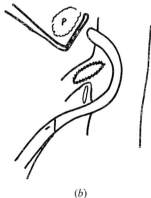

(b)

Fig. 17.19. Superior mesenteric thromboendarterec-tomy.

(a) By the closed method using a loop stripper inserted below the level of the pancreas.

(b) Open endarterectomy behind the mobilised pancreas with lateral clamping of the aorta from beneath the left renal vein.

sclerosed, calcified, or adherent, there are dangers of poor exposure, incomplete clearance of the proximal end of the endarterectomised segment, and of dis-integration of the outer layer at is junction with the aorta. As in reconstruction of the innominate and left subclavian near the aorta, this accident may be extremely difficult to correct with the limited access to the aorta which is all that is necessary in the favourable case. Endarterectomy of the SMA may be closed or open.

Closed Endarterectomy

This is the simpler method. With the type of plaque that separates freely and cleanly, it should be easy to remove the obstruction within the proximal SMA through a short arteriotomy lower down in the free zone, using either a Watson-Cheyne dissector or a Vollmar loop stripper (Fig. 17.19a). It is often un-necessary to suture the distal edge of the intimal layer.

A vein patch is preferable for the closure of the arteriotomy at this situation (Fig. 17.13), for it should give good late patency, and in an artery of this small diameter will be under no great strain.

Open Endarterectomy

The body of the pancreas is lifted up on a broad retractor to provide a good working space around the SMA origin. This is the key to success in an operation of considerable potential difficulty. In-feriorly is the left renal vein, which may require mobilising downwards, and above is the splenic vein, which comes freely upwards and forwards with the pancreas (Fig. 17.19b). A curved lateral clamp should now be placed on the aorta at least 1 cm from the SMA origin. Direct vision endarterectomy and patching may now be completed, using flat knitted dacron, the best choice for these local conditions of high flow and high tension on the repair.

2. BY-PASS GRAFTING TO THE FREE SEGMENT OF THE SMA

With surgeons of wide experience, there is preference for this well-tried, adaptable technique in the correc-tion of proximal mesenteric occlusion. Of 18 cases reported in 1965 it had been chosen in 12 [29]. In the total experience of Morris and his colleagues in Houston, Texas, up till 1966 there were 31 successful cases (including some with aneurysm), in most of which the by-pass method was used [112].

This operation owes its leading position to its limited, selective interference with the two main arteries concerned, and the relative simplicity of exposure, possible because of their control by lateral clamping (*see also* Chapter 3, p. 65). Either auto-genous saphenous vein (Fig. 17.20) or 8 mm knitted

Inferior Mesenteric Ischaemia

Much of what has been said about ischaemia of the mid-gut loop applies equally to the hind-gut. Though as a clinical problem it is less common, it is easier to recognise; and because the lesions produced are limited and mostly less acute in comparison with most of those due to small bowel ischaemia, they can often be successfully treated by well-timed operation along general surgical lines without the need for an arterial procedure. Moreover, these lesions generally simulate those of common, non-vascular conditions, with ample evidence in most cases of their site, and of the need for intervention.

Most cases are of the arteriosclerotic hypotensive type (*see* p. 376) but some are associated with rheumatoid arthritis [95, 103], pheochromocytoma [132A], and the contraceptive pill [24A].

There is good clinico-pathological correlation between the three main types of hind-gut ischaemia [93] (Table 17.7).

EFFECTS OF ISCHAEMIA UPON THE COLON
[12, 86A, 95, 131, 146]

Mucosal damage occurs early; the submucosal vessels become engorged, and soon, multiple haemorrhages occur, producing the raised, rounded lesions ('thumb-prints' and 'pseudo-tumours') now recognised radiologically and in excised specimens as being due to this same cause. This lesion may fully resolve or it may go on to ulceration, transverse ridging, and stricture. Damage to the muscle coat is later and less severe.

The typical sites for colon ischaemia are at the splenic flexure [95] and the recto-sigmoid [131]. Defects in the marginal artery have been demonstrated arteriographically from anatomical causes [56] or arterial disease [95, 146]. These two areas then, represent the limits of the inferior-mesenteric territory most at risk. In the worst cases the whole distal colon becomes gangrenous.

Table 17.7. The Inferior Mesenteric Syndromes

	Acute gangrenous infarction	*Ischaemic segmental colitis*	*Recoverable local ischaemia*
Causes	Inferior mesenteric or middle colic occlusion Period of hypotension Heart failure Clostridia Aortic thrombosis Aortography Aortic surgery	Identical, though colon survives because of better collateral inflow; plus better general condition of patient	The same in milder forms; also atheromatous embolism
Diagnosis	An abdominal catastrophe Recognised at laparotomy or post-mortem	Pain, diarrhoea, bleeding Evidence of sigmoidoscopy, barium enema, or laparotomy Variable length of colon is engorged, thickened and with oedematous mesentery, especially splenic flexure and rectosigmoid	The same
Effects and outcome	Necrosis of part or whole of hind-gut (including rectum, after aortic surgery)	Rectum unaffected Submucosal haemorrhages, ('thumb-printing' and pseudo-tumours on barium X-ray) Later, ulceration and transverse ridging. Bowel contracted and rigid; local stricture; colostomy unhealthy; or colon anastomosis may leak	Same clinical and radiological appearances, though less severe and fully reversed within a few weeks

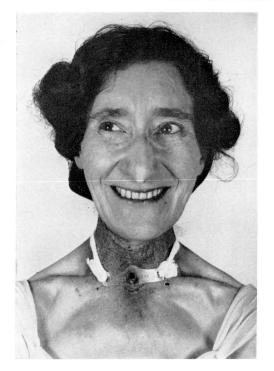
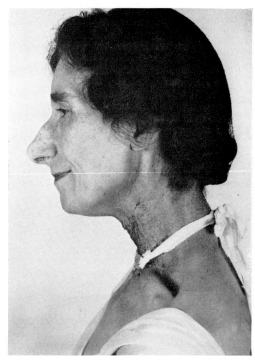

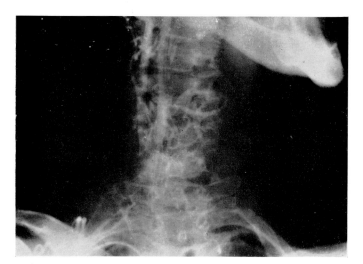

Fig. 17.26. Free sigmoid autografting for pharyngeal replacement. Early recovery with full swallowing and well-being at fourteen days.

Filling of inferior mesenteric and its arcades on carotid arteriography.

postoperative period, and early swallowing function was good on the 7th day. Her clinical condition and carotid arteriogram on the 14th day are shown in Fig. 17.26.

Perfusion of the specimen, and later infusion of the patient with heparin and low molecular weight dextran, probably helped to maintain the patency of the veins and arteries respectively. The use of 7/0 arterial sutures proved an advantage over the earlier trials with 5/0.

This patient continues with normal swallowing and free from recurrence over seven years later.

REFERENCES

1. Aakhus, T. (1966) The value of angiography in superior mesenteric artery embolism. *Brit. J. Radiol.*, **39**, 928.
2. Abrahams, D. G. and Parry, E. H. O. (1962) Hypertension due to renal artery stenosis caused by abdominal aortic aneurysm. *Circulation*, **26**, 104.
2A. Amsterdam, E. A., Couch, N. P., Christlieb, A. R., Harrison, J. H., Crane, C., Dobrzinsky, S. J. and Hickler, R. B. (1969) Renal-vein renin activity in the prognosis of surgery for reno-vascular hypertension. *Amer. J. Med.*, **47**, 860.
3. Atwill, W. H., Boyarsky, S. and Glenn, J. F. (1968) Effect of adrenalectomy on the course of experimental renovascular hypertension. *Amer. J. Surg.*, **115**, 755.
4. Baird, R. J., Yendt, E. R. and Firor, W. B. (1965) Anuria due to acute occlusion of the artery to a solitary kidney. Successful treatment by operative means. *New Eng. J. Med.*, **272**, 1012.
5. Baker, G. P., Page, L. B. and Leadbetter, G. W. (1962) Hypertension and renovascular disease: a follow-up study of 23 patients, with an analysis of factors influencing the results of surgery. *New Eng. J. Med.*, **267**, 1325.
6. Beecher, H. K., Simeone, F. A., Burnett, C. H., Shapiro, S. L., Sullivan, E. R. and Mallory, T. B. (1947) The internal state of the severely wounded man on entry to the most forward hospital. *Surgery*, **22**, 672.
6A. Benraad, H. B., Benraad, T. J. and Kloppenborg, P. W. C. (1969) Transient hypertension caused by renal segmental artery occlusion. *Brit. med. J.*, **4**, 408.
7. Bergan, J. J., Gilliland, V., Troop, C. and Anderson, M. C. (1964) Hyperkalemia following intestinal revascularisation. *J. Amer. med. Assoc.*, **187**, 17.
8. Berger, R. L. and Byrne, J. J. (1961) Intestinal gangrene associated with heart disease. *Surg. Gynec. Obstet.*, **112**, 529.
9. Bernatz, P. E. (1960) Necrosis of the colon following resection for abdominal aortic aneurysms. *Arch. Surg.*, **81**, 373.
10. Blalock, A., Levy, S. E. and Cressman, R. D. (1939) Experimental hypertension. The effects of unilateral renal ischemia combined with intestinal ischemia on the arterial blood pressure. *J. Exp. Med.*, **69**, 833.
11. Boley, S. J., Schwartz, S., Lash, J. and Sternhill, V. (1963) Reversible vascular occlusion of the colon. *Surg. Gynec. Obstet.*, **116**, 53.
12. Boley, S. J., Krieger, H., Schultz, L., Robinson, K., Siew, F. P., Allen, A. C. and Schwartz, S. (1965) Experimental aspects of peripheral vascular occlusion of the intestine. *Surg. Gynec. Obstet.*, **121**, 789.
13. Braunwald, E. and Chidsey, C. A. (1965) The adrenergic nervous system in the control of the normal and failing heart. *Proc. Roy. Soc. Med.*, **58**, 1063.
14. Brawley, R. K., Roberts, W. C. and Morrow, A. G. (1966) Intestinal infarction resulting from non-obstructive mesenteric arterial insufficiency. *Arch. Surg.*, **92**, 374.
15. Brittain, R. S. and Earley, T. K. (1963) Emergency thrombo-endarterectomy of the superior mesenteric artery: report of four cases. *Ann. Surg.*, **158**, 138.
16. Brolin, I. and Paulin, S. (1964) Abnormal communications between splanchnic vessels. *Acta. Radiol.* **2**, [*Diagn.*], p. 460.
16A. Brom, B., Bank, S., Marks, I. N., Milner, G. and Baker, P. (1969) Ischaemic colitis, gastric ulceration and malabsorption in a case of primary amyloidosis. *Gastroenterol.*, **57**, 319.
17. Brown, J. J., Davies, D. L., Lever, A. F. and Robertson, J. I. S. (1966) Renin and angiotensin. A survey of some aspects. *Postgrad. Med. J.*, **42**, 153.
18. Brown, J. J., Owen, K., Peart, W. S., Robertson, J. I. S. and Sutton, D. (1960) The diagnosis and treatment of renal-artery stenosis. *Brit. med. J.*, **ii**, 327.
19. Bruetsch, W. L. (1965) Rheumatic nephrosclerosis, with special reference to rheumatic endarteritis. *Circulation*, **31**, 805.
20. Carron, D. B. and Douglas, A. P. (1965) Steatorrhoea in vascular insufficiency of the small intestine: five cases of polyarteritis nodosa and allied disorders. *Quart. J. Med.*, **34**, 331.
21. Carter, D. and Einheber, A. (1966) Intestinal ischemic shock in germ-free animals. *Surg. Gynec. Obstet.*, **122**, 66.
22. Carter, R., Vannix, R., Hinshaw, D. B. and Stafford, C. E. (1959) Acute inferior mesenteric vascular occlusion, a surgical syndrome. *Amer. J. Surg.*, **98**, 271.
23. Chiene, J. (1868) Cited by Marston, A. (1964) in: Patterns of intestinal ischaemia [93].
24. Chinaglia, A. (1964) Distinguishing painful abdominal syndrome in patients suffering from a polypoid pillow in the common liver artery: arteriotomy, recovery. *J. Cardiovasc. Surg.*, **5**, 375.
24A. Cotton, P. B. and Thomas, M. L. (1971) Ischaemic colitis and the contraceptive pill. *Brit. med. J.*, **3**, 27.
24B. Crummy, A. B., Whittaker, W. B., Morrissey, J. F. and Cossman, F. P. (1971) Intestinal infarction secondary to retroperitoneal fibrosis. *New Eng. J. Med.*, **285**, 28.
25. d'Abreu, F. and Strickland, B. (1962) Developmental renal-artery stenosis. *Lancet*, **ii**, 517.
26. Danaraj, T. J., Wong, H. O. and Thomas, M. A. (1963) Primary arteritis of aorta causing renal artery stenosis and hypertension. *Brit. Heart J.*, **25**, 153.
26A. Danford, R. O. (1971) The splanchnic vasoconstrictive effect of digoxin and its reversal by glucagon. In *Vascular Disorders of the Intestine*. (Ed. Boley, S. J.) London: Butterworths, p. 421.
27. D'Angelo, G. J., Ameriso, L. M. and Tredway, J. B. (1963) Survival after mesenteric arterial occlusion

by treatment with low molecular weight dextran. *Circulation*, **27**, 662.

28. Daniel, W. J., Mohamed, S. D. and Matheson, N. A. (1966) Treatment of mesenteric embolism with dextran 40. *Lancet*, **i**, 567.

29. Dardik, H., Seidenberg, B., Parker, J. G. and Hurwitt, E. S. (1965) Intestinal angina with malabsorption treated by elective revascularisation. *J. Amer. med. Assoc.*, **194**, 1206.

30. Davies, E. R. and Sutton, D. (1965) Hypertension and multiple renal arteries. *Lancet*, **i**, 341.

31. DeBakey, M. E., Morris, G. C., Morgen, R. O., Crawford, E. S., and Cooley, D. A. (1964) Lesions of the renal artery. *Amer. J. Surg.*, **107**, 84.

32. DeCamp, P. (1963) Surgical treatment of renovascular hypertension cited by Kaufman, J. J. (1965) [68].

33. Demos, N. J., Bahuth, J. J. and Urnes, P. D. (1962) Comparative study of arteriosclerosis in the inferior and superior mesenteric arteries: with a case report of gangrene of the colon. *Ann. Surg.*, **155**, 599.

34. DeMuth, W. E. (1962) Mesenteric vascular occlusion in children. *J. Amer. med. Assoc.*, **179**, 130.

35. Derrick, J. R. and Logan, W. D. (1958) Mesenteric arterial insufficiency. *Surgery*, **44**, 823.

36. Derrick, J. R. (1962) Clinical and pathological variability in patients with constriction of the superior mesenteric artery. *Surgery*, **52**, 309.

37. Douglas, D. M., Lowe, K. G. and Mitchell, R. G. (1959) Hypertension and unilateral renal disease treated by nephrectomy. *Brit. Heart J.*, **21**, 361.

38. Dowling, R. H. and Booth, C. C. (1966) Functional compensation after small-bowel resection in man. Demonstration by direct measurement. *Lancet*, **ii**, 146.

39. Dunbar, J. D., Molnar, W., Beman, F. F. and Marable, S. A. (1965) Compression of the celiac trunk and abdominal angina. Preliminary report of 15 cases. *Amer. J. Roent.*, **95**, 731.

40. Dunphy, J. E. (1936) Abdominal pain of vascular origin. *Amer. J. med. Sci.*, **192**, 109.

41. Drapanas, T. and Bron, K. M. (1966) Stenosis of the celiac artery. *Ann. Surg.*, **164**, 1085.

42. Eastcott, H. H. G. and Simpson, J. F. (1965) Colonic reconstruction of the pharynx. *Lancet*, **i**, 1067.

42A. Edwards, A. J., Hamilton, J. D., Nichol, W. D., Taylor, G. W. and Dawson, A. M. (1970) Experience with coeliac axis compression syndrome. *Brit. med. J.*, **1**, 342.

43. Ende, N. (1958) Infarction of the bowel in cardiac failure. *New Eng. J. Med.*, **258**, 879.

44. Fine, J., Frank, E. D., Ravin, H. A., Rutenberg, S. H. and Schweinburg, F. B. (1959) The bacterial factor in traumatic shock. *New Eng. J. Med.*, **260**, 214.

45. Fogarty, T. J. and Fletcher, W. S. (1966) Genesis of nonocclusive mesenteric ischemia. *Amer. J. Surg.*, **111**, 130.

45A. Foster, J. H., Oates, J. A., Rhamy, R. K., Klatte, E. C., Burko, H. C. and Michaelakis, A. M. (1969) Hypertension and fibromuscular dysplasia of the renal arteries. *Surgery*, **65**, 157.

46. Freeman, N. E., Leeds, F. H., Elliott, W. G. and Roland, S. I. (1954) Thromboendarterectomy for hypertension due to renal artery occlusion. *J. Amer. Med. Assoc.*, **156**, 1077.

47. Fry, W. J. and Kraft, R. O. (1963) Visceral angina. *Surg. Gynec. Obstet.*, **117**, 417.

48. Geyer, J. R. and Poutasse, E. F. (1962) Incidence of multiple renal arteries on aortography. *J. Amer. med. Assoc.*, **182**, 120.

49. Gilfillan, R. S., Smart, W. R. and Bostick, W. L. (1956) Dissecting aneurysm of the renal artery. *Arch. Surg.*, **73**, 737.

50. Glotzer, D. J. and Glotzer, P. (1966) Superior mesenteric embolectomy. Report of two successful cases using the Fogarty catheter. *Arch. Surg.*, **93**, 421.

51. Goldblatt, H., Lynch, J., Hanzal, R. F. and Summerville, W. W. (1934) Studies on experimental hypertension. I. The production of persistent elevation of systolic blood pressure by means of renal ischemia. *J. Exp. Med.*, **59**, 347.

51A. Gomes, M. M. R. and Bernatz, P. E. (1970) Aorto-iliac occlusive disease. Extension cephalad to origin of renal arteries, with surgical considerations and results. *Arch. Surg.*, **101**, 161.

52. Gooding, R. A. and Couch, R. D. (1962) Mesenteric ischemia without vascular occlusion. *Arch. Surg.*, **85**, 186.

53. Green, H. D. and Kepchar, J. H. (1959) Control of peripheral resistance in major systemic vascular beds. *Physiol. Rev.*, **39**, 617.

54. Green, H. D., Deal, C. P., Bardhanabaedya, S. and Denison, A. B. (1955) The effects of adrenergic substances and ischemia on the blood flow and peripheral resistance of the canine mesenteric vascular bed before and during adrenergic blockade. *J. Pharm. Exp. Therap.*, **113**, 115.

55. Greever, C. J. and Watts, D. T. (1959) Epinephrine levels in the peripheral blood during irreversible hemorrhagic shock in dogs. *Circulation Res.*, **7**, 192.

56. Griffiths, J. D. (1961) Extramural and intramural blood-supply of colon. *Brit. med. J.*, **i**, 323.

57. Grosh, J. L., Mann, R. H. and O'Donnell, W. M. (1965) Nonthrombotic intestinal infarction in heart disease. *Amer. J. med. Sci.*, **250**, 613.

58. Guilfoil, P. H. (1963) Inferior-mesenteric-artery syndrome after translumbar aortography. *New Eng. J. Med.*, **269**, 12.

59. Hawkins, C. F. (1957) Jejunal stenosis following mesenteric-artery occlusion. *Lancet*, **ii**, 121.

60. Hejnal, J., Hejhal, L., Firt, P. and Michal, V. (1965) Surgical management of vasorenal hypertension. *J. Cardiovasc. Surg.*, **6**, 400.

61. Hodson, C. J. (1957) Renal arteriography in hypertension. *Proc. Roy. Soc. Med.*, **50**, 539.

62. Holley, K. E., Hunt, J. C., Brown, A. L., Kincaid, O. W. and Sheps, S. G. (1964) Renal artery stenosis: a clinical-pathologic study in normotensive and hypertensive patients. *Amer. J. Med.*, **37**, 14.

63. Hsiung, J., Miao, T., Ch'en, C., Chang, J., Miao, C.

and Chao, S. (1965) An investigation into hypertension due to renal tuberculosis. *Chinese med. J.*, **84**, 327.

64. Hsiung, J. (1966) Surgical treatment of renovascular hypertension. *Chinese med. J.*, **85**, 29.

65. Hudgson, P., Pearce, J. M. S. and Yeates, W. K. (1967) Renal artery stenosis with hypertension and high haematocrit. *Brit. med. J.*, **i**, 18.

66. Hurwitz, R., Campbell, R. W., Gordon, P. and Haddy, F. J. (1961) Interaction of serotonin with vasoconstrictor agents in the vascular bed of the denervated dog forelimb. *J. Pharm. Exp. Therap.*, **133**, 57.

67. Hwang, W. and Liu, L. S. (1962) Constrictive arteritis of the aorta and its branches. *Chinese med. J.*, **81**, 526.

67A. Jago, R. H. (1971) Superior mesenteric embolectomy. *Brit. J. Surg.*, **58**, 628.

68. Kaufman, J. J. (1965) Results of surgical treatment of renovascular hypertension: an analysis of 70 cases followed from 1 to 6 years. *J. Urol.*, **94**, 211.

68A. Kaufman, J. J., Lupu, A. N., Franklin, S. and Maxwell, M. (1970) Diagnostic and predictive value of renal-vein renin activity in renovascular hypertension. *J. Urol.*, **103**, 702.

69. Kennedy, A. C., Luke, R. G., Briggs, J. D. and Stirling, W. B. (1965) Detection of renovascular hypertension. *Lancet*, **ii**, 963.

70. Kincaid-Smith, P. (1955) Vascular obstruction in chronic pyelonephritic kidneys and its relation to hypertension. *Lancet*, **ii**, 1263.

71. Kobold, E. E. and Thal, A. P. (1963) Quantitation and identification of vasoactive substances liberated during various types of experimental and clinical intestinal ischemia. *Surg. Gynec. Obstet.*, **117**, 315.

71A. Kock, N. G., Tibblin, S. and Schenk, W. G. (1970) Hemodynamic responses to glucagon. An experimental study of central visceral and peripheral effects. *Ann. Surg.*, **171**, 373.

71B. Kock, N. G., Tibblin, S. and Schenk, W. G. (1971) Modification by glucagon of the splanchnic vascular responses to activation of the sympathicoadrenal system. *J. Surg. Research*, **1**, 12.

71C. Lacombe, M. (1970) The surgical treatment of renal artery embolism with anuria. *Surg. Gynec. Obstet.*, **133**, 419.

72. Laufman, H. (1950) Experimental evidence of factors concerned in the eventual recovery of strangulated intestine: effects of massive penicillin therapy. *Surgery*, **28**, 509.

73. Laufman, H., Nora, P. F. and Mittelpunkt, A. I. (1964) Mesenteric blood vessels: advances in surgery and physiology. *Arch. Surg.*, **88**, 1021.

74. Lavender, J. P. (1957) Hypertension and tuberculous renal lesions. *Brit. med. J.*, **i**, 1221.

75. Lawrence, J. R., Doig, A., Knight, I. C. S., MacLaren, I. F. and Donald, K. W. (1964) Renal artery stenosis without renal ischaemia. *Lancet*, **i**, 62.

76. Leading article (1965) Irreversible shock. *Lancet*, **i**, 255.

76A. Leading Article (1971) Compression of the coeliac axis. *Brit. med. J.*, **4**, 378.

77. Lepley, D., Mani, C. J. and Ellison, E. H. (1962) Superior mesenteric venous occlusion. A study using low molecular weight dextran to prevent infarction. *J. Surg. Res.*, **2**, 403.

78. Li, C., Chiang, H., Liu, C. and Chang, T. (1964) Acute superior mesenteric vascular occlusion: report of a case successfully treated by local use of Regitine. *Chinese med. J.*, **83**, 59.

79. Lillehei, R. C. and MacLean, L. D. (1958) The intestinal factor in irreversible endotoxin shock. *Ann. Surg.*, **148**, 513.

80. Lillehei, R. C. (1957) The intestinal factor in irreversible hemorrhagic shock. *Surgery*, **42**, 1043.

81. Lillehei, R. C., Longerbeam, J. K., Bloch, J. H. and Manax, W. G. (1964) The nature of irreversible shock: experimental and clinical observations. *Ann. Surg.*, **160**, 682.

81A. Lindberg, E. F., Grinnan, G. L. B. and Smith, L. (1970) Acalculous cholecystitis in Viet Nam casualties. *Ann. Surg.*, **171**, 152.

82. Ljungqvist, A. and Wallgren, G. (1962) Unilateral renal artery stenosis and fatal arterial hypertension in a newborn infant. *Acta paediat.*, **51**, 575.

83. Luke, R. G., Briggs, J. D., Kennedy, A. C. and Stirling, W. B. (1966) The isotope renogram in the detection and assessment of renal artery stenosis. *Quart. J. Med.*, **35**, 237.

83A. MacMahon, H. E. (1972) Systemic scleroderma and massive infarction of intestine and liver. *Surg. Gynec. Obstet.*, **134**, 10.

84. Malvin, R. L. (1965) Hypertension resulting from renal arterial injection of microspheres. *Nature*, **206**, 938.

85. Marable, S. A., Molnar, W. and Beman, F. M. (1966) Abdominal pain secondary to celiac axis compression. *Amer. J. Surg.*, **111**, 493.

86. Marable, S. A., Moore, F. T. and Schieve, J. F. (1966) Treatment of hypertension associated with the solitary ischemic kidney. *New Eng. J. Med.*, **275**, 1278.

86A. Marcuson, R. W. and Forman, J. A. (1971) Ischaemic disease of the colon. *Proc. Roy. Soc. Med.*, **64**, 1080.

87. Marrash, S. E., Gibson, J. B. and Simeone, F. A. (1962) A clinicopathologic study of intestinal infarction. *Surg. Gynec. Obstet.*, **114**, 323.

88. Marston, A. (1962) The bowel in shock. The role of mesenteric arterial disease as a cause of death in the elderly. *Lancet*, **ii**, 365.

89. Marston, A. (1962) The bowel in shock. *Lancet*, **ii**, 881.

90. Marston, A. (1962) Massive infarction of the colon demonstrated radiologically. *Brit. J. Surg.*, **49**, 609.

91. Marston, A. (1963) Causes of death in mesenteric arterial occlusion: I. Local and general effects of devascularisation of the bowel. *Ann. Surg.*, **158**, 952.

92. Marston, A. (1963) Causes of death in mesenteric arterial occlusion: II. Observations on revascularisation of the ischemic bowel. *Ann. Surg.*, **158**, 960

93. Marston, A. (1964) Patterns of intestinal ischaemia. *Ann. Roy. Coll. Surg. Eng.*, **35**, 151.

94. Marston, A. (1966) Clinical features of ischaemic colitis. *Proc. Roy. Soc. Med.*, **59**, 882.

94A. Marston, A. (1971) Intestinal angina. *Proc. Roy. Soc. Med.*, **64**, 1079.

95. Marston, A., Pheils, M. T., Thomas, M. L. and Morson, B. C. (1966) Ischaemic colitis. *Gut*, **7**, 1.

96. Martorell, R. (1963) Spontaneous rupture of the superior mesenteric artery. *Ann. Surg.*, **157**, 292.

97. Mavor, G. E. (1959) Stenosis of the superior mesenteric artery. *Postgrad. med. J.*, **35**, 558.

98. Mavor, G. E. and Lyall, A. D. (1962) Superior mesenteric artery stenosis treated by iliac-mesenteric arterial bypass. *Lancet*, **ii**, 1143.

99. Mavor, G. E., Lyall, A. D., Chrystal, K. M. R. and Tsapogas, M. (1962) Mesenteric infarction as a vascular emergency. *Brit. J. Surg.*, **50**, 219.

100. Mavor, G. E., Lyall, A. D., Chrystal, K. M. R. and Proctor, D. M. (1963) Observations on experimental occlusion of the superior mesenteric artery. *Brit. J. Surg.*, **50**, 536.

101. Mavor, G. E. (1963) In *Indications and Techniques in Arterial Surgery* (Ed. Martin, P.) Edinburgh and London: E. & S. Livingstone, p. 71.

102. Maxwell, M. H. and Prozan, G. B. (1962) Renovascular hypertension. *Prog. Cardiovasc. Dis.*, **5**, 81.

103. McGovern, V. J. and Goulston, S. J. M. (1965) Ischaemic enterocolitis. *Gut*, **6**, 213.

104. Meier, A. L. and Waibel, P. (1964) Mesenteric artery occlusion with intestinal gangrene. *Arch. Surg.*, **88**, 181.

105. Menser, M. A., Dorman, D. C., Reye, R. D. K. and Reid, R. R. (1966) Renal-artery stenosis in the rubella syndrome. *Lancet*, **i**, 790.

106. Mikkelsen, W. P. (1957) Intestinal angina; its surgical significance. *Amer. J. Surg.*, **94**, 262.

107. Mikkelsen, W. P. and Berne, C. J. (1962) Intestinal angina. *Surg. Clin. N. Amer.*, **42**, 1321.

108. Miller, D. R. and O'Farrell, T. P. (1965) Perforation of the small intestine secondary to necrotising vasculitis (Periarteritis Nodosa). *Ann. Surg.*, **162**, 81.

109. Milliken, J., Nahor, A., and Fine, J. (1965) A study of the factors involved in the development of peripheral vascular collapse following release of the occluded superior mesenteric artery. *Brit. J. Surg.*, **52**, 699.

110. Morris, G. C., Crawford, E. S., Cooley, D. A. and DeBakey, M. E. (1962) Revascularisation of the celiac and superior mesenteric arteries. *Arch. Surg.*, **84**, 95.

111. Morris, G. C., DeBakey, M. E., Crawford, E. S., Cooley, D. A. and Zanger, L. C. C. (1966) Late results of surgical treatment for renovascular hypertension. *Surg. Gynec. Obstet.*, **122**, 1255.

112. Morris, G. C., DeBakey, M. E. and Bernhard, V. (1966) Abdominal angina. *Surg. Clin. N. Amer.*, **46**, 919.

113. Musa, B. U. (1965) Intestinal infarction without mesenteric vascular occlusion. A report of 31 cases. *Ann. Int. Med.*, **63**, 783.

114. Nahor, A., Milliken, J., and Fine, J. (1966) Effect of celiac blockade and dibenzyline on traumatic shock following release of occluded superior mesenteric artery. *Ann. Surg.*, **163**, 29.

115. Nelson, L. E. and Kremen, A. J. (1950) Experimental occlusion of the superior mesenteric vessels with special reference to the role of intravascular thrombosis and its prevention by heparin. *Surgery*, **28**, 819.

116. Orr, T. G., Lorhan, P. H. and Kaul, P. G. (1954) Mesenteric vascular occlusion. A report of two cases. *J. Amer. Med. Assoc.*, **155**, 648.

117. Owen, K. (1963) In *Indications and Techniques in Arterial Surgery* (Ed. Martin, P.) Edinburgh and London: E. & S. Livingstone, p. 76.

117A. Owen, K. (1967) Kongress der Internationalen Gesellschaft für Urologie. München.

118. Palubinskas, A. J. and Wylie, E. J. (1961) Roentgen diagnosis of fibromuscular hyperplasia of the renal arteries. *Radiology*, **76**, 634.

119. Payan, H., Levine, S., Bronstein, L. and King, E. (1965) Subtotal ischemic infarction of colon simulating ulcerative colitis. *Arch. Path.*, **80**, 530.

120. Peart, W. S. (1965) The renin-angiotensin system. *Pharmac. Rev.*, **17**, 143.

121. Peart, W. S. (1959) Hypertension and the kidney. I. Clinical, pathological and functional disorders, especially in man. *Brit. med. J.*, **ii**, 1353.

121A. Perdue, G. D. and Smith, R. B. (1969) Atheromatous microemboli. *Ann. Surg.*, **169**, 954.

122. Pope, C. H. and O'Neal, R. M. (1956) Incomplete infarction of ileum simulating regional enteritis. *J. Amer. Med. Assoc.*, **161**, 963.

123. Postlethwait, R. W., Hernandez, R. R., and Dillon, M. L. (1964) Hepatic artery lesions. *Ann. Surg.*, **159**, 895.

124. Poutasse, E. F. (1961) Diagnosis and treatment of occlusive renal artery disease and hypertension. *J. Amer. Med. Assoc.*, **178**, 1078.

125. Ranger, I. and Spence, M. P. (1962) Superior mesenteric artery occlusion treated by ileo-colic aortic anastomosis. *Brit. med. J.*, **ii**, 95.

126. Rees, R. S. O. (1966) Aortography in hypertension. *Amer. Heart J.*, **71**, 420.

127. Rob, C. G. and Owen, K. (1956) Ligation of both the coeliac axis and superior mesenteric artery with survival of the patient. *Brit. J. Surg.*, **44**, 247.

128. Rob, C. (1966) Surgical diseases of the celiac and mesenteric arteries. *Arch. Surg.*, **93**, 21.

129. Rob, C. and Snyder, M. (1966) Chronic intestinal ischemia: a complication of surgery of the abdominal aorta. *Surgery*, **60**, 1141.

130. Roberts, J. C., Moses, C. and Wilkins, R. H. (1959) Autopsy studies in atherosclerosis: I, II, and III. *Circulation*, **20**, 511, 520, 527.

131. Roberts, W. M. (1965) Ischaemic lesions of the colon and rectum. *South African J. Surg.*, **3**, 141.

132. Robertson, P. W., Klidjian, A., Hull, D. H., Hilton, D. D. and Dyson, M. L. (1962) The assessment and treatment of hypertension. New views on essential hypertension. *Lancet*, **ii**, 567.

132A.Rosati, L. A. and Augur, N. A. (1971) Ischaemic enterocolitis in pheochromocytoma. *Gastroenterol.*, **60**, 581.

133. Rosch, P. J. (1959) Gastrointestinal bleeding in pheochromocytoma and following the administration of norepinephrine (Arterenol). *Arch. Int. Med.*, **104**, 175.

134. Rosenberg, J. C. (1964) Circulating serotonin and catecholamines following occlusion of the superior mesenteric artery. *Ann. Surg.*, **160**, 1062.

135. Schwartz, C. J. and White, T. A. (1964) Stenosis of renal artery: an unselected necropsy study. *Brit. med. J.*, **ii**, 1415.

136. Schwartz, D. T. (1965) Relation of superior-mesenteric-artery obstruction to renal hypertension. A review of 56 cases. *New Eng. J. Med.*, **272**, 1318.

137. Seedat, Y. K. and Pooler, N. R. (1965) Vascular occlusion presenting as chronic diarrhoea with intermittent claudication. *Brit. J. Med.*, **i**, 497.

138. Serebro, H. (1965) A diagnostic sign of carcinoma of the body of the pancreas. *Lancet*, **i**, 85.

139. Serjeant, J. C. B. (1965) Mesenteric embolus treated with low-molecular-weight dextran. *Lancet*, **i**, 139.

140. Serrallach-Mila, N., Paravisini, J., Mayol-Valls, P., Alberti, J., Casellas, A. and Nollas-Panadés, J. (1965) Renal autotransplantation. *Lancet*, **ii**, 1130.

141. Shanahan, M. X. and Steedman, P. K. (1963) Inferior mesenteric artery occlusion. *Brit. J. Surg.*, **50**, 533.

142. Shaw, R. S. and Rutledge, R. H. (1957) Superior-mesenteric-artery embolectomy in the treatment of massive mesenteric infarction. *New Eng. J. Med.*, **257**, 595.

143. Shaw, R. S. and Maynard, E. P. (1958) Acute and chronic thrombosis of the mesenteric arteries associated with malabsorption. *New Eng. J. Med.*, **258**, 874.

144. Sheiner, N. M., Palayew, M. J., and Sedlezky, I. (1966) Gas in the portal vein: a report of two cases. *Canad. med. Assoc., J.* **95**, 611.

145. Shenoi, P. M., Smits, B. J. and Davidson, S. (1966) Massive removal of small bowel during criminal abortion. *Brit. med. J.*, **ii**, 929.

146. Shippey, S. H. and Acker, J. J. (1965) Segmental infarction of the colon demonstrated by selective inferior mesenteric angiography. *Amer. J. Surg.*, **109**, 671.

147. Short, D. W., Kennedy, A. C., Luke, R. G. and Mackey, W. A. (1965) Renovascular hypertension in aortic arch syndrome due to Takayasu's arteritis. *Brit. J. Surg.*, **52**, 963.

148. Simpson, J. F. (1966) Some facets of hypopharyngeal surgery. *J. Laryngol. Otol.*, **80**, 1077.

148A.Smellie, W. A. B., Vinik, M. and Hume, D. M. (1969) Angiographic investigation of hypertension complicating human renal transplantation. *Surg. Gynec. Obstet.*, **128**, 963.

149. Smith, H. W. (1956) Unilateral nephrectomy in hypertensive disease. *J. Urol.*, **76**, 685.

150. Smith, R. (1966) Pancreatic arterial disease. Personal communication.

151. Spencer, F. C., Stamey, T. A., Bahnson, H. T. and Cohen, A. (1961) Diagnosis and treatment of hypertension due to occlusive disease of the renal artery. *Ann. Surg.*, **154**, 674.

152. Starer, F. and Sutton, D. (1958) Aortic thrombosis, *Brit. med. J.*, **i**, 1255.

153. Steiness, I. (1965) Hypertension due to renal artery obstruction in Eskimo girl: case of primary arteritis of aorta. *Brit. med. J.*, **ii**, 1291.

154. Stewart, G. D., Sweetman, W. R., Westphal, K. and Wise, R. A. (1960) Superior mesenteric embolectomy. *Ann. Surg.*, **151**, 274.

154A.Stewart, R. H., Dustan, H. P., Kiser, W. S., Meany, T. F., Straffon, R. A. and McCormack, L. J. (1970) Correlation of angiography and natural history in evaluation of patients with renovascular hypertension. *J. Urol.*, **104**, 231.

155. Stoney, R. J. and Wylie, E. J. (1966) Recognition and surgical management of visceral ischemic syndromes. *Ann. Surg.*, **164**, 714.

156. Sutton, D., Brunton, F. J. and Starer, F. (1961) Renal artery stenosis. *Clinical Radiol.*, **12**, 80.

157. Sutton, D., Brunton, F. J., Foot, E. C. and Guthrie, J. (1963) Fibromuscular, fibrous, and non-atheromatous renal artery stenosis and hypertension. *Clin. Radiol.*, **14**, 381.

158. Sutton, D. (1966) Arteriography and renal artery stenosis. *Postgrad. med. J.*, **42**, 183.

159. Sutton, R. A. L. and Rosenheim, M. L. (1967) Coeliac axis stenosis. *Proc. Roy. Soc. Med.*, **60**, 139.

160. Szilagyi, E. (1963) Cited by Laufman, H., *et al.* (1964) in Mesenteric blood vessels [73].

161. Texter, E. C., Merrill, S., Schwartz, M., Van Derstappen, G. and Haddy, F. J. (1962) Relationship of blood flow to pressure in the intestinal vascular bed of the dog. *Amer. J. Physiol.*, **202**, 253.

162. Thomas, J. F. and Jordan, G. L. (1965) Massive resection of small bowel and total colectomy: use of reversed segment. *Arch. Surg.*, **90**, 781.

163. Thomas, R. G. and Levin, N. W. (1961) Ureteric irregularity with renal artery obstruction. A new radiological sign. *Brit. J. Radiol.*, **34**, 438.

164. Trippel, O. H., Bergan, J. J., Simon, N. M. and O'Conor, V. J. (1964) Bilateral simultaneous renal endarterectomy. *Arch. Surg.*, **88**, 818.

165. Uricchio, J. F., Calenda, D. G. and Freedman, D. (1954) Mesenteric vascular occlusion: an analysis of 13 cases with a report of 2 cases with survival following extensive intestinal resection. *Ann. Surg.*, **139**, 206.

166. Van Zyl, J. J. W. and Du Toit, F. D. (1966) Superior mesenteric artery occlusion treated by common iliac-ileocolic anastomosis. *Brit. J. Surg.*, **53**, 522.

166A.Wade, O. L. and Bishop, J. M. (1962) *Cardiac Output and Regional Blood Flow.* Oxford: Blackwell.

167. Webb, W. R. and Hardy, J. D. (1962) Relief of abdominal angina by vascular graft. *Ann. Int. Med.*, **57**, 289.

168. Wilson, S. (1963) Mesenteric arteriosclerosis; incidence and distribution of plaques and stenoses. Personal communication.

169. Wolf, B. S. and Marshak, R. H. (1956) Segmental infarction of the small bowel. *Radiology*, **66,** 701.

170. Wylie, E. J. and Wellington, J. S. (1960) Hypertension caused by fibromuscular hyperplasia of the renal arteries. *Amer. J. Surg.*, **100,** 183.

171. Yates-Bell, J. G. (1959) Nephrectomy in cases of hypertension. *Brit. med. J.*, **ii,** 1371.

172. Zuidema, G. D. (1961) Surgical management of superior mesenteric arterial emboli. *Arch. Surg.*, **82,** 267.

173. Zuidema, G. D., Reed, D., Turcotte, J. G. and Fry, W. J. (1964) Superior mesenteric artery embolectomy. *Ann. Surg.*, **159,** 548.